T0203165

BSAVA Manual of Rabbit Surgery, Dentistry and Imaging

Editors:

Frances Harcourt-Brown
BVSc DipECZM(Small Mammal) FRCVS
RCVS Recognized Specialist in Rabbit Medicine and Surgery
European Recognized Veterinary Specialist in
Zoological Medicine (Small Mammal)
30 Crab Lane, Harrogate, North Yorkshire HG1 3BE

and

John Chitty
BVetMed CertZooMed MRCVS
Anton Vets, Unit 11, Anton Mill Road, Andover,
Hampshire SP10 2NJ

Published by:

British Small Animal Veterinary Association
Woodrow House, 1 Telford Way,
Waterwells Business Park, Quedgeley,
Gloucester GL2 2AB

A Company Limited by Guarantee in England
Registered Company No. 2837793
Registered as a Charity

Republished 2016, 2018, 2020, 2021, 2022
Copyright © 2022 BSAVA

Illustrations on pages 10, 11, 30, 70, 73, 105, 117–19, 120–1, 139, 144, 150–2,
159, 169, 170, 172, 188, 191, 199–202, 205, 211, 228, 233, 240, 248–51, 288–90,
315, 319, 322–4, 356, 392–3 and 407–8 were drawn by S.J. Elmhurst BA Hons
(www.livingart.org.uk) and are printed with her permission.

A catalogue record for this book is available from the British Library.

ISBN 978-1-905319-41-1

The publishers, editors and contributors cannot take responsibility for information
provided on dosages and methods of application of drugs mentioned or referred to
in this publication. Details of this kind must be verified in each case by individual
users from up to date literature published by the manufacturers or suppliers of
those drugs. Veterinary surgeons are reminded that in each case they must follow
all appropriate national legislation and regulations (for example, in the United
Kingdom, the prescribing cascade) from time to time in force.

Printed in the UK by Severn, Gloucester GL2 5EU – a carbon neutral printer
Printed on ECF paper made from sustainable forests

17841PUBS22

Other titles in the BSAVA Manuals series:

Manual of Avian Practice: A Foundation Manual
Manual of Backyard Poultry Medicine and Surgery
Manual of Canine & Feline Abdominal Imaging
Manual of Canine & Feline Abdominal Surgery
Manual of Canine & Feline Advanced Veterinary Nursing
Manual of Canine & Feline Anaesthesia and Analgesia
Manual of Canine & Feline Behavioural Medicine
Manual of Canine & Feline Cardiorespiratory Medicine
Manual of Canine & Feline Clinical Pathology
Manual of Canine & Feline Dentistry and Oral Surgery
Manual of Canine & Feline Dermatology
Manual of Canine & Feline Emergency and Critical Care
Manual of Canine & Feline Endocrinology
Manual of Canine & Feline Endoscopy and Endosurgery
Manual of Canine & Feline Fracture Repair and Management
Manual of Canine & Feline Gastroenterology
Manual of Canine & Feline Haematology and Transfusion Medicine
Manual of Canine & Feline Head, Neck and Thoracic Surgery
Manual of Canine & Feline Musculoskeletal Disorders
Manual of Canine & Feline Musculoskeletal Imaging
Manual of Canine & Feline Nephrology and Urology
Manual of Canine & Feline Neurology
Manual of Canine & Feline Oncology
Manual of Canine & Feline Ophthalmology
Manual of Canine & Feline Radiography and Radiology:
 A Foundation Manual
Manual of Canine & Feline Rehabilitation, Supportive and
 Palliative Care: Case Studies in Patient Management
Manual of Canine & Feline Reproduction and Neonatology
Manual of Canine & Feline Shelter Medicine: Principles of Health
 and Welfare in a Multi-animal Environment
Manual of Canine & Feline Surgical Principles: A Foundation Manual
Manual of Canine & Feline Thoracic Imaging
Manual of Canine & Feline Ultrasonography
Manual of Canine & Feline Wound Management and Reconstruction
Manual of Canine Practice: A Foundation Manual
Manual of Exotic Pet and Wildlife Nursing
Manual of Exotic Pets: A Foundation Manual
Manual of Feline Practice: A Foundation Manual
Manual of Practical Animal Care
Manual of Practical Veterinary Nursing
Manual of Practical Veterinary Welfare
Manual of Psittacine Birds
Manual of Rabbit Medicine
Manual of Rabbit Surgery, Dentistry and Imaging
Manual of Raptors, Pigeons and Passerine Birds
Manual of Reptiles
Manual of Rodents and Ferrets
Manual of Small Animal Practice Management and Development
Manual of Wildlife Casualties

For further information on these and all BSAVA publications please visit our website:
www.bsava.com

RELATED TITLES

BSAVA Manual of Rabbit Medicine

Edited by Anna Meredith and Brigitte Lord

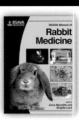

- The 'rabbit friendly practice'
- Neoplasia and endocrine disease covered
- Approaches to common conditions
- In-depth information for practitioners
- Useful appendices
- Client handouts

BSAVA Manual of Exotic Pet and Wildlife Nursing

Edited by Molly Varga, Rachel Lumbis and Lucy Gott

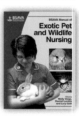

- Husbandry and biology
- Ward design and management
- Inpatient care
- Nursing clinics
- Useful forms and questionnaires
- Client handouts

Contents

Contributors

Livia Benato DVM CertZooMed MRCVS
School of Veterinary Medicine, College of Medicine,
Veterinary Medicine and Life Sciences (MVLS),
University of Glasgow, Bearsden Road,
Glasgow G61 1QH

Brendan Carmel BVSc MVS MANZCVS (Unusual Pets) GDipComp
Warranwood Veterinary Centre,
2/1 Colman Road, Warranwood,
Victoria 3134, Australia

John Chitty BVetMed CertZooMed MRCVS
Anton Vets, Unit 11, Anton Mill Road,
Andover, Hampshire SP10 2NJ

Will Easson BVMS MRCVS
12 Maes Y Grug, Church Village, Pontypridd,
Mid Glamorgan CF38 1UN

Sally Everitt BVSc MSc(VetGP) PhD
Scientific Policy Officer, BSAVA

Michael Fehr DVM PhD DipECZM (Small Mammal)
*European Recognized Veterinary Specialist in
Zoological Medicine (Small Mammal)*
Clinic for Exotic Pets, Reptiles, Pet and Feral Birds,
Hannover Veterinary University, Buenteweg 9,
D- 30559 Hannover, Germany

Nicki Grint BVSc PhD DVA DiplECVAA MRCVS
Cave Veterinary Specialists, George's Farm,
West Buckland, Nr Wellington,
Somerset TA21 9LE

Frances Harcourt-Brown BVSc DipECZM (Small Mammal) FRCVS
*RCVS Recognized Specialist in Rabbit Medicine
and Surgery*
*European Recognized Veterinary Specialist in
Zoological Medicine (Small Mammal)*
30 Crab Lane, Harrogate,
North Yorkshire HG1 3BE

Nigel Harcourt-Brown BVSc FRCVS
30 Crab Lane, Harrogate,
North Yorkshire HG1 3BE

Craig Hunt BVetMed CertSAM CertZooMed MRCVS
Chine House Veterinary Hospital, Sileby Hall,
Cossington Road, Sileby, Loughborough,
Leicestershire LE12 7RS

Vladimír Jekl DVM PhD DipECZM (Small Mammal)
*European Recognized Veterinary Specialist in
Zoological Medicine (Small Mammal)*
Avian and Exotic Animal Clinic,
Faculty of Veterinary Medicine, University of
Veterinary and Pharmaceutical Sciences Brno,
Palackého 1–3, 61242 Brno, Czech Republic

Cathy Johnson-Delaney DVM DABVP-Avian DABVP-Exotic Companion Mammal
Avian and Exotic Animal Medical Center,
Kirkland, WA 98034, USA

Emma Keeble BVSc Diploma Zoological Medicine (Mammalian) MRCVS
*RCVS Recognized Specialist in Zoo and Wildlife
Medicine*
The Royal (Dick) School of Veterinary Studies,
Easter Bush Campus, Midlothian EH25 9RG

Sorrel J. Langley-Hobbs MA BVetMed DSAS(O) DipECVS MRCVS
Department of Veterinary Medicine,
University of Cambridge, Madingley Road,
Cambridge CB3 OES

Angela M. Lennox DVM DABVP-Avian DABVP-Exotic Companion Mammal
Avian and Exotic Animal Clinic of Indianapolis,
9330 Waldemar Road, Indianapolis,
IN 4626, USA

William GV Lewis BVSc CertZooMed MRCVS
Orchid Veterinary Surgery, 309 Ongar Road,
Brentwood, Essex

Alessandro Melillo DVM
Roma, Italy

Anna Meredith MA VetMB PhD CertLAS DZooMed MRCVS
Professor of Zoological and Conservation Medicine,
Head of Exotic Animal and Wildlife Service,
Royal (Dick) School of Veterinary Studies,
University of Edinburgh, Hospital for Small Animals,
Easter Bush Veterinary Centre, Roslin,
Midlothian EH25 9RT

Aidan Raftery MVB CertZooMed CBiol MSB MRCVS
Avian and Exotic Animal Clinic,
221 Upper Chorlton Road, Whalley Range,
Manchester M16 0DE

Sharon Redrobe BSc(Hons) BVetMed CertLAS
DZooMed MRCVS
RCVS Specialist in Zoo & Wildlife Medicine
Zoological Director, Twycross Zoo, Burton Road,
Atherstone, Warwickshire CV9 3PX

Richard Saunders BSc BVSc MRCVS CBiol MSB
DZooMed (Mammalian)
Veterinary Department, Bristol Zoo Gardens,
Clifton, Bristol BS8 3HA

Nico J. Schoemaker DVM PhD DipECZM (Small
Mammal & Avian) DipABVP-Avian
*European Recognized Veterinary Specialist in
Zoological Medicine (Small Mammal)*
Division of Zoological Medicine, Department of
Clinical Sciences of Companion Animals,
Faculty of Veterinary Medicine, Utrecht University,
Yalelaan 108, 3584 CM Utrecht, The Netherlands

Molly Varga BVetMed DZooMed MRCVS
*RCVS Recognized Specialist in Zoo and Wildlife
Medicine*
Cheshire Pet Medical Centre, Holmes Chapel,
Cheshire CW4 8AB

Stefanie Veraa DVM DipECVDI
Division of Diagnostic Imaging, Department of
Clinical Sciences of Companion Animals,
Utrecht University, Yalelaan 108, 3584 CM Utrecht,
The Netherlands

Foreword

Publication of this latest BSAVA Manual dealing solely with rabbits indicates how much our knowledge of the veterinary care of this species has advanced. I contributed a chapter on Rabbits to an early BSAVA Exotic Pets Manual in the 1980s, and again in 1995. These sections were intended to provide veterinary surgeons with everything they needed to know about rabbits. When the *BSAVA Manual of Rabbit Medicine and Surgery* was published five years later, the amount of knowledge available, and the application of this information in veterinary practice had increased dramatically. Six years after that, a second edition expanded this information still further.

This new Manual represents a milestone in the development of rabbit medicine and surgery, since the information needed to deal with rabbits in veterinary practice can no longer be encompassed in a single volume. A companion volume dealing with rabbit medicine is in preparation, and together these manuals will provide an invaluable resource for busy practitioners.

As with other BSAVA Manuals, the various sections of the text are well illustrated, informative, readily accessible and, most importantly, written by colleagues with an excellent understanding of their subject. Rabbit owners expect high standards of care for their pets and this text will greatly assist practitioners in delivering this care. Some of the techniques described will no doubt seem challenging, but the clear descriptions of the surgical approaches will encourage colleagues to transfer experience gained in other species and apply this to rabbits.

I congratulate the editors on providing such an excellent contribution to the veterinary care of rabbits, and I am sure this volume will become indispensible to our colleagues in small animal practice.

Paul Flecknell MA VetMB PhD DECLAM DLAS DECVA(Hon) DACLAM(Hon) FRCVS
Comparative Biology Centre
University of Newcastle

Preface

Rabbits are now the third most commonly kept pet in the UK and make up a considerable component of the work of any small animal practice. As a consequence, knowledge of rabbit medicine and surgery has had to grow rapidly in the past decade, in a manner not dissimilar to the situation seen with cats in the 1970s and '80s. Since the second edition of the *BSAVA Manual of Rabbit Medicine and Surgery* was published in 2006, the volume of published knowledge and field experience has increased to the extent that a single Manual will no longer suffice.

This book presents the major surgical and dental issues that are so common in rabbits yet do not receive full coverage elsewhere.

The first part of the Manual consists of two chapters on anaesthesia and analgesia. Rabbits have an unjust reputation for being poor surgical candidates; Chapter 1 explains how this has come about and explains how to achieve greater success with rabbit anaesthesia, as well as providing practical advice on different regimes for different situations/risk levels. Being prey species, reduction of pain and stress is vital for achieving surgical success in rabbit surgery. The analgesia chapter therefore covers not just chemical pain relief but also hospitalization and postoperative care.

The second part of the Manual covers imaging techniques. Radiography is an essential tool in diagnosis and surgical planning and so five chapters are devoted to general and specific radiographic techniques and interpretation. Chapters follow on other imaging techniques (ultrasonography, endoscopy, CT and MRI) which are achieving ever-increasing prominence in rabbit practice.

The third part covers surgical techniques in the rabbit. General principles of rabbit surgery, as compared to the more familiar pet species, are discussed, as well as specific surgical techniques and procedures. These cover basic techniques such as neutering, and progress to more specialized techniques in each organ system. Soft and hard tissue surgery are covered in this section. Extensive use is made of 'Operative Techniques' that allow detailed coverage (in words and pictures) of specific surgical procedures.

The final section of the Manual is devoted to probably the most common problems seen in rabbit practice – dental disease and abscessation. As would be expected for such a complex and difficult syndrome, comprehensive coverage is given to the aetiology and pathogenesis of dental disease and the techniques required for a full dental examination and evaluation.

Treatment of both cheek tooth overgrowth and dental abscesses encompasses many controversies and the editors have made no attempt to draw a veil over these. Instead, many different techniques are described and the reader is encouraged to draw their own conclusions as to the correct methods to use in each case.

This book could not have been produced without a lot of help. We are very grateful to all the authors for their time, patience and hard work. We are particularly grateful to the BSAVA publishing team for all their encouragement and technical assistance – the unseen work without which no book could be produced. Excellent drawings have been produced by Samantha Elmhurst and these greatly enhance the text.

Finally, the editors would like to thank their families for tolerating their long-term absence from family life, and for all their support and encouragement.

Frances Harcourt-Brown and John Chitty
July 2013

Anaesthesia

Nicki Grint

Rabbits may require sedation or anaesthesia for a variety of reasons. Neutering of male and female rabbits is now commonplace in general practice, as is dental treatment. Clinical cases may also require sedation or anaesthesia for investigation or treatment of various conditions. This chapter details specific considerations for rabbit anaesthesia, and also includes an overview of sedative, anaesthetic and analgesic drugs which may be used in this species.

Comparative risk of anaesthesia

Rabbits are famed for being high-risk candidates for anaesthesia. This infamy is only partially deserved; a recent study by Brodbelt *et al.* (2008) identified that 1 in 72 rabbits die within 48 hours of anaesthesia, compared with 1 in 601 dogs and 1 in 419 cats. When data from healthy rabbits (ASA classification of 1 or 2; Figure 1.1) were assessed separately, the mortality rate was 1 in 137 healthy rabbits (compared with 1 in 1840 dogs and 1 in 893 cats). Rabbits with systemic disease or injury increasing their risk category to an ASA classification of 3 or more also have an increased risk of perianaesthetic death, at 1 in 14 (compared with 1 in 75 dogs and 1 in 71 cats). Of the cases reported, 6% died during induction of anaesthesia, 30% during maintenance of anaesthesia, with the remaining 64% of animals dying in the postoperative period. The majority of these animals died in the first 3 hours after the end of anaesthesia. Almost 60% of deaths had no known cause, with the majority of the remaining cases dying from cardiovascular or pulmonary complications. Understanding

that rabbits with systemic disease need to be anaesthetized differently from healthy rabbits, and improving vigilance in the postoperative period, will greatly increase the general practitioner's success in anaesthetizing these animals.

Although there is still scope for substantial improvement in these mortality figures, the statistics for healthy rabbits dying under anaesthesia improved over the 18 years previous to the study by Brodbelt *et al.* (2008). The first UK study of this kind suggested an overall death rate of 1 in 28 in rabbits (Clarke and Hall, 1990). This improvement is encouraging and suggests that veterinary surgeons and nurses are becoming increasingly familiar with this species in their day-to-day work, with the rabbit now the third most commonly anaesthetized pet in the UK (Brodbelt *et al.*, 2008). This is also coupled with the release into the market of anaesthetic and sedative drugs with wider safety profiles.

When anaesthetizing rabbits several factors should be considered.

- **Underlying disease**. Many rabbits that are presented for anaesthesia are not in full health. Malnourishment and dehydration (common in rabbits requiring dental treatment) should be identifiable on clinical examination. However, some conditions, such as subclinical respiratory disease caused by pasteurellosis, may be present but not apparent on clinical examination. This disease can affect the rabbit's ability to oxygenate its tissues during anaesthesia, and may also progress to a clinical infection postoperatively.

Grade	Categorization	How it should influence anaesthesia
1	A normal healthy patient	Standard protocols should apply with routine monitoring
2	A patient with mild systemic disease	Standard protocols may still apply with additional monitoring
3	A patient with severe systemic disease	Thorough stabilization should be performed before anaesthesia is attempted. Intravenous catheterization, fluid therapy and airway protection are strongly advised
4	A patient with severe systemic disease that is a constant threat to life	As for grade 3. Owners should be fully briefed as to additional anaesthetic risk. Doses for CCPR should be calculated and the first dose drawn up
5	A moribund patient who is not expected to survive without the operation	As for grade 4

1.1 American Society of Anesthesiologists (ASA) classification system (adapted) and how it should influence anaesthesia. (Source: www.asahq.org)

- **Poor husbandry and feeding practices** can produce obese rabbits. These rabbits can be poor candidates for anaesthesia due to their high resting heart rates and predisposition to developing hypertension and cardiac hypertrophy. They will be more prone to oxygen desaturation, owing to a reduction in their functional residual capacity, especially when turned into dorsal recumbency. All drug doses should be based on the rabbit's lean bodyweight; particular attention should be paid to cardiovascular monitoring and pre-oxygenation; and oxygen supplementation is advised to offset potential hypoxaemia.
- **Lack of expertise.** Although rabbits are the third most commonly anaesthetized pet there are still veterinary staff who are unfamiliar or lacking in confidence with the anaesthesia of this species. The dissimilarities in anatomy and physiology between rabbits and other small animal species

(Figure 1.2) also make extrapolation of techniques and dosages inappropriate. When presented with an unfamiliar species to anaesthetize, many veterinary surgeons will look to textbooks for anaesthetic protocols. Until recently, doses of drugs listed in many texts were taken from studies based on experimental animals that were specific-pathogen-free and of a higher health status than pet rabbits. The drug requirements and doses required to produce sedation and anaesthesia for rabbits being anaesthetized in everyday veterinary practice will often be much lower than those used in biomedical research. In recent years, more and more studies have been published based on data from pet rabbits of a similar health status to those seen in general practice; several of these papers are referred to in the anaesthetic protocols section below.

Differences	Implications for anaesthesia
Respiratory system	
Glottis size is smaller per unit bodyweight than in dogs and cats	A range of ET tubes should be prepared, and the sizes chosen should be slightly smaller than would fit a cat or dog of the same bodyweight
Limited gape with larger incisors and fleshier tongue than dogs and cats	Visualization for ET intubation can be more challenging
Minute volume, alveolar ventilation and metabolic oxygen demand are higher than in larger animals	Fresh gas flow calculations should be based on a minute volume of 250 ml/kg/min instead of 200 ml/kg/min. Uptake of volatile agents is faster. Lower tolerance of hypoxaemia
Smaller tidal volume than dogs and cats	Smaller tidal volumes of 6–8 ml/kg should be used during IPPV
Thoracic cavity is smaller in comparison to rest of body	Abnormalities such as abdominal distension, pleural effusion, etc. that can compromise thoracic excursions will have a significant impact on the rabbit's respiratory efforts
Cardiovascular system	
Blood volume is approximately 60 ml/kg *versus* 90 ml/kg in dogs	Even small blood losses may be of more consequence in a rabbit
Limited collateral circulation in the myocardium	May be more prone to myocardial hypoxaemia and arrhythmias
Daily fluid maintenance is 100–120 ml/kg/day – higher than that of dogs and cats	Maintenance fluid therapy is 4–5 ml/kg/h *versus* 2 ml/kg/h in dogs and cats
Gastrointestinal system	
Complex digestive physiology of hindgut fermenters compared to monogastrics (dogs and cats)	Disruption of physiology perianaesthesia, e.g. starvation, untreated pain, can lead to gastrointestinal stasis
Well developed and anatomically arranged cardiac sphincter prevents vomiting	Rabbits should not be fasted prior to anaesthesia – there is no risk of vomiting at induction
Higher metabolic rate	Greater requirements for metabolic substrates, so may be prone to hypoglycaemia, etc. during longer anaesthetics
Pharmacokinetics and pharmacodynamics	
Higher surface area to volume ratio than larger animals	Allometric scaling (arithmetic relationship of biological function to body mass) means that drug dosages will be higher on a mg/kg basis
Higher metabolic rate	Many drugs will have a shorter duration of action
Higher levels of atropinase in some strains of rabbit	Atropine will be ineffective in these rabbits; if an anticholinergic is required, glycopyrrolate should be used

1.2 Some anatomical and physiological differences between the rabbit and larger animals.

- **Size.** Although rabbit breeds can range in size, from dwarfs to giant French Lops, most rabbits presented for anaesthesia will be of a small size. Anaesthetic techniques such as intravenous cannulation and endotracheal intubation are therefore more precise procedures, but can be easily mastered with practice. Small rabbits will not be able to tolerate high levels of resistance and dead space in the anaesthetic breathing systems used to deliver volatile agents and oxygen. In general terms, a smaller animal has a higher metabolic rate. Metabolism requires several driving forces, e.g. glucose and oxygen, and rabbits have higher demands for these substrates than larger animals. A smaller animal will have a higher surface area to volume ratio than a larger animal; having a relatively larger surface area tends to make the animal more susceptible to heat loss under anaesthesia. Hypothermia is common in small animal anaesthesia in general, but may be more pronounced in smaller species such as the rabbit.
- **Endotracheal (ET) intubation.** In addition to their small size, ET intubation in the rabbit can be made more challenging by a variety of other factors. Rabbits have a narrow gape, which makes visualization of the larynx difficult, and the view is also obscured by the long incisors and fleshy tongue. Laryngospasm (similar to that seen when attempting ET intubation in the cat) can be encountered, and may be influenced by the choice of anaesthetic protocol. The glottis of the rabbit is relatively small compared with that of other species of a similar weight, and therefore the practitioner should be prepared to insert a slightly smaller diameter ET tube than they would use for a cat of the same bodyweight. Iatrogenic respiratory mucosal damage is a potential consequence of ET intubation, as with any species, but can be avoided by the use of clean, contaminant-free tubes and handling the rabbit gently (especially when turning it) when intubated.
- **Pain.** Rabbits are a prey species and so will be unwilling to show signs of pain, especially when housed with cats, dogs and other animals they may see as predators. Pain assessment in rabbits is in its infancy, but our ability to recognize pain

behaviours is improving, and pain assessment should be carried out regularly (see Chapter 2).
- **Gastrointestinal system.** Rabbits are classed as hindgut fermenters: they use microbes for the digestion of food in their large caecum and proximal colon. Rabbits can develop ileus postoperatively, and factors that may increase the likelihood of this include starvation and alteration of diet. As gut motility is governed by the parasympathetic nervous system, sympathetic stimulation resulting from stress, anxiety, fear and pain will all slow gut motility. Simple husbandry choices such as housing away from predator species in a quiet calm environment, not starving before anaesthesia, and ensuring adequate analgesia, should limit the likelihood of gut stasis. The choice of anaesthetic and analgesic drugs has also been suggested to influence the development of ileus. Tympany, due either to gut stasis or intestinal obstruction, can have deleterious effects during anaesthesia, increasing pressure on the diaphragm and thus affecting the rabbit's ability to ventilate and reducing its functional residual lung capacity. Aortocaval compression can also occur when the rabbit is turned into dorsal recumbency, owing to pressure on the vessels from the tympanic gut content.
- **Authorization of drugs.** There are few anaesthetic, sedative and analgesic drugs authorized in the UK for use in the rabbit. Authorization indicates that the product has undergone rigorous clinical testing in this particular species by the drug manufacturing company, as required by UK law. While authorized drugs should be used whenever possible, it is often necessary to follow the prescribing cascade. Many drugs that are not authorized in the rabbit have been used successfully over many years for rabbit anaesthesia, with clinical research published on the relevant protocols (see Figure 1.3 for examples). Practitioners are encouraged to refer to Figure 1.4, which contains notes relating to pre-anaesthetic, analgesic and sedative drugs, with an indication as to whether the drug is currently authorized or not.

Pre-anaesthetic medication	Induction of anaesthesia	Reference
	Ketamine 15 mg/kg + midazolam 3 mg/kg i.m.	Grint and Murison (2008)
	Ketamine 15 mg/kg + medetomidine 0.25 mg/kg i.m. or s.c.	Grint and Murison (2008) Orr *et al.* (2005)
	Ketamine 15 mg/kg + medetomidine 0.5 mg/kg s.c.	Orr *et al.* (2005)
Fentanyl/fluanisone 0.1 ml/kg i.m.	Propofol i.v. to effect (mean dose 2.2 mg/kg)	Martinez *et al.* (2009)
Fentanyl/fluanisone 0.1 ml/kg i.m.	Midazolam i.v. to effect (mean dose 0.7 mg/kg)	Martinez *et al.* (2009)
Buprenorphine 0.03 mg/kg i.m.	Alfaxalone 2–3 mg/kg i.v.	Grint *et al.* (2008)

1.3 Pre-anaesthetic medication and induction doses from studies on pet rabbit populations.

Drug	Drug type	Notes	Dosage	Authorized for use in rabbits in the UK?
Acepromazine	Phenothiazine	Produces sedation and some anxiolysis. No antagonist available. Several sites of action, including alpha-1 adrenoceptor blockade which causes vasodilation. Highly protein-bound. Undergoes hepatic metabolism and then excretion in urine and bile	0.1–1 mg/kg s.c. or i.m.	No
Medetomidine	Alpha-2 adrenergic agonist	Can be combined with opioids and with ketamine for more profound sedation. Produces anxiolysis, profound sedation and analgesia. Also causes: muscle relaxation; bradycardia; blood pressure effects (initial hypertension, then reduction in blood pressure to near normal or slight hypotension); reduction in gastrointestinal tract motility; increased uterine activity; and diuresis. Metabolized in the liver, and excreted in the urine. Atipamezole is an antagonist specifically for medetomidine (and dexmedetomidine, below; suggested doses 0.5–1 mg/kg s.c. or i.m.)	80–100 µg/kg s.c. or i.m.	No
Dexmedetomidine	Alpha-2 adrenergic agonist	Active enantiomer of medetomidine. Similar effects to those described for medetomidine	25 µg/kg i.m.	No
Pethidine	Full µ agonist opioid	Causes histamine release and must not be given intravenously. Tends to increase heart rate in mammals. Mild sedation and good analgesia produced. Schedule 2 Controlled Drug	5–10 mg/kg s.c. or i.m. q2–3h	No
Butorphanol	Mixed agonist–antagonist opioid	κ agonist and µ antagonist. Produces analgesia and good sedation. Reverses respiratory depression produced by fentanyl/fluanisone (Flecknell *et al.*, 1999)	0.1–0.5 mg/kg s.c. q4h	No
Buprenorphine	Partial µ agonist opioid	Produces analgesia and moderate sedation. Longer lasting than other opioids. Increases duration of ketamine + medetomidine anaesthesia (Murphy *et al.*, 2010). Reverses respiratory depression produced by fentanyl/fluanisone (Flecknell *et al.*, 1999). Produces mild respiratory depression but little cardiovascular change (Shafford and Schadt, 2008). Schedule 3 Controlled Drug	0.01–0.05 mg/kg i.m., s.c. or i.v.	No
Morphine	Full µ agonist opioid	Provides sedation and analgesia. Produces some histamine release. Tends to produce slight bradycardia. Schedule 2 Controlled Drug	2–5 mg/kg i.m. or s.c. q2–4h	No
Midazolam	Benzodiazepine	Twice as potent as diazepam. Water-soluble so can be given intramuscularly or intranasally. Produces anxiolysis and sedation. Not analgesic. Anticonvulsant and also causes skeletal muscle relaxation. Few cardiovascular and respiratory effects. Binds to GABA$_A$ receptors. Highly protein-bound. Undergoes hepatic metabolism before urinary and biliary elimination	0.2–2 mg/kg i.m. or i.v.	No
Diazepam	Benzodiazepine	Half as potent as midazolam but otherwise similar effects. Not water soluble and so should not be injected intramuscularly or subcutaneously (will cause pain and be of low bioavailability)	1 mg/kg i.v. or per rectum	No
Fentanyl/fluanisone	Combination of butyrophenone (fluanisone) and full µ agonist opioid (fentanyl)	Butyrophenones will cause sedation and vasodilation via alpha-1 adrenergic blockade. Fentanyl produces sedation, analgesia and some respiratory depression. Can produce full anaesthesia if combined with benzodiazepine. Sequential analgesia produced if buprenorphine administered. Schedule 2 Controlled Drug	0.2–0.5 ml/kg i.m.	Yes

1.4 Pre-anaesthetic medications commonly used in rabbits. Drug doses are taken from the *BSAVA Small Animal Formulary*, 7th edn.

Pre-anaesthetic preparation

All animals should be assessed and stabilized as fully as possible before they are anaesthetized.

Assessment

Assessment should be carried out by the veterinary surgeon, and should include a full clinical examination and history taking. Clinical examination should include:

- Mucous membrane colour
- Assessment of hydration (Figure 1.5)
- Thoracic auscultation: should encompass the whole thorax, paying particular attention to the sternal area or immediately lateral to it, where many murmurs can be auscultated
- Assessment of peripheral pulse quality (from the auricular artery).

Percentage dehydration	Clinical signs
<5%	History of fluid loss, e.g. diarrhoea, but no evidence of mucous membrane dryness or skin tenting
5%	Mild skin tenting and mucous membrane dryness
7%	Increased skin tenting, dry mucous membranes, possible sunken globes, pulse quality acceptable
10%	Increased skin tenting, dry mucous membranes, sunken globes, decreased pulse quality
12%	As for 10%, but altered level of consciousness, may now be bradycardic
15%	As for 12%, but moribund

1.5 Assessment of dehydration in mammals.

Routine pre-anaesthetic blood screening is not warranted in healthy patients. A thorough clinical examination and history taking will be more pertinent to the anaesthetic choices than routine biochemistry and haematology. If abnormalities are identified on clinical examination or the history suggests underlying illness, investigations should be performed to gain all relevant information before proceeding to general anaesthesia. Pre-anaesthetic assessment using conscious capnography can identify individuals with respiratory compromise. This is performed by connecting a capnograph (see section on Monitoring below) to a small ET tube connector and positioning it in the nostril of the conscious rabbit (with or without topical local anaesthetic). Elevated carbon dioxide levels suggest pneumonia, even when the rabbit's respiratory pattern appears normal.

Stabilization
Rabbits that are not in ASA class 1 or 2 should be stabilized as fully as possible. Examples include: correcting dehydration with fluid therapy; antibiosis; and treatment to improve lung function if pneumonia is present.

Fluid therapy
The fluid deficit which needs to be restored can be calculated by multiplying bodyweight in kilograms by the percentage dehydration. For example, if a 2 kg rabbit is 10% dehydrated, its fluid deficit is estimated as 200 ml. This fluid deficit can be corrected over the same timeframe as that over which the fluid loss was estimated to have happened.

Up to 60 ml/kg (equivalent to one blood volume) can be supplied over 1 hour to extremely hypovolaemic patients. These fluids should be given intravenously or via the intraosseous route. Rabbits that are in hypovolaemic shock may be bradycardic (unlike cats and dogs, which tend to mount a tachycardia), hypothermic and hypotensive. Blood pressure monitoring (using the Doppler technique – see later) can be used to help assess the response to fluid therapy.

Fluid therapy can be administered via a variety of routes. Mildly dehydrated animals can be given slurry diets orally, which will provide water and food. Small animal patients have an extensive potential subcutaneous space which can be utilized for the administration of crystalloid fluids, although only mild dehydration should be corrected by this route. Complete absorption of subcutaneous fluid can take 6–8 hours. In the case of moderate to marked dehydration, absorption of subcutaneous fluid will be slower, if it occurs at all. Suggested volumes vary between authors, but are between 10 and 20 ml/kg per site, or 30–50 ml per rabbit.

Intravenous access
Securing intravenous access is recommended for anaesthesia (other than for very short procedures) and high-risk sedation procedures. Once in place, cannulas should not be removed until the rabbit has recovered fully from anaesthesia. Intravenous cannulation allows pre-anaesthetic medications and induction agents to be given accurately, avoiding the drug being deposited outside the vein. Intravenous fluid therapy can be used perioperatively, and it facilitates 'topping up' of injectable anaesthetic agents, analgesics and any other intravenous drugs. In addition, having intravenous access allows emergency drug administration during any critical incident.

Intravenous cannulas that are commonly used in rabbits tend to be made of polyurethane and are usually 22 or 24 G. The larger the diameter of cannula (i.e. the lower the gauge) that can be placed, the easier the fluid or drug administration will be, owing to lower resistance to flow. In the rabbit, cannulas are usually placed in the marginal ear vein. Cannulation is facilitated by the use of a local anaesthetic cream (such as EMLA) applied to a clipped area over the insertion site, and covered with an occlusive dressing (such as cling film or Opsite Flexigrid), 30–40 minutes before cannula placement. Most rabbits will leave this dressing alone (especially if it is covered with a cohesive bandage and secured with adhesive tape to the base of the ear) for the prescribed time. For a step-by-step guide to cannulation see Technique 1.1.

Most cannulas can be removed once the rabbit has recovered fully from anaesthesia. Cannulas that are left in place when they are not required will act as potential sites for infection. They can also subdue rabbits, which appear to dislike the weight of the dressings. If the cannula needs to be left *in situ* for clinical reasons, it can be maintained for up to 2–3 days as long as it is checked regularly, i.e. the dressing is unwrapped and the cannula checked for patency and for evidence of infection and flushed with heparinized saline at least twice daily.

If the rabbit's peripheral veins are particularly small (due to the size of the rabbit or vasoconstriction), the following techniques may be useful. First, EMLA cream may vasodilate the vascular bed, facilitating visualization of the veins. If using a 24 G cannula, it should first be pre-flushed with heparinized saline, because the bore of the cannula is often so narrow that a clot will occlude the internal diameter and prevent blood flowing back. If the peripheral circulation is poor, sometimes blood will not flow back into the cannula hub. If this is suspected, the cannula should be threaded off the stylet and flushed to ensure correct positioning. If the cannula is lying outside the vein, a second attempt should be made more proximal to the ear base. If cannulation of a marginal ear vein is unsuccessful, the cephalic vein can be cannulated; it is usually of a slightly larger diameter. Making a small 'cut down' with a scalpel blade over the vein and retracting the skin either side to aid visualization of the vessel may help when establishing intravenous access in rabbits with peripheral shutdown. An alternative method, if intravenous access is unsuccessful, involves intraosseous cannulation, either into the greater trochanter of the humerus or femur, or into the tibial crest.

Preventing heat loss

Prevention of hypothermia can be achieved by passive or active methods. Passive techniques involve insulation, i.e. wrapping any areas not exposed for surgery with thermal material or bubble wrap. Reduction of evaporative heat loss can be achieved by maintaining a high ambient theatre temperature, and minimizing the area of the surgical clip and volume of surgical scrub used. Reducing heat and moisture loss from the respiratory tract can also be of use in preventing hypothermia. In large rabbits that are of an appropriate size, a rebreathing system can be used to deliver volatile agents and carrier gases. Partial rebreathing of the exhaled gases will ensure that some of the moisture and heat are retained, alongside the water and heat generated by the reaction of soda lime with carbon dioxide. Non-rebreathing systems will be used for most rabbits and cold dry gases tend to exacerbate hypothermia. Heat–moisture exchangers (HMEs) can be placed between the ET tube and the breathing system to warm and humidify the inspired gases. They are available in a variety of sizes but will increase the amount of breathing system dead space and resistance. Paediatric versions are available and are most appropriate for use in the rabbit.

Warming a rabbit 'pre-induction' is a very useful technique to prevent heat loss during the first hour of anaesthesia. Active warming should continue through anaesthesia and into recovery. Rabbits can be actively warmed using heated mats, wheat bags and heat lamps. Given that unconscious or sedated rabbits are unable to move away from the source of heat, direct contact against the skin should be avoided to prevent thermal burns. Circulating warm air or warm water blankets can also be used to good effect, maintaining or even increasing a rabbit's body temperature during surgery. Intravenous fluids can be gently warmed during infusion, as can surgical preparation solutions and lavage fluids.

Feeding

Rabbits cannot vomit and can therefore be fed up to the point of premedication; this will maintain glucose levels, sustain body heat production as a byproduct of metabolism, and minimize the risk of gut stasis.

Pre-anaesthetic medication

Pre-anaesthetic medications are used to sedate and calm animals before anaesthetic induction. Pre-anaesthetic medication is used for a variety of reasons:

- To reduce anxiety in the patient, making it more amenable to handling for intravenous cannulation and induction of anaesthesia. Rabbits can be easily stressed, and struggling before anaesthesia can result in fracturing of vertebrae, catecholamine-induced arrhythmias, or difficulty placing the intravenous cannula. Stress is also a contributing factor to gut stasis and may influence the distribution and action of certain anaesthetic drugs
- To smooth the induction of anaesthesia and reduce the induction dose needed
- To smooth the maintenance phase of anaesthesia and reduce the percentage of volatile agent required
- To smooth the recovery from anaesthesia
- To provide pre-emptive analgesia
- To provide muscle relaxation.

Once the drug has been administered, the rabbit should be left undisturbed for the expected time of onset of action of the drug, to achieve the best effect. During this time the animal should be monitored unobtrusively.

Drugs that have been used as premedicants in rabbits include acepromazine, benzodiazepines, alpha-2 adrenergic agonists and opioids. Notes on these drugs can be found in Figure 1.4, which includes drug dosages suggested by the *BSAVA Small Animal Formulary*. Drug choice will depend on the health status of the animal, and the familiarity of the practitioner with different drugs. For example, depth of sedation will be greatest with alpha-2 adrenergic agonists and these are appropriate drugs to give to rabbits in ASA classes 1 and 2. However, opioids and benzodiazepines, which are less sedative and have fewer cardiovascular effects, are more appropriate for less healthy rabbits.

While the breed of rabbit can have an influence on the drug doses required, dosages (on a mg/kg basis) tend to be higher in rabbits than in dogs and cats. This is due to allometric scaling, because rabbits have a higher surface area to volume ratio.

As noted above, few premedicants are authorized for use in the rabbit in the UK. One authorized premedicant is a neuroleptanalgesic combination of fentanyl and fluanisone, marketed under the trade name Hypnorm. It is a Schedule 2 Controlled Drug. Fluanisone is a butyrophenone and produces sedation and cardiovascular effects similar to those of the phenothiazine drugs (e.g. acepromazine). Fentanyl, an opioid, produces sedation and analgesia, but also some respiratory depression. By itself, Hypnorm produces poor muscle relaxation, and so it is often co-administered with a benzodiazepine. The administration of buprenorphine after this neuroleptanalgesic combination produces 'sequential analgesia' – where the partial antagonism of the fentanyl reduces respiratory depression, but does not completely discontinue analgesia. The combination of Hypnorm and a benzodiazepine provides good sedation and is recommended for rabbits in ASA classes 1 and 2. However, recovery from anaesthesia, while smooth, can be prolonged, and therefore the author recommends this protocol for cases anaesthetized early in the day or those that are to be hospitalized overnight.

Atropine is an antimuscarinic drug that elevates the heart rate and reduces respiratory secretions. The author does not recommend the use of this drug in rabbits for routine pre-anaesthetic medication, because increasing their already fast heart rate further may impair myocardial oxygenation. In addition, drier, more viscous respiratory secretions can block small airways. Ileus may also occur after atropine administration owing to the effect of the drug on the parasympathetic drive of gut motility. In addition, rabbits produce a high level of atropinases, which means that any effects of atropine are short lived. If an anticholinergic is needed for any reason, e.g. to treat a vasovagal reflex, glycopyrrolate (0.1 mg/kg s.c.) should be used instead.

Pre-oxygenation

Given that pet rabbits often have subclinical respiratory infections and that ET intubation can take time, pre-oxygenation before induction of anaesthesia is of great value. Supplying a high fraction of inspired oxygen will delay desaturation if any problems occur during induction and ET intubation.

An effective and practical method is to administer the oxygen via facemask for 5 minutes. A clear Perspex mask is recommended (Figure 1.6) so that the anaesthetist can observe the colour of the rabbit's mucous membranes. Using a mask with a rubber diaphragm to create a seal will increase the level of inspired oxygen and these should be used in rabbits that are sufficiently sedated. However, lightly sedated or fully conscious rabbits may struggle if attempts are made to pre-oxygenate with a tight-fitting mask. Stress is counterproductive and therefore a balance may have to be sought whereby the fraction of inspired oxygen is increased moderately using a looser-fitting mask, but without undue stress to the rabbit.

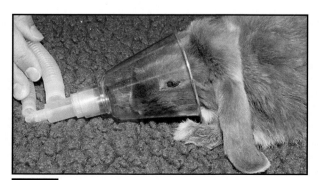

1.6 Administration of oxygen using a facemask.

Alternatives such as flow-by oxygen (i.e. holding an oxygen source in front of the rabbit's head) provide levels of inspired oxygen only just higher than room air, and any pre-oxygenation achieved by placing a rabbit in an oxygen tent is soon lost when the rabbit is lifted out of the oxygen tent for induction; these techniques are therefore not recommended for pre-oxygenation.

Induction of anaesthesia

Anaesthesia can be induced by intravenous, intramuscular, subcutaneous or inhalational drug administration. All of these techniques have relative advantages and disadvantages (Figure 1.7).

Intravenous	Intramuscular	Inhalation
Can be titrated to effect	Whole dose is given, unable to give to effect	Can be titrated to effect
Effect usually shorter	Effect usually longer	Effect usually shorter
Needs intravenous access	No special equipment needed	Anaesthetic machine, volatile agent, mask and oxygen needed
No pollution potential	No pollution potential	Environmental pollution potential
Rapid induction	Slower induction	Slower induction
Accurate weight needed	Accurate weight needed	Accurate weight not needed

1.7 Relative advantages and disadvantages of different induction techniques.

Induction using injectable agents

- Intravenous cannulation will facilitate the slow administration of intravenous induction agents 'to effect', which is preferred to a rapid bolus dose.
- The author administers intramuscular injections into the lumbar epaxial muscles. Injections of anaesthetic and sedative drugs into the muscle of the hindlimbs have led to self-mutilation in some rabbits. Many drugs (e.g. alpha-2 adrenergic agonists, ketamine, opioids, acepromazine) are suitable for mixing with another drug in the same syringe to limit the number of injections given and to increase the volume of injectate, because very small volumes may not be absorbed well. Very large volumes of injectate can produce discomfort, and current recommendations are to limit the volume to 0.25 ml/kg for an intramuscular injection, and 0.5 ml/kg for other routes (Diehl *et al.*, 2001).
- Several drug combinations can be effective when given by the subcutaneous route. The onset of action will usually be slower, but the discomfort on injection is reduced for the rabbit, and therefore this route is preferred if either intramuscular or subcutaneous injections are available.

Various injectable agent combinations have been used in pet rabbits (Figure 1.8) which the author has found useful in her rabbit patients. Further information on individual drugs can be found in Figure 1.4.

Induction using inhalational agents

Inhalational induction using a vaporized volatile anaesthetic can be carried out using a facemask (with diaphragm) or an induction chamber. There are advantages and disadvantages of this technique over injectable techniques (see Figure 1.7). Disadvantages of inhalational induction include a slower time to loss of consciousness compared with intravenous induction. In addition, inhalational induction can potentially create atmospheric pollution and therefore effective scavenging is mandatory.

The main reason that this method is not recommended by the author is that it can be very stressful for the patient. Rabbits appear to find inhalational agents aversive, and can struggle violently if induced with no premedication or sedation (Flecknell *et al.*, 1999). Therefore the author prefers to use injectable anaesthesia for rabbits in ASA classes 1 and 2, and in general does not recommend the use of inhalation induction unless the rabbit is very obtunded through illness or moderately to deeply sedated with premedication. Inhalational inductions can be useful in rabbits in ASA classes 3 to 4 because, if properly managed, the cardiovascular effects of the volatile agents tend to be less marked than with injectable agents. In addition, unlike injectable agents, volatile agent induction can be stopped immediately and the gases will be excreted very quickly as they are exhaled; cases of overdose are therefore easy to rectify if the drug in question is a volatile agent.

Chambers *versus* facemasks

Induction chambers can be specially constructed or made from plastic boxes. The box should have a tight seal with an entry and exit portal. A pipe from the fresh gas flow of the anaesthetic machine should be plugged into the entry portal (preferably at the bottom of the chamber), and a scavenging hose should be connected to the exit portal (at the top of the chamber). All connections should be tight, to avoid leaks of volatile agent which will pollute the atmosphere. Smaller chambers are preferable to larger ones, because gas concentrations will change more rapidly after changing the dialled percentage on the vaporizer. In addition, some authors suggest that a close-fitting chamber in which the rabbit has contact with the walls appears to produce fewer stress-associated behaviours.

Initially, a high flow of oxygen should be introduced into the chamber to acclimatize the patient to the environment and pre-oxygenate them. Stress may also be reduced by adding some of the animal's bedding to the chamber, to provide some familiar smells and textures. Volatile agent can then be added incrementally. This is preferable to the sudden administration of a high percentage of volatile agent, which may cause the rabbit to hold its breath. The higher the fresh gas flow of carrier gas, the faster these changes in volatile agent percentage will be made. Volatile agent should be administered until the rabbit loses its righting reflex. At this point, the volatile agent should be discontinued, the chamber flushed with oxygen and the animal removed. If additional volatile agent is required, this can be administered by facemask.

Inhalational induction using a mask is an alternative technique, although breath-holding, leading to hypoxia, hypercapnia and bradycardia, can develop

Drug	Drug type	Notes	Authorized for use in rabbits in the UK?
Propofol	Substituted phenol	Intravenous administration only. Non-irritant if injected perivascularly. Acts at $GABA_A$ receptors. 98% protein-bound. No inherent analgesia. Apnoea can occur after injection. Hypotension may occur due to vasodilation and myocardial depression. Faster recovery from anaesthesia than with ketamine or thiopental	No
Alfaxalone	Neurosteroid	Solubilized in cyclodextrin. Intravenous or intramuscular administration. Non-irritant. Acts at $GABA_A$ receptors. 30% protein-bound. No inherent analgesia. Apnoea often occurs after intravenous induction. Tachycardia often seen after induction as a reflex response to hypotension	No
Ketamine	Phencyclidine derivative	Produces dissociative anaesthesia, characterized by light sleep and immobility. Intravenous or intramuscular administration. Intramuscular administration often painful. Poor muscle relaxation. Profound analgesia (especially effective against somatic pain and chronic pain). Antagonist at NMDA receptor. Active cranial nerve reflexes remain. Needs to be combined with other drugs (e.g. benzodiazepines or alpha-2 adrenergic agonists) to produce good quality anaesthesia. Slower onset of action than other induction agents. May produce increase in heart rate and blood pressure due to sympathetic nervous system stimulation	No
Etomidate	Short-acting hypnotic agent	Produces minimal cardiovascular or respiratory effects so ideal for the haemodynamically compromised patient. Solubilized in propylene glycol and therefore may cause thrombophlebitis, pain on injection and haemolysis. Can lead to short-term primary adrenal suppression, so corticosteroid synthesis is reversibly inhibited. Often administered after benzodiazepine premedication to improve muscle relaxation	No

1.8 Injectable induction agents commonly used in rabbits.

(Flecknell *et al.*, 1996). This technique also produces more environmental pollution than a chamber induction. The use of clear plastic masks with rubber seals will minimize environmental contamination with waste gases. As with chamber inductions, acclimatizing the animal using higher flow rates of oxygen will be of benefit, especially if the animal proceeds to hold its breath. The percentage of volatile agent can then be increased until the patient becomes unconscious. Occasionally, patients may show signs of involuntary excitement as they progress through the stages of anaesthesia. A small dose of intravenous induction agent can be used to stop this excitement; this smaller intravenous dose will have fewer cardiovascular effects than the full intravenous dose required to induce anaesthesia. Figure 1.9 summarizes the relative advantages and disadvantages of masks *versus* chambers for induction of anaesthesia.

Facemask	Induction chamber
Cheaper outlay for equipment	Purpose-built chambers are more expensive
Environmental pollution greater	Potential for environmental pollution is present but less than with mask
Faster change in inspired percentage after dial on vaporizer is changed	Slower change in inspired percentage after dial on vaporizer is changed, and rate of change dependent on fresh gas flow
Lower fresh gas flow required	Higher fresh gas flow required
Can cause stress to rabbit owing to restraint, application of tight-fitting mask and odour of volatile agent	Can cause stress to rabbit owing to unfamiliar surroundings and materials, high fresh gas flow and odour of volatile agent
If involuntary excitement is seen, a small intravenous dose of induction agent is more easily given	Unable to gain direct access to rabbit if involuntary excitement is witnessed

1.9 Some advantages and disadvantages of inhalational induction techniques.

Agents

All volatile agents can be used for inhalation induction, but the ideal agent would have the following properties:

* Non-irritant
* Pleasant taste and smell
* Does not induce respiratory depression
* No arrhythmias produced if adrenaline is released
* Rapid onset of action.

Of all the agents currently available, sevoflurane is the author's inhalation induction drug of choice, because its low blood gas solubility produces a fast induction, and it has a more pleasant odour and causes less respiratory mucosal irritation than isoflurane. However, significant periods of apnoea can still occur with sevoflurane. If the rabbit does become stressed, sevoflurane, in contrast to halothane, will not sensitize the myocardium to catecholamine-induced arrhythmias. Nitrous oxide will hasten the speed of anaesthetic induction, owing to its 'second gas effect', and can be added to the fresh gas flow to produce a 50:50 mixture with oxygen.

> **PRACTICAL TIP**
> Caution should be employed when interpreting blood biochemical analysis if blood samples have been drawn after the rabbit has been sedated or anaesthetized. Significant alterations in plasma cholesterol, triglycerides, lactate dehydrogenase (LDH), aspartate transaminase (AST), alanine aminotransferase (ALT), urea and creatinine are observed after administration of certain anaesthetics, including ketamine + diazepam and ketamine + xylazine. Therefore it is recommended that blood for biochemical analysis is drawn before anaesthesia.

Airway protection

Airway protection is recommended for all anaesthetized rabbits, except for the shortest procedures, where a mask may be sufficient. If a mask is employed for any length of time, hypercapnia, hypoxaemia and airway obstruction can develop (Bateman *et al.*, 2005).

Endotracheal tubes

An ET tube maintains a patent airway and prevents airway obstruction. The tube acts as a conduit to provide oxygen, volatile agents and other carrier gases to the patient's lungs, and to remove waste gases including carbon dioxide. As the volatile agent bypasses the olfactory parts of the respiratory mucosa when delivered down the ET tube, breath-holding (caused by the rabbit responding to the smell of the volatile agent) will be avoided. As well as delivering gases, ET intubation will prevent contamination of the environment with volatile agent pollutants. Intermittent positive pressure ventilation (IPPV) of a patient's lungs will be facilitated if an ET tube is in place.

ET tubes come in a variety of sizes and materials, including red rubber, polyvinyl chloride (PVC) and silicone. Tubes with internal diameters of 2.0–5.5 mm can be used, depending on the rabbit's size. Most small animal tubes are cuffed; the cuff, once inflated, creates a seal between the tube and the tracheal wall to prevent dilution of inspired gases with room air, prevent environmental pollution and provide additional airway protection from aspiration of fluid or debris. However, most ET tubes used in rabbits are uncuffed owing to the small laryngeal size and difficulty of intubation. Tubes should be lubricated to aid intubation. The author recommends a silicone-type spray, because jelly lubricant can block the end of small ET tubes.

Intubation techniques: Intubation via the oral route should only be attempted once general anaesthesia has been induced. The larynx is easily traumatized and therefore the tube should never be forced if any resistance is felt. Forcing the tube may produce oedema, swelling and haemorrhage, which will cause post-extubation airway occlusion. Some authors advocate the use of topical lidocaine applied to the larynx to prevent the laryngospasm that may result from ET intubation attempts. Intubation can take a little longer to perform in rabbits than in dogs and cats, especially while the practitioner is learning the technique, and therefore pre-oxygenation by mask for 2–3 minutes is suggested before intubation is attempted.

The larynx of the rabbit can be visualized with the aid of an endoscope, an otoscope or a paediatric laryngoscope (Wisconsin size 1 blade) in larger rabbits. A rigid endoscope is easier to use than a flexible endoscope, and a step-by-step guide can be seen in Technique 1.2. If a laryngoscope or otoscope is used, it is often helpful to place the rabbit in dorsal recumbency to aid visualization of the larynx. Often, with direct visualization, a stylet or canine urinary catheter can be introduced into the trachea initially, and then the ET tube can be 'railroaded' over this (see Technique 1.3). An alternative technique of ET intubation is the 'blind' method, where the anaesthetist relies on hearing breath sounds coming through the ET tube as the tube is advanced (see Technique 1.4).

The correct placement of any ET tube or supraglottic airway device (see below) can be confirmed by a variety of methods; the most reliable is detection of carbon dioxide on a capnograph with each breath. If a capnograph is not available, watching the reservoir bag on the breathing system once connected (for excursions in time with breathing), feeling for breath coming from the end of the tube or watching for condensation to form in time with each breath in clear tubes are alternative methods. The compression of a rabbit's chest to feel for breath coming from the end of the tube is not recommended and can lead to false results.

ET intubation is recommended for dental work because it protects the airway from fluid and debris. Orotracheal intubation can still be used, with the ET tube pushed to one side to allow access. An alternative is nasotracheal intubation, which leaves the oral field free while still providing airway protection and ensuring delivery of anaesthetic gases and oxygen. It has been described in the rabbit (Stephens DeValle, 2009; see Technique 1.5) and was found to be easier to perform than orotracheal intubation in the study population. Stephens DeValle suggests that this was because the rabbit is an obligate nasal breather, with the epiglottis naturally entrapped on the dorsal surface of the soft palate. This provides a conduit for air to move from the nasopharynx to the trachea, and so passage of a tube from the nasopharynx instead of the oropharynx should be easier to perform. Other authors had previously raised concerns about the introduction of pathogens from the nasopharynx. Although no respiratory infections were observed after intuba-tion in the specific-pathogen-free study rabbits (Stephens DeValle, 2009), the risk may be increased in the pet rabbit population.

Laryngeal mask airway (LMA) device

LMAs have also been used to maintain the airway in rabbits. A laryngeal mask is a tube (with a connector that is attached to the breathing system) and an inflatable cuff that sits over the larynx (Figure 1.10 and Technique 1.6). The advantages of this technique, when compared with ET intubation, are that

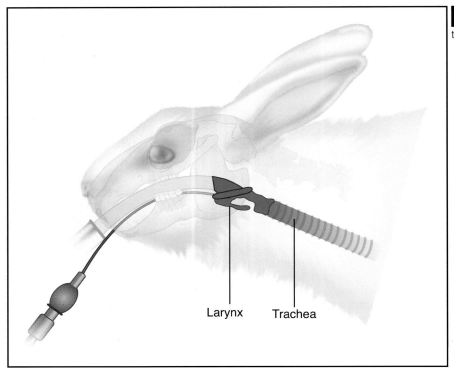

1.10 A laryngeal mask airway (LMA) device sits over the larynx of the rabbit.

Larynx   Trachea

it is reportedly easier to master and less induction agent is required for placement. LMAs are available in a range of sizes; size 1 will fit rabbits >4 kg in bodyweight. This technique is therefore unsuitable for smaller rabbits, and may also be more difficult to perform in older rabbits owing to the length of their incisors. The cuff on the LMA can be inflated, although lingual cyanosis caused by vascular compression of the tongue may be seen. The degree of airway security lies between that obtained by the mask and ET intubation. Use of IPPV is possible using LMAs; however, inflation of the stomach with air (and possible gastro-oesophageal reflux) is a potential outcome.

Supraglottic airway device

A recent addition to the products available for airway protection in rabbits is a supraglottic airway device, which uses a non-inflatable soft gel cuff to create a seal over the glottis (Figure 1.11). Unlike the LMA it incorporates an oesophageal seal to prevent aspiration of any gastric reflux. The range comes in six sizes, with the smallest designed to fit rabbits down to 600 g in bodyweight.

Maintenance of anaesthesia

Some of the induction protocols may produce anaesthesia for sufficient time for short procedures to be carried out, although oxygen should always be supplemented. If volatile agents are to be used for the maintenance of anaesthesia (Figure 1.12), an ideal agent for the rabbit would be of low blood solubility (e.g. isoflurane, sevoflurane or desflurane), leading to a faster recovery from anaesthesia. Minimum alveolar concentrations (MACs) in rabbits are higher than those in dogs and cats. Knowing the MAC for individual volatile agents will guide the choice of vaporizer settings (Figure 1.12).

Nitrous oxide

Nitrous oxide (N_2O) is an anaesthetic gas, usually used as a carrier gas alongside oxygen in a ratio of either 50:50 or 60:40 N_2O to oxygen. It is a potent analgesic, although its potency in the rabbit is half that in humans. It has been shown to inhibit increases in blood pressure in response to stimulation under anaesthesia. Adding N_2O to the carrier gas mixture reduces the MAC of other volatile agents needed. Another potential benefit is the 'second gas effect', which hastens the uptake of the second gas (i.e. the volatile agent) by increasing the concentration gradient of the second gas. Clinically, this translates to a faster induction of anaesthesia.

Some authors are concerned about the use of N_2O in rabbits. One reason is the potential for accumulation of gas in the gastrointestinal tract of the rabbit if administered for long periods; N_2O accumulates quickly in air-filled spaces because it replaces nitrogen more quickly than it can diffuse out of the space. The author regularly uses N_2O in rabbits, however, because a rabbit's guts are not air-filled, and so tympany should not be a problem. If during anaesthesia abdominal tympany should occur, N_2O can be discontinued.

There are some situations in which the author would not use N_2O:

- Owing to the speed of accumulation of N_2O in air-filled spaces, increasing their volume substantially and quickly, the use of this gas should be avoided in rabbits with certain clinical conditions, e.g. gastric tympany following aerophagia

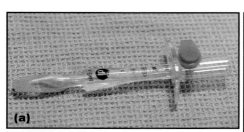

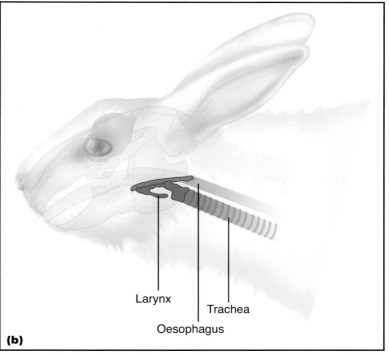

1.11 **(a)** The V-gel supraglottic airway device for rabbits. **(b)** Positioning of a supraglottic airway device. Whereas an LMA forms a seal over the larynx, the V-gel seals the oesophagus while the hole lies over the larynx. (Photo © John Chitty)

Larynx

Trachea

Oesophagus

Effect	Halothane	Isoflurane	Sevoflurane	Desflurane
Respiratory depression	+	++	++	++
Vasodilation	+	++	++	++
Myocardial depression	++	+	+	+
Arrhythmogenic effect	+	–	–	–
Blood gas solubility	High	Low	Low	Very low
Minimum alveolar concentration	1.08% [a]	2.49% [b]	3.7% [c]	8.9% [d]
Liver metabolism	Moderate	Very low	Low	Very low
Odour/taste	Acceptable	Unpleasant	Acceptable	Acceptable
Hepatic blood flow	–	++	+	+

1.12 Volatile agents used for maintenance of anaesthesia in rabbits. Key: – = reduced; + = increased. [a] Shi *et al.*, 1985; [b] Turner *et al.*, 2006; [c] Scheller *et al.*, 1988; [d] Doorley *et al.*, 1988.

- Including N_2O as a carrier gas will decrease the percentage of oxygen inspired by the patient, which may be detrimental to some patients with respiratory disease
- If a rabbit is suffering from clinical respiratory problems, N_2O should not be used.

Given that rabbits are often affected by subclinical respiratory disease, pulse oximetry should always be used to ensure adequate oxygen saturation. It is recommended, at the end of the anaesthetic maintenance period, to provide oxygen via the breathing system after the volatile agent and N_2O have been discontinued. This will prevent any possibility of 'diffusion hypoxia', a theoretical sequel to N_2O use, and will limit environmental pollution.

Breathing systems

During maintenance of anaesthesia, breathing systems are used to deliver anaesthetic agents and carrier gases to the rabbit. They are also integral to the removal of waste gases and carbon dioxide (CO_2) produced by the patient to the scavenging system. Breathing systems with large amounts of resistance and dead space should be avoided in small patients. Resistance is conferred by valves, narrow bore hosing, and soda lime. Breathing system dead space is defined as the volume of the breathing system between the rostral borders of the teeth and the division between the inspiratory and expiratory gas flows of the breathing system.

Anaesthetic gases should be delivered via non-rebreathing systems to all but the largest rabbits. Non-rebreathing systems rely on high fresh gas flows to 'sweep' CO_2 out of the breathing system, ensuring that the patient breathes in only fresh gas. Fresh gas flow calculations should be based on a higher minute volume than for dogs and cats, approximately 250 ml/kg/min. The minute volume is then multiplied by a 'circuit factor' to produce the fresh gas flow. These 'circuit factors' will depend on the non-rebreathing system chosen, which in turn depends on the rabbit's bodyweight (Figure 1.13).

Rebreathing systems, e.g. circle systems, can be used for large rabbits (lean weight >10 kg). They use soda lime to remove CO_2 from the patient's exhaled gases. Once the CO_2 has been removed (scrubbed) from the exhaled gases, some of the remaining exhaled gas can be rebreathed. The resistance of the circle is higher than that of non-rebreathing systems owing to the number of valves and the soda lime. The adsorption of CO_2 means that fresh gas flow requirements are lower in rebreathing systems than in non-rebreathing systems. Oxygen at ≥5–10 ml/kg/min (equivalent to the metabolic oxygen demand of most mammals) is

Breathing system	Circuit factor	Resistance	Dead space	Patient weight range	IPPV
Ayre's T-piece with Jackson–Rees modification	2.5–3	Low	Low	<10 kg	Yes
Bain	2.5–3	Low	Low	5–15 kg	Yes
Mini-Lack	1–1.5	Low	Low	<10 kg	No
Lack	1–1.5	Medium	Low to medium	>10 kg	No
Magill	1–1.5	Medium	Low to medium	>10 kg	No

1.13 Breathing systems.

added as fresh gas flow to match the amount that the rabbit is consuming.

Oxygen is the usual carrier gas delivered by the breathing system. If N_2O is used as a carrier gas, it should be delivered at between 50 and 66% of the gas mixture. N_2O can be used in circle systems, as long as the fraction of inspired oxygen is monitored, and remains above 30%.

Intermittent positive pressure ventilation (IPPV)

This technique should be used during anaesthesia if the rabbit's thorax is open (e.g. during thoracotomy), or if neuromuscular blocking drugs or other drugs that produce apnoea are used. IPPV is also used to deepen planes of anaesthesia rapidly, to aid in reducing end-tidal CO_2 tensions if hypercapnia is present, and may improve oxygenation if pulse oximeters display an S_pO_2 reading of <90%. It can be performed either manually or automatically using a ventilator. Given the small size of most rabbits, paediatric bellows or valves should be used with the ventilators. Ventilators can be pressure- or volume-limited (i.e. the ventilator stops delivering the breath when either a preset volume or pressure is reached). The author recommends pressure-limited ventilators, to reduce the risk of ventilator-induced injury to the lung, and because pressure can be a more useful parameter to measure when an uncuffed ET tube is used (some volume of gas may leak around the tube). Approximate tidal volumes of 4–6 ml/kg (Gillett, 1994) should be administered at a rate of 20–30 breaths per minute. Peak inspiratory pressures should be set between 12 and 15 cmH$_2$O. CO_2 tensions should be monitored, and the rate and tidal volume adjusted to maintain normocapnia (35–45 mmHg). A ratio of inspiratory to expiratory time of approximately 1:3 should be used.

If manual IPPV is employed (by squeezing the reservoir bag on the breathing system), a Bain, Ayre's T-piece with Jackson–Rees modification (for small rabbits), or circle breathing system (for larger rabbits) should be used. Mapelson A classified breathing systems such as the Lack, mini-Lack or Magill are unsuitable for a prolonged period of IPPV. The valve of the breathing system should be closed, the bag squeezed, and the valve then re-opened for the expiratory pause. The rabbit's chest should be observed during the breath, to ensure that the chest excursion is equal to or slightly greater than a normal spontaneous breath. Over-inflation of the lungs caused by squeezing the bag should be avoided, because it may lead to a tension pneumothorax and other lung damage.

At the end of IPPV, the rabbit may be apnoeic if end-tidal CO_2 is too low because, unless the rabbit has chronic respiratory disease, CO_2 will be the drive for ventilation. If apnoea occurs, IPPV should continue but at a slower rate, allowing accumulation of CO_2. Hypothermia will often develop more quickly if IPPV is undertaken, and the temperature should be monitored and warming devices used as described below.

Neuromuscular blocking agents

Neuromuscular blocking drugs can be administered to block acetylcholine at the neuromuscular junction, and produce flaccid paralysis of all skeletal muscles. They may be used during anaesthesia for several reasons: to produce a central, akinetic eye for ocular surgery; to produce excellent muscle relaxation to aid certain surgical procedures; or for use during thoracotomy to facilitate IPPV. Intercostal muscles and the diaphragm will also be relaxed and spontaneous ventilation will stop, therefore it is mandatory that the trachea is intubated and IPPV carried out while the rabbit is under neuromuscular blockade. Jaw tone, eye position, pedal withdrawal reflex and respiratory rate will no longer be useful aids to assess the depth of anaesthesia. However, if the rabbit is at a light depth of anaesthesia under neuromuscular blockade an increase in blood pressure and heart rate may be seen, and lacrimation or salivation observed.

In addition to the provision of IPPV, if neuromuscular blockade is going to be undertaken it is recommended that facilities for monitoring the depth of the blockade are available. This is done using a peripheral nerve stimulator, with electrodes positioned over the ulnar nerve on the forelimb or the peroneal nerve on the hindlimb. Different twitch patterns (e.g. train-of-four) can be used to assess the depth of blockade. Ventilation should continue until all four twitches have returned to an equal magnitude. Antagonism of neuromuscular blocking drugs can be performed once the first twitch in the train-of-four pattern has returned. Antagonists of anticholinesterase, such as neostigmine and edrophonium, will increase the concentration of acetylcholine at the neuromuscular junction. Additional muscarinic effects (i.e. brady-arrhythmia), which may be ob-served after administration of the antagonists, can be prevented by the co-administration of an antimuscarinic such as glycopyrrolate.

Maintenance fluid therapy

Fluid therapy should be used perioperatively if a rabbit is suspected of being dehydrated or hypovolaemic. Ideally, hydration and volume status will have been assessed (see Figure 1.5) and corrected before anaesthesia is attempted. In addition to restoring any fluid deficit (see earlier), the rabbit's maintenance fluid therapy rate of 4 ml/kg/h needs to be added to the amount infused. This is a higher maintenance rate than used for dogs and cats, reflecting a higher fluid requirement.

Crystalloids can be given perianaesthetically by the intraperitoneal route. Fluid absorption from this site will be quicker than from the subcutaneous site; however, there is a risk of organ perforation and peritonitis. Injection into the right posterior quadrant of the abdomen avoids the bladder and the caecum. The author does not give glucose-containing fluids by either intraperitoneal or subcutaneous routes to avoid abscessation, which is a potential consequence.

Fluid therapy will be most effective when administered intravenously or intraosseously through an indwelling cannula. The additional benefits of intravenous cannulation have been detailed earlier. When correcting fluid deficits via this route, the rate of infusion and type of fluids given depend on what type and amount of fluid has been lost and over what time period. During anaesthesia, in an animal that is normovolaemic, crystalloid fluid therapy should be administered at 6 ml/kg/h. This rate is greater than the maintenance rate of 4 ml/kg/h, which replaces sensible and insensible losses, because the rabbit's blood pressure needs to be supported during anaesthesia to compensate for evaporative losses from the respiratory system and the vasodilatory and myocardial depressant action of several sedative and anaesthetic drugs. Marked hypotension has been reported in clinically healthy rabbits anaesthetized with 'routine' anaesthetic protocols (Harvey and Murison, 2010). If the rabbit is undergoing surgery, especially where body cavities are opened, the intravenous fluid therapy rate should be increased to 10 ml/kg/h to compensate for greater evaporative fluid losses and haemorrhage.

Excessive blood loss during surgery should be monitored and the amount of blood lost estimated. This can be done by weighing swabs and drapes and subtracting their dry weight, and by measuring the amount of bloody fluid in the suction device before subtracting the volume of saline flush used. Once the amount of blood lost is known, the percentage blood lost should be calculated, assuming that a rabbit's blood volume is approximately 60 ml/kg. While rabbit-specific data are not available, the author extrapolates from the values for dogs and cats and uses the following as a guide:

- If blood loss is >10% of blood volume, this should be corrected with crystalloid fluid, giving three times the amount lost
- If blood loss is >15% of blood volume, in addition to crystalloids, colloids can be administered at a rate equal to the volume of blood lost
- If blood loss is >20% of blood volume, this requires blood product replacement to maintain oxygen-carrying capacity.

Monitoring anaesthesia

Maintaining anaesthetic records shows that due care and attention has been paid to the animal during anaesthesia. Records should be filled out in indelible ink, contemporaneously (i.e. at the same time as the anaesthetic). All drugs administered from pre-anaesthetic medication through to recovery from anaesthesia should be recorded. The minimum parameters recorded should be the respiratory rate and heart rate. If any other monitoring devices are being used, the data they generate should also be recorded.

Anaesthetic monitoring must be continuous, and in some cases should start after the animal has received its pre-anaesthetic medication. It should also carry on well into the recovery phase. Although different types of monitoring equipment are available, there is no substitute for 'hand and eye' monitoring.

'Hand and eye' monitoring

- Peripheral pulses, e.g. auricular, metacarpal or pedal pulses, should be palpated when possible; the author finds the middle auricular artery the easiest to palpate. A good quality pulse (i.e. fairly 'bouncy' and not easy to compress) palpated peripherally will demonstrate good perfusion to the extremities. Palpation of a femoral pulse is less useful because this is a more central pulse.
- Mucous membrane colour can be assessed from the gums, conjunctiva and external genitalia.
- At surgical depths of anaesthesia, the eye should rotate ventromedially, and the rabbit should retain a sluggish palpebral reflex. Ketamine-based anaesthetics, however, tend to produce a more central eye.
- Both the chest and the reservoir bag of the breathing system should be observed for tidal volume movement. Observation of both ensures that the ET tube and breathing system are patent and securely connected. Observation of the chest will alert the anaesthetist to abnormal ventilatory patterns such as paradoxical and abdominal ventilation.
- Assessment of jaw tone as an indicator of depth of anaesthesia may be of limited use in the rabbit because of its narrow gape.
- Movement of the ears when lightly touching the inside of the pinnae suggests a light plane of anaesthesia.
- The presence and strength of the dorsal pedal reflex can be used to gauge depth of anaesthesia; however, it is observed to be present until very deep planes of anaesthesia are achieved (Hall *et al.*, 2001).

Pulse oximetry

Pulse oximetry is a non-invasive, continuous monitor of the percentage of arterial haemoglobin oxygen saturation (S_pO_2). The probe on a pulse oximeter has a light-emitting diode on one side and a photodetector on the other. Oxyhaemoglobin and deoxyhaemoglobin absorb light differently, so the amount of light transmitted through the tissue bed (e.g. the tongue) and reaching the photodetector on the other side will depend on the proportions of oxyhaemoglobin and deoxyhaemoglobin present.

A pulse oximeter will indicate three things: the haemoglobin oxygen saturation (S_pO_2) as a percentage; the pulse rate in beats per minute; and, if there is sufficient peripheral perfusion, the machine will detect a pulse. Some pulse oximeters will produce a pulse waveform, although some of these models will expand this waveform to fit the screen, which can be misleading. Pulse oximetry is not an indicator of whether an animal is ventilating adequately; for this assessment to be made a capnograph must be used to measure end-tidal CO_2.

- Oxygen haemoglobin saturation should be ≥95%.
- A value of <95% is considered to represent moderate hypoxia and a value of <90% indicates profound hypoxia. Action should be taken in both of these circumstances.

Pulse oximetry is recommended during rabbit anaesthesia because of the high prevalence of subclinical respiratory conditions that may affect oxygenation. Pulse oximeter probes can be placed on a variety of locations in rabbits, including the tongue, the ear or between the digits. Lingual probes tend to be the most reliable in the author's experience, but may not be appropriate for procedures such as dentistry. Readings may not be accurate if the tissue is excessively pigmented or hairy. Pulse oximetry may fail in rabbits with poor peripheral perfusion (including after administration of alpha-2 adrenergic agonists) or if the spring of the probe is very tight and causes local ischaemia. Several veterinary-specific pulse oximeter models have been successfully validated in rabbits. Some general practices use second-hand machines from human hospitals; these monitors will struggle to register the high heart rates often observed in rabbits.

Capnography

Capnometry is the monitoring of the partial pressure or concentration of CO_2 in respiratory gases. Capnography is the graphical representation of the measured CO_2. The amount of CO_2 in respiratory gases is measured continuously by a capnometer, using infrared light absorption. There are two types of analyser: sidestream and mainstream.

- A sidestream analyser will aspirate gas from a connector between the ET tube and the breathing system, to be analysed in the main body of the monitor (Figure 1.14).
- A mainstream system will perform the analysis at a site between the ET tube and the breathing system.

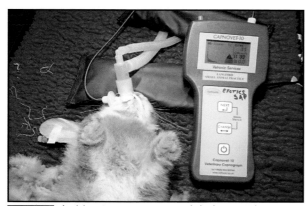

1.14 A side-stream capnograph being used to monitor end-tidal carbon dioxide during anaesthesia in a rabbit.

For rabbit anaesthesia, the connector that represents the lowest increase in dead space should be chosen. Dead space tends to be less with sidestream monitors, but many mainstream capnographs come with a choice of connectors, including paediatric sizes.

The end-tidal carbon dioxide ($ETCO_2$) values can be displayed simply as numbers, usually in pressure units (mmHg or kPa) but some may also display as a percentage. CO_2 is produced as a byproduct of metabolism and is eliminated from the body by the lungs. A capnograph therefore provides information about CO_2 production, perfusion of the lungs, alveolar ventilation, respiratory patterns, and elimination of CO_2 from the breathing system.

Normocapnia (i.e. a normal $ETCO_2$ value) is 35–45 mmHg. Common reasons for hypo- and hypercapnia are listed in Figure 1.15. Hypocapnia may be observed during anaesthesia of a rabbit if the patient has a very small tidal volume. One of the occasions when capnography is invaluable in anaesthetic monitoring is in the case of cardiac arrest, because this is often the first monitor to identify a problem. If circulation slows or stops, the blood cannot deliver the CO_2 (which is a waste product from cells) to the lungs to be eliminated, and so a sudden decrease in CO_2 levels should prompt a check of the rabbit's pulse.

Zero level
• Oesophageal intubation
Sudden decrease to zero
• Airway obstruction • Airway disconnection • Ventilator failure • Capnograph malfunction • Obstructed aspirating tube • Apnoea • Cardiac or respiratory arrest
Hypocapnia
• Airway leak • Severe cardiovascular disturbance • Hyperventilation • Hypothermia • Vasoconstriction • Low aspirating flow rates • Fresh gas contamination • Large physiological dead space • Small tidal volume
Hypercapnia
• Hypoventilation • Increased rate of metabolism • Rebreathing

1.15 Causes of changes in $ETCO_2$.

Oesophageal stethoscope

This simple and relatively inexpensive piece of monitoring equipment is used to monitor heart rate, although respiratory sounds are also often heard. Stethoscope ear pieces are attached to a long tube of soft plastic. The tube is available in varying diameters and the narrowest should be used in rabbits. In the smallest rabbits, sometimes even a narrow-bore tube is too large to share the pharynx with an ET tube, and this piece of monitoring equipment may not be suitable. In larger rabbits, after pre-measuring the length of the tube to the point of the elbow, the oesophageal stethoscope should be passed down the oesophagus in the anaesthetized patient (only if the trachea has already been intubated). When passed to the pre-measured point, its tip should lie just over the heart base and transmit heart sounds up to the ear pieces.

Blood pressure

Measurement of arterial blood pressure is one of the most useful measures of cardiovascular function, especially as rabbits may be severely hypotensive during anaesthesia (Harvey and Murison, 2010). Arterial blood pressure can be measured either invasively (directly) or non-invasively (indirectly).

Direct measurement

Direct arterial blood pressure measurement requires the placement of an intra-arterial cannula. This technique is rarely performed in general practice because it is more involved than indirect techniques, requires monitors with invasive blood pressure measuring capabilities, and there are possible adverse consequences of the cannulation. However, in severely hypotensive rabbits, this technique is likely to be the only accurate method of blood pressure measurement. In the rabbit this is most easily achieved using the auricular artery, which runs along the middle of the ear. Arterial cannulation is painful and should be performed when the animal is anaesthetized; or the skin above the site may be desensitized by the application of a local anaesthetic cream. The cannula and its attachments must be placed aseptically and secured well, because dislodgement of any part will result in the formation of a large haematoma, air embolism or severe blood loss.

The cannula is connected via non-compliant, saline-filled extension tubing to a pressure transducer device that converts the pulsatile pressure signal into a numerical value on a monitor. Pressures are measured against a reference level (level of the heart), and devices to record pressure need to be 'zeroed' to atmospheric pressure. Electronic transducers can convert the numerical values into waveforms. Alternatively aneroid manometers can be attached to the extension tubing and values read from the deflection of the needle.

Non-invasive measurement

These techniques utilize a cuff to occlude the blood flow to an appendage by increasing the inflation pressure to a level higher than systolic blood pressure. As the cuff is gradually deflated, the resumption of the arterial blood flow is detected by a variety of methods. The width of the cuff should be 40% of the circumference of the appendage that it is to be fitted around.

Of the non-invasive techniques, Doppler blood pressure measurement (Figure 1.16) is the author's preferred method for use in the rabbit, and a step-by-step guide is given in Technique 1.7. The Doppler technique uses sound waves emitted from a probe. If the sound waves are reflected back by a moving structure (e.g. arterial wall or blood cells), an audible signal ('whoosh') will be heard. In the rabbit the

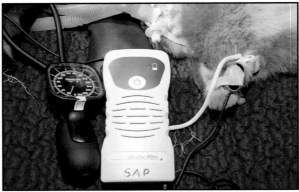

1.16 Indirect measurement of blood pressure using the Doppler technique.

Doppler technique has been shown to underestimate systolic blood pressure by an average of 5 mmHg (±9 mmHg) and to overestimate mean blood pressure by an average of 10 mmHg (±8 mmHg) (Harvey and Murison, 2010).

Oscillometric blood pressure monitors are automated; they can be programmed to measure blood pressure at set intervals and display the results digitally, alongside a pulse rate. The cuff will usually have an arrow indicating which part of the cuff should overlie the pulse. After the cuff is in place the machine inflates and deflates the cuff cyclically, and sensors detect pressure changes in the cuff during its deflation as pulsatile flow returns to the appendage. In the rabbit, positioning the cuff over the forelimb produces more accurate readings than positioning the cuff over the hindlimb; data suggest that oscillometric measurements are less accurate when the blood pressure is high than when it is in the normal range or low (Ypsilantis et al., 2005).

Electrocardiography

An electrocardiogram (ECG) indicates the electrical activity of the heart but gives no information on whether the heart is beating effectively. The electrodes of the ECG need to triangulate over the heart. In small animals they are conventionally placed on the two forelimbs and the left hindlimb. They can be attached using crocodile clips (preferably atraumatic) or sticky pads, and spirit or ultrasound gel is used to improve the conductance of the electrical signal. Excessive application of the conductive substance will quickly cool the rabbit during anaesthesia.

Body temperature

Body temperature can be monitored using thermometers, thermistors or thermocouples. While thermometers are most common in veterinary practice, temperature probes inserted into the nasopharynx, oesophagus or rectum (Figure 1.17) are thermistor-based. In these devices, the current flowing is proportional to the resistance in the circuit, which is affected by the temperature. Oesophageal temperature reflects that of the heart, and is a 'core' temperature. The rectal temperature is commonly used because it is easy to perform and relatively safe, but it is more of a peripheral measurement.

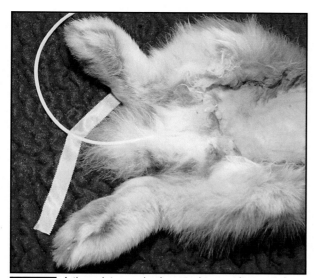

1.17 A thermistor probe inserted to monitor rectal temperature continuously in an anaesthetized rabbit.

Complications during anaesthesia

Hypothermia

Hypothermia can be common during anaesthesia of rabbits, and if it occurs will contribute to morbidity and mortality. Anaesthesia generally depresses the 'thermostat' in the hypothalamus of the central nervous system, and thereby reduces the patient's ability to thermoregulate. Anaesthesia also prevents the animal from moving around, shivering and huddling if it becomes hypothermic, all of which it would normally do while conscious either to generate body heat or to avoid heat loss. Many of the drugs used during anaesthesia also cause peripheral vasodilation and thereby influence heat loss. This is exacerbated by the clipping of large patches of fur (reducing insulation), followed by the use of scrub preparations and spirit which further increase evaporative heat loss. The rabbit is at high risk of developing hypothermia during anaesthesia owing to its small size and large surface area to volume ratio.

Marked hypothermia influences anaesthetic drug behaviour: metabolism of injectable drugs is slowed, and the MAC values of volatile agents are reduced. If any drugs are injected subcutaneously, uptake may be delayed or reduced as a result of poor peripheral perfusion. Heart rate and respiratory rate can also decrease in response to hypothermia.

It is easier to prevent heat loss than to re-warm a rabbit. Measures to prevent hypothermia are described earlier in the section on Pre-anaesthetic preparation.

Cardiopulmonary arrest

If the rabbit is of ASA status 4 or 5 and cardiopulmonary arrest during anaesthesia is a possibility, initial doses of emergency drugs should be drawn up and be readily available before anaesthesia is commenced. Owing to the small volumes needed, the drugs may need to be diluted for accurate dosing.

If respiratory arrest is observed and the rabbit's trachea is intubated, the first step should be to check that the tube is patent and has not become dislodged or blocked with secretions or debris. After patency has been confirmed, IPPV using 100% oxygen and an appropriate breathing system can be applied (at 20–30 breaths per minute) until spontaneous ventilation returns. During this time, administration of the volatile agent should be discontinued and specific antagonists for any components of the anaesthetic protocol (e.g. atipamezole for alpha-2 adrenergic agonists; naloxone for opioids; flumazenil for benzodiazepines) should be administered. If the rabbit's trachea is not intubated, the head and neck should be extended and the tongue pulled forwards (to move the base of the tongue away from the epiglottis) before oxygen is supplied using a mask. IPPV using a tight-fitting mask may inflate the lungs, but it also tends to inflate the stomach. In smaller rabbits, gentle manual compression of the thorax (at 20–30 breaths per minute) using the thumb and forefinger may aid movement of gas in and out of the lungs. Doxapram (10 mg/kg i.v. or sublingually) is a central respiratory stimulant and may increase rate and depth of breathing, but it also increases oxygen demand so should be used with caution.

If cardiac arrest occurs, in addition to the steps described above, cardiac compressions should be undertaken at approximately 100 compressions per minute. The anaesthetist's thumb and forefinger should compress the chest directly over the heart using a regular rhythm. During abdominal or thoracic procedures the surgeon can perform direct manual compressions of the heart (through the diaphragm if the abdominal cavity is open). If an ECG is available the heart rhythm should be monitored and emergency drugs can be administered as appropriate (Figure 1.18). Ideally, drugs should be administered intravenously; if this is done through a peripheral cannula, it should be followed by a bolus of crystalloid to ensure that the drugs enter the central circulation. If no intravenous cannula is in place, the drugs listed in Figure 1.18 can be administered down the ET tube, followed by IPPV to help the drug distribute into the alveoli to be absorbed by the pulmonary circulation.

Arrhythmia	Drug	Dose
Asystole	Adrenaline	0.1 ml/kg of 1 in 10,000
	Vasopressin	0.8 IU/kg
Ventricular fibrillation	Lidocaine	1–2 mg/kg
	Vasopressin	0.8 IU/kg
Tachyarrhythmias	Propranolol	0.1 mg/kg
Bradyarrhythmias	Glycopyrrolate	0.1 mg/kg

1.18 Emergency drugs for cerebrocardiopulmonary resuscitation (CCPR). Doses taken from Flecknell (1996) and Lichtenberger (2007).

Recovery from anaesthesia

The immediate recovery period after anaesthesia is of high risk for any patient, because the sedative and physiological effects of the drugs administered are still in place, but monitoring and supportive therapies such as oxygen and fluid therapy are usually removed at this time. Recent research (Brodbelt *et al.*, 2008) has highlighted that the first 3 hours after anaesthesia is the greatest risk period, with 60% of anaesthesia-related rabbit deaths occurring during this time.

Rabbits should be allowed to recover from anaesthesia in a warm (20–25°C), calm environment away from predator species (e.g. cats, dogs, ferrets, birds of prey). They should be placed on absorbent bedding, but sawdust should be avoided because it may occlude nostrils and irritate eyes. The ET tube should be removed when swallowing is first seen.

Immediate assessment should be made to ensure adequate airflow, because laryngospasm can potentially occur after extubation. If no airflow is felt, the rabbit's head and neck should be extended and oxygen administered by mask while preparing to re-anaesthetize and re-intubate.

Regular checks on the rabbit's level of consciousness, mucous membrane colour, and pulse and respiratory rates should be made until the rabbit is moving well around the kennel. Temperature checks should be made every 15–30 minutes until the rabbit's rectal temperature has reached 38°C. Warming techniques should still be employed to prevent further progression of hypothermia while the rabbit is still sedated and unable to move around. If the rabbit is known to have respiratory disease, oxygen provision should be continued into recovery by mask or piped into an oxygen tent or incubator. Monitoring devices that are sufficiently mobile to be transferred to the recovery kennel can be used, although probe sites may need to be changed as the rabbit regains consciousness. Intravenous cannulas should remain in place until the rabbit has fully recovered from anaesthesia to facilitate administration of any emergency drugs or further analgesia, and to continue intravenous fluid therapy. Short-acting anaesthetic drugs or those with specific antagonists (Figure 1.19) should be chosen wherever possible, because the sooner rabbits are moving around after anaesthesia, the sooner they will be able to maintain their own body temperature. It must be remembered, however, that administration of an antagonist will also stop any analgesic effect associated with the agonist, e.g. alpha-2 adrenergic agonists.

Food should be offered as soon as the rabbit can maintain sternal recumbency, lift its own head and swallow. Early feeding will lessen the risk of ileus and provide a source of glucose. Analgesia should also be continued into the postoperative period, although opioid-based drugs may sedate the rabbit and hypothermia may redevelop. As complications can be avoided by judicious monitoring, this should not prevent the veterinary surgeon from continuing analgesia into the postoperative period. Once the rabbit is more alert and moving around, frequent handling and disturbances may cause stress, depending on how used the rabbit is to such handling. At this stage monitoring should become remote, albeit still frequent.

Rabbits that are not eating or passing faeces 24 hours after anaesthesia should be returned to the practice for appropriate treatment.

Anaesthetic considerations for specific cases

Whilst anaesthesia should be tailored to the individual rabbit using the information gained by pre-anaesthetic assessment (especially when it is of ASA class 3 or higher), there are additional considerations for specific scenarios that may be encountered in general practice.

Anaesthetizing the rabbit with respiratory tract disease

- Assess the rabbit's ability to oxygenate its tissues and to ventilate before anaesthesia using capnography (see earlier for details) and pulse oximetry (place the probe on the ear or paw). If S_pO_2 is <90% on room air and $ETCO_2$ is >45 mmHg, anaesthesia should be postponed if possible to allow stabilization and treatment, e.g. antibiosis.
- Ensure a stress-free environment.
- Place an intravenous catheter after the use of topical local anaesthetic.
- Pre-oxygenate by mask.
- Use an opioid with or without benzodiazepine premedication intravenously, followed by an intravenous induction agent to effect.
- Intubate the trachea so that IPPV is possible if necessary.
- Maintain with inhalation agents delivered in 100% oxygen. Do not use nitrous oxide.
- Choose a breathing system appropriate to the size of the rabbit, suitable for IPPV with low resistance to breathing.
- Monitor cardiovascular and respiratory parameters (especially S_pO_2 and $ETCO_2$) throughout anaesthesia. Intervene if S_pO_2 drops below 95% and $ETCO_2$ increases above 50 mmHg with IPPV (with or without suction of the ET tube; see below).

Drug	Antagonist for	Dose
Atipamezole	Medetomidine	1 mg/kg
Flumazenil	Midazolam or diazepam	0.1 mg/kg
Naloxone	µ opioid agonists	0.03 mg/kg

1.19 Drugs that can be used to antagonize certain sedative and anaesthetic agents (data from Baumgartner *et al.*, 2010). The doses given are for subcutaneous administration; however, if rapid recovery from anaesthesia is necessary, such as in CCPR, intravenous administration can also be used.

- Monitor (using the capnograph trace and movement of the rebreathing bag) for occlusion of the ET tube with secretions.
- Keep to a minimum the time the rabbit spends in dorsal recumbency.
- Maintain normothermia.
- Supplement oxygen and monitor S_pO_2 during recovery from anaesthesia.

Anaesthetizing the rabbit with chronic dental disease in poor condition

- Assess hydration status and body condition. Feed the rabbit a slurry diet before anaesthesia; this should also correct mild dehydration.
- If more than mildly dehydrated, admit for intravenous fluid therapy to restore fluid deficit before anaesthesia.
- Premedicate the rabbit with an opioid, with or without benzodiazepine, followed by intravenous induction agent to effect.
- Intubate the trachea, either orotracheally or nasotracheally.
- Maintain anaesthesia with a volatile agent in oxygen, with or without nitrous oxide.
- Employ multimodal analgesia.
- Continue with fluid therapy intraoperatively.
- Monitor body temperature and maintain normothermia.
- Ensure good airway protection, including the use of a pharyngeal pack in larger rabbits, and apply suction to the pharynx before allowing the rabbit to recover from anaesthesia.
- Check blood glucose levels if a long dental procedure is necessary.
- Keep the rabbit warm and comfortable in recovery; encourage it to eat as soon as possible.

Anaesthesia for the long-duration orthopaedic case

- The anaesthetic protocol will depend on the circumstances surrounding the orthopaedic repair. If the fracture was due to a traumatic injury, remember to check for associated injuries, e.g. bladder damage, pneumothorax.
- Chose a protocol encompassing multimodal analgesia, including local anaesthetic techniques if possible.
- If the anaesthetic is of a long duration, shorter-acting analgesics (e.g. opioids) may need topping up.
- Check blood glucose levels every 60–90 minutes.
- Use intravenous fluid therapy at 5–10 ml/kg/h.
- Ensure ET intubation, because using a mask for this length of time will not maintain an airway sufficiently.
- Monitor body temperature and maintain normothermia.
- Ensure good positioning and padding of the rabbit's body.
- Lubricate the rabbit's eyes periodically.

Anaesthesia for thoracotomy to treat thymoma

- Assess the rabbit's ability to ventilate and to oxygenate its tissues (see above); thymoma often has a mass effect and diminishes lung capacity.
- Place an intravenous catheter.
- Calculate and draw up the first doses of emergency drugs.
- Use an opioid, with or without benzodiazepine, for intravenous premedication.
- Pre-oxygenate for 5 minutes before induction.
- Induce anaesthesia with an intravenous induction agent to effect.
- ET intubation is essential.
- Use a multimodal analgesia approach including local anaesthetic techniques. Non-steroidal anti-inflammatory drugs (NSAIDs) should be administered post anaesthesia once hypotension is less of a risk.
- Monitoring should include pulse oximetry and capnography, an ECG and blood pressure monitoring.
- Ensure that IPPV is performed during the entire time the thoracic cavity is open.
- Neuromuscular blockade can be used at much lower doses (start with one-tenth of the recommended dose and titrate from there using peripheral nerve stimulator monitoring). It is unknown whether thymomas in rabbits cause the same myasthenia gravis effects as those in dogs and cats, which make affected dogs and cats very sensitive to neuromuscular blockers.
- The surgical approach may be via sternotomy or lateral thoracotomy. If the rabbit is turned into dorsal recumbency for sternotomy, the mass may cause aortocaval compression and reduce blood pressure.
- Fluid therapy should involve crystalloids at 10 ml/kg/h to start with. Colloids may be needed if hypotension is seen.
- Some thymomas are very invasive, and blood loss may occur. Quantify, calculate the percentage blood loss and administer different fluid types as necessary.
- Vasovagal reflexes (sudden bradycardia caused by retraction of structures) may be seen. The surgeon should stop traction immediately and, if bradycardia persists, glycopyrrolate should be administered.
- The chest should be drained of air after the thorax has been closed. If a chest drain has been placed it can be used to give intrapleural analgesia.
- Continue monitoring, oxygen supplementation and fluid therapy into recovery.

Acknowledgements

The author thanks Georgina Herbert and Elisa Bortolami for their comments on the manuscript, and Tracy Dewey and Colin Blakey for assistance with photography.

References and further reading

Bateman L, Ludders JW, Gleed RD and Erb HN (2005) Comparison between facemask and laryngeal mask airway in rabbits during isoflurane anesthesia. *Veterinary Anaesthesia and Analgesia* **32**, 280–288

Baumgartner C, Bollerhey M, Ebner J *et al.* (2010) Effects of medetomidine-midazolam-fentanyl IV bolus injections and its reversal by specific antagonists on cardiovascular function in rabbits. *Canadian Journal of Veterinary Research* **74**, 286–298

Brodbelt DC, Blissitt KJ, Hammond RA *et al.* (2008) The risk of death: the Confidential Enquiry into Perioperative Small Animal Fatalities. *Veterinary Anaesthesia and Analgesia* **35**, 365–373

Clarke KW and Hall LW (1990) A survey of anaesthesia in small animal practice. AVA/BSAVA report. *Journal of Veterinary Anaesthesia* **17**, 4–10

Coulter CA, Flecknell PA and Richardson CA (2009) Reported analgesic administration to rabbits, pigs, sheep, dogs and non-human primates undergoing experimental surgical procedures. *Laboratory Animals* **43**, 232–238

Diehl KH, Hull R, Morton D *et al.* (2001) A good practice guide to the administration of substances and removal of blood, including routes and volumes. *Journal of Applied Toxicology* **21**, 15–23

Doorley BM, Waters SJ, Terrell RC and Robinson JL (1988) MAC of I-653 in beagle dogs and New Zealand White rabbits. *Anesthesiology* **69**, 89–91

Flecknell P (1996) Anaesthesia and analgesia for rodents and rabbits. In: *Handbook of Rodent and Rabbit Medicine*, ed. K Laber-Laird, MM Swindle and P Flecknell, pp. 219–237. Pergamon, Oxford

Flecknell PA, Cruz IJ, Liles JH and Whelan G (1996) Induction of anaesthesia with halothane and isoflurane in the rabbit: a comparison of the use of a face mask or an anaesthetic chamber. *Laboratory Animals* **30**, 67–74

Flecknell PA, Rougham JV and Hedenqvist P (1999) Induction of anaesthesia with sevoflurane and isoflurane in the rabbit. *Laboratory Animals* **33**, 41–46

Gillett CS (1994) Select drug dosages and clinical reference data. In: *The Biology of the Laboratory Rabbit, 2nd edn*, ed. PJ Manning *et al.*, pp. 468–472. Academic Press, Waltham, MA

Grint NJ and Murison PJ (2008) A comparison of ketamine-midazolam and ketamine-medetomidine combinations for induction of anaesthesia in rabbits. *Veterinary Anaesthesia and Analgesia* **35**, 113–121

Grint NJ, Smith HE and Senior JM (2008) Clinical evaluation of alfaxalone in cyclodextrin for the induction of anaesthesia in rabbits. *Veterinary Record* **163**, 395–396

Hall LW, Clarke KW and Trim CM (2001) Anaesthesia of birds, laboratory animals and wild animals. In: *Veterinary Anaesthesia, 10th edn*, ed. LW Hall *et al.*, pp. 463–479. WB Saunders, London

Harvey L and Murison P (2010) Comparison of direct and Doppler arterial blood pressure measurements in rabbits during isoflurane anaesthesia. Abstract presented at Spring AVA Conference, Cambridge, UK, 30–31 March 2010

Lichtenberger M (2007) Case-based approach to the emergent exotic small mammal patient. In: *Proceedings of the 56th Società Culturale Italiana Veterinari per Animali da Compagnia (SCIVAC) Congress, Rimini, Italy*, pp. 335–340

Martinez MA, Murison PJ and Love E (2009) Induction of anaesthesia with either midazolam or propofol in rabbits premedicated with fentanyl/fluanisone. *Veterinary Record* **164**, 803–806

Murphy KL, Roughan JV, Baxter MG and Flecknell PA (2010) Anaesthesia with a combination of ketamine and medetomidine in the rabbit: effect of premedication with buprenorphine. *Veterinary Anaesthesia and Analgesia* **37**, 222–229

Orr HE, Roughan JV and Flecknell PA (2005) Assessment of ketamine and medetomidine anaesthesia in the domestic rabbit. *Veterinary Anaesthesia and Analgesia* **32**, 271–279

Scheller MS, Saidman LJ and Partridge BL (1988) MAC of sevoflurane in humans and the New Zealand White rabbit. *Canadian Journal of Anaesthesia* **35**, 153–156

Shafford HL and Schadt JC (2008) Respiratory and cardiovascular effects of buprenorphine in conscious rabbits. *Veterinary Anaesthesia and Analgesia* **35**, 326–332

Shi WZ, Fahey MR, Fisher DM *et al.* (1985) Laudanosine (a metabolite of atracurium) increases the minimum alveolar concentration of halothane in rabbits. *Anesthesiology* **63**, 584–588

Stephens DeValle JM (2009) Successful management of rabbit anesthesia through the use of nasotracheal intubation. *Journal of the American Association of Laboratory Animal Science* **48**, 166–170

Turner PV, Kerr CL, Healy AJ and Taylor WM (2006) Effects of meloxicam and butorphanol on minimum alveolar concentration of isoflurane in rabbits. *American Journal of Veterinary Research* **67**, 770–774

Ypsilantis P, Didilis VN, Politou M *et al.* (2005) A comparative study of invasive and oscillometric methods of arterial blood pressure measurement in the anesthetized rabbit. *Research in Veterinary Science* **78**, 269–275

TECHNIQUE 1.1:
Placing a marginal ear vein cannula

1 Clip a strip of hair over the marginal ear vein (unfolded edge of the ear).

2 If the catheter is to be placed in a conscious rabbit, apply EMLA cream, without rubbing it in, over the length of the vein. Cover with an occlusive dressing.

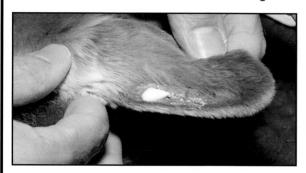

3 After 30–40 minutes, wipe off the cream and prepare the site aseptically with an antibacterial solution.

4 Choose a site relatively distal to the ear base, with an easily visible section of marginal ear vein.

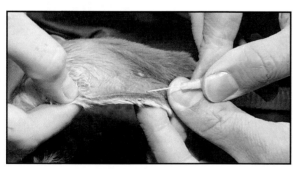

5 Pre-flush a 24 or 26 G cannula with heparinized saline.

6 Advance the catheter through the skin into the vessel until blood is seen in the hub of the cannula.

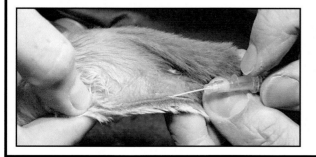

7 Advance both the stylet and cannula together for a further millimetre. This will ensure that the end of the cannula is sitting entirely within the vessel lumen.

8 Holding the stylet still, run the cannula off the stylet until the hub of the cannula meets the skin.

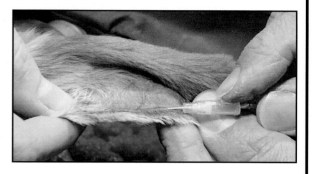

9 Remove the stylet and place the bung in the cannula.

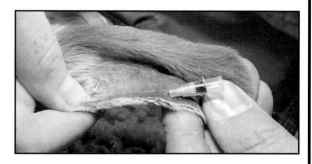

10 Pass adhesive tape between the skin and the cannula and then wrap it once or twice over the hub, ensuring that the skin–catheter junction is covered.

11 Flush the cannula with saline to check for accurate placement.

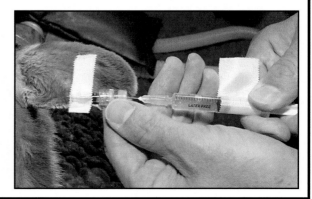

TECHNIQUE 1.2:
Placing an ET tube with the assistance of a rigid endoscope

The tube can either be inserted alongside the endoscope, or slid over the endoscope (as shown here). The latter approach will only work with larger diameter ET tubes (e.g. internal diameter 3 mm).

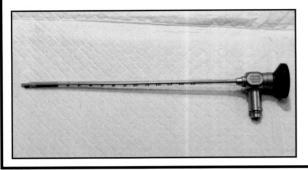

1 Advance the endoscope into the rabbit's mouth until the larynx is visualized. As the rabbit is an obligate nasal breather, the epiglottis will usually be entrapped on the dorsal aspect of the soft palate.

2 Exert gentle dorsal pressure on the soft palate to free the epiglottis; the glottal opening should now be visible.

3 Slowly and gently advance the bevel of the ET tube between the arytenoids into the trachea.

4 Remove the endoscope.

5 Secure the ET tube in place.

TECHNIQUE 1.3:
Placing an ET tube under direct visualization

1 Place the rabbit in either sternal or dorsal recumbency with head and neck extended.

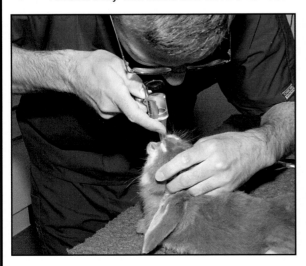

2 Gently retract the tongue to one side of the mouth.

3 Use an otoscope or laryngoscope (Wisconsin size 1 blade for larger rabbits) to visualize the larynx.

4 Place the introducer or stylet (e.g. dog urinary catheter) into the larynx.

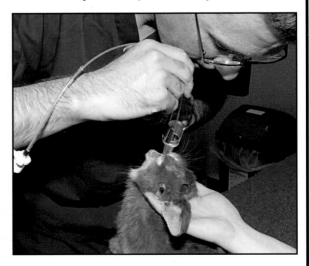

5 Remove the otoscope or laryngoscope from the mouth.

TECHNIQUE 1.3 continued:
Placing an ET tube under direct visualization

6 Railroad the ET tube over the introducer, into the larynx.

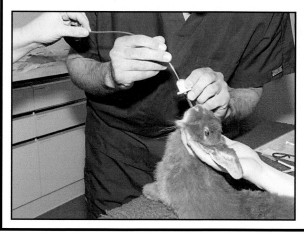

7 Check for breath sounds from the end of the tube. Condensation may be seen in clear tubes.

8 Secure the tube in place.

TECHNIQUE 1.4:
Intubating a rabbit's trachea using the 'blind' technique

1 Hold the rabbit in sternal recumbency with the head and neck extended in a straight line.

2 Stand to one side of the rabbit facing forwards with your non-dominant side next to the rabbit.

3 With your dominant hand, introduce the tube into the side of the rabbit's mouth and advance it towards the larynx.

4 Either listen to the end of the tube or position the end of the tube so that you can feel the rabbit's breath on the side of your face.

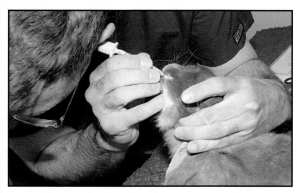

5 Once the tube has been advanced a sufficient distance, which suggests that it is close to the larynx, drip topical lidocaine (up to 4 mg/kg) down the tube. The lidocaine can be dispersed onto the larynx by blowing down the tube; this should be performed without touching the end of the tube with the mouth, to prevent absorption of spilt lidocaine.

6 If the rabbit's respiratory rate is sufficiently slow, advancement through the larynx should be attempted at inspiration.

7 If the breath sounds disappear as the tube is advanced, oesophageal intubation should be suspected. Withdraw and redirect the tube.

8 When tracheal intubation is successful, breath sounds will usually become louder, and the rabbit may cough suddenly.

9 Hold the tube firmly so it is not displaced by coughing, and secure it in place with white open-weave bandage behind the rabbit's head.

TECHNIQUE 1.5:
Performing nasotracheal intubation

1 Choose an ET tube of sufficiently small diameter to advance through the nares, and long enough to extend past the glottis. (Stephens Devalle (2009) used a tube with an internal diameter of 2–2.5 mm and length 14.5 cm in rabbits of 3–5.5 kg bodyweight.)

2 Place the rabbit in dorsal recumbency.

3 Grasp the maxillary arches of the rabbit with your non-dominant hand.

4 Position the rabbit's head so it is dorsiflexed.

5 Lift the nasal fold and, with your dominant hand, advance the tube medially and ventrally towards the nasal septum and hard palate.

6 If the tube is not passing easily, do not force the tube but withdraw it slightly and redirect.

7 Check the tube for condensation; this suggests endotracheal placement.

8 Place a butterfly of tape around the end of the tube next to the connector, and suture to the dorsum of the rabbit's nose.

TECHNIQUE 1.6:
Placing a laryngeal mask airway (LMA) in a rabbit

1 Select a suitably sized LMA. A size 1 LMA will fit a 4 kg rabbit.

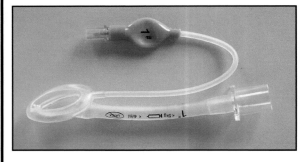

2 Ensure the cuff of the LMA is deflated.

3 With the rabbit in sternal recumbency, hold the rabbit's tongue gently with one hand, and with the other insert the LMA into the rabbit's mouth.

4 Advance the LMA towards the rabbit's pharynx, keeping it centred and parallel to the hard palate.

5 Once resistance is felt (and there may be signs of respiratory obstruction at this point, e.g. stridor or stertor) move the LMA slowly rostrally until clear breath sounds are heard.

6 Secure the tube in place and attach a breathing system. Reservoir bag excursions should be obvious for each breath.

TECHNIQUE 1.7:
Performing Doppler blood pressure measurement in a rabbit

1 Palpate a pulse on a limb of the rabbit (usually metacarpal or metatarsal).

2 Clip the hair from over the area where the pulse is palpable.

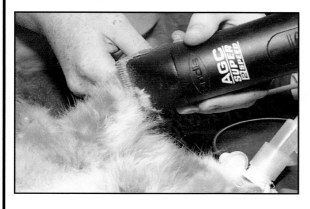

3 Apply some water-based gel to the Doppler probe and also apply it over the pulse site.

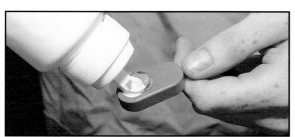

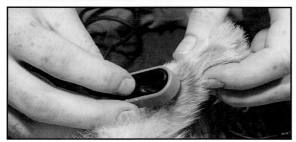

4 Reposition the probe until you hear the 'whoosh' sound associated with blood flow.

5 Tape the probe in place.

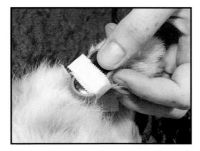

6 Proximal to the probe, wrap and secure a blood pressure cuff around the limb (the width of the cuff should be approximately 40% of the circumference of the limb).

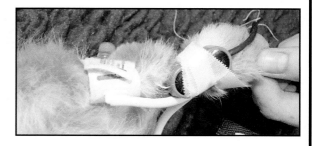

7 Attach the sphygmomanometer to the cuff.

8 Pump the bulb on the sphygmomanometer until the 'whoosh' sounds disappear.

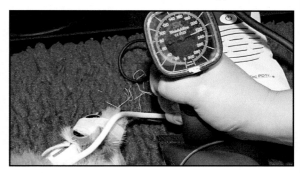

9 Slowly deflate the cuff (using a lever next to the bulb) until the 'whoosh' sounds return.

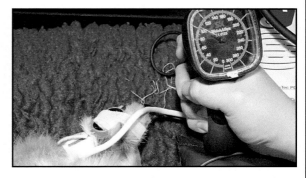

10 Record this value as systolic blood pressure.

11 Repeat this process a further two times and take the average of the three values.

12 Between recordings, leave the cuff deflated.

2

Analgesia and postoperative care

Cathy A. Johnson-Delaney and Frances Harcourt-Brown

Analgesia

Rabbits are often used as animal models for aspects of pain and anaesthesia, not only to provide good care for the laboratory rabbit, but also to increase understanding of the pharmacology for other species. It is often from the field of laboratory animal medicine that practitioners can gain information for use in the companion rabbit. The field of analgesia is continuously changing as a better understanding of pain and anaesthesia is attained.

Effects of pain

Pain causes an endocrine stress response with release of cortisol, catecholamines and other stress hormones. This stress response has many undesirable physiological effects, such as activation of the complement cascade, cytokine systems and the arachidonic acid cascade, and activation of the sympathetic nervous system (Barter, 2011). Pain can affect several organ systems, with serious interrelated results that can be fatal if left untreated. Examples include:

- **Cardiac effects:** tachycardia, dysrhythmias, vasoconstriction, altered cardiac output and increased myocardial oxygen demand, which can alter organ perfusion and organ function
- **Gastrointestinal effects:** anorexia and reduced gut motility can cause dehydration and negative energy balance that can result in hepatic lipidosis and fatty infiltration of the kidneys
- **Respiratory effects:** changes in respiratory rate and reduced tidal volume may intensify any existing respiratory compromise and affect oxygenation of organs
- **Metabolic effects:** disorders of fluid, electrolyte and acid–base balance, such as ketoacidosis, can be the indirect result of pain on organ systems. Hyperglycaemia is a response that can be measured to assess the degree of pain. It can rise to levels as high as 20–30 mmol/l in response to painful conditions such as intestinal obstruction, ureteral obstruction or enterotoxaemia (Harcourt-Brown and Harcourt-Brown, 2012). Catabolism, delayed wound healing and lowered immune response may be the result of chronic pain.

Assessment of pain in rabbits

The word 'pain' is derived from the Latin *poena*, or penalty. The Committee on Taxonomy Association for the Study of Pain defines pain as 'unpleasant sensory and emotional experience associated with actual or potential tissue damage'. As a prey species, rabbits mask signs of pain so the signs may be very subtle (Figure 2.1). Obvious signs of illness are a bad prognostic indicator and are only seen in rabbits with life-threatening illness (Figure 2.2). Otherwise, effective assessment is very difficult and investigators have struggled to find a reliable scoring system because rabbits tend to 'freeze' and remain immobile in the presence of an observer. Video footage has shown that a rabbit's behaviour is very different if someone is in the room with it (Leach *et al.*, 2009). In the absence of any reliable indicators of pain, it is safer to expect that any procedure or disease that would be likely to cause pain in a human will also cause pain in a rabbit.

Acute pain
• Freezing (remaining motionless for long periods of time)   • Twitching (rapid fur movement on the back)   • Wincing (rapid backward movement associated with eye closing and swallowing)   • Staggering (partial loss of balance)   • Flinching (rapid upward body jerks for no reason)   • Pressing (pushing abdomen towards floor)   • Very slow postural adjustments, and shuffling (walking at very slow pace)   • Piloerection   • Hiding   • Vocalization   • Loud grinding of teeth   • Pale eyes (if albino)
Chronic pain
• Reduced activity   • Failure to groom   • Reduced food and/or water intake   • Changed posture, tucking of abdomen, tensing of muscles   • Lameness   • Attempting to hide   • Aggressiveness   • Reduced faeces   • Reluctance to move   • Air boxing or licking a limb excessively

2.1 Signs of pain in rabbits. (Adapted from Kohn *et al.* (2007) and Leach *et al.* (2009))

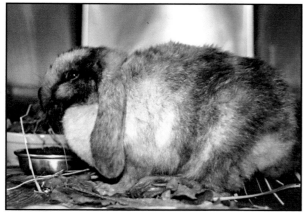

2.2 This rabbit was suffering from acute enterotoxaemia. He died, and post-mortem examination showed a severely inflamed caecum. The hunched posture, unresponsiveness, piloerection, immobility and desire to hide are typical signs of pain.

Pre-emptive analgesia
Current understanding of the mechanism of pain indicates that surgical incisions and other painful stimuli induce changes within the central nervous system (CNS) that may later contribute to post-operative pain. The 'noxious stimulus-induced sensitization' can be pre-empted by the administration of analgesics prior to tissue injury (Hawkins, 2006). Pre-emptive analgesia may be provided by opiates, non-steroidal anti-inflammatory drugs (NSAIDs) and/or local anaesthetics which block sensory noxious stimuli and transmission to the CNS. This decreases the overall potential for pain and will improve both the short-term and long-term recovery of the patient (see Chapter 1).

Non-pharmacological pain management
There are many simple non-pharmacological steps that can be taken to reduce pain in rabbits. Examples include:

- Treating the condition that is causing the pain (e.g. immobilizing a fractured limb or removing a dental spur) – this is the most effective way to prevent and relieve pain
- Gentle tissue handling and good technique during surgery (see Chapter 11)
- Placing skin sutures that are comfortable and not under tension – these will be less painful than sutures that are too tight
- Preventing infection with good aseptic technique
- Controlling infection with antibiotics or other antimicrobial therapy
- Providing good postoperative care such as soft, clean bedding and accessible food and water.

Pharmacological pain management
The plan for pharmacological pain management must take into consideration the severity, extent and duration of the painful condition. The route of administration may be an additional consideration and may depend on whether the patient is hospitalized or treatment takes place at home. Sources of acute

pain include surgical procedures, trauma and a variety of medical conditions, such as inflammation due to dental disease or otitis. Chronic pain sources include osteomyelitis associated with dental disease, arthritis or other degenerative orthopaedic processes. Medications that are used for pain management should address the problem being treated. The patient needs to be assessed on a regular basis for adjustment.

There are five main classes of drug used for acute pain management:

- Local anaesthetics
- Alpha-2 agonists
- NSAIDs
- Opioids
- Miscellaneous agents such as N-methyl-D-aspartate (NMDA) receptor antagonists, serotonin reuptake inhibitors and calcium channel antagonists.

Local anaesthetics
Local anaesthetics block ion channels, which prevents the generation and conduction of pain impulses. Analgesia is achieved by the abolition of neural input to the CNS. Lidocaine and bupivacaine are the two most commonly used agents. They can be applied topically, by infiltration of the tissue, or administered by injection directly into a joint, regionally as a nerve block, or intrathecally by epidural or subarachnoid injection. Local anaesthesia can be used as an adjunct to general anaesthesia to reduce the amount of anaesthetic that is used. It may also reduce postoperative analgesic requirements.

During surgery, incisional line blocks and local nerve blocks are relatively easy to administer.

Wound infiltration can provide immediate pain relief in a conscious rabbit to aid in the physical examination process. Lidocaine at 2–4 mg/kg and bupivacaine at 0.5–1 mg/kg can be used for any local infiltration or nerve block. Ropivacaine at 1.5 mg/kg has also been used.

A topical cream formulation of 2.5% lidocaine and 2.5% prilocaine (EMLA) may be used on the skin prior to puncture for blood sampling or catheter placement. It must remain in contact with the skin for up to 1 hour for maximum effectiveness.

Spinal administration of local anaesthetic drugs has been studied in laboratory rabbits (Hughes et al., 1993; Malinovsky et al., 1997). It has been used for Caesarean section in laboratory rabbits to study the fetus during parturition (Kero et al., 1981). There is a major difference in the spinal cords of rabbits and some other mammals (Chitty, 2007). The spinal cord ends and the cauda equina begins in the midsacral region rather than the caudal lumbar region, so it is probable that administration of a spinal injection results in subarachnoid rather than epidural injection. The best site for injection is into the subarachnoid space between the dura mater and pia mater at L6/L7 (Figure 2.3; see also Chapter 3). Laboratory studies suggest that a volume of 0.2 ml/kg is optimal. Lidocaine (0.2%), lidocaine

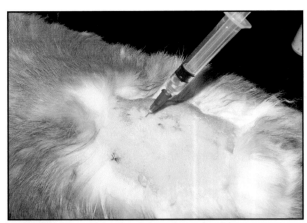

2.3 Site of injection into subarachnoid space. The subarachnoid space can be used to deliver local anaesthetics or morphine. The injection is given at L6/L7. The landmarks are the iliac crests (X) and the spinous processes (●). Prepared vertebrae showing the intervertebral space are shown in Technique 3.1.

with adrenaline (0.2%) or bupivacaine (0.5%) can be used. These doses produce sensory loss, loss of weight-bearing ability and flaccid paralysis. The effects of lidocaine are rapid in onset (1–3 minutes) and last 30–40 minutes. Bupivacaine is longer acting, and used at a lower dose may cause minimal motor effects. Both the epidural and subarachnoid blocks should be utilized only if the rabbit is fully anaesthetized because inability to move the hindlimbs can be extremely stressful.

Local anaesthetics can have dose-related toxic side effects on both the nervous system and the cardiovascular system, so doses should always be calculated.

Non-steroidal anti-inflammatory drugs

NSAIDs have anti-inflammatory, analgesic and anti-pyretic activity. They can be used in combination with opiates and other pure analgesic medications. When used in combination with opioids, a lower dose of opioid may be used because there seems to be a synergistic action. Usually NSAIDs are used alone for the management of mild to moderate acute or chronic pain, particularly in chronic inflammation such as osteomyelitis associated with dental disease. While the onset of action of the NSAIDs may be fairly long, the dosing interval is also long, making compliance easier for owners. The oral form is particularly useful for extending postoperative pain control for several days. Side effects in other species include renal dysfunction, hepatic dysfunction, gastrointestinal ulceration and inhibition of platelet function. If NSAIDs are administered prior to surgery, the risk of side effects is increased by the hypotension induced by general anaesthesia. In rabbits, side effects of NSAIDs have not been reported in the literature, although they have been studied extensively.

Meloxicam: Meloxicam is a popular choice of NSAID for rabbits because the oral preparation is palatable

and easy for owners to administer. Meloxicam blocks cyclo-oxygenase 2 (COX2)-related prostaglandins and in dogs has fewer gastrointestinal side effects (such as gastric ulceration) than some other NSAIDs. The pharmacokinetics of oral meloxicam in rabbits have been published (Carpenter *et al.*, 2009). Turner *et al.* (2006) gave doses of 0.3 mg/kg (the canine dose) and 1.5 mg/kg to rabbits as single doses, or repeated doses for 5 days. No adverse effects were seen. Maximum plasma levels were achieved 6–8 hours after dosing and decreased to near undetectable levels by 24 hours, indicating rapid metabolism and clearance in rabbits. The efficacy of meloxicam in reducing signs of pain after ovariohysterectomy has also been studied. Leach *et al.* (2009) showed that a high dose of meloxicam (1 mg/kg) followed by 0.5 mg/kg q24h induced a degree of analgesia but recommended that an additional opioid analgesic should be given. Cooper *et al.* (2009) showed that meloxicam (0.2 mg/kg q24h) was as effective as buprenorphine (0.03 mg/kg q12h) in reducing postoperative pain and preventing gut stasis. As a result of these studies and the variation in dose rates, there is a wide range of anecdotal dose rates for meloxicam. In view of the rapid metabolism of meloxicam in rabbits, one author (FHB) uses 0.2 mg/kg q12h for acute pain and combines meloxicam with an additional analgesic, such as tramadol or buprenorphine. Once-daily dosing of meloxicam is recommended for long-term analgesia, e.g. for patients with spondylosis.

Opioids

These drugs are the mainstay of analgesia for moderate to severe pain. Those most commonly used include buprenorphine, butorphanol, morphine and fentanyl. Many have been investigated, with the pharmacology reported in the laboratory animal literature. The controlled work has been done in New Zealand White rabbits, and many practitioners find that other breeds may react slightly differently to the drugs. Opioids act centrally but have been shown to have some peripheral effect in inflamed tissues (Barter, 2011). Most opioids must be used parenterally, owing to their poor oral bioavailability due to the first-pass effect through the liver. Opioids as a group cause varying levels of sedation in rabbits, with buprenorphine causing the least and butorphanol and μ agonists the most. In other species, opioids can cause decreased gastrointestinal motility. In rabbits, with the exception of intrathecal morphine, there appear to be no adverse effects of opioids on gut motility. If there are, they are outweighed by their analgesic effect, which suppresses the adrenergic response to pain, i.e. pain is more likely than opoids to reduce gut motility.

Buprenorphine: Buprenorphine is a popular choice of opioid analgesic. It is a slow-onset, long-acting opiate, acting as a partial μ agonist. Its κ activity is poorly defined. It may exhibit a plateau of effectiveness for analgesia, with higher doses providing no additional analgesia or duration of action. Its effects persist for 7 hours after administration.

Butorphanol: Butorphanol is a mixed agonist/antagonist with relatively low μ receptor activity and strong agonist κ receptor activity. It does not appear to produce dose-related respiratory depression, unlike other μ receptor agonists. It is short-acting (2–4 hours), requiring frequent dosing to maintain adequate pain control. It does have some sedative effects, making it excellent as part of the pre-emptive analgesia combination for preoperative medication.

Morphine: Morphine is a μ receptor agonist that is used to manage acute pain in other species, although it is not generally used in rabbits. Preservative-free morphine has been used as an epidural analgesic in rabbits (Barter, 2011). The onset of effect is slow (up to 1 hour) but the duration of action is long (up to 20 hours). Although this agent may be useful for rabbits undergoing orthopaedic procedures or extensive surgery, there are no clinical reports of its use at the time of writing.

Fentanyl: Fentanyl is a potent μ agonist with a short duration of action. In combination with fluanisone (Hypnorm), it is used for sedation or as a premedicant (see Chapter 1) and its potent analgesic properties can be very beneficial. If fentanyl alone is used as an analgesic, it is most commonly used as a transdermal patch, although in rabbits this may result in variable plasma levels. This is in part due to the rapidity of hair growth in rabbits, which results in the patch not maintaining contact. The highest dosages are reached 12–24 hours after patch application. The drug can have a sedative effect, so the rabbit must be closely monitored. The patch should also be covered to prevent the rabbit removing and/or eating it.

Miscellaneous analgesics

Alpha-2 adrenergic agonists: The alpha-2 adrenergic agonists have analgesic properties as well as sedative, muscle relaxant and sympatholytic activity (see Chapter 1). They are easily reversible and are frequently used as pre- or intraoperative agents, reducing general anaesthetic requirements.

Ketamine: Ketamine is primarily used for the induction and maintenance of general anaesthesia, generally in combination with a sedative. Other uses include sedation and analgesia, although its specific analgesic properties in rabbits have not been determined.

Tramadol: Tramadol has multiple actions, including μ opioid receptor agonist activity and serotonin and noradrenaline reuptake inhibitory activity. It also has alpha-2 adrenergic agonist activity. The pharmacokinetics of oral and intravenous administration in rabbits shows great variability in plasma levels with the active metabolite, *O*-desmethyltramadol, likely to be responsible for some of the effects. Plasma levels start to fall 8 hours after administration. Adverse effects are not reported, even using dose rates of up to 10 mg/kg i.v. and 11 mg/kg orally in laboratory investigations (Kuek *et al.*, 2005; Souza *et al.*, 2008).

A therapeutic dose of tramadol for rabbits has not been established, despite its widespread use for acute and chronic pain in this species. One author (FHB) uses a dose rate of 5 mg/kg q8h s.c. or i.v., in combination with an NSAID such as meloxicam. Oral administration for chronic pain is also useful for rabbits with incurable conditions such as osteoarthritis.

Pain management in specific conditions/situations

Critical illness
A critically ill rabbit may have non-specific aches and pains from multiple systems. Frequently this includes the gastrointestinal system. Gas and fluid distension may be extremely painful, although the rabbit may just sit with its feet tucked under its body and its muscles tense (see Figure 2.2). A benzodiazepine relaxant, such as midazolam, can help to address the muscle tension and anxiety associated with the condition. Administration of an opioid such as buprenorphine, or even a fentanyl patch, will address the gastrointestinal pain. Pain management must be accompanied with fluid therapy and nutritional support to prevent gastrointestinal stasis or worsening of any gastrointestinal hypomotility.

Dyspnoea
Respiratory disease and prolonged dyspnoea may contribute to thoracic muscle fatigue and actual airway pain. Again, a benzodiazepine may help to alleviate muscle tension and anxiety, allowing the rabbit to relax and breathe more deeply. An NSAID would be the medication of choice because its anti-inflammatory properties can benefit the airways.

Painful eye
Ophthalmic conditions can be treated topically using direct anaesthesia (such as proxymetacaine) and/or an NSAID such as flurbiprofen.

Caesarean section
This procedure is rare in general practice. Pre-emptive pain management should include an anxiolytic coupled with an opioid. An epidural anaesthetic/analgesic is indicated for prevention of abdominal pain. Incisional anaesthesia/analgesia should be used. One author (CJD) has used sterile lidocaine gel on the uterus where the incision is made. It has not interfered with involution after delivery and oxytocin injection. Postoperative analgesia can be achieved with an NSAID such as meloxicam or carprofen, which will not sedate the kits or slow the doe's gastrointestinal system.

Routine surgery
Pre-emptive pain management needs to be designed for the type of surgery to be performed, and the medications need to be effective for the duration. In general, a multi-modal analgesia/anaesthesia method should be used (see Chapter 1). The combination of drugs used for premedication may include a benzodiazepine and an opioid to help with sedation.

Incisional blocks can be applied wherever surgery is to be performed. Patients requiring surgery on the cornea or conjunctival tissues may benefit from an ophthalmic local anaesthetic.

Dentistry

After the rabbit has been anaesthetized, local nerve blocks can be performed depending on which teeth are going to be worked on and how invasive the dentistry will be.

After dental procedures, oral pain should be considered, as well as muscle strain that can accompany the prolonged stretching with equipment used to expose the oral cavity. Extensive burring can expose innervated dentine.

Opioids and NSAIDs can be continued for longer if dentistry is invasive or if teeth have been extracted. If no invasive oral surgery was performed, administration of an NSAID for 24–48 hours is sufficient.

Regional nerve blocks for dentistry

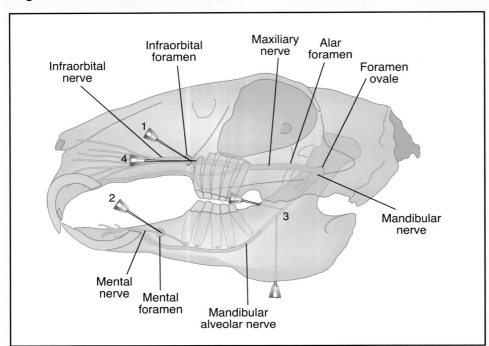

Sites of needle insertion for dental nerve blocks numbered below.

Regional nerve blocks can be used for dentistry. Local anaesthetic is either introduced around the nerve by inserting a needle through a foramen to access the nerve or by identifying the course of the nerve in the soft tissue from anatomical landmarks. For dental nerve blocks to be effective, the section of nerve that supplies the apices of the teeth must be blocked, otherwise it is only the soft tissue that is anaesthetized. Lidocaine alone or with bupivacaine for prolonged analgesia/anaesthesia can be used effectively. A tract should be laid down as close to where the nerve exits the skull as possible.

Block 1: For maxillary incisors, the infraorbital nerve is blocked as it exits the skull through the infraorbital foramen at approximately the level of cheek tooth 1 (red arrow). The approach is dorsally from the buccal gingival area of the mouth.

Block 2: The mandibular incisors can be blocked by laying down a line over the mental foramen on the mandible (green arrow). This lies just craniad to the mandibular cheek teeth. The approach is through the gingiva.

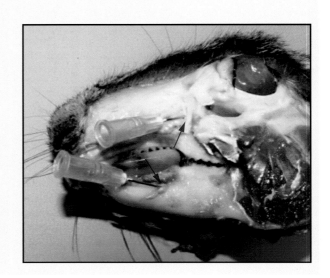

Block 3: The mandibular cheek teeth can be blocked by laying down a tract over the mandibular alveolar nerve close to the mandibular foramen (white arrow) that lies slightly lateral to the last cheek tooth from inside the oral cavity, but this can be difficult to identify due to the narrow gape of rabbits.

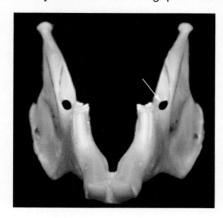

Abscess surgery

Superficial abscesses may benefit from a local anaesthetic block encompassing the incisional area as well as the deep 'stalk'. Once the abscess is debrided, it may be necessary to apply a local anaesthetic to the tissue connecting the abscess pocket to the body prior to full excision of the tissue. Postoperatively, an opioid with or without a benzodiazepine can be used to keep the rabbit relaxed. Follow-up analgesia can be achieved with an NSAID, such as meloxicam, in combination with an opioid, such as buprenorphine or tramadol. Deep abscesses may require multimodal analgesia/anaesthesia along with local anaesthesia of the area itself. Instillation of local anaesthetic (e.g. daily bupivacaine) into the abscess cavity can be effective and aids cleansing of the cavity to remove any residual necrotic or infected tissue (see Chapter 29).

Orthopaedic pain

Joint pain due to conditions such as spondylosis, spondylitis or arthritis tends to be chronic. For many, use of an NSAID long term or as needed is sufficient. Use of tramadol or an opioid is added on an 'as needed' basis. Owners can be taught to recognize signs of pain and administer the stronger analgesic as needed. Acute orthopaedic pain, such as from an injury, fracture or luxation, requires opioids, although rabbits generally also need a benzodiazepine initially because immobility in a prey species is associated with fear and anxiety. Ring blocks or local infusion of lidocaine and/or bupivacaine can reduce the need for higher-dose opioids. Knowledge of the nerves to the area can help with placement of the blocks (see Chapter 22). Following correction of the fracture or luxation, the rabbit should be continued on NSAIDs and, initially postoperatively, on an opioid. The NSAID may be continued as needed until resolution.

An alternative approach has been described (Lichtenberger, 2007). The site of the foramen is approximately 2–5 mm distal to the third cheek tooth so a needle is 'walked along' the medial aspect of the mandible and inserted alongside the bone to the depth of the nerve. Care is required to avoid other nerves and blood vessels.

Block 4: The maxillary cheek teeth are usually blocked individually by 'splash blocks', i.e. individual injections through the gingiva into the periodontal ligaments and alveolar tissue. A major regional nerve block is impossible from inside the oral cavity. However, in large rabbits the maxillary nerve can be accessed by a 'caudal infraorbital' strategy (Lichtenberger, 2007). A needle is advanced 1–2 cm into the infraorbital foramen and aspirated to ensure the retrobulbar venous sinus has not been perforated. Firm digital pressure is applied to the rostral end of the infraorbital canal as the local anaesthetic is injected.

Postoperative care

The goal of appropriate postoperative care is to return the rabbit to acceptable physical and behavioural parameters. This includes the parameters listed in Figure 2.4, as defined by Weaver *et al.* (2010). Good postoperative care is essential to restore a rabbit to good health, and there are many factors to consider.

Behaviour	Description
Sitting	Fully balanced on hindlimbs, forelimbs or both. Appears relaxed, abdomen not hunched
Sprawled	Reclined in sternal or half-lateral recumbency, relaxed. Limbs extended horizontally
Travelling	Moving around pen, walking or hopping. May include looking at/sniffing ground if food in abnormal place, or novel item found
Foraging and intake	Sniffing or rummaging in food, eating, drinking
Grooming	Paws or mouth washing any part of body. Relaxed. Scratching, licking. Watch for incisional licking, over-grooming (indication of irritation and/or pain?)
Rearing up	Stand up using hindlimbs or staying on all fours and looking/sniffing upwards in air. Ears upright
Playing with toys	Interacting with cage furnishings or toys
Frolicking	Hops, jumps rapidly, may do 'binky' (fling self into air)
Stool	Ideally return to normal output quantity and normal quality as soon as possible
Urination	Within a short time after anaesthesia, and normal volume in first 12 hours postoperatively

2.4 Desirable postoperative behavioural and physical parameters in rabbits.

A stress-free environment

On recovery from an anaesthetic (see also Chapter 1), the rabbit should be placed in a dim, quiet area for recovery, away from the noise and smells of predator species (e.g. dogs and cats). This is often not the situation in a busy small animal practice. Proximity of humans, bright lights, unfamiliar surroundings, noises from machinery, bandages, tubing, collars and splints can all be stressful for an animal whose instinct is to hide in a burrow if it is stressed or in pain. A quiet corner in a kennel area where a member of the nursing staff can keep a vigilant eye on the patient is needed.

Maintaining body temperature

In rabbits, it is important to maintain optimal body temperature during surgery and postoperatively (Sikoski *et al.*, 2007). A forced-air heating device or a combination of heating platforms, water blankets, paediatric incubator or heat pads should be available for rabbits recovering from anaesthesia, and their temperature should be monitored closely until they are normothermic and ambulatory. A low body temperature can prolong recovery but hyperthermia can also be a risk, so discretion is required in determining which rabbits require additional heat and which do not. The rabbit should be housed on a towel or padded surface and turned regularly until it is in sternal recumbency and moving on its own.

Careful observation

Careful observation is vital for good postoperative care and begins as soon as the rabbit starts to recover from the anaesthetic. It is necessary to observe rabbits closely during this period to make sure they are warm enough and that any intravenous fluids are being administered at the correct rate. Overperfusion is a risk. Another problem is the rabbit moving and kinking the giving set so no fluid goes into the vein. Monitoring the rabbit's breathing is important. If the airway is occluded, e.g. by food, blood or pus in the larynx, their response is not to cough or show respiratory effort; instead they stop breathing and may die. Positioning them so they have a clear airway is therefore essential.

Hospitalization

Once the rabbit has recovered from the anaesthetic, a decision must be taken on whether it should be allowed home. Rabbits may be hospitalized for a number of reasons:

- **Careful observation** of appetite, demeanour and faecal output (e.g. postoperatively, for anorexic rabbits or those with diarrhoea)
- **Repeated radiography and/or blood sampling** (e.g. moving ureteral stones or suspected intestinal obstruction)
- **Provision of analgesia.** Multi-modal analgesia may require injections several times a day with opioids. Observation is needed to assess the degree of pain and efficacy of analgesia in order to formulate a treatment plan

- **Prevention of gut stasis.** It is vital that rabbits have food passing through their digestive tract. Prokinetic therapy and nutritional support are often needed and are life-saving (see later). Although many owners are able to syringe-feed their rabbits, many are unable or unwilling to do so
- **Fluid therapy.** Intravenous or subcutaneous fluid therapy is indicated for some conditions
- **Medication.** In addition to analgesics, antibiotics and prokinetics, other medication, such as topical eye, ear or nose drops, may be needed that is hard for the owner to administer
- **Wound cleaning.** Effective wound cleaning is an important part of successful treatment of abscesses. The procedure may be required twice daily and can be an unpleasant experience for the owner. Many prefer to leave the rabbit in the hospital so the nursing staff can take care of it
- **Restricted activity.** It is sometimes important that a rabbit is cage-rested, e.g. after orthopaedic surgery or for non-surgical treatment of ataxia or lameness
- **Provision of special bedding.** Some neurological cases (e.g. those with severe head tilt) benefit from bedding that prevents them from rolling and offers some protection if they do
- **Re-bandaging or re-dressing.** For example, rabbits with sore hocks may benefit from wound re-dressing daily
- **Bladder emptying.** Repeated manual expression of the bladder may be indicated for some neurological or urinary tract diseases.

A lot will depend on the type of surgery that has taken place, and also the owner. Although many owners believe they can manage their rabbit at home, it can be a mistake to discharge a rabbit too soon. If the rabbit is bright, alert and eating postoperatively it is safe to send it home, although an information sheet describing the postoperative care that is needed and the signs of gut stasis that the owners should look out for is extremely useful. If there is any doubt about the owner's ability to observe and care for their rabbit, hospitalization is preferable so the nursing staff can observe the rabbit carefully, ensure that all medication is given, provide nutritional support, provide analgesia and comfort, and attend to any wounds effectively.

Observation of the hospitalized rabbit

If the rabbit is to be hospitalized for any length of time, a cage in a quiet area with a litter tray, a range of palatable foods, good quality hay and water from a bowl are advisable (Figure 2.5). An enclosed area for the rabbit to move around in while its demeanour and recovery are observed is beneficial (Figure 2.6). If the space is available, an indoor run is ideal (Figure 2.7).

Careful observation is important for hospitalized rabbits, and the observer needs to be familiar with normal rabbit behaviour and be able to recognize signs of pain or stress as well as signs of good health (see Figures 2.1, 2.2 and 2.6). Water and food intake can be measured and recorded in addition to the type, nature and quantity of faeces

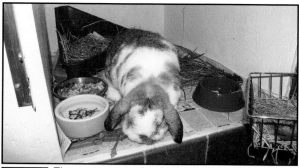

2.5 There are many simple steps that can be taken to reduce stress and improve recovery in hospitalized rabbits. A kennel in a quiet place away from unfamiliar noise and the sight and smell of other animals is ideal. Provision of a wide range of favourite foods, including fresh grass and dandelions, will tempt rabbits to eat, although food may need to be shredded or grated for rabbits with dental problems. Good quality hay or dried grass should be freely available and the use of racks or jars will reduce contamination. Water should be provided in a bowl, rather than a sipper bottle, which can reduce water intake (Tschudin *et al.*, 2011). A litter tray is beneficial, especially for housetrained rabbits.

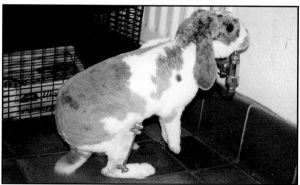

2.6 This rabbit is showing many positive behavioural signs that indicate that he has recovered well from surgery to repair a fractured tibia. He has come out of his cage to investigate the surroundings and is scent-marking the radiator. His fur is groomed and he is weight-bearing.

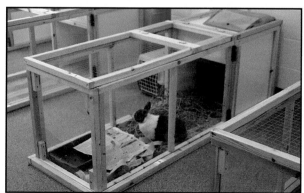

2.7 Indoor rabbit runs. These enable rabbits to express most of their normal behaviours. The runs should be tall enough to allow the rabbit to stand and provide sufficient length for limited exercise – particularly useful for rabbits with gut stasis. The run is built from perspex/plastic, enabling easy cleaning and disinfection. A darkened 'house' provides security. Seeing other rabbits in neighbouring runs also helps to provide mental security. (© John Chitty)

that are passed. The observer needs to be able to distinguish among hard faecal pellets, caecotrophs and diarrhoea and know what the normal size and shape of hard faeces should be. Saving faeces for the attending veterinary surgeon to examine is recommended if there is any doubt about whether they are normal or not. The amount and nature of urine output can also be observed by examining the contents of the litter tray or bedding.

Preventing wound interference

For all rabbits that have undergone surgery, post-operative observations need to be frequent to ensure that there is no incisional bleeding or dehiscence, and that the rabbit is not chewing or licking the surgical site excessively. Comfortable incisions with no tension on the wound are more likely to be left alone, although some rabbits, usually healthy young rabbits undergoing neutering, will interfere with their wound postoperatively. Steps may be required to prevent wound interference, and there are several options.

> ### Options for preventing wound interference
>
> Most rabbits will leave wounds alone, although their incisors (if they are healthy) are normally used for biting through fibrous stems so they are sharp and effective at cutting and can easily bite through skin sutures. Painful wounds or those under tension are most likely to cause patient interference from constant licking, nibbling, chewing and self-mutilation. Several steps can be taken to prevent a vicious cycle (uncomfortable wound → chewing/licking → inflammation → uncomfortable wound) starting.
>
> - **Comfortable wound repair.** Placing sutures that do not cause tension so the wound is comfortable is the most important method of preventing patient interference.
> - **Effective analgesia.**
> - **Subcuticular sutures, staples and/or tissue glue** can be used to avoid the need for skin sutures, which are the most likely to be removed.
> - **Local anaesthesia.** If a rabbit seems to be uncomfortable and/or is bothering the surgical site, a local nerve block with lidocaine/ bupivacaine can be performed or topical lidocaine/prilocaine (EMLA) cream can be applied to painful wounds.
> - **Blunting incisors.** Some rabbits, usually healthy young rabbits undergoing neutering, will interfere with their wound postoperatively, no matter how comfortable the wound is. One author (FHB) blunts the incisors of likely candidates for wound interference by smoothing <1 mm from the sharp tips with the surface (not the edge) of a diamond cutting disc before the rabbit recovers from anaesthesia. The sharp tips grow back within a week, by which time the wound will have healed.   ▶

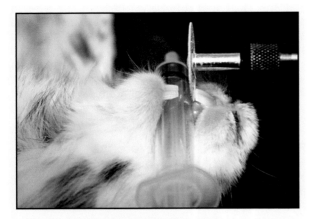

- **Vests for premature babies.** Tiny vests for human babies can be useful to protect wounds and prevent patient interference in rabbits. They are more comfortable and less stressful than Elizabethan collars and do not prevent caecotrophy. They are easily available and can be laundered.

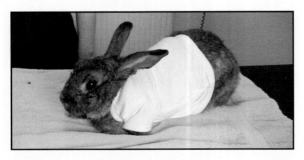

- **Body stockings.** Body stockings ('onesies') are now available commercially for use with rabbits and can provide a comfortable and secure way of preventing self-trauma.
- **Elizabethan collars.** In the authors' opinion, Elizabethan collars are seldom or never required to prevent wound interference. Wearing an Elizabethan collar is stressful for rabbits and can cause anorexia in its own right. It restricts their normal field of vision, prevents prehension of caecotrophs and can rub on the ears. Soft collars that are tied around the neck and flapped down over the shoulders may be used for wounds in some positions and these appear to be well tolerated (see Chapter 11).

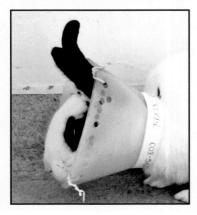

Bedding, litter trays and companions

Bedding
Comfortable bedding is beneficial for rabbits. At home, many pet rabbits spend much of their time on a bed of hay and appreciate the same bedding during their stay at a veterinary surgery, although storing and disposing of hay can cause practical problems. Long strands of hay are not a good idea for bedding paretic rabbits because they can get their legs caught and entwined in the hay. Towels or fleecy beds can be used as alternatives but may be chewed. As a general rule, synthetic fibre is not a good idea for rabbits that chew because it is not broken down in the digestive tract and could accumulate and cause an obstruction; cotton towels are preferable. Sawdust or wood shavings are generally unsatisfactory because they are messy and the small particles can easily adhere to wounds or faeces.

Litter trays
Most rabbits prefer to defecate and urinate in the same place and many rabbit patients are house-trained to use a litter tray and will use one if they are hospitalized. Most owners are prepared to provide litter material. Alternatively, hay over newspaper is satisfactory.

Companions
Many rabbit patients have left a bonded companion at home. Hospitalizing the companion has advantages and disadvantages. The advantages are that the rabbit patient will appreciate companionship and there will be no reintroduction problems once he or she goes home; some rabbits, especially females, can become aggressive towards a rabbit that they have not seen for a few days. The disadvantage is that it is not possible to know how much the patient is eating and defecating. A compromise is to hospitalize both rabbits but to separate them at night and keep them together during the day when they can be observed easily.

Preventing gut stasis
Gut stasis is a real risk for any rabbit that has had surgery. It is a potentially fatal condition that may be triggered by any pain or stress because stimulation of the sympathetic nervous system inhibits gut motility and reduces appetite. Left untreated, gut stasis can result in death a few days after the anaesthetic. Slow gut motility and reduced food intake decrease the absorption of sugars, starches and volatile fatty acids from the digestive tract and result in a negative energy balance, so adipose tissue is broken down as an energy source instead. This releases free fatty acids (FFAs) that are transported to the liver where they are oxidized as an energy source. Oxidation of FFAs releases ketones and causes ketoacidosis, which is a problem for rabbits because they lack some renal metabolic pathways that correct acidosis. In addition, if large amounts of FFAs are present in the liver a metabolic bottleneck

occurs which results in fatty infiltration and hepatic degeneration, and ultimately causes liver failure and death. Obese rabbits or those with a high energy demand, such as pregnant or lactating does, are most susceptible to death from hepatic lipidosis.

The clinical signs of gut stasis are:

- Anorexia
- Reduced or absent faecal output, perhaps with small hard faecal pellets
- Progressively quiet demeanour
- Firm small stomach, both radiographically and palpably
- Reduced amount of ingesta in the gastrointestinal tract.

Without treatment, a number of additional problems can develop. Gastric ulcers are common. Slow gut motility also results in fermentation of the intestinal contents and accumulation of gas, especially in the caecum and proximal colon. Gas distension causes pain, which reduces gut motility further. Gas shadows can be seen radiographically (see Chapters 7 and 14).

Food and good postoperative care are essential to prevent gut stasis. At the end of surgery, if a rabbit has not eaten well prior to the procedure, or is likely to have problems eating postoperatively, food can be instilled directly into the stomach via a feeding tube (see Technique 2.1). The only occasion when this procedure should be avoided is at the end of surgery to treat gastric dilation, when the food can ferment and cause problems because paralytic ileus may be present (see Chapter 14).

Nutritional support

Tempting foods

Good hay, freshly picked grass and dandelions or palatable vegetables such as kale, spring cabbage or carrot tops are good for tempting rabbits to eat postoperatively, and a supply can be kept in stock. Otherwise, it is a good idea for owners to leave some favourite foods with their rabbit or to fill in a menu sheet so the nursing staff know what the rabbit likes to eat. Some rabbits will eat as soon as they recover from anaesthesia, despite extensive surgery. Others refuse to eat, despite minimal surgery. House rabbits may not eat just because they are away from home. Rabbits that have dental problems may only be able to eat softened, grated or shredded foods and it is important to know this when preparing the rabbit's food.

Syringe feeding is necessary for any rabbit that does not eat or is struggling to eat because of dental problems. Various foods are available for syringe feeding (e.g. Oxbow Critical Care, Supreme Science Recovery). One author (FHB) likes to mix some baby cereal (e.g. Heinz cereal for babies aged 4–6 months) with the food because it is fruit-flavoured and palatable; it also has no lumps and goes through a syringe easily. Leaving the mixture for 10 minutes or so seems to improve the texture, but leaves the larger particles of fibre that can assist gut

motility. Approximately 10–20 ml/kg of the mixture four times daily is a satisfactory amount. Syringe feeding (Figure 2.8) requires patience but is a safe way to provide food and fluids, which are essential to prevent (or treat) gut stasis.

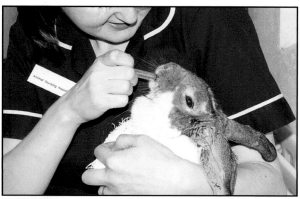

2.8 Syringe feeding is a safe and effective way to provide food and fluids to a rabbit that is reluctant to eat on its own. It can be used for any rabbit that has not eaten well. The majority of rabbits will accept syringe feeding. There are several methods of restraint. Wrapping them in a towel and cradling them is often successful. A relaxed attitude and patience is required to administer the food into the diastema and wait for the rabbit to swallow it between mouthfuls.

Feeding tubes

Very occasionally, syringe feeding is impossible and an alternative method of providing nutrition becomes necessary. Examples include rabbits with jaw fractures or iatrogenic damage to the oral cavity during dentistry. In these rabbits nasogastric, naso-oesophageal or oesophagostomy tubes may be used. Although percutaneous endoscopic gastrostomy (PEG) tubes have been used for enteral nutritional support in rabbits (Smith *et al.*, 1997), the technique does not appear to be as useful in rabbits as it is in dogs and cats. It is difficult to pass an endoscope through the rabbit's mouth and pharynx and to obtain a good endoscopic view because the stomach always contains some food and is never empty.

Naso-oesophageal and nasogastric tubes: A feeding tube can be placed through the nose, pharynx and oesophagus to administer nutritional support. The tube is generally kept in place by suturing it to the nares and/or skin. The tip of the tube can be placed in the oesophagus or in the stomach. Although these tubes permit easy administration of liquid food, they have some disadvantages. It is impossible to administer long particles of fibre through naso-oesophageal or nasogastric tubes without blocking them, so only liquid or finely ground food can be administered, which does not stimulate gut motility. The nasal mucosa of rabbits is very sensitive; therefore inserting the tube and suturing it to the nostril can be stressful, even after the administration of local anaesthetic drops or gel. Sedation is beneficial. Placing the tube can damage the nasal mucosa and cause epistaxis. It is contraindicated in rabbits with upper respiratory tract problems.

Nasogastric or naso-oesophageal tubes also carry a risk of iatrogenic complications such as inhalation pneumonia, gastric reflux, oesophagitis and stricture if food or gastric contents enter the oesophagus (Powers, 2006). After the tube has been placed, an Elizabethan collar may or may not be necessary to prevent the rabbit removing the tube. Elizabethan collars add to the stress level of the rabbit, and prevent caecotrophy. Both the tube and the collar can be stressful for some rabbits, which increases the risk of anorexia and gut stasis.

Tube placement: Paediatric tubes (4–8 French) are suitable for this purpose, or customized veterinary products are available in various sizes. A closed-end tube minimizes trauma to the nasal passages. Additional holes in the side of the tube may be necessary to prevent it becoming occluded with food.

1. Local anaesthetic is instilled into the nostril. Sufficient time (2–3 minutes) is allowed to elapse for the anaesthetic to take effect before the tube is introduced.
2. Prior to insertion, the tube is measured against the rabbit and marked to give an idea of the position of the tip as the tube is being placed.
3. The tube is then lubricated and placed by grasping and elevating the rabbit's head and introducing the tube into the middle meatus, where it is directed slightly ventrally and medially. To minimize the risk of introducing the tube into the trachea, the head is flexed as the tube passes through the nasopharynx. Swallowing may be noted as the tube enters the pharynx. Occasionally resistance is encountered in the nasal passage due to an elongated tooth root. In this instance, the other nostril can be tried.
4. After placement, it is important to ensure that the tube is not placed in the trachea before introducing food. Listening for breath sounds in the tube or attaching a syringe and aspirating can be helpful. If the end of the tube is in the trachea, air is aspirated. If the end is in the oesophagus or stomach, there will be resistance and negative pressure. A lateral radiograph may be necessary to confirm correct placement of the tube.

Oesophagostomy tubes: To place an oesophagostomy tube:

1. A 1 cm incision is made, under general anaesthesia, 5 mm from the midline just anterior to the larynx on the left-hand side.
2. A tube is passed through the oral cavity into the oesophagus and down to the stomach. Soft feeding tubes designed for oesophagostomy in cats are suitable for this purpose.
3. The tube is grasped with artery forceps through the mouth and pushed against the wall of the distal oesophagus to cause a bulge under the skin incision. The muscle overlying the bulge is carefully incised using the hard tip of the artery forceps in the pharynx as a guide.

4. The oesophageal wall is incised and the oral end of the stomach tube exteriorized through the incision.
5. The tube is then anchored at the oesophageal incision. It may be gently bandaged around the neck or it can be run through the subcutaneous tissues to emerge at the base of the ear, where it is anchored with skin sutures so the end is accessible for administration of food. An advantage of this technique is that the tubes are large enough to administer fibrous foods without blocking. The tube should be flushed through with water after each feed. It is possible for rabbits to eat and drink with these tubes in place and an Elizabethan collar may not be necessary.

Prokinetic therapy

Prokinetic therapy is indicated for those rabbits that are not passing hard faeces or are only passing small ones. Different medications are available in different countries. In the UK, domperidone (0.5 mg/kg q12h), cisapride (0.5 mg/kg q12h) or metoclopramide (0.5 mg/kg q6–8h) are used.

Anti-ulcer therapy

Gastric ulcers are a common post-mortem finding in anorexic rabbits. They are impossible to diagnose during life, so ranitidine (5 mg/kg orally q12h), which is available as a palatable paediatric syrup and also has some prokinetic properties, is recommended to be given alongside prokinetic therapy for all anorexic rabbits.

References and further reading

Barter LS (2011) Rabbit analgesia. *Veterinary Clinics of North America: Exotic Animal Practice* **14**, 93–104
Carpenter JW, Pollock CG, Koch DE and Hunter RP (2009) Single and multiple-dose pharmacokinetics of meloxicam after oral administration to the rabbit (*Oryctolagus cuniculus*). *Journal of Zoo and Wildlife Medicine* **40**, 601–606
Chitty J (2007) The subarachnoid space: Its clinical relevance in rabbits. *Journal of Exotic Pet Medicine* **16**, 179–182
Cooper CS, Metcalfe-Pate KA, Barat CE, Cook JA and Scorpio DA (2009) Comparison of side effects between buprenorphine and meloxicam used postoperatively in Dutch Belted rabbits. *Journal of the American Association for Laboratory Animal Science* **48**, 279–285
Harcourt-Brown FM and Harcourt-Brown SF (2012) Clinical value of blood glucose measurement in pet rabbits. *Veterinary Record* **170**, 674
Hawkins MG (2006) The use of analgesics in birds, reptiles, and small exotic mammals. *Journal of Exotic Pet Medicine* **15**, 177–192
Hughes PJ, Doherty MM and Charman WN (1993) A rabbit model for the evaluation of epidurally administered local anaesthetic drugs. *Anaesthesia and Intensive Care* **21**, 298–303
Kero P, Thomasson B and Soppi A (1981) Spinal anaesthesia in the rabbit. *Laboratory Animals* **15**, 347–348
Kohn SD, Martin TE, Foley PI *et al.* (2007) Guidelines for the assessment and management of pain in rodents and rabbits. *Journal of the American Association for Laboratory Animal Science* **46**, 97–108
Kuek A, Kadioglu Y and Celebi F (2005) Investigation of the pharmacokinetics and determination of tramadol in rabbit plasma by a high performance liquid chromatography-diode array detector method using liquid-liquid extraction. *Journal of Chromatography* **B816**, 203–208
Leach MC, Allweiler S, Richardson C, *et al.* (2009) Behavioural effects of ovariohysterectomy and oral administration of meloxicam in laboratory housed rabbits. *Research in Veterinary Science* **87**, 336–347
Lichtenberger M (2007) Anesthetic cases in exotics. Part 1. *Proceedings of the SCIVAC Congress, Rimini, Italy*

Malinovsky J, Bernard J, Baudrimont M, Dumand J and Lepage J (1997) A chronic model for experimental investigation of epidural anaesthesia in the rabbit. *Regional Anaesthesia and Pain Medicine* **22**, 80–85

Powers LV (2006) Techniques for drug delivery in small mammals. *Journal of Exotic Pet Medicine*, **15**, 201–209

Sikoski P, Young RW and Lockard M (2007) Comparison of heating devices for maintaining body temperature in anesthetized laboratory rabbits (*Oryctolagus cuniculus*). *Journal of the American Association for Laboratory Animal Science* **46**, 61–63

Smith DA, Olson PO and Matthews KA (1997) Nutritional support for rabbits using the percutaneously placed gastrotomy tube: a preliminary study. *Journal of the American Animal Hospital Association* **33**, 48–54

Souza MJ, Greenacre CB and Cox SK (2008) Pharmacokinetics of orally administered tramadol in domestic rabbits (*Oryctolagus cuniculus*). *American Journal of Veterinary Research* **69**, 979–982

Tschudin A, Clauss M, Codron D and Hatt JM (2011) Preference of rabbits for drinking from open dishes versus nipple drinkers. *Veterinary Record* **168**, 190

Turner PV, Chen HC and Taylor WM (2006) Pharmokinetics of meloxicam in rabbits after single and repeat oral dosing. *Comparative Medicine* **56**, 53–67

Weaver LA, Blaze CA, Linder DE, Andrutis KA and Karas AZ (2010) A model for clinical evaluation of perioperative analgesia in rabbits (*Oryctolagus cuniculus*). *Journal of the American Association for Laboratory Animal Science* **49**, 845–851

TECHNIQUE 2.1 ➜

TECHNIQUE 2.1:
Instilling food into the stomach prior to recovery from anaesthesia

Rabbits that were having problems eating prior to anaesthesia or those that may have painful mouths postoperatively (e.g. after abscess removal or incisor extraction) often benefit from a stomach full of food to stimulate gut motility and to provide fluid and nutrition at the end of surgery. Oral medications can be administered at the same time. The procedure avoids the need for syringe feeding as soon as the rabbit regains consciousness after its anaesthetic, and gives it time to recover and respond to any treatment that it has had. Syringe feeding can then be delayed for several hours or even overnight depending on the condition of the rabbit.

Positioning

The rabbit is placed in lateral recumbency. If it is intubated the ET tube can be left in place.

Assistant

No assistant is necessary.

Equipment

- 20 ml or 30 ml syringes containing 20–25 ml/kg of liquid food (e.g. Oxbow Critical Care, Supreme Science Recovery Diet).
- Any oral medications that need to be given.
- A 20–30 cm length of soft tube that will fit on to the end of the syringe. A feeding tube or piece of giving set tubing works well.

Approach

1 Measure the tube against the body and mark the distance from the nose to the last rib on the tube.

2 Pass the tube through the mouth into the oesophagus and into the stomach.

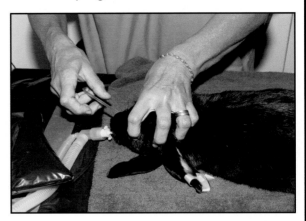

3 Minimal force should be used on the stomach tube, but slight resistance may be felt as it passes through the cardia. Insertion can be accomplished without a gag, with or without an ET tube in place. If the mouth is gently held closed, a lightly anaesthetized rabbit cannot chew through the tube.

4 Check that the tube is not in the trachea, which is impossible if the rabbit is intubated but possible if it is not. Tracheal intubation is unlikely but easily detected by a change in breathing pattern, the presence of breath sounds and condensation in the tube and an inability to pass the tube past the level of the bronchi. If there is any doubt, withdraw the tube and try again.

5 Instil liquid feed plus any oral medication followed by 2–3 ml of air or water to push the contents of the tube into the stomach.

6 Withdraw the tube gently.

3

Principles of radiography

Vladimir Jekl

Radiography is the most commonly used diagnostic tool in veterinary practice and has an important role in the diagnosis of rabbit diseases. It is non-invasive and provides the clinician with a large amount of information. Radiological studies should always follow the full clinical examination. The goal of these studies is to confirm disease, exclude disease, or discover new information. Proper patient positioning is crucial to achieving images of diagnostic quality.

Equipment

Radiographic machines
Due to the relatively small size of rabbits, particularly their legs, the radiographic equipment should be capable of producing 300 milliamperes (mA) and obtaining a minimum exposure time of 0.02 seconds with a kilovoltage peak (kVp) setting between 35 and 70 kVp. There are three main types of X-ray machine available:

- Hand-held portable X-ray units
- Dental X-ray units
- Conventional mobile or wall/ceiling-mounted X-ray units.

Portable machines are ideal for the veterinary surgeon in mobile practice as they can be transported to the client's premises and set up anywhere within reach of a power supply. A new portable X-ray system, which operates at a fixed 60 kV and 2.3 mA, has a focal spot distance of 0.4 mm and a source-to-object distance of 20 cm with variable exposure times (0.01–0.99 s). The relatively low mA capacity makes movement blur more likely than with more powerful machines. Dental X-ray machines may also have fixed kV options. The advantages of hand-held and dental X-ray machines are a simultaneous mA and kV output, and small focal spot-to-film distance (20–30 cm), which is adequate for radiography of small body regions (e.g. teeth, skull, joints, appendicular skeleton) and creates minimal scatter radiation.

Conventional X-ray units have higher output capabilities than portable units and most are capable of producing diagnostic views of the larger structures (e.g. thorax, abdomen) in the rabbit. The cassette is placed on the table top and the X-ray head manoeuvred to achieve a focal spot-to-film distance of 70–100 cm. The focal spot should be as small as possible in order to achieve sharp images (0.4 mm). Close collimation around the area of interest helps to decrease scatter radiation and maximize detail.

The appropriate selection of amperage, exposure time and kVp results in a radiographic image with the correct density, contrast and detail of anatomical structures. The optimal kilovoltage for rabbits is in a fixed range of approximately 65 kVp. As there are a number of different types of radiographic machine available, stable technique and exposure charts for particular anatomical regions of the rabbit should be established to standardize and expedite the radiographic examination.

PRACTICAL TIP
Radiography charts for young animals should have kVp ranges 5–10% lower than those of the corresponding adult animal because of incomplete bone mineralization. This prevents overexposure and increases visualization of soft tissue structures.

Conventional films and screens
Obtaining excellent radiographs with optimal contrast and detail is essential in rabbits. Determining the most desirable speed is a major factor in the selection of a film–screen system. The combination of a standard film and an intensifying screen with a number of 100 is recommended.

More detailed images can be obtaining by using ultraslow-speed, single-emulsion mammography films. These films provide enhanced soft and hard tissue detail, resulting in sharp, non-grainy images, and are therefore especially useful in rabbits.

Despite the fact that slow-speed screens and films require longer exposure times than regular screens/films, they are rarely affected by patient motion caused by breathing.

- High quality, detailed images can be achieved using settings of 300 mA, an exposure time of 0.1 s and 40–70 kVp.
- When using double-sided films, good quality images can be obtained using settings of 300 mA, an exposure time of 0.01 s and 40–70 kVp.

Non-screen films are commonly used in dental radiography and to image distinct anatomical areas to provide the greatest possible detail. Due to the small size of the anatomical region being examined, and therefore the small area being irradiated, grids are not generally used for imaging pet rabbits.

Digital radiography

Digital radiography shows great promise for the replacement of conventional radiography, as computer-generated images provide superior detail and allow post-processing adjustments in tissue density and contrast. Digital radiography (Figure 3.1) is filmless and provides the final image on a computer screen.

There are two general types of digital radiography: computed radiography (CR; also known as indirect digital radiography) and direct digital radiography (DDR).

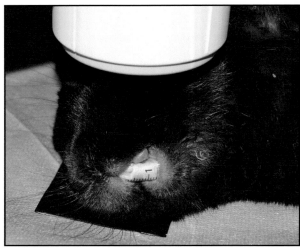

3.1 Computed digital radiography is commonly used, especially for dental radiography. This rabbit is positioned for a lateral extraoral view of the skull. The open mouth allows evaluation of the occlusal surfaces. A piece of a 2 ml syringe can be cut – approximately 1 cm in length – so that it fits between the incisors.

Factors that vary amongst digital systems include the efficiency of the detector for identifying incident X-ray protons, dynamic range, spatial resolution, noise and contrast resolution.

When evaluating the image quality of a system, the matrix size of the digital image (pixel limited resolution), spatial resolution (the smallest line pairs that can be seen as separate structures) and image depth (the number of shades of grey that can be displayed) should be considered. The designation for a digital image indicates the matrix size and image depth. Based on the above factors, the recommended parameters for images of rabbit patients are:

* >5 megapixels
* >22 line pairs per mm (22 LP/mm = 1100 dpi)
* >12-bits of greyscale (12-bit = 4096; 16-bit = 65,536 shades of grey).

The computer hardware includes a user computer workstation with professional medical monochromatic monitors, which can display 3061 unique shades of grey. Post-processing image software may vary between companies and includes various tools that can be used to enhance the final images and allow optimal interpretation.

Digital Imaging and Communications in Medicine (DICOM) radiographic images contain information about the patient as well as about the equipment used to produce the image embedded within the file. The image can never be separated from this information by mistake.

Conventional *versus* digital radiography

Conventional film–screen radiography has many limitations compared with digital radiography. However, in rabbit medicine, mammography films for thoracic and abdominal radiography still provide better detail than most digital systems, although post-processing adjustments are not possible. Use of dental radiography and new CR systems (e.g. CR-7 Vet Automatic Image Plate Scanner) is very promising due to the optimal radiographic images obtained of the rabbit skull, teeth and appendicular skeleton.

Radiation safety rules

Radiation safety rules should be established and all individuals involved in diagnostic imaging should be closely monitored for any possible exposure. If there is a need to use manual restraint, risk assessments and appropriate protective equipment (e.g. aprons, gloves) should be agreed in advance with the practice's Radiological Protection Advisor. **No part of the human body, even wearing protective equipment, should be placed within the primary beam.** A chart or book of suitable exposure times for the machine that is used should be available, to ensure that these are kept to a minimum and repeated exposures due to incorrect technique are avoided.

Patient restraint

Restraint of the conscious rabbit requires practice and can be useful in selected situations (see Chapter 14 and Appendix 4) although optimal positioning is not always possible due to patient activity. In the author's opinion, anaesthesia or sedation should be used for restraint whenever possible. Sandbags, sponges, tapes or other restraining devices for patient positioning can be used. Sedation and anaesthesia for radiographic procedures is discussed in Chapter 1.

Patient positioning

Manipulating the position of the patient and the radiographic beam to improve visualization of lesions and abnormalities can maximize the diagnostic information obtained. In general, when determining patient position, the lesion should be placed as close as possible to the X-ray film to minimize the lesion-to-film distance and blurred contours caused by magnification. However, the reverse applies if the lesion is located within the lungs because the dependent lobes are poorly aerated and lesions might therefore be overlooked. Radiography of the whole body is not generally recommended due to the differences in radiographic settings required to obtain optimal images of the skull, thorax and abdomen.

The appropriate cassette, film and/or sensor size should be selected for the examination and properly positioned. No artefacts or foreign objects should hamper visualization of the normal and abnormal anatomical structures. Positioning aids should be radiotransparent. Endotracheal tubes can interfere with the structures being imaged, particularly on dorsoventral (DV) or ventrodorsal (VD) views of the skull or thoracic cavity, so it may be preferable to perform radiography following patient sedation but prior to intubation.

Skull radiography

Ideally, radiography of the head should be performed in all cases of suspected dental or skull disease. An understanding of the anatomy of the skull and teeth is crucial (see Chapters 4 and 24). Radiographs should be obtained with the rabbit under general anaesthesia because even slight changes in positioning can cause severe anatomical distortion on the image and thus misinterpretation. Oxygenation is required throughout the procedure. If a facial mass is present, cotton wool or a foam wedge should be used for positioning.

Conventional DV, right lateral, two lateral oblique and rostrocaudal views are usually obtained. Digital dental radiographs are particularly useful when evaluating dental disease. In the author's experience, a combination of intraoral and extraoral views is preferable as this allows interpretation of even subtle pathological changes. Placing the patient in dorsal recumbency to obtain a VD view can impair respiration and rabbits should be returned to sternal recumbency as soon as possible.

The tympanic bullae, temporomandibular joint and teeth can be assessed by positioning the head at an angle. The tympanic bullae are best examined using DV and left and right 40 degree lateral oblique views. The temporomandibular joint is best visualized using a 90 degree rostrocaudal view. Left lateral, DV and VD views allow evaluation of the relationship between the mandible and skull, and examination of the integrity of the margins of the mandibular and maxillary bones. The anatomical structures that can be seen on different views are summarized in Figure 3.2. Complete symmetry on the final radiograph indicates optimal positioning.

Dorsoventral and ventrodorsal views

For a DV view, the rabbit is placed in sternal recumbency with its mandible resting on the cassette or sensor (Figure 3.3). The position of the head is maintained by using a bandage placed over the

Radiographic view	Anatomical structures that can be examined
Dorsoventral (DV)	Skull (shape, opacity, fractures); tympanic bullae; mandibular premolars and molars; periodontal space of the maxillary second molar; relationship between the skull and mandible
Ventrodorsal (VD)	As for dorsoventral view, but better for nasal cavity; recommended in cases of mandibular abscesses
Lateral	Skull (shape, opacity, fractures); relationship between the skull and mandible; incisors, premolars and molars (apical and occlusal surfaces, tooth length, shape and curvature, fractures, resorptive lesions); nasolacrimal duct (better with contrast studies); hyoid bone (calcification)
Lateral oblique	Tympanic bulla; mandibular rami; incisors, premolars and molars (apices and reserve crown)
Rostrocaudal	Temporomandibular joint; incisors; premolars and molars (apical and occlusal surfaces); nasal cavity

3.2 Skull radiography: anatomical structures seen on different views.

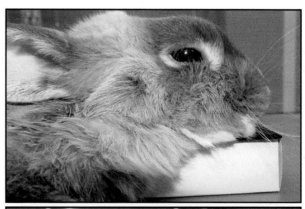

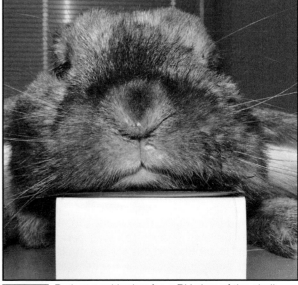

3.3 Patient positioning for a DV view of the skull. The rabbit is positioned on the X-ray film and a small box is placed below the mandible to support the head. The patient position can be evaluated from the front, where an imaginary medial head line should be perpendicular to the table.

dorsal cervical region. Alternatively, a small box can be placed below the mandible to support the head. The pinnae need to be positioned away from the area of interest. The forelimbs are taped cranially or left without fixation. Exact positioning is achieved by gentle manipulation of the head to ensure that the interdental incisor space, nasal philtrum and the middle of the area between the eyes are in a straight line. The X-ray beam is centred on the middle of the imaginary connecting line between the medial canthus of each eye. Complete symmetry on the final radiograph indicates optimal positioning.

A VD view is obtained with the patient in dorsal recumbency. The head is extended and either taped or held in place using a bandage. The ventral margins of the mandible should be parallel with the cassette. Symmetry between the left and right side of the head should always be evaluated. The X-ray beam is centred on the middle of the imaginary connecting line between the medial canthus of each eye. If the rostral part of the nasal cavity or the maxillary incisors and premolars need to evaluated, the mandible is gently displaced laterally to allow visualization.

Rostrocaudal view
For a rostrocaudal view, the rabbit is placed in dorsal recumbency with the head positioned so that the nose is pointing upwards and the long axis of the head is perpendicular to the X-ray film (Figure 3.4). The rabbit can be placed in a trough. The forelimbs are positioned parallel to the thorax and the head is supported with a foam wedge or bandage. The mouth is closed (an open mouth view does not provide any additional information about the teeth, tympanic bullae or other bony structures). The X-ray beam is centred in the middle of the imaginary connecting line between the medial canthus of each eye.

Lateral view
For a lateral view, the rabbit is placed in either left or right lateral recumbency, depending on the localization of the lesion. If the rabbit is undergoing screening for dental pathology, the right lateral position is recommended as a standard view. Cotton wool or a foam wedge is used to support the nose and head in a position where the nasal philtrum is parallel to the X-ray film and the rami of the mandible, tympanic bullae, incisors and all other bilateral anatomical structures are superimposed. The pinnae and forelimbs are left in a normal position or taped away from the skull to prevent superimposition. The occlusal surface of the premolars and molars can be assessed by opening the mouth slightly using a plastic syringe (see Figure 3.1) or a bandage. The X-ray beam is centred on the medial canthus of the eye. Exact superimposition of the tympanic bullae and mandibles on the final radiograph indicates optimal positioning.

Lateral oblique view
For a lateral oblique view, the rabbit is placed in either left or right lateral recumbency, depending on

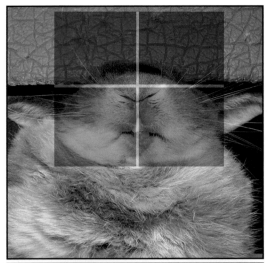
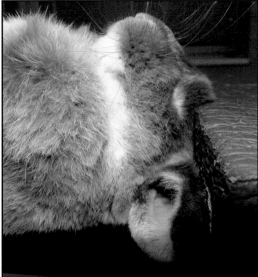

3.4 Patient positioning for a rostrocaudal view of the skull. The rabbit is placed in dorsal recumbency with its nostrils pointing upwards. The head is supported with a foam wedge. The X-ray beam should be centred on the middle of the imaginary connecting line between the medial canthus of each eye.

the part of the head under examination. The mouth is closed or held open either with a syringe inserted between the incisors or with a bandage. A foam wedge is placed under the mandible to elevate the nose slightly and rotate the head at a 30–40 degree angle; alternatively, the X-ray tube can be adjusted to the desired angle (Figures 3.5 and 3.6). To minimize image distortion, the rotation should not be excessive. The X-ray beam is centred on the medial canthus of the eye.

Dental radiography
Digital radiography has advantages compared with conventional radiography because of the enhanced image resolution and detail. Small dental films or digital sensors (20 x 30 mm; 20 x 40 mm; 27 x 54 mm) can be used for intraoral radiography. The use of specialized rabbit and rodent intraoral plates is recommended for mandibular cheek teeth. Larger

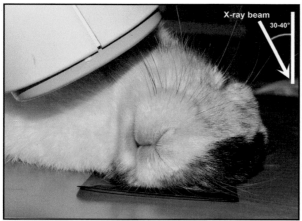

3.5 Patient positioning for a lateral oblique view of the skull. The rabbit is placed in lateral recumbency; the mouth may be closed or held open. The X-ray tube is then adjusted through a 20–40 degree angle.

films (30 x 40 mm; 57 x 76 mm) are used for extraoral radiography. Correct film placement within the oral cavity is difficult in rabbits that weigh <1 kg. However, with the use of small films or specialized rabbit intraoral sensors, as well as additional views, it is possible to evaluate all incisors, premolars and molars precisely, even in small patients.

Intraoral views

Parallel technique: The parallel technique, which is performed with the rabbit in lateral recumbency, requires that the film and long axis of the tooth are parallel to each other and that the X-ray beam is directed perpendicular to the X-ray sensor. This technique can be used for assessment of the occlusal surface of the maxillary and mandibular premolars and molars (Figure 3.7). It is also possible to evaluate the whole crown of the mandibular molars.

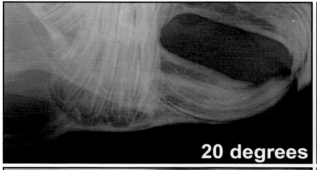

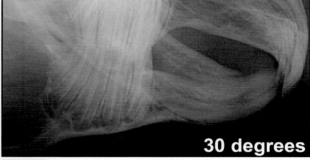

3.6 Lateral oblique views of the left mandible of the rabbit in Figure 3.5. Note that in the 40 degree view a larger part of the premolar and molar reserve crowns can be seen compared with the 20 degree view.

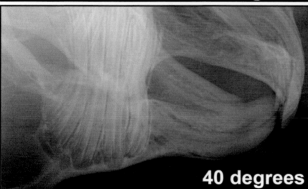

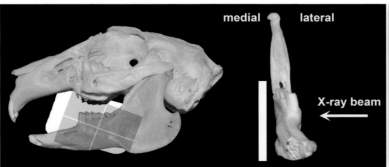

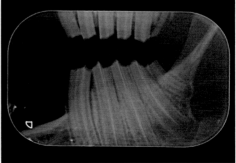

3.7 Intraoral dental radiograph of the left mandibular arcade obtained using the parallel technique. All the tooth structures and the alveolar bone are visible in high detail. The last two molars were examined. For a detailed examination of the premolar apices, the film would need to be slightly repositioned. (Indirect digital radiography; film size = 20 x 30 mm; scanner = Durr CR 7 VET)

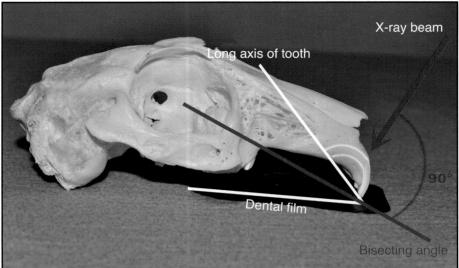

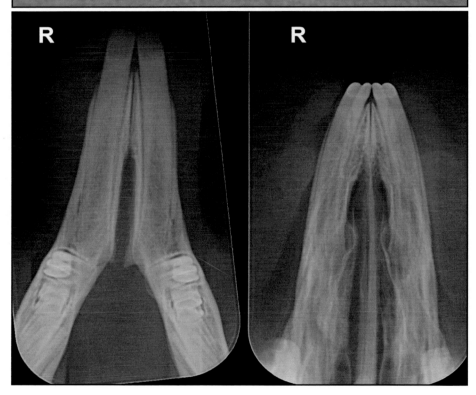

3.8 Intraoral dental radiographs of the mandibular incisors (left) and maxillary incisors (right) obtained using the bisecting angle technique. The maxillary peg teeth are missing in this patient. (Indirect digital radiography: film size = 27 x 54 mm; scanner = Durr CR 7 VET)

Bisecting angle technique: A bisecting angle technique can be performed with the rabbit in sternal or lateral recumbency. Only the mandibular incisors can be examined with the patient in dorsal recumbency. The bisecting angle technique overcomes the difficulties of obtaining accurate images of teeth with different shapes and superimposition by surrounding structures (Figure 3.8). In rabbits, it is impossible to place a film parallel to the maxillary incisors, premolars and molars, so the X-ray beam is centred on the area of interest and perpendicular to the bisecting angle (the angle which bisects the angle created by the long axis of the tooth and the sensor). Due to the relatively high curvature of the maxillary incisors and the very long anatomical roots, the final image is foreshortened.

Extraoral views
Extraoral dental radiography can be used for examination of the maxillary premolars and molars. The animal is placed in lateral recumbency with the X-ray sensor positioned just underneath the check teeth. With this technique, conventional left lateral, left lateral oblique and DV views can be obtained.

Thoracic radiography
Patient positioning for thoracic radiography is particularly important because any errors that occur cannot be subsequently corrected. Although some rabbits permit a complete radiographic study of the thorax with minimal restraint, many require sedation or anaesthesia. Sedation with benzodiazepines is recommended to alleviate anxiety and fear. Heavy

sedation or general anaesthesia may result in pulmonary or cardiac artefacts (e.g. congestion of the pulmonary parenchyma and partial atelectasis of the lung closest to the cassette).

Thoracic radiographs should be taken using a high kVp and low mA to maximize the latitude of contrast and to allow the examiner to identify vascular, interstitial and bronchial structures. The highest mA and fastest exposure time should be used to minimize respiratory motion artefacts and avoid overexposure. Timing the exposure is important. It is optimal to take the radiograph during the slight pause at the end of full inspiration, as this helps decrease motion-related blurring and increases inherent thoracic contrast due to the increased volume of air. In rabbits in respiratory distress, timing the exposure relative to respiration is difficult. In cases where the rabbit is intubated, radiographs taken during assisted positive pressure inspiration can be helpful in differentiating subtle lung abnormalities. Rabbits with distended abdominal organs should be placed on the X-ray cassette with the thoracic region elevated; however, the thorax should still be parallel to the cassette.

Standard thoracic radiographic examinations include the right lateral, left lateral, DV and VD views. The X-ray beam is centred on the mid-thorax at the level of the cardiac silhouette and collimated to include the entire thoracic cavity. The thoracic inlet to the most caudal part of the caudodorsal lung field, including the whole diaphragm, should be visible in the field of view. The field of view should be enlarged to the second or third lumbar vertebra if all 12 ribs are to be evaluated. The cervical portion of the trachea can also be included in the field of view, or a separate radiograph of the cervical region can be obtained. In a radiograph taken at peak inspiration, the caudodorsal aspect of the lung is caudal to the ninth thoracic vertebra. Separation of the cardiac silhouette from the diaphragm is not commonly seen due to the fat localized in this region.

Dorsoventral and ventrodorsal views

Significant respiratory compromise may occur if a rabbit is placed in dorsal recumbency when the stomach or caecum is greatly distended, so a DV view (Figure 3.9) is preferred. A VD view is indicated for evaluation of the cranial mediastinum, lungs,

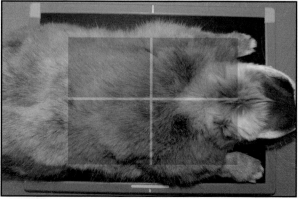

3.9 Patient positioning for a DV view of the thorax. The X-ray beam is centred on the area of interest.

caudal vena cava and for cases of pleural effusion. The DV view is the standard view for most accurate assessment of the position of the heart (the cardiac apex is in its normal position). The forelimbs and hindlimbs should be gently pulled forward and caudally, respectively, so that the soft tissues of the brachium and scapulae are not superimposed over the cranial thorax. Care should be taken not to twist the legs. The vertebral column should be superimposed on the sternum throughout the entire length of the thorax. It should be in a straight line and the ribs should be symmetrical in shape and position.

Lateral view

When a left or right (Figure 3.10) lateral radiograph is described, the terminology refers to the recumbent position of the patient. Selecting the appropriate patient position depends on the location of the expected pathology. Conscious rabbits may respond to restraint by arching the spine, which results in thoracic misalignment. The vertebral column and sternum should be parallel with the cassette or table. The forelimbs and hindlimbs should be pulled slightly cranially and caudally, respectively. Care must be taken to ensure that they are parallel, in order to avoid rotation of the thorax or spine.

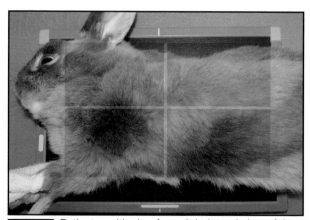

3.10 Patient positioning for a right lateral view of the thorax. The X-ray beam is centred on the area of interest.

If auscultation reveals abnormalities in a particular thoracic quadrant, the patient should be positioned so that the normal side is closer to the X-ray film. When the rabbit is in lateral recumbency, the lung parenchyma closest to the cassette cannot inflate completely, due to compression by the structures above it, which results in suboptimal lung contrast as a result of the relative lung collapse and decreased parenchymal inflation. If no abnormalities are detected or the thorax is being examined for suspected pulmonary lesions, both left and right lateral views should be obtained to avoid making a false negative diagnosis and to assess any subtle pathological changes. The cardiac silhouette is typically more oval and relatively smaller on right lateral views than on left lateral views.

In addition to changing the position of the patient, the vertical X-ray beam can be oriented horizontally with the patient in a standing position in cases of pleural effusion. Other radiographic views of the thorax that can be helpful include lateral oblique views to evaluate the ribs, mediastinal or pleural abnormalities.

Evaluation

Thoracic radiographs can be challenging to evaluate and easy to over-interpret. The thoracic cavity is small compared with the abdominal cavity and large amounts of intrathoracic fat are often present. The thymus is located within the cranial mediastinum and persists throughout the life of the rabbit. The cranial lung lobes are small and commonly superimposed by mediastinal fat. The caudal lung lobes have pronounced vasculature. The cranial border of the heart, which is located between the second/third and fifth/sixth intercostal spaces, is less distinct due to the presence of the thymus. Cardiac size is evaluated based on vertebral heart score. The interpretation of thoracic radiographs is described in detail in Chapter 5.

Abdominal radiography

Standard abdominal radiographic examinations include VD and right lateral views. For a VD view, the thorax of the rabbit can be placed in an adjustable trough, with the forelimbs fixed cranially and the hindlimbs taped caudally to achieve a proper midline/lateral position and to avoid superimposition of the soft tissues over the caudal abdomen. In some cases (large rabbits or thin animals), a foam wedge should be placed under the sternum to avoid axial rotation. The X-ray beam is centred on the mid-abdomen, and the caudal thorax and the whole of the pelvis should be included in the field of view. The entire abdomen, ventral, dorsal and lateral soft tissue margins, including the gluteal musculature and perianal region, should be visible on the radiograph. When evaluating a radiograph for symmetry, the position of the spine and pelvis can be used to determine whether the abdomen was straight or at an oblique angle.

Evaluation

The stomach is usually clearly visible because it contains ingesta, hair and small amounts of gas. Loops of small intestine may also be seen, due to the liquid nature of their contents. The largest organ in the abdomen is the caecum, which should be filled with ingesta. Rounded faecal pellets are often visible in the rectum or distal colon. The ventral margin of the liver may be identified in the region of the xyphoid cartilage. The spleen is small and not visible. The urinary bladder is usually obvious, especially when it is distended with urine or filled with sediment, which is radiopaque. The uterus is located between the colon and the urinary bladder. The bean-shaped kidneys are approximately 30 x 20 x 10 mm and located within the retroperitoneal space. The kidneys are embedded in adipose tissue in the region of T11–T13 (right kidney) or L2–L4 (left kidney). The renal pelvis and renal processes do not exceed 2–4 mm in diameter. The ureters are not visible unless there is

pathology. Other retroperitoneal organs include the adrenal glands, aorta, caudal vena cave, lymphatic vessels and loose connective tissue. Artefacts that can affect abdominal radiographs include shadows caused by nipples, skin folds, wet and dirty hair, and subcutaneous fluid and air.

Limb radiography

Scapula

For a mediolateral view, the patient is placed in lateral recumbency with the affected forelimb closest to the X-ray film. The affected limb is extended cranially and traction is applied. The head, neck and contralateral forelimb are flexed and pulled away from the region of interest to prevent superimposition. The X-ray beam is centred on the neck of the scapula.

For a caudocranial view, the rabbit is placed in dorsal recumbency with the forelimb extended cranially and secured in position with sandbags and a bandage. The forelimb to be examined can be abducted slightly from the body of the patient. The X-ray beam is centred on the scapula.

Shoulder joint

For mediolateral and caudocranial views, the patient is placed in lateral recumbency (as for radiographic assessment of the scapula). The X-ray beam is centred on the shoulder joint.

Humerus

For a mediolateral view, the patient is placed in lateral recumbency with the affected forelimb extended cranially and traction is applied. The head, neck and contralateral forelimb are flexed and pulled away from the region of interest to prevent superimposition.

For a craniocaudal view, the patient is placed in dorsal recumbency with the affected forelimb extended caudally so that the humerus is parallel with the table. The X-ray beam is centred to the middle of the diaphysis. It should be noted that an image magnification is caused by the greater object-to-film distance. A caudocranial view can be obtained using a horizontal X-ray beam, but is not commonly used.

Elbow joint

For a mediolateral view, the patient is placed in lateral recumbency with the forelimb either extended (120 degrees), flexed (90 degrees) or maximally flexed. The X-ray beam is centred on the medial epicondyle.

For a craniocaudal view, the patient is placed in sternal recumbency with the affected forelimb pulled cranially (Figure 3.11). The antebrachium is positioned parallel to the table. Taping the elbow joint in place may prevent rotation. The head is elevated and retracted away from the affected limb. The X-ray beam is directed distoproximally at a 10–20 degree angle and is centred on the medial epicondyle.

Other special views that can be used to evaluate the anconeal process and humeral condyles include extended supinated mediolateral, craniolateral–caudomedial oblique, craniomedial–caudolateral oblique and distomedial–proximolateral oblique views.

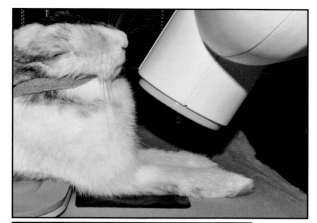

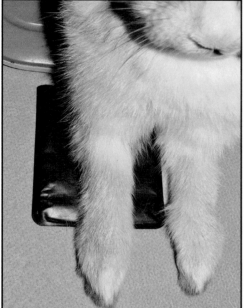

3.11 Patient positioning for a craniocaudal view of the elbow joint. The head is elevated and retracted away from the affected limb. The X-ray beam is directed distoproximally at a 10–20 degree angle and is centred on the medial epicondyle.

Antebrachium

For a lateral view, the patient is placed in lateral recumbency with the forelimb extended and the carpus slightly flexed to prevent supination. The head, neck and contralateral forelimb are flexed and pulled away from the region of interest to prevent superimposition.

For a craniocaudal view, the patient is placed in sternal recumbency with the affected forelimb pulled as cranially as possible and taped in place. A sandbag or other positioning aid is used to support the caudal part of the elbow. The X-ray beam is centred to the middle of the antebrachium.

Carpus, metacarpus and digits

For a lateral view, the patient is placed in lateral recumbency with the affected forelimb closest to the X-ray film. The carpus is hyperflexed, slightly flexed (90 degrees) or extended. For an accurate evaluation of the digits, each individual digit should be taped in a different place to avoid superimposition.

For a dorsopalmar view, the patient is placed in sternal recumbency with the affected forelimb extended cranially and fixed in place, so that the carpus, metacarpus and all digits are parallel with the X-ray film (Figure 3.12). If the claws are long, it is recommended that they are trimmed before the procedure. It is advisable to tape the digits in place. The X-ray beam is centred on the region of interest.

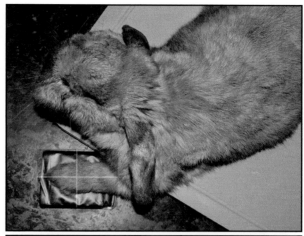

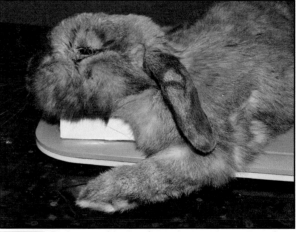

3.12 Patient positioning for a dorsopalmar view of the metacarpus and digits. The rabbit is in sternal recumbency with the elbow joint positioned ventral to the body, allowing the carpus, metacarpus and digits to be parallel with the cassette without any anatomical distortion.

Pelvis and hip

For a lateral view, the patient is placed in left lateral recumbency with the left hindlimb positioned slightly caudal to the right hindlimb. An optimal view is obtained when a sandbag or sponge is placed between the stifle joints to achieve proper positioning. The X-ray beam is centred on the hip joint.

For a VD view (Figure 3.13), the patient is placed in dorsal recumbency with both pelvic limbs extended caudally and taped tightly with gauze, in a similar manner to evaluating hip dysplasia in dogs. The X-ray beam is centred on the midpoint of an imaginary line between the hip bones.

A mediolateral view is recommended for the assessment of a single hip joint. The patient is

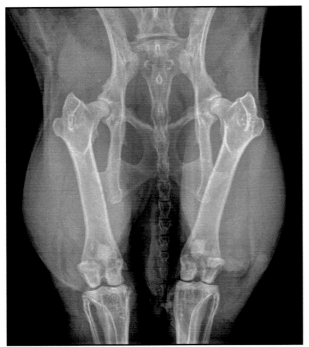

3.13 VD view of the pelvis with craniocaudal view of both femurs.

placed in lateral recumbency with the affected limb closest to the X-ray film. The contralateral limb is retracted away and the X-ray beam is centred on the affected hip joint.

Other views of possible diagnostic value for the evaluation of hip joints in rabbits include: VD view with flexed limbs ('frog leg' view); VD view with the hindlimbs flexed (distraction view); and VD view with limbs extended (fulcrum position). Patient positioning for these views is described in radiographic texts for dogs and cats (see *BSAVA Manual of Canine and Feline Musculoskeletal Imaging*).

Femur

For a lateral view, the patient is placed in lateral recumbency with the affected limb extended and taped in position. The contralateral limb is retracted away to prevent superimposition. The X-ray beam is centred on the middle of the femoral diaphysis. Both proximal and distal joints should be included in the final radiograph.

For a craniocaudal view, the patient is placed in dorsal recumbency (as described for radiographic assessment of the pelvis). Correct positioning is ensured by taping the leg or tying the leg with gauze. The X-ray beam is centred to the middle of the femur diaphysis.

Stifle

For a lateral view, the patient is placed in lateral recumbency with the affected knee joint closest to the X-ray film. The contralateral limb is retracted away to prevent superimposition.

For a caudocranial view, the patient is placed in sternal recumbency with both legs extended caudally and individually fixed using an elastic bandage

or tape. The X-ray beam is centred on the knee joint. The optimal position of the femorotibial joint is with the midline of the patella within the femoral trochlear groove, which is superimposed on the femoral long axis and aligned with the trochlear notch. The medial and lateral femoral condyles should be symmetrical to the femoral long axis and the fibulotibial joint space clearly outlined.

Tibia, fibula, tarsus, metatarsus and digits

For a mediolateral view, the patient is placed in lateral recumbency with the affected limb closest to the X-ray film. The tarsus can be hyperflexed, slightly flexed (90 degrees) or extended. For an accurate evaluation of the digits, each individual digit should be taped in a different place to avoid superimposition (Figure 3.14).

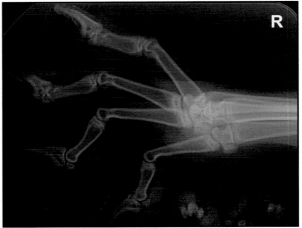

3.14 Mediolateral view of the right hind paw of a rabbit. The image is achieved by taping each individual digit in a different position. The rounded opacities are soil particles embedded in the rabbit's fur and the radiodense lines at the bottom of the image are produced by the tape. (Indirect digital radiography: film size = 57 x 76 mm; scanner = Durr CR 7 VET)

For a plantodorsal view, the patient is placed in sternal recumbency (Figure 3.15) in the same manner as for assessment of the stifle. The X-ray beam is centred on the region of interest.

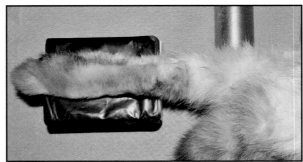

3.15 Patient positioning for a plantodorsal view of the right metatarsus. The rabbit is placed in sternal recumbency with both legs extended caudally. Each leg can be fixed in position using an elastic bandage or tape. The lateral aspect of the stifle needs to be supported to stabilize the leg. The X-ray beam is centred on the area of interest.

Contrast studies

The use of contrast media enhances or allows visualization of organs surrounded by tissue of the same radiopacity, providing information about the size, shape and position of a particular organ and surrounding tissues.

Contrast media

In general, there are two categories of contrast agents.

Positive contrast media

Positive contrast media are more radiopaque than the surrounding organs or tissues.

The most commonly used contrast medium for evaluation of the gastrointestinal tract is barium sulphate, which is an insoluble and inert medium that is not absorbed by the gastrointestinal mucosa. Barium sulphate is commercially available as a suspension paste or powder or as barium-impregnated spheres. Barium sulphate paste allows examination of the oesophageal wall, whereas the suspension allows evaluation of the stomach, intestine, caecum and colon. Due to its chemical properties, barium sulphate can induce granulomatous inflammation when inspired or introduced into the thoracic or abdominal cavities as a result of leakage through a perforation in the gastrointestinal wall. In rabbits, fine particulate matter is selectively moved into the caecum by motility of the hindgut, which can cause problems if large amounts of barium are used, caecal motility is reduced or the rabbit is dehydrated. Caecal impaction can also occur.

Organic iodine positive contrast media are used for the evaluation of numerous organ systems. In clinical veterinary practice, radiographic contrast studies in rabbits are performed to visualize the urogenital system, vertebral column, nasolacrimal duct, ear canal, joints, fistulae and cardiovascular system. Non-ionic water-soluble agents (e.g. iohexol, iopamidol and iomeprol) are used in these studies. Agents with low osmolality and low viscosity (e.g. iomeprol) are preferred for myelography.

Calcium salts are radiopaque and can act as a natural contrast medium in rabbits. Calcium is excreted into the urine and can outline the bladder. Dystrophic mineralization can reveal areas of degenerative tissue and ectopic mineralization can outline organs such as the aorta (see Chapter 5).

Negative contrast media

Negative contrast media (i.e. air, oxygen, carbon dioxide) are radiolucent and commonly used in other species for evaluation of the stomach and urinary bladder. Optimal tissue contrast and mucosal detail are achieved when negative contrast media are used together with a small amount of a positive contrast medium. Negative contrast studies are not often performed in rabbits, although the gas that is naturally produced in the gastrointestinal tract can be of value in outlining the stomach and/or intestines (see Chapters 7 and 14).

Views

There are numerous radiographic studies performed in rabbits which involve the use of contrast media. The most commonly used are described below. The indications, contraindications and side effects of these studies are summarized in Figure 3.16.

Radiographic study	Indications	Contraindications	Possible adverse effects
Excretory urography	Urinary system morphology; assessment of obstructed urinary flow; dysuria; haematuria; abnormal biochemical parameters (urea, creatinine, phosphorus); suspected bladder herniation	Oliguria; dehydration	Hypotension
Dacryocystography	Epiphora; facial mass in the orbital or nasal area		Possible inhalation of the contrast medium (mostly non-significant)
Gastrointestinal tract contrast study	Unidentified abdominal masses; suspected intramural/extramural gastrointestinal tract stenosis; assessment of gastrointestinal tract position; herniation; evaluation of gastric mucosa	Mechanical obstruction; gastrointestinal tract wall perforation; dehydration; respiratory distress	Obstipation by retention of contrast medium in the caecum
Canalography	External ear canal stenosis; impossible to perform endo-otoscopy		Possible inhalation of the contrast medium through the Eustachian tube
Myelography	Confirmation, exact localization and degree of compression of spinal and other neural structures within the vertebral column	Neural inflammation	Seizures and collapse (associated with cerebellomedullary cistern puncture); spinal cord puncture; subdural contrast medium administration; epidural contrast medium leakage

3.16 Indications, contraindications and possible adverse effects for particular radiographic contrast studies.

Excretory urography

Survey radiography sometimes provides insufficient information with regard to upper urinary tract disorders. The kidneys are usually well visualized because of the presence of large amounts of adipose tissue, but the ureters are not normally seen. Intravenous pyelography is a minimally invasive procedure used to define anatomical structures and make qualitative assessments of kidney function by outlining the collecting system. The resultant images provide valuable and detailed information about the size, shape and position of the kidneys as well as the density of the parenchyma. The size, shape and position of the ureters can also be evaluated.

Indications

Indications for intravenous pyelography include a wide variety of disorders, such as haematuria, polyuria, abdominal pain, gait disorders, suspected obstruction of the urinary tract, traumatic abdominal injury and rupture or pathological termination of the urinary tract. Intravenous pyelography can also be performed with fluoroscopy (i.e. a radiograph is converted into a real-time video image).

Considerations

Intravenous pyelography can be affected by the hydration status, glomerular filtration rate and renal concentrating ability of the patient. The contrast material used in the procedure can affect urinalysis by increasing the specific gravity, altering cellular morphology and creating unusual crystals. Thus, urinalysis as well as urinary tract ultrasonography and urinary culture should be performed prior to contrast medium administration. The rabbit should be well hydrated before the procedure. If a patient presents with oliguria or anuria due to low urine flow, the administration of contrast medium is not recommended. Fluids should be administered intravenously and subcutaneously following the procedure to maintain diuresis and the patient closely monitored. Oxygenation is also recommended.

Patient preparation

In dogs, it is recommended to evacuate the colon using laxatives. Laxatives are not recommended for rabbits, due to their herbivorous nature and specific digestive physiology; however, withholding food for 2 hours prior to the imaging study can be of benefit. Based on the author's experience, if a rabbit is kept outside, it should be moved indoors at least a day before the examination to prevent it from eating grass with radiopaque soil or feeding from the ground surface. The kidney function of the patient should be evaluated and the rabbit should be well hydrated. A bolus of crystalloids should be administered prior to the contrast medium to reduce the risk of adverse kidney effects.

Procedure

A bolus of iodinated contrast medium (iohexol, iomeprol: 300–400 mg iodine/ml; 600–1200 mg/kg) should be administered intravenously or intraosseously. Immediately following contrast medium administration, VD and right lateral radiographs should be taken. As the contrast material is processed by the kidneys, a series of images should be obtained to determine the actual size of the kidneys and evaluate the collecting system as it begins to empty. Particular views should be repeated at 1, 5, 10 and 15 minutes following contrast medium administration. In cases of kidney failure, the amount of contrast medium administered should be increased to ensure adequate visualization. In addition, a pneumocystogram can also be performed to allow better visualization of the ureters and bladder.

Evaluation

The excretory urogram can be divided into two phases:

* Nephrogram – opacification of the functional renal parenchyma
* Pyelogram – opacification of the renal pelvis, pelvic recesses and ureters.

These phases should be evaluated separately. Kidney, pelvis and ureteral lumen measurements are determined on right lateral and VD views (Figure 3.17). Good visualization of the kidneys depends on the presence of retroperitoneal fat surrounding them. The kidney should appear homogenous but,

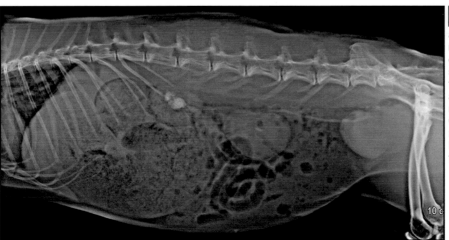

3.17 Right lateral view of the pyelographic phase of an excretory urogram taken 5 minutes after the administration of contrast medium. Renal opacity is still visible, which indicates a functional problem. The kidneys are of different sizes and there are nephroliths within the right kidney. Only the left ureter is visible. The radiopaque areas dorsal to the bladder represent regions of fatty tissue calcification.

on rare occasions, the cortex may be more radiopaque than the medulla in the initial radiographs. The normal kidney should be radiopaque within 10–60 seconds following contrast medium administration. Renal function is evaluated by the degree of opacification and fading patterns. The pyelogram of a normal functioning kidney is more radiopaque than the pyelogram of a diseased organ. The time taken for contrast medium to appear in the renal pelvis, ureters and urinary bladder varies, but in general the ureters should be visible within 5–10 minutes following administration. The ureters are seen as two radiopaque lines parallel with the vertebral column. The diameter of the ureteral lumen can vary with peristaltic movement, but should not exceed 2 mm in size.

Abnormal findings on intravenous pyelography relate to changes in the number, topographical location, size, shape and structure of the kidneys and ureters, and whether they empty into an abnormal region. Chronic kidney disease can be seen as changes in the size of the kidney, diffuse parenchymal opacity and size of the renal pelvis and its recesses. Focal opacification can be caused by cysts, hydronephrosis and granulomas. Hydronephrosis is characterized by dilation of the renal pelvis, renal diverticula and, on occasion, ureteral dilation. In rabbits, uroliths are generally radiopaque; however, small uroliths may not be visible and can cause ureteral obstruction. Ectopic ureters are rare in rabbits.

Dacryocystography

Contrast examination of the nasolacrimal duct is easy to perform and can reveal the degree of distension of the duct and localize the site of an obstruction (usually extraluminal). Complete clinical, intraoral and ophthalmological examinations, including cytological and/or bacteriological testing if necessary, should be performed prior to the procedure. Nasolacrimal duct flushing should precede dacryocystography.

Procedure

General anaesthesia, with the use of systemic and local analgesics (see Chapter 2), is recommended for the initial examination and irrigation of the nasolacrimal duct. For dacryocystography, the patient is placed in lateral recumbency with the affected side uppermost to facilitate contrast medium administration. The rabbit should be placed on the X-ray cassette, with its head fixed in position, prior to initiating the procedure. Dacryocystography is performed using 0.5–1 ml of iodine contrast medium (iohexol, iomeprol: 300–400 mg iodine/ml). The concentrated solution results in better final images than diluted preparations. Gentle pressure only should be applied during nasolacrimal duct irrigation. There is a risk of nasolacrimal duct rupture if high pressure is applied during the procedure (see Chapter 28). Based on the author's experience, initial administration of a small amount of contrast medium (0.3–0.5 ml) is recommended to prevent inhalation and superimposition within the nasolacrimal duct. Right lateral (Figure 3.18) and DV radiographs

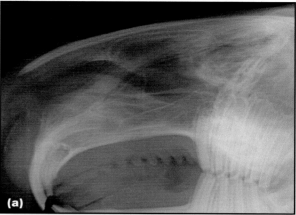

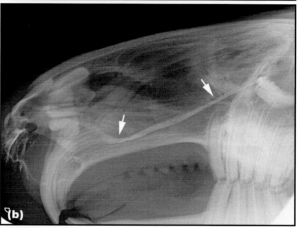

3.18 **(a)** Pre-contrast and **(b)** post-contrast right lateral radiographs of the normal nasolacrimal duct in a rabbit. The arrows indicate the tortuous route of the contrast medium. A small amount of the contrast medium (iomeprol) can be seen in the nasal cavity.

should be taken immediately. Following the procedure, application of a protective eye gel containing retinol and anti-inflammatory drugs is recommended to protect the superficial eye structures.

Evaluation

Abnormal findings on dacryocystography include partial or complete obstruction of the nasolacrimal duct, duct distension, skull fractures and apical maxillary teeth pathology.

Gastrointestinal tract contrast study

Survey right lateral and VD radiographs should be obtained prior to the contrast study.

Indications

A contrast radiographic study of the gastrointestinal tract is performed in cases where pathology of the oesophagus, stomach, intestines, caecum or colon is suspected. These studies are contraindicated in cases of suspected mechanical obstruction of the gastrointestinal tract or gastrointestinal wall perforation. Gastrointestinal contrast studies are not recommended in patients with ileus, in obvious respiratory distress, or that are severely dehydrated or anaemic.

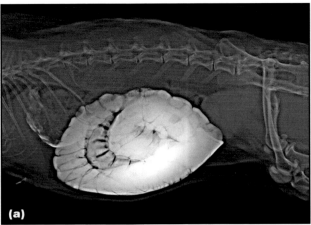
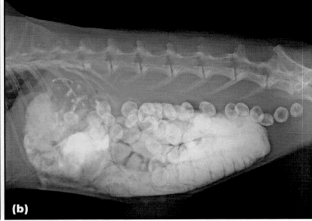

3.19 Lateral radiographs of two rabbits with **(a)** scrotal and **(b)** ventral abdominal herniation. (a) This radiograph was taken 4.5 hours after contrast medium administration. The contrast medium is located mainly in the caecum and proximal colon. (b) This radiograph was taken 5.5 hours after contrast medium administration. The contrast medium is distributed throughout the gastrointestinal tract. No part of the small intestines, caecum or colon is involved within the herniated tissue in either case.

Procedure

As gastrointestinal tract contrast studies are not commonly used for the assessment of gastrointestinal transit time, the use of sedation or short-term anaesthesia is possible. Barium sulphate (10–15 mg/kg of a 30% suspension) is the most commonly used contrast medium for gastrointestinal tract studies. Iopamidol (oral formulation) can also be used to evaluate the gastrointestinal tract without any negative effects associated with leakage or problems with caecal impaction. Contrast media should be administered orally or via a gastric tube. Food should be offered throughout the whole contrast study. Left and right lateral and VD views are recommended for assessment of the gastrointestinal organs. Radiographs should be obtained immediately and then at 15, 30, 60, 120, 240 and 360 minutes following contrast medium administration.

Evaluation

Different parts of the gastrointestinal tract can be evaluated with respect to position, lumen, content and function. Contrast studies can reveal the presence of intraluminal masses and mural or extramural lesions. The gastrointestinal tract can also be displaced by intrathoracic or intra-abdominal masses. Liver lobe masses or liver enlargement often cause caudodorsal displacement of the stomach. If the stomach wall and liver margins are barely visible, contrast gastrography is helpful to confirm liver enlargement, especially when ultrasonographic examination is difficult to achieve. Gastric peristalsis and gastric emptying may also be observed directly during fluoroscopy with the use of positive contrast media.

The normal gastrointestinal tract transit time in rabbits is between 17 and 91 hours, depending on diet composition (especially fibre) and the amount of ingesta present in the tract. Transit time can also be altered by the chemical and physical properties of the ingesta as well as gut motility, patient hydration, medication and the type of contrast agent. The reference range for gastrointestinal emptying time in rabbits is wide, and so interpretation is problematic or almost impossible. Gastric emptying should begin within 15–30 minutes following the administration of barium, although some contrast material may remain in the stomach even after 5–24 hours due to the presence of fur and ingesta. Contrast medium may be seen in the caecum 40 minutes after administration and within 1–3 hours it can be filled. The presence of contrast medium in the colon may be seen 5–12 hours following administration (Figure 3.19).

Canalography

Canalography is a contrast radiographic technique used to examine the ear canal, especially in cases of suspected tympanic membrane perforation. This technique is commonly used when the tympanic membrane cannot be examined using an otoscope or endoscope due to a stricture, or when other imaging methods (e.g. computed tomography (CT) and MRI) are not available. Survey radiographs should be obtained prior to the contrast study (Figure 3.20a).

Procedure

A dose of 1 ml of a non-diluted positive contrast agent (iomeprol) is instilled into the external ear canal and gently massaged to allow the fluid to reach the tympanic membrane. The external ear canal can be plugged with cotton wool to prevent leakage of the contrast media. VD, DV and 40 degree lateral oblique views should be obtained to visualize the tympanic bulla and external ear canal. If the contrast medium reaches the tympanic bulla, the membrane is perforated (Figure 3.20b). If cerumen or pus is present in the external ear canal, it can be gently flushed with saline. False-negative results can be obtained if a large amount of pus is present. The rabbit should be intubated to prevent aspiration of excessive fluid through the ruptured membrane into the pharynx via the Eustachian tube.

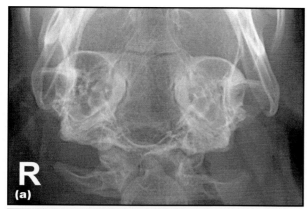

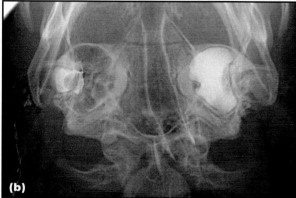

3.20 **(a)** Pre-contrast and **(b)** post-contrast DV radiographs showing the ear canals in a rabbit. The tympanic membrane in the right ear is intact, whereas the left tympanic bulla is completely filled with contrast medium, indicating that the membrane is perforated.

Myelography

Lateral and VD survey radiographs should be taken prior to myelography to ensure proper patient positioning and exposure. Cerebrospinal fluid (CSF) should also be collected before myelography, as contrast agents can alter its composition. CSF sampling is relatively straightforward in rabbits and can be achieved via a cisternal or lumbar subarachnoid puncture (see Technique 3.1). CSF analysis may be useful to investigate a disease process or to make a definitive diagnosis.

Indications

Possible vertebral column disorders that can be identified on radiography and investigated using myelography include vertebral fractures/luxations, congenital vertebral anomalies, vertebral neoplasia, spondylosis and infectious conditions such as discospondylitis (see Chapter 6).

Procedure

The procedure for myelography is described in Technique 3.1.

Evaluation

A list of differential diagnoses can be established based on the myelographic pattern. There are three types of pattern:

- Extradural – attenuation, thinning or deviation of the contrast medium column
- Intradural–extramedullary – golf tee appearance of the contrast medium column
- Intramedullary – circumferential attenuation of the contrast medium column.

Lesions that cause an extradural pattern include vertebral fractures/luxations, extradural haemorrhage, disc protrusion or extrusion with spinal cord compression, epidural infection, vertebral neoplasia and other extradural neoplasia. An intradural–extramedullary pattern is uncommon and typically seen with space-occupying lesions within the subarachnoid space. An intramedullary pattern occurs when the lesion is located within the spinal cord parenchyma. Possible causes include parenchymal inflammation, intramedullary haemorrhage and intramedullary neoplasia.

The advantages of myelography are that it is relatively inexpensive, the entire spinal cord can be evaluated relatively quickly, and it delineates extradural lesions well. The disadvantage is that the anatomy of an individual rabbit may make myelography difficult or even impossible. Possible complications range from transient exacerbation of clinical signs to paralysis and even death. In addition, despite the relatively high sensitivity for localizing a lesion within the vertebral column in rabbits, it is better to use radiography in conjunction with other imaging methods (e.g. magnetic resonance imaging, MRI) to provide optimal information on lateralization of the lesion, the extent and degree of spinal cord compression and the presence of concurrent lesions (see Chapter 9).

Indications for advanced imaging

CT and MRI can provide valuable information about pathological lesions in organs and their surrounding structures. MRI is particularly useful for the evaluation of soft tissue, including the nervous system. CT provides important information about bony structures and is commonly used in cases of odontogenic abscesses (see Chapter 9).

Radiographic interpretation

When viewing radiographs, the reviewer should create a mental three-dimensional (3D) image of the area of interest, so, ideally, a minimum of two orthogonal views should be available for evaluation (Figure 3.21). A successful examination of a radiograph must be systematic in order to ensure that all parts are evaluated (Figure 3.22). X-ray identification (i.e. left *versus* right side labelling) should have been performed during the radiographic exposure, using radiodense markers. The process of radiographic interpretation includes:

- Determination of patient position and whether the examined area has been correctly identified
- Verification of adequate diagnostic imaging quality (radiographic technique, artefacts)

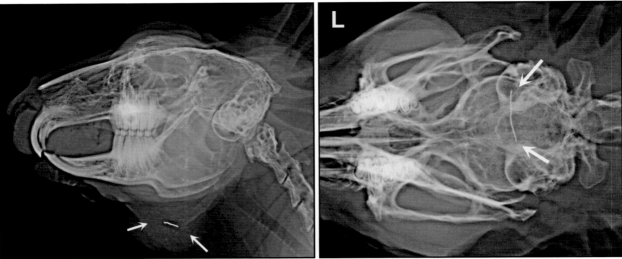

3.21 Lateral and VD radiographs of the head of a rabbit showing swelling of the soft tissues (an abscess) in the ventral mandibular area due to foreign body (wire) penetration (arrowed). The length of the wire on the lateral radiograph measured 1 cm, whereas on the VD radiograph it measured 3.5 cm.

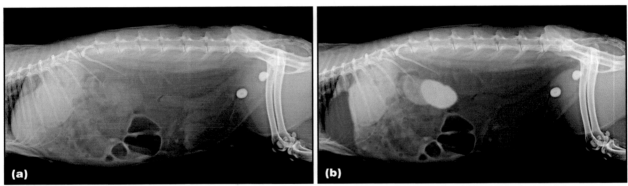

3.22 Right lateral radiograph of the abdomen of a rabbit. All parts of the radiograph should be evaluated to determine whether the features are normal or if there is abnormal pathology. In this case, apart from the obvious urolithiasis (two cystoliths), the uterus is enlarged and the caecum contains gas. The final diagnoses were obesity, cystolithiasis, uterine adenocarcinoma and ileus. The image in **(b)** has been coloured to show the positions of the colon (blue), kidneys (yellow), liver (brown) and uterus (red).

- Thorough evaluation focusing on anatomy and topography (e.g. the physes of different long bones and vertebrae close at different ages; Figure 3.23)
- Description of all abnormalities (e.g. organ position, variation in size, shape and number, changes in radiopacity, alterations in architectural pattern and changes in function)
- Formulation of a list of differential diagnoses ranked in order of likelihood
- A written report with proposed further diagnostic procedures or a treatment plan. This can be included in the patient's record.

Artefacts and pitfalls

A radiographic artefact is a feature in an image that masks or mimics a clinical feature, impairs image quality or obscures an abnormality. Possible artefacts encountered in rabbit imaging are similar to those seen with other companion animals (see Figure 3.14). The most common radiographic pitfalls are associated with exposure factors, collimation inaccuracy and improper patient positioning.

Epiphyseal line	Age at radiographic physeal closure (weeks)
Distal epiphyseal line of the femur	20–23
Proximal epiphyseal line of the tibia	21–32
Distal epiphyseal line of the tibia	20–32
Proximal epiphyseal line of the fibula	23–32
Proximal epiphyseal line of the ulna	17–30
Distal epiphyseal line of the ulna	26–32
Proximal epiphyseal line of the radius	13–19
Distal epiphyseal line of the radius	30–32
Vertebral physes	32–44

3.23 Radiographically apparent physeal closure of selected rabbit bones. (Data from Heikel, 1960; Kaweblum *et al.*, 1994)

References and further reading

Armbrust LJ (2009) Comparing types of digital capture. *Veterinary Clinics of North America: Small Animal Practice* **39**, 677–688

Bischoff MG and Kneller SK (2004) Diagnostic imaging of the canine and feline ear. *Veterinary Clinics of North America: Small Animal Practice* **34**, 437–458

Böhmer E (2005) Radiographic examination in rabbits and rodents (gastrointestinal tract, urinary organs, spinal cord). Part 2: contrast medium radiography of particular organ systems (passage, urography, myelography). *Tierärztliche Praxis Ausgabe Kleintiere Heimtiere* **33**, 207–216

Böhmer E (2010) *Zahnheilkunde bei Kaninchen und Nagern.* Schauttauer, Stuttgart

Boulocher CB, Viguier ER, Da Rocha *et al.* (2010) Radiographic assessment of the femorotibial joint of the CCLT rabbit experimental model of osteoarthritis. *BMC Medical Imaging* **10**, 3–9

Capello V and Lennox AM (2008) *Clinical Radiology of Exotic Companion Mammals.* Blackwell Publishing, Ames, IA

Capello V and Lennox AM (2011) Diagnostic imaging of the respiratory system in exotic companion mammals. *Veterinary Clinics of North America: Exotic Animal Practice* **14**, 369–389

Chitty J (2007) Clinical techniques: the subarachnoid space – its clinical relevance in rabbits. *Journal of Exotic Pet Medicine* **16**, 179–182

Daniel GB (2009) Digital imaging. *Veterinary Clinics of North America: Small Animal Practice* **39**, 667–676

Gracis M (2008) Clinical technique: normal dental radiography of rabbits, guinea pigs and chinchillas. *Journal of Exotic Pet Medicine* **17**, 78–86

Hammond G, Sullivan M, Posthumus J and King A (2010) Assessment of three radiographic projections for detection of fluid in the rabbit tympanic bulla. *Veterinary Radiology & Ultrasound* **51**, 48–51

Harcourt-Brown F (2002) *Textbook of Rabbit Medicine.* Reed Education and Professional Publishing, Oxford

Heikel HA (1960) On ossification and growth of certain bones of the rabbit; with a comparison of the skeletal age in the rabbit and in man. *Acta Orthopedica Scandinavica* **29**, 171–184

Heuter KJ (2005) Excretory urography. *Clinical Techniques in Small Animal Practice* **20**, 39–45

Kaweblum M, Aguilar MC, Blancas E *et al.* (1994) Histological and radiographic determination of the age of physeal closure of the distal femur, proximal tibia, and proximal fibula of the New Zealand white rabbit. *Journal of Orthopedic Research* **12**, 747–749

Knipe MF (2007) Principles of neurological imaging of exotic animal species. *Veterinary Clinics of North America: Exotic Animal Practice* **10**, 893–907

Krautwald-Junghanns M-E, Pees M, Reese S and Tully T (2011) *Diagnostic Imaging of Exotic Pets: Birds, Small Mammals and Reptiles.* Schlütersche, Hannover

Latham C (2005) Practical contrast radiography: 1. Contrast agents. *In Practice* **27**, 348–352

Lennox AM (2008) Clinical technique: small exotic companion mammal dentistry – anesthetic considerations. *Journal of Exotic Pet Medicine* **17**, 102–106

Marini RP, Foltz CJ, Kersten D *et al.* (1996) Microbiologic, radiographic and anatomic study of the nasolacrimal duct apparatus in the rabbit (*Oryctolagus cuniculus*). *Laboratory Animal Science* **46**, 656–662

Morgan JP (1993) *Techniques of Veterinary Radiography, 5th edn.* Iowa State University Press, Ames, IA

Owens JM and Biery DN (1999) *Radiographic Interpretation for the Small Animal Clinician, 2nd edn.* Williams and Williams, Baltimore

Redrobe S (2001) Imaging techniques in small mammals. *Seminars in Avian and Exotic Pet Medicine* **10**,187–197

Thrall DE (2002) *Textbook of Veterinary Diagnostic Radiology, 4th edn.* Elsevier Saunders, Philadelphia

Whittington JK and Bennet RA (2011) Clinical technique: myelography in rabbits. *Journal of Exotic Pet Medicine* **20**, 217–221

Widmer WA (2008) Acquisition hardware for digital imaging. *Veterinary Radiology & Ultrasound* **49**, S2–S8

Wiggs RB and Lobprise HB (1997) *Veterinary Dentistry: Principles and Practice.* Lippincot-Raven, Philadelphia

Wright MA, Balance D, Robertson ID and Poteet B (2008) Introduction to DICOM for the practicing veterinarian. *Veterinary Radiology & Ultrasound* **49**, S14–S18

TECHNIQUE 3.1 →

TECHNIQUE 3.1:
Myelography

Positioning

- Lateral recumbency for cerebrospinal fluid (CSF) collection and cisternal administration of contrast medium. The head of the rabbit should be flexed at 90 degrees to the neck to increase the dorsal exposure of the foramen magnum. Care must be taken not to kink the endotracheal tube.
- For a right-handed person, it is easiest to place the patient in right lateral recumbency with the head to the right. This position facilitates handling and spinal needle manipulation.

Preparation

- General anaesthesia and intravenous access are required.
- Analgesia and fluid therapy should be provided as needed.
- The surgical field should be clipped and prepared aseptically. The use of sterile drapes is recommended.

Assistant

An assistant is not required.

Equipment

- 22–23 G spinal needle
- Contrast medium (e.g. iohexol, iopamidol, iomeprol)
- Extension set with a 1 or 2 ml syringe

Surgical technique

Cisternal puncture

1 Insert a spinal needle into the dorsal midline of the atlanto-occipital region, approximately midway between the external occipital protuberance and the craniodorsal tip of the dorsal spine of the axis, just cranial to the cranial wings of the atlas.

2 Slowly introduce the needle until the subarachnoid space is entered, which may be felt as a sudden loss of resistance or seen as the appearance of CSF within the needle hub after stylet removal.

3 Collect approximately 0.3–1 ml of CSF into a collection tube either passively or using gentle aspiration with a 1 ml syringe.

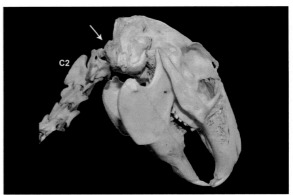

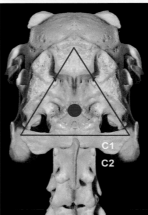

Lateral and dorsal views of cisterna magna puncture in the rabbit. A needle is inserted into the dorsal midline of the atlanto-occipital region (white arrow), approximately in the middle (blue spot) of a triangle connecting the dorsal tip of the occipital protuberance and the lateral wings of the atlas (C1) vertebra. The correct position is located cranial to the craniodorsal tip of the dorsal spine of the axis (C2) vertebra.

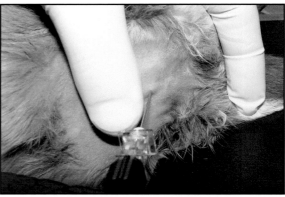

A spinal needle is introduced into the cisterna magna where a slight depression can be palpated.

TECHNIQUE 3.1 continued:
Myelography

Lumbar puncture

1 Gently flex the spine and insert the spinal needle in a cranioventral direction just caudal to the dorsal spinal processes of L6 or L7, where the intervertebral space is relatively wide (see Figure 2.3). Alternatively, the subarachnoid space can be punctured through the spinal canal as rabbits do not have a typical cauda equina. In these cases, slight jerking movements of the hindlimbs may be seen but these are not significant.

2 A slight resistance is felt as the needle passes through the dura and arachnoid mater and enters the subarachnoid space. If excessive resistance is encountered, the needle should be repositioned. CSF is not always visible within the needle hub following stylet removal.

3 Passively collect a small amount of CSF into a collection tube.

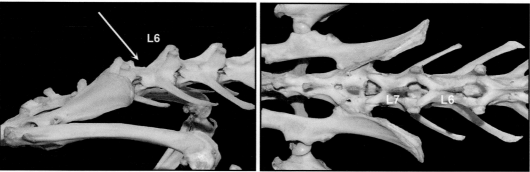

Lateral and dorsal views of lumbar puncture in the rabbit. The needle (white arrow) is inserted in a cranioventral direction just caudal to the dorsal spinal process of L6.

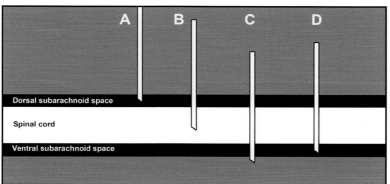

Spinal canal and spinal needle position. **A** = correct position. **B** = spinal cord puncture; the needle should be repositioned dorsally or ventrally. **C** = the needle should be slightly retracted to achieve subarachnoid puncture. **D** = correct position.

Contrast medium administration

Radiography can be used to confirm correct placement of the needle. Fluoroscopy can be used to direct needle placement, confirm subarachnoid contrast medium flow and localize the site of contrast medium administration during injection.

1 Attach an extension set with a syringe filled with contrast medium to the spinal needle to prevent needle dislocation and contrast study failure.

2 Inject non-ionic iodinated contrast medium into the subarachnoid space to delineate the spinal cord and identify any compression or distortion. A dose of 50–100 mg of iodine/kg (usually equivalent to 0.2–0.4 ml/kg of the contrast medium, depending on the iodine concentration) should be used.

TECHNIQUE 3.1 continued:
Myelography

3 Immediately following the contrast medium injection, obtain left lateral and VD views of the area of interest. Oblique and dynamic (flexed) views may also be of benefit, particularly for circumferential lesion localization.

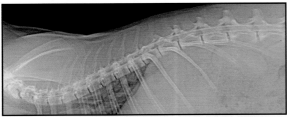

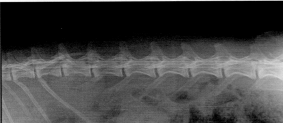

Lateral myelograms of a rabbit with hindlimb paresis. No abnormalities were evident. When taking a myelogram it is advisable to include at least two or three regions (cervical, thoracic, lumbar) within the field of view to obtain as much information as possible.

Postoperative management

- The patient should be monitored for at least 24 hours following the procedure for the presence of neurological signs.
- Analgesia and fluid therapy should be provided as needed.

Pitfalls and adverse effects

- Lumbar myelography is more technically demanding than cervical myelography, but it is more likely to reveal thoracolumbar lesions because the contrast medium injection can be performed with a reduced risk of seizures.
- Risks and complications associated with myelography include transient or permanent neurological damage, which can result from improper needle placement and patient reactions secondary to the contrast medium injection.
- With cisterna magna puncture/contrast medium injection, the needle can be advanced too far and the patient can be injured by a direct puncture to the brainstem.
- Intrathecal contrast medium injection has been reported to exacerbate neurological deficits and may cause seizures. Transient seizures are controlled with benzodiazepines.
- Passing the needle through the lumbar spinal parenchyma results in transitional hindlimb paresis.

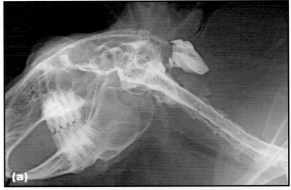

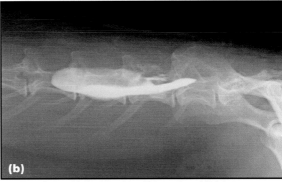

(a) During a cisterna magna puncture, high pressure was applied, resulting in contrast medium passing into the ventricles of the brain (cadaver specimen). This volume of contrast medium in the CSF of a live rabbit will cause seizures or even death. **(b)** Myelogram showing leakage of the contrast medium into the surrounding soft tissues as a result of inadequate needle placement.

4

Radiographic interpretation of the skull

Aidan Raftery

Radiographs of the skull can provide important diagnostic and prognostic information; however, positioning and exposure have a huge impact on the interpretation. General anaesthesia is usually required to prevent movement artefacts (see Chapter 3). The aims of skull radiography are to identify disease, formulate treatment plans or further diagnostic plans, and monitor progress. Other diagnostic techniques may be needed to provide additional information.

High-quality radiographs are essential for correct interpretation. Incorrect exposure or developing, or incorrect, inadequate or insufficient views may result in an incorrect or overlooked diagnosis. As with a clinical examination, the entire radiograph should be examined in a systematic approach. Focusing just on areas where there is obvious abnormality should be avoided, as should focusing on areas of suspicion from the history and physical examination. It is also important to try to avoid jumping to a diagnosis when interpreting a radiograph. The changes visible (size, shape, location, margination and opacity) should always be recorded; the conditions (pathological and anatomical variations) that could cause these radiographic changes can then be considered.

PRACTICAL TIPS
- The orientations in which radiographs are viewed should be standardized so as to develop a mental image of the normal:
  - Lateral images should always be viewed with the rostral aspect to the left
  - Dorsoventral (DV) and ventrodorsal (VD) views should be viewed with the rostral aspect pointing upwards. Conventionally, the DV and VD views are viewed with the left side to the viewer's right, and this is how they are printed in most radiology reference books.
- Skull radiographs require the highest quality viewing monitor for digital images or the best quality viewing box, ideally with a spotlight for better evaluation of overexposed areas of the radiograph.
- A collection of normal skull radiographs should be established to use as reference material for comparison.

Rabbits have very fragile skeletons. In wild rabbits the skeleton is 9% of total bodyweight (in comparison a cat's skeleton makes up 13% of its bodyweight). Domestication and breeding selection have reduced this further in rabbits, to between 6% in larger breeds, where there was greater genetic selection for more muscle, and 7–8% in dwarf rabbits (Reese and Fehr, 2009). Rabbit bones will appear much thinner when compared with those of other species, especially the dog and cat with which most veterinary practitioners are more familiar.

Indications for skull radiography

Dental disease is the most common indication for radiography in rabbits. Clinical signs that may lead to a suspicion of dental disease include swellings on the mandible or maxilla, anorexia, abnormalities of mastication, and bruxism. Established dental disease, where there is malocclusion, clinical crown elongation, occlusal surface abnormalities, loose teeth or teeth with pustular material draining from the alveolus, should be further evaluated by radiography. The reserve crowns of the incisors should be evaluated radiographically prior to extraction to identify any fractures of tooth or bone, and any other pathology that would render extraction to be contraindicated. Epiphora and/or dacrocystitis are often related to dental disease and are indications for radiography. Contrast studies of the nasolacrimal duct may be necessary to identify the site and underlying cause (see Chapters 3 and 28).

Upper respiratory tract disease is the second most common indication for skull radiography in the rabbit. Clinical signs that suggest that radiography should be part of the investigation include uni- or bilateral nasal discharge, sneezing, and increased respiratory sounds associated with narrowing of the airways of the upper respiratory tract.

Disease processes that may involve the bony orbit are also indications for skull radiography. Exophthalmos is the most common presenting sign. Abnormal positioning of one eye, normal eye position but difficulty in retropulsing the eye, strabismus, chemosis, prolapse of the third eyelid or of the Harderian gland, and visual impairment where there is an optical nerve neuropathy are less common clinical signs for which radiography is indicated. Epiphora and dacrocystitis have already been mentioned under signs that may be associated with dental disease; however, the underlying aetiology could be ocular disease. Ultrasonography is also a very useful diagnostic technique for investigation of disease of the eye and the bony orbit (see Chapter 8).

Neurological signs for which skull radiography is indicated include seizures, head tilt, vestibular signs, personality changes, nystagmus, ataxia, deficient palpebral closure, drooling, facial asymmetry, one ear lying down, drooping or retracted lip, incoordination and any other cranial nerve deficits identified, for example deviation of the tongue.

Cases of otitis externa where there is suspicion of otitis media or interna should be investigated radiographically. If a bulging tympanic membrane is found, this also warrants radiographic investigation.

A history of trauma, abnormal temporomandibular joint movement, facial pain, any palpable swelling, deformity, asymmetry of the skull and the investigation of any non-specific clinical signs may also be indications for skull radiography in the rabbit.

Radiographic anatomy and interpretation

Dental anatomy

Normal dental anatomy is rarely seen in rabbits presented at veterinary surgeries. Most rabbits, except the very young, have some radiographic signs of dental disease. It is important to be familiar with the normal, however, in order to be able to fully evaluate the abnormal.

The examination should start rostrally, at the incisors, noting the shape of their occlusal surfaces and how they have worn. The layer of enamel on the labial surface of the primary incisors results in a 45-degree chisel shape. The tips of the mandibular incisors should be between the 1st and 2nd maxillary incisors when at rest. The 2nd maxillary incisors should not be chisel-shaped. These are missing in some rabbits. The occlusal surface of the mandibular incisors should line up roughly with a line that follows the curvature of the mandible (Figure 4.1). Elongation, and increased or decreased curvature of the crown, can also be gauged using this imaginary line. The primary maxillary incisors are more curved than the mandibular incisors (Figure 4.2). The enamel of the incisors should be seen to be smooth, especially on the labial surfaces. The pulp cavity can be used as a measure of eruption.

Normally, as the tooth grows, dentine slowly fills in the pulp cavity. If the growth rate is slower than normal, or even arrested, the pulp cavity will be reduced or even absent (see Figure 4.1 for the normal anatomy; Figure 4.7, later, shows the pulp cavity when tooth growth has been arrested). A more rapid growth rate than normal will result in the pulp cavity being close to or even beyond the gingival margin, as in cases where the incisors are not occluding and there is no negative pressure on growth (see Figure 4.6). This is clinically significant if reduction of the height of the clinical crown is planned. The apices of the mandibular incisors are just rostral to the first cheek teeth (see Figure 4.1). The apices of the 1st maxillary incisors are at the junction between the incisive and maxillary bones of the diastema. Each should be at least the diameter of its apex away from the diastema. The lamina dura is visualized as a more radiopaque line of denser bone demarcating the alveolus. At the area of the apex there should be room between the tooth and the lamina dura for the germinal tissue. The periodontal space is the more radiolucent line between the tooth and the lamina dura.

The cheek teeth should be evaluated next. With the mandible in the resting position, i.e. with the incisors in normal occlusion on a lateral view, the occlusal plane of the cheek teeth should be seen as a zigzag line, as in Figure 4.10. The rostrocaudal view can also be used to evaluate the occlusal plane of the cheek teeth (Figure 4.3). The apices of the cheek teeth are more difficult to visualize because of the superimposition of the contralateral side. Lateral oblique views allow a clearer view of the apices. The tympanic bullae are also separated on this view (Figure 4.4). Both a right and a left oblique lateral view are required to visualize all the apical areas. As with the incisors, the lamina dura should be seen as a smooth thin curved radiopaque line; the space between the lamina dura and the tooth represents the periodontal ligaments and, at the end of the tooth, the germinal tissues.

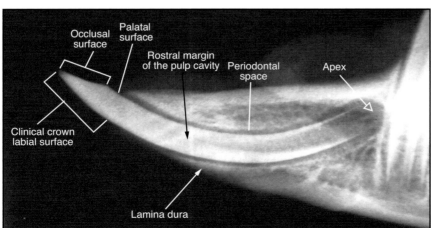

4.1 Detail of the mandibular incisor. The solid white arrow marks the more radiodense line of the lamina dura, the wall of the dental alveolus. The line of the occlusal surface of the mandibular incisors is a continuation of the line of the diastema. Note the normal position of the apex in relation to the 1st mandibular cheek tooth and the normal distance between the apical end of the tooth and the lamina dura in this radiograph (open arrow). The black arrow indicates the normal coronal extent of the pulp cavity, extending for approximately two-thirds the length of the tooth. (© Aidan Raftery)

Labels on figure: Occlusal surface; Palatal surface; Rostral margin of the pulp cavity; Periodontal space; Apex; Clinical crown labial surface; Lamina dura

The mandibular cheek teeth should show at least the same distance between the tooth and the lamina dura as between the lamina dura and the line of the ventral cortex of the mandible. Evaluating the maxillary teeth for apical elongation is more difficult because there is no similar reference point. Various guidelines have been proposed, although all have their limitations. Elongation of teeth at the apices will result in loss of the normal appearance in this area and loss of the line of the lamina dura.

Many clinicians evaluate the height of the clinical crowns of the cheek teeth by projecting the line of the maxillary diastema and the mandibular diastema rostrally. This line should be converging to meet in front of the rabbit's nose. If these lines are parallel or diverging, the most common reason is elongation of the clinical crowns of the cheek teeth (Figure 4.5). There are, however, normal skulls where this guideline does not work.

On the right and left lateral oblique views an attempt should be made to identify each of the cheek teeth separately. There are five mandibular cheek teeth and six maxillary cheek teeth on each side. The 5th mandibular cheek tooth is significantly smaller, while the 2nd and 3rd are less curved than the others (Figure 4.6). The 1st maxillary cheek tooth is smaller and shorter than the others, and the 6th is shorter still. The apex of the 3rd maxillary cheek tooth usually extends beyond those of its neighbours (see Figure 4.5). A longitudinal ridge, which is an enamel infolding, should be visible from the apex to the occlusal surface of each tooth. This should be a smooth unbroken line, where not obscured by superimposition. The extent of the pulp cavity is not easily seen in the cheek teeth. In the oblique views, where rotation frees the distal part of the tooth from superimposition by the contralateral side, the pulp cavity can be more easily evaluated just proximal to the apices. The degree of curvature of the teeth and the size of the interproximal spaces should also be noted.

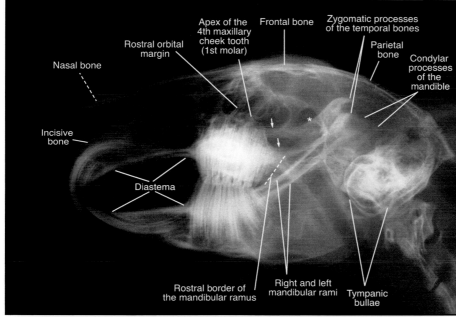

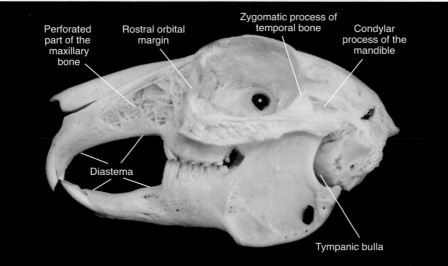

4.2 Lateral views of the skull and mandible showing important anatomical landmarks. Solid arrows mark the temporal processes of the zygomatic bones (right and left). The dotted line marks the rostral border of the mandibular ramus, the coronoid process. The asterisk marks the orbital foramen. Note: this radiograph is not a true lateral view, which is why there are two lines around the tympanic bullae and two zygomatic processes of the temporal bone. (Radiograph © Aidan Raftery; skull model image courtesy of Frances Harcourt-Brown)

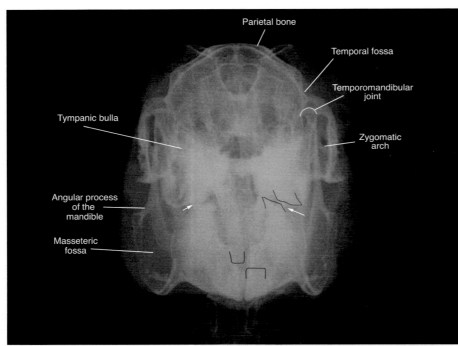

Parietal bone

Temporal fossa

Temporomandibular joint

Zygomatic arch

Tympanic bulla

Angular process of the mandible

Masseteric fossa

4.3 Rostrocaudal views of the skull showing the occlusal plane of the cheek teeth (arrows). The maxillary and mandibular cheek teeth are outlined in red. The maxillary and mandibular incisors are outlined in blue. The temporomandibular joints are also seen on this view (yellow line). (Radiograph © Aidan Raftery; skull model image courtesy of Frances Harcourt-Brown)

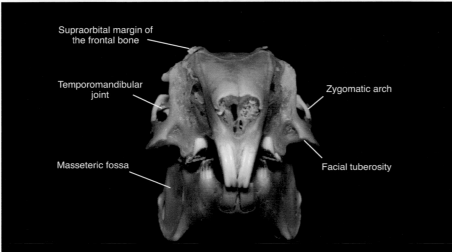

Supraorbital margin of the frontal bone

Temporomandibular joint

Zygomatic arch

Masseteric fossa

Facial tuberosity

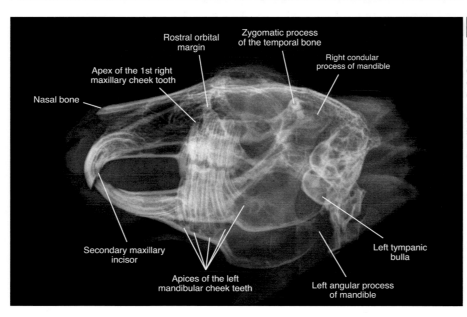

Rostral orbital margin

Zygomatic process of the temporal bone

Right condular process of mandible

Apex of the 1st right maxillary cheek tooth

Nasal bone

Secondary maxillary incisor

Apices of the left mandibular cheek teeth

Left tympanic bulla

Left angular process of mandible

4.4 Lateral oblique views of the skull. This radiographic view allows the mandibular cheek teeth apices on one side and the maxillary cheek teeth apices on the contralateral side to be projected free from superimposition by the opposite sides. (Radiograph courtesy of Matthew Baraclough) (continues) ▶

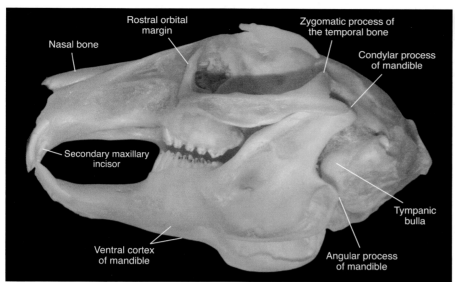

4.4 (continued) Lateral oblique views of the skull. (© Aidan Raftery)

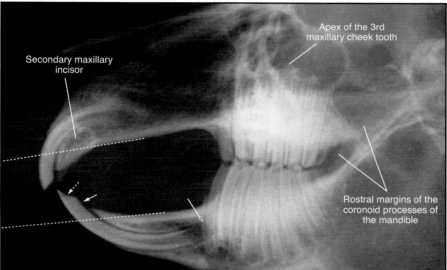

4.5 Converging diastema as a measure of normal clinical crown height. Elongation of the mandibular incisors is shown by the closed arrow. Elongation of the mandibular incisor apices occurs behind the 1st mandibular cheek teeth. There is an abnormal angle to the occlusal surface of the mandibular incisors (dotted arrow). Although still converging, the lines of the diastema (dashed lines) are moving closer to parallel, indicating elongation of the clinical crowns of the cheek teeth. (© Aidan Raftery)

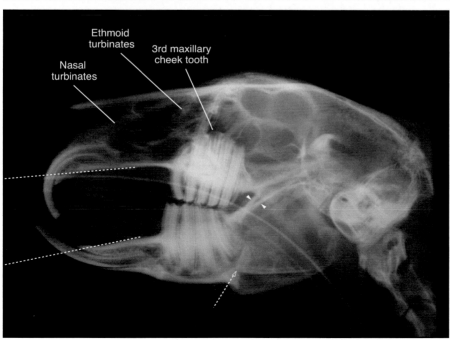

4.6 A fracture of the mandible can be seen just caudal to the 5th cheek tooth (dotted arrow) in this radiograph of a 3-year-old neutered female Dwarf Lop that had been attacked by a dog. The ramus of the mandible is displaced ventrally (solid arrowheads), which has resulted in incisor malocclusion. The upper and lower sides of the diastema (dotted lines) should be convergent or parallel and not diverging as here. The 2nd maxillary incisors are missing. This is common in dwarf rabbits. Each cheek tooth should be identified and evaluated separately. The 3rd maxillary cheek tooth is often the longest. There is elongation of the clinical crowns of all teeth, together with malocclusion of the incisors. The pulp cavity is more proximal in the incisors than normal, indicating a more rapid growth rate. (Courtesy of Frances Harcourt-Brown)

Upper respiratory tract

Upper respiratory tract disease is a common indication for radiography in rabbits. The lateral and DV views are the most useful. The area of the nasal and ethmoid turbinates and the areas of the nasal cavity where air provides good negative contrast should be evaluated (see Figure 4.6). The surrounding structures should also be evaluated for pathological processes that may be affecting the nasal cavity. The nasal turbinates are in the rostral area of the nasal cavity and have a linear pattern caused by the delicate bony scrolls and their surrounding air. Loss of the linear pattern is seen when the air spaces between the turbinate bones fill up with accumulated exudate, reducing the contrast between bone and surrounding material. There is often destruction of the nasal turbinates, which is seen as an area of decreased radiopacity. In some cases of chronic upper respiratory tract disease there may be mixed areas of increased and decreased radiopacity. Localized chronic disease may sometimes show radiographically as focal radiodense lesions where there has been mineralization of chronic inflammatory or neoplastic tissue. Comparison of a lesion on different views will be necessary to localize it. These lesions can be further investigated by rhinoscopy and/or computed tomography (CT) (see Chapters 9 and 10). The ethmoid turbinates are seen as a more irregular pattern of thin radiopaque lines caudal to the nasal turbinates (see Figure 4.6). The radiographic appearance of pathological changes is broadly similar to that described for the nasal turbinates.

Paranasal sinuses

Sinusitis is a common sequel to chronic upper respiratory tract disease. Diagnosis is difficult and the condition is often chronically undiagnosed. The clinical signs are similar to those of chronic rhinitis, and the findings on rhinoscopy will raise the suspicion of sinusitis. Skull radiology will identify clinically significant chronic sinusitis, but CT scans are better at identifying mild sinusitis. However, because of cost considerations, radiology currently plays an important part in the diagnosis and management of sinusitis for most patients. The exception is sinusitis of the sphenoidal sinus, which is much more difficult to identify by conventional radiography.

Owing to the anatomy of the dorsal conchal sinus and the maxillary sinus, inflammatory exudates tend to accumulate in the ventral recess of the maxillary sinus, it being the most ventral sinus compartment. It has no gravitational drainage. Drainage relies on the normal functioning of the ciliary system and occurs against gravity. On lateral radiographs the ventral recess of the maxillary sinus can be visualized, if it is filled with inflammatory exudates, as a thick linear area of increased radiopacity projecting from the area of the apex of the primary maxillary incisors to the angle between the ethmoid turbinates and the apex of the 1st maxillary cheek tooth (Figure 4.7). In less severe cases, when the recess is not filled with accumulated exudate, it may be visualized as a semi-opaque line. DV views are not as useful, but an increased soft tissue density on one side will help to localize the lesion. Pathology within the nasal cavities may obscure the contrast, and changes in the sinuses may be more difficult to recognize. Sinus puncture with the collection of diagnostic samples for culture and sensitivity is the gold standard for the diagnosis of sinus diseases (see Chapter 16).

The ear

The DV view is the best view for evaluating the tympanic bullae, although they are superimposed on the temporal petrous bone. The other advantage of the DV or VD views is that both bullae are visible and directly comparable with the same exposure development factors (Figure 4.8).

Lateral views result in superimposition of the tympanic bullae and are therefore of limited value for evaluating them; also each bulla cannot be compared easily with the contralateral one. The lateral oblique views separate most of the structure of the bullae from superimposition. However, the tympanic

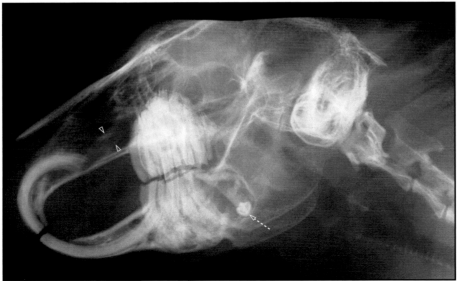

4.7 The maxillary sinus is visible because it is filled with inflammatory exudate (open arrowheads). This rabbit has more advanced dental disease, with mineralization of areas of chronic inflammation (dotted arrow). There is remodelling of the ventral cortex of the mandible as the apices of the cheek teeth elongate. Malocclusion of the incisors is present, and the pulp cavity is reduced in size, indicating slow or arrested growth. The maxillary sinus is also visible in Figure 4.6. (© Aidan Raftery)

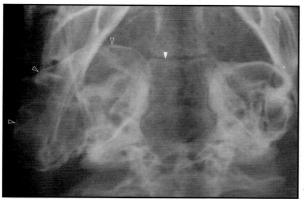

4.8 Detail of the DV view of chronically diseased tympanic bullae with extensive remodelling of the lateral and rostral walls of the tympanic bulla, most severe on the right side (open arrowheads). The spheno-occipital fissure is marked by a closed arrowhead. (© Aidan Raftery)

bullae are not completely free from superimposition until 30 degrees of rotation from the lateral is obtained along the long axis. The upper tympanic bulla still overlies the cranium at this point (King *et al.*, 2002a). The rostrocaudal view with the mouth open is used in the dog and cat to evaluate

the tymphanic bullae; however, the rabbit jaw will only open 20–25 degrees, which is not sufficient to prevent superimposition of the jaws on the bullae (King *et al.*, 2002b).

On the DV view the bones of the external acoustic meatus can be seen extending laterally from the tympanic bulla. The rostral border of the tympanic bulla should be seen as a thin curved arc of bone, which should not extend past the spheno-occipital fissure (see Figure 16.19). The lateral extent of the bulla should not be superimposed on the angular process of the mandible. With disease this bone may become irregular, thicker in some areas and thinner in others. There may be remodelling, with extra bone laid down extending rostrally, with the bulla appearing irregular and larger than that on the opposite side. It often also extends to overlap the angular process of the mandible (Figure 4.9). Occasionally it can extend rostrally past the spheno-occipital fissure. The air density within the tympanic bulla may be partially or completely replaced with a soft tissue density, and occasionally the bulla may be partly or completely filled with bone density. This may represent neoplasia or mineralization resulting from a chronic inflammatory process.

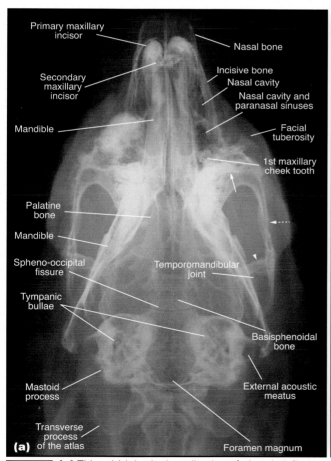

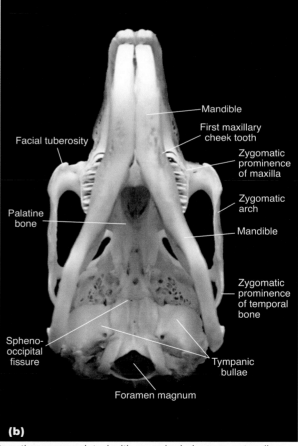

4.9 **(a)** This rabbit had mineralization of chronic inflammatory tissue associated with an apical abscess extending from the right 1st and 2nd maxillary cheek teeth. The zygomatic process of the temporal bone is marked with a solid arrowhead. The temporal process of the zygomatic bone is marked with a dotted arrow. The 2nd maxillary cheek tooth has an elongated apex and is marked with a solid arrow. The bulla is normal. **(b)** Skull model image of the same view. (Radiograph © Aidan Raftery; skull model image courtesy of Frances Harcourt-Brown)

If there is disease of the external ear canal, the bony external acoustic meatus may not be visible as a consequence of its destruction or the external ear canal being filled with soft tissue density. The diameter of the external ear canal at that level is often increased (see Figure 4.8).

When otitis media is diagnosed the radiographs should also be evaluated for concurrent upper respiratory tract disease. Otitis media can be secondary to upper respiratory tract infections with access gained up the auditory tube. Disease of the inner ear is rarely appreciated radiographically unless it is an extension of otitis media.

Canalography is a contrast technique used to evaluate the patency of the tympanic membrane (see Chapter 16).

The eye and associated structures
Radiographic evaluation of ocular disease is limited to the evaluation of other structures that are affecting the eye. Apical abscessation affecting the 5th or 6th maxillary cheek tooth is a common cause of exophthalmia. Caudal extension of an infection in the maxillary sinus is also seen as a cause of exophthalmia. Space-occupying lesions in the thoracic cavity can increase blood pressure, causing bilateral exophthalmia due to congestion of the orbital venous sinus. In the case of exophthalmia caused by increased blood pressure, skull radiographs will be non-diagnostic.

On the lateral view the rostral margin of the bony orbit is formed by the zygomatic prominence of the maxilla and can usually be seen as a curved line of increased density starting at the apex of the 2nd maxillary cheek tooth. The caudal border is not delineated but is roughly dorsal to the zygomatic process of the temporal bone. The orbital foramen should be clearly visible (see Figure 4.2). These structures may appear as double lines, depending on positioning. When an apical abscess is causing

exophthalmia it may be visible on the radiograph as a delineated area of increased soft tissue density extending caudally and dorsally, often partially obscuring the optic foramen.

On the DV view the eye can be seen as a soft tissue density in the area bounded by the zygomatic arch. The lateral margin of the orbit is not normally visible beyond the soft tissues on the zygomatic arch.

The nasolacrimal duct is often partially or completely blocked at some point by secondary disease processes, most commonly by pathology at the apices of the maxillary teeth. At the level of the apex of the primary maxillary incisors the nasolacrimal duct narrows and makes a right angled bend. This is the most common area affected by dental disease. It also runs in close association with the apical areas of the rostral cheek teeth, and any pathology causing bone remodelling at this level can also affect the duct. Upper respiratory tract infections where thick exudates are produced may also interfere with the duct as will any condition causing scarring just inside the nose. Exudates in the nasal cavities will obscure the detail of the nasal turbinates.

Nasolacrimal duct contrast studies will help to identify the site of obstruction (Figure 4.10). Occasionally the nasolacrimal duct will rupture through its medial wall into the maxillary sinus. This is more common when there are attempts to cannulate the duct with suture material (see Chapter 16).

The temporomandibular joint
Visualization of the temporomandibular joint radiographically is difficult in the rabbit. It can be seen in the DV view but the vertical ramus of the mandible is superimposed (Figure 4.11). Rostrocaudal views with the mouth closed give the most clinically useful views of the temporomandibular joint. Both sides are visible on the same view, so they can be

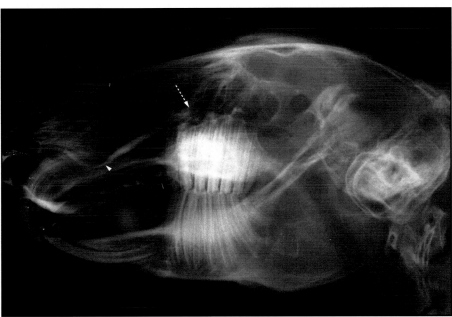

4.10 Nasolacrimal duct contrast study. The dotted arrow marks the end of the first narrow section. After this the duct is approximately 2 mm in diameter until the area of the apex of the primary maxillary incisor. At this point, which is marked by a solid arrowhead, the duct narrows to approximately 1 mm in diameter, makes a 90-degree bend medially and traverses to exit several millimetres caudal to the mucocutaneous junction at the alar fold. Note the normal occlusal plane of the cheek teeth. (© Aidan Raftery)

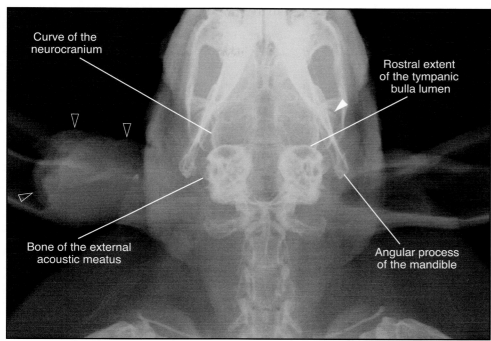

Curve of the
neurocranium

Rostral extent
of the tympanic
bulla lumen

Bone of the external
acoustic meatus

Angular process
of the mandible

4.11 DV view showing the temporomandibular joint (solid arrowhead). This rabbit also has a fibrosarcoma filling the distal part of the right external ear canal (margins marked with open arrowheads). (© Aidan Raftery)

compared (see Figure 4.3). The temporomandibular joint is very mobile and the position of the lower jaw in relation to the skull will affect its radiological appearance (see Figures 4.8 and 4.9).

The skull and mandible

Diseases of other areas of the skull and the mandible are less common. Figures 4.2, 4.3, 4.4 and 4.9 illustrate important landmarks of the anatomy of the skull which will allow lesions to be localized and any changes in appearance from the normal to be described. Generally, both the lateral and DV views should be evaluated. A useful landmark, seen in most rabbits, is the spheno-occipital fissure (see Figure 4.9). This is visualized on the DV view as a small linear gap between the basisphenoidal bone rostrally and the occipital bone caudally. In other species this area is ossified in adults. The rostrocaudal view is useful when evaluating the upper part of the cranium and the zygomatic arches (see Figure 4.3).

Fractures due to trauma are the most common abnormal findings on examination of these areas of the skull and mandible (see Figure 4.6). Neoplasia is a relatively rare finding on rabbit skull radiographs. Differentiation of neoplasia from osteomyelitis and other bony lesions is difficult using radiography alone. Deep biopsy and histopathology is necessary for a definitive diagnosis. A biopsy specimen obtained from the periphery of a lesion may incorrectly appear to be reactive bone. Comparison of different views can provide information on the invasiveness of the lesion. Deeper lesions that are difficult to biopsy can have repeat radiographs taken 10–14 days later for comparison. Most neoplasms will have changed in appearance and grown, whereas most other bony lesions will not have changed. Mineralization of chronic inflammatory

tissue is commonly seen. This is most commonly seen as a consequence of chronic dental disease (see Figures 4.7 and 4.9). Hydrocephalus is occasionally seen in young rabbits. In these cases there will be enlargement of the head circumference due to doming of the bones of the neurocranium as a result of the increased intracranial pressure (Figure 4.12).

Renal disease is the main differential diagnosis when there is a generalized increase in bone density. Calcification of the hyoid bone is also seen with renal disease (see Figure 29.29) (Harcourt-Brown, 2007).

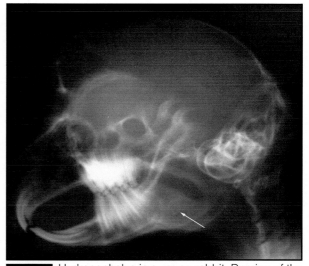

4.12 Hydrocephalus in a young rabbit. Doming of the bones of the neurocranium is evident in this 7-week-old rabbit. The owner reported that it had been born with an abnormally shaped head. The normal diamond-shaped hyoid bone is identified by the white arrow. (Courtesy of Sergio Silvetti)

References and further reading

Harcourt-Brown F (2007) Radiographic signs of renal disease in rabbits. *Veterinary Record* **160**, 787–794

King AM, Cranfield F, Hall J, Hammond G and Sullivan M (2010a) Radiographic anatomy of the rabbit skull with particular reference to the tympanic bulla and temporomandibular joint. Part 1: Lateral and long axis rotational angles. *The Veterinary Journal* **186**, 232–243

King AM, Cranfield F, Hall J, Hammond G and Sullivan M (2010b) Radiographic anatomy of the rabbit skull, with particular reference to the tympanic bulla and temporomandibular joint. Part 2: Ventral and dorsal rotational angles. *The Veterinary Journal* **186**, 244–251

Lamming GE, Woollam DHM and Millen JW (1954) Hydrocephalus in young rabbits associated with maternal vitamin A deficiency. *British Journal of Nutrition* **8**, 363–369

Reese S and Fehr M (2009) Radioanatomy. Skeletal system. In: *Diagnostic Imaging of Exotic Pets*, ed. M Krautwalds-Junghanns *et al.*, pp. 158–159. Schlütersche, Hannover

5

Radiographic interpretation of the thorax

Brendan Carmel

The unique anatomical features and small thorax of the rabbit make interpretation of radiographic images of this species a challenge, even for experienced veterinary surgeons. Despite the challenge, the fundamentals of radiography apply to rabbits as they do to any other species, and attention to details such as equipment selection, correct patient positioning and restraint are essential in order to obtain worthwhile images. Chapter 3 outlines equipment, positioning and restraint methods and Chapter 1 provides information on sedation and anaesthesia; these aspects will not be discussed here.

Indications for thoracic radiography

Indications for thoracic radiography of the rabbit include:

- Investigation of trauma patients
- Dyspnoea
- Tachypnoea (increased respiratory rate)
- Other respiratory signs such as sneezing, wheezing or nasal discharge
- Dysphagia (difficulty in swallowing)
- Collapse/syncope
- Lethargy or exercise intolerance
- Coughing
- Evaluation of suspected cardiac abnormalities:
  - Murmurs
  - Dysrhythmias
  - Cardiomegaly
- Other potential signs of cardiovascular disease such as peripheral perfusion deficits, jugular pulse abnormalities, exophthalmos
- As an aid for diagnostic procedures, for example nasogastric, endotracheal or thoracic tube placement
- Evaluation of thoracic skeletal abnormalities such as rib fractures or disc disease (see also Chapter 6)
- Investigation of suspected intrathoracic masses. Non-respiratory signs that may suggest mediastinal masses include:
  - Exophthalmos
  - Sebaceous adenitis
- Screening of rabbits diagnosed previously with neoplasia, for example uterine adenocarcinoma, mammary neoplasms
- Investigation of chronic weight loss.

Special considerations

- In contrast to dogs and cats, the thorax of the rabbit is small in relation to the large abdomen. Severe acute thoracic injury is more likely to be fatal in a rabbit, although chronic injuries are sometimes seen as incidental findings on thoracic radiographs. For example, a rabbit with a chronic diaphragmatic hernia survived for a prolonged period of time with no apparent signs of illness (Stauber *et al.*, 2006).
- It can be difficult to differentiate signs of respiratory or cardiac disease from physiological stress responses such as tachypnoea. A thorough clinical examination and detailed patient history will help to determine whether the clinical signs and/or patient evaluation indicate the need for thoracic radiography. Additional procedures such as conscious capnography may help to distinguish cardiorespiratory disease from stress and/or pain responses. The gas exchange results are likely to be abnormal if cardiorespiratory disease is present.
- Sedation or general anaesthesia is required to obtain good quality radiographs of the rabbit thorax in almost all cases. Many patients with thoracic disease are severely compromised and chemical or physical restraint methods must be carefully selected and balanced against the risks involved. If a sedative is to be used, one that has minimal cardiovascular effects, e.g. midazolam, should be considered.
- As with any species, radiographs of the chest should ideally be taken during inhalation to limit artefacts and help interpretation of normal and abnormal findings. This is particularly important with rabbits because of their small chest cavity. However this may be difficult to achieve owing to their rapid respiratory rate. Anaesthetized and intubated rabbits can have their lungs gently inflated during chest radiography to aid interpretation.

Views, positioning and normal anatomy

At least one lateral and a dorsoventral (DV) or ventrodorsal (VD) view are required to assess the thoracic cavity adequately. Obtaining a DV radiograph of the chest can be less stressful for a severely compromised patient and can often be done quickly without using sedation.

Right and left lateral views

The lateral views optimize visualization of the thoracic skeleton, heart and lung fields. Obtaining both a left and a right lateral view can help to differentiate structures or lesions within the thoracic cavity, such as mediastinal masses or abnormalities of the left or right lung lobe that may not be apparent with one view.

Right lateral recumbency is preferred if only one lateral view is taken, because this is the most commonly used standard lateral view. If possible, the forelegs should be retracted cranially to help prevent superimposition of the scapulae over the cranial portion of the thoracic cavity. However, this can restrict chest movement and may compromise breathing and so needs to be performed with caution. The structures that can be seen on the lateral view of the thorax are shown in Figure 5.1.

VD and DV views

In conjunction with the lateral views, the VD and DV views allow more complete assessment of the thoracic cavity, including greater differentiation of some portions of the lung fields (Figure 5.2). A DV view provides more information than a VD view because the thoracic structures sit in their natural positions, allowing assessment of pathology, such as effusion, to be performed more readily.

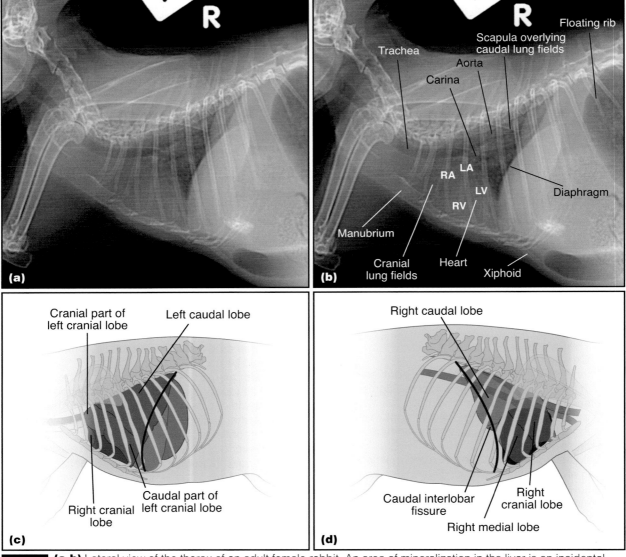

5.1 **(a,b)** Lateral view of the thorax of an adult female rabbit. An area of mineralization in the liver is an incidental finding on this radiograph; it is in the region of the gall bladder. Post-mortem examination of similar cases has shown dilation of the extrahepatic bile ducts, filled with mucinous material containing mineralized cellular debris. LA = left atrium; LV = left ventricle; RA = right atrium; RV = right ventricle. **(c)** Diagram of the left lateral view of the thorax, showing the lung lobes. **(d)** Diagram of the right lateral view of the thorax, showing the lung lobes. (a,b Courtesy of the University of Melbourne Veterinary Hospital)

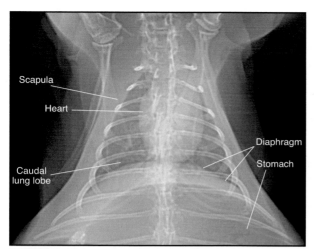

5.2 VD thoracic radiograph of the same rabbit as shown in Figure 5.1. Note the relatively large heart in comparison to the thoracic cavity. (Courtesy of the University of Melbourne Veterinary Hospital)

Normal anatomy

Normal thoracic anatomy and radiographic features in the rabbit are detailed below.

- There are 12 (rarely 13) thoracic vertebrae. The costal cartilages of the first seven (true) ribs articulate directly with the sternum, and the remaining ribs have either attached costal cartilages or are floating ribs. The sternum is comprised of seven sternebrae, with the manubrium the most cranial and the xiphoid process and cartilage the most caudal.
- Intrathoracic fat deposits are common, especially in obese patients.
- The aorta and cranial vena cava are usually visible.
- The diaphragm is long and slopes cranioventrally, which results in a short craniocaudal thoracic field.
- The silhouette of the liver usually obscures much of the dorsal diaphragmatic lung field.
- The trachea is clearly visible entering the thoracic cavity. The cartilage rings are often mineralized and visible within the tracheal wall. The trachea runs dorsally in the thoracic cavity, almost parallel with the thoracic vertebrae.
- The carina lies at the 4th or 5th intercostal space.
- The lungs have three main lobes, cranial, middle and caudal, with the left cranial lobe much smaller than the right owing to the position of the heart. The left cranial lobe is divided into cranial and caudal sections by a fold. There is an accessory lobe of the right lung on the mediastinal aspect. The cranial lung lobes can be difficult to visualize because they are relatively small.
- The thymus persists in the adult rabbit and lies ventral to the heart, extending forward into the thoracic inlet. It often obscures the cranial lung fields and the cranial border of the heart.

- The cardiac silhouette is large and approximately triangular in shape. The heart is normally located between the 3rd or 4th and the 6th pair of ribs, situated cranioventrally and occupying a relatively large volume of the thoracic cavity. It has a relatively upright position on the lateral view. The presence of pericardial fat, especially in obese animals, can obscure the outline.

Radiographic features of thoracic diseases that can be diagnosed using radiography

Pneumonia

Pneumonia in the rabbit carries a poor prognosis because most infections are chronic and clinical signs are often not apparent until the disease has progressed significantly. Widespread lung involvement is usually present owing to the thin pleurae and lack of septa dividing the lung lobes in the rabbit; pneumonia in other mammals may be more localized.

Interstitial or alveolar patterns are seen radiographically with pneumonia in the rabbit (Figure 5.3). Alveolar patterns are characterized as increased

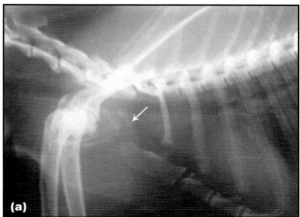

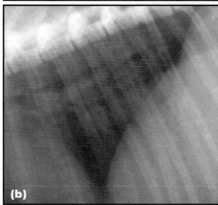

5.3 **(a)** Pneumonia in a neutered adult male dwarf rabbit that presented with severe dyspnoea. The suprahamate process is visible in the cranial thorax (arrow). This is a bony projection jutting out at right angles to the acromion process of the scapula. **(b)** An enlarged view of the caudal lung fields, which exhibit increased pulmonary densities typical of an alveolar pattern. Such patterns are characterized as increased pulmonary densities, which are patchy in appearance on this radiograph.

pulmonary densities, sometimes patchy in appearance, which may partially obscure the cardiac silhouette. Interstitial patterns seen with pneumonia in the rabbit are mostly hazy and diffuse. The lung lobe margins may be indistinct and air bronchograms and lobar consolidation are also possible. Intrathoracic fat can be misinterpreted as a pulmonary abscess or pneumonia.

Further investigation

When pneumonia is suspected or diagnosed from thoracic radiographs, signs of concurrent upper respiratory tract disease should be searched for on radiographs of the neck and head. Obtaining a sample from the respiratory tract for bacterial culture and sensitivity testing is recommended, because identification of the causative organism(s) and selecting appropriate antibiotics will increase the chance of successful treatment. The bacteria causing the pneumonia may be difficult to culture and a 'no growth' result is not uncommon. Fine-needle aspiration (FNA) from the chest is often the safest method for obtaining a sample for culture or cytology and is surprisingly well tolerated by rabbits. Bronchoalveolar lavage is more difficult and carries a risk in the rabbit.

Fine-needle aspiration

In rabbits FNA is preferable to bronchoalveolar lavage. Samples can be aspirated from sites identified on thoracic radiographs, or guided by ultrasonography. Specimens can be collected for visual examination, laboratory analysis, cytology and/or culture and sensitivity testing.

1. Restrain the rabbit in a normal sitting position.
2. Clip and surgically scrub the area of interest.
3. Local anaesthesia may be applied to the skin, although many rabbits tolerate the procedure without it.
4. Use a 22–25 G needle attached to a 3 or 5 ml syringe.
5. Gently insert the needle in the direction of the suspected lesion.
6. Apply suction to the syringe to obtain the sample.
7. Place the sample on to a glass slide for examination. Note that sometimes the sample is only present in the needle hub. If this is the case, attach an air-filled syringe to the hub and gently squirt the contents on to a glass slide.
8. Fluid from effusions can be placed into a sterile sample tube.

Metastatic disease

The typical radiographic feature of pulmonary metastases is the presence of multiple interstitial nodular densities within the thoracic cavity. These may be well or ill defined and may coalesce, merging with neighbouring densities and obscuring the heart in some cases. Elevation of the trachea can also be present.

An example of metastatic disease in the rabbit is uterine adenocarcinoma (Figure 5.4). Adenocarcinoma of the uterus is the most commonly reported neoplasm of the female rabbit. The incidence increases with age, and pulmonary metastases carry a grave prognosis. Thoracic radiography is advisable in all rabbits with suspected uterine abnormalities to assess the prognosis before considering surgery. Ovariohysterectomy is curative if metastasis has not occurred (see Chapter 12). Metastases may not be visible at the time of surgery or on survey thoracic radiographs; therefore regular repeat thoracic and abdominal survey radiographs, at least every 6 months, may be taken in any suspect cases after neutering has been performed.

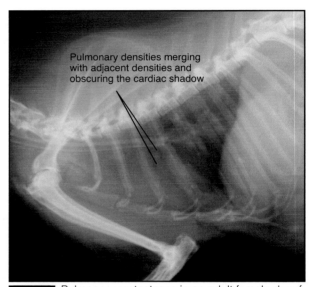

5.4 Pulmonary metastases in an adult female dwarf rabbit. Diffuse pulmonary densities are present (some merging with adjacent densities) and obscure the heart silhouette. An ovariohysterectomy had been performed to remove a uterine adenocarcinoma several months previously, at which time there were no pulmonary changes evident on survey radiographs. Also note the prominent cartilaginous tracheal rings and the tip of the endotracheal tube at the bronchial bifurcation. The rabbit was given a hopeless prognosis and euthanased after this radiograph was taken.

Further investigation

Metastatic masses in the chest are usually secondary, so it is critical to look elsewhere for the primary source of the neoplasm. Ultrasonography of the chest and abdomen, together with survey abdominal radiography, is recommended. A complete blood count, looking for a high white cell count or abnormal cells, and a biochemistry panel to detect any organ dysfunction can help to detect metastatic disease in other organs and determine treatment options and prognosis. Although costly, magnetic resonance imaging (MRI) or computed tomography (CT) may be worth considering. Obtaining a fine-needle aspirate (see above) of the thoracic mass, ideally with ultrasound guidance, will often enable cytological confirmation of the neoplasm.

Mediastinal masses

Mediastinal masses are relatively common in rabbits (see Chapter 19). Thymoma and thymic lymphoma are the most frequently encountered. Bilateral exophthalmos is commonly reported in rabbits with thymoma and is thought to occur as a consequence of compromise of vascular return to the heart. Sebaceous adenitis is a common paraneoplastic syndrome that is often seen in association with thymic masses.

Visualization of small thymic masses radiographically can be difficult in rabbits because the thymus persists into adulthood and there is a danger of misdiagnosing a normal thymus as pathogenic. The presence of intrathoracic fat, especially in obese animals, can be a further complication. Large thymic tumours can be seen radiographically because the cranial mediastinal mass obscures the heart (effacement) and the cranial lung lobes. The heart may be displaced caudally. The thymic mass is sometimes large enough to occupy the entire cranial thoracic cavity. Elevation of the trachea is also typically seen (Figure 5.5). Pleural effusion may be apparent in some cases.

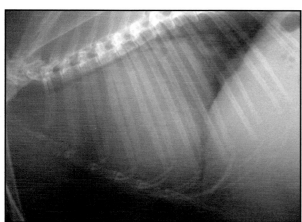

5.5 A cranial mediastinal mass in an adult male dwarf rabbit. Note the severe compression and elevation of the trachea, and the poor outline (effacement) of the heart silhouette caused by the thoracic mass.

Pulmonary abscesses and thymic cysts can also result in mediastinal masses. Mineralization of mediastinal masses can give them a distinct radiographic appearance.

Further investigation

Differentiating the cause of mediastinal masses seen on radiographs can be difficult. Ultrasound examination and advanced imaging such as MRI may be of use to differentiate among abscesses, cysts and solid tumours. FNA (see above) may be helpful. Surgery for mediastinal tumours is feasible and is described in Chapter 19.

Cardiac disease

Valvular disease, idiopathic hypertrophic cardiomyopathy and myocarditis have all been reported in rabbits. The right atrioventricular valve has only two cusps; hence the term 'tricuspid' should not be used. Congenital heart abnormalities include ventricular septal defects (Voros *et al.*, 2011). Clinical signs of cardiac disease are variable and may include lethargy, collapse, and respiratory signs such as tachypnoea or dyspnoea. There may be no clinical signs of illness or congestive heart failure may result in pulmonary oedema or pleural effusion.

The thoracic cavity of the rabbit is small compared with that of other species and the heart is relatively large, so a diagnosis of cardiomegaly must be made with caution. Radiographic measurements of cardiac size have been undertaken in a small number of apparently healthy rabbits (Onuma *et al.*, 2010). Right lateral radiographs were taken at the point of inspiration in a group of non-sedated rabbits; cardiac size was measured and related to bodyweight and gender. The authors found significant differences in the long axis (LA), short axis (SA) and vertebral heart size (VHS), and concluded that these values should prove useful as diagnostic indices for cardiac disease in rabbits (Figure 5.6). Although it is yet to be determined whether increased VHS measurement correlates with cardiac disease in rabbits, there is clinical evidence that this is the case. Obvious cardiomegaly is sometimes present in rabbits with cardiac disease (Figure 5.7). Other radiographic changes in cardiac disease may include rounding of the cardiac borders, elevation of the trachea, pulmonary vascular enlargement and interstitial or alveolar patterns.

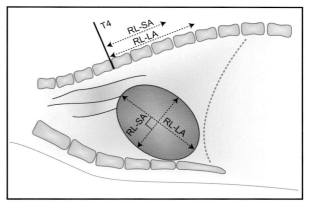

5.6 Vertebral heart score. A study by Onuma *et al.* (2010) determined long axis (LA) values of 4.22 ± 0.25 cm and vertebral heart score (VHS) of 7.55 ± 0.38 cm for rabbits <1.6 kg, and LA values of 4.48 ± 0.3 cm and VHS of 7.99 ± 0.5.8 cm for disease-free rabbits ≥1.6 kg. Note: these measurements are for right lateral radiographs. SA = short axis.

Further investigation

Electrocardiography and echocardiography studies are recommended for any rabbit with suspected cardiovascular disease. Blood pressure measurements can help to complete the diagnostic picture. A paediatric cuff applied to the proximal tarsus or carpus can be used to record systolic blood pressure, with a normal reading for a rabbit being 90–135 mmHg (Orcutt, 2006). See Chapter 1 for more information on blood pressure measurement.

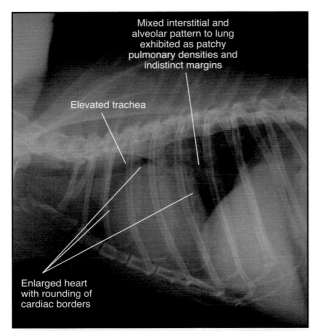

Mixed interstitial and alveolar pattern to lung exhibited as patchy pulmonary densities and indistinct margins

Elevated trachea

Enlarged heart with rounding of cardiac borders

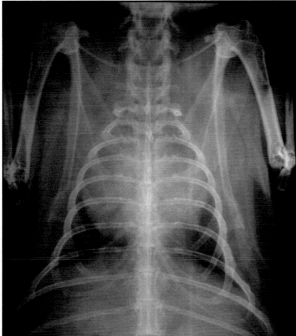

5.7 Lateral and DV views of the thorax of an 8-year-old mixed-breed rabbit with cardiomegaly, which presented with exercise intolerance and lethargy. The rabbit improved on furosemide and benazepril but died suddenly 3 weeks later. (Courtesy of Frances Harcourt-Brown)

Aortic mineralization

Mineralization of the aorta may be seen on thoracic radiographs (Figure 5.8). Clinical signs include those of cardiac disease, seizures and/or chronic renal failure (polydipsia, weight loss). In pet rabbits, mineralization of the aorta is usually associated with chronic renal disease (Harcourt-Brown, 2007) which is often linked with *Encephalitozoon cuniculi* infection. In rabbits, calcium metabolism is regulated by renal excretion rather than intestinal uptake, and

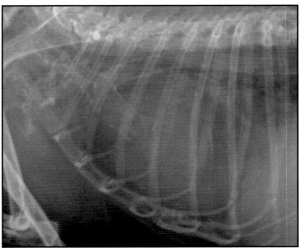

5.8 Lateral thoracic radiograph of a 4-year-old mini-lop rabbit, showing extensive mineralization of the aortic arch and other vessels in the cranial chest, including the subclavian arteries. There is also cardiomegaly, elevation of the trachea, and interstitial and alveolar patterns indicating pulmonary oedema. (Courtesy of Frances Harcourt-Brown)

therefore advanced renal disease impairs calcium (and phosphorus) excretion. This can result in high blood calcium and phosphorus values and ectopic mineralization of tissues, especially the aorta and skeleton. Osteosclerosis may be seen in the vertebral bodies (see Chapter 6) or the hyoid bone (see Figure 29.29). Vitamin D toxicity, which increases intestinal absorption of calcium, can also result in aortic mineralization.

In laboratory rabbits, aortic mineralization can be induced by stomach-tube feeding with very large amounts of calcium and vitamin D (Kamphues *et al.*, 1986). Aortic mineralization can also be seen in cases of arteriosclerosis, which is defined as any condition characterized by thickening and loss of elasticity of the arterial walls (Saunders and Rees Davies, 2005). The type of mineralization, for example calcification, cannot be determined radiographically. Lipid deposits in arteries result in atherosclerosis, a form of arteriosclerosis, and develop as a result of abnormal cholesterol metabolism. Rabbits are used as laboratory models of arteriosclerosis, which can be induced by feeding a high-cholesterol diet.

Further investigation

A full blood panel, including calcium, phosphorus, urea and creatinine, should be performed. Serology for *E. cuniculi* exposure may be useful. Survey radiographs of the whole body are recommended to determine whether there are any other areas of mineralization. Critical assessment of the diet is important to ensure limited but adequate intake of calcium and phosphorus.

Spinal deformities

Spinal deformities such as kyphosis, scoliosis, vertebral spondylosis or spondylitis may be found as an incidental finding on thoracic radiographs. These conditions can cause pain and other problems such as chronic perineal scalding due to leakage of urine or faeces, reduced mobility, tachycardia or respiratory noises, or an inability to groom properly (see Chapter 6). If spinal deformities are seen on thoracic radiographs and the rabbit is suspected to be in pain or suffering from reduced mobility, a trial of medical treatment may be beneficial. A trial of an analgesic or anti-inflammatory agent for several days to weeks is used, and the response to treatment (increased mobility, return to normal behavioural patterns) indicates that the deformity may have been painful for the rabbit.

References and further reading

Capello V and Lennox AM (2008) *Clinical Radiology of Exotic Companion Mammals.* Wiley-Blackwell, Iowa
Gibbs C and Hinton MH (1981) Radiographic examination of the rabbit. 1. The head, thorax and vertebral column. *Journal of Small Animal Practice* **22**, 687–703
Harcourt-Brown F (2002) Cardiorespiratory disease. In: *Textbook of Rabbit Medicine*, pp. 324–334. Butterworth-Heinemann, Oxford
Harcourt-Brown F (2007) Radiographic signs of renal disease in rabbits. *Veterinary Record* **160**, 787–794
Kamphues VJ, Carstensen P, Schroeder D, *et al.* (1986) Effect of increasing calcium and vitamin D supply on calcium metabolism in rabbits. *Journal of Animal Physiology and Nutrition* **50**, 191–208 [Article in German with an English summary]
O'Malley B (2005) *Clinical Anatomy and Physiology of Exotic Species.* Elsevier Saunders, Edinburgh
Onuma M, Ono S, Ishida T, Shibuya H and Sato T (2010) Radiographic measurement of cardiac size in 27 rabbits. *Journal of Veterinary Medical Science* **72**, 529–531
Orcutt C (2006) Cardiovascular disorders. In: *BSAVA Manual of Rabbit Medicine and Surgery, 2nd edn*, ed. A Meredith and P Flecknell. pp. 96–103. BSAVA Publications, Gloucester
Popesko P, Rajtova V and Horak J (1992) *A Colour Atlas of Anatomy of Small Laboratory Animals. Volume 1: Rabbit, Guinea Pig.* Wolfe, London
Reusch B (2005) Investigation and management of cardiovascular disease in rabbits. *In Practice* **27**, 418–425
Saunders RA and Rees Davies R (2005) Cardiovascular disease. In: *Notes on Rabbit Internal Medicine*, pp. 91–93. Blackwell Publishing, Oxford
Stauber E, Finch N and Caplazi P (2006) Diaphragmatic kidney hernia in a rabbit. *Exotic DVM* **8**, 11–12
Voros K, Seehusen F, Hungerbuhler S, Meyer-Lindenberg A and von der Hoeh H (2011) Ventricular septal defect with aortic valve insufficiency in a New Zealand White rabbit. *Journal of the American Animal Hospital Association* **47**, e42–e49
Wolvekamp P and Oschwald CH (1991) Rabbit. In: *Atlas of Diagnostic Radiology of Exotic Pets*, ed. GA Rubel *et al.* pp. 26–51. WB Saunders, Philadelphia

6

Radiographic interpretation of the vertebral column

Craig Hunt

The rabbit has a relatively delicate skeleton, which accounts for 6–8% of total bodyweight compared with 13% in a similarly sized cat. However, the rabbit has increased hindlimb musculature designed for explosive running. These two anatomical traits place the rabbit at increased risk of spinal fractures and luxations if improperly handled or allowed to kick out, twist or struggle. Poor husbandry and diet may compound the problem, with osteoporosis being common in rabbits confined to hutches and fed cereal-type mixes.

Being a prey species, the rabbit has a tendency to hide pain and illness very well; clinical signs of pain (see Chapter 2) and disease may be very subtle and easily missed by both the owner and the attending veterinary surgeon. Complex digestive physiology and unique renal physiology may compound the effects of spinal disease; conversely, spinal pathology may have a direct impact on normal functioning of these two systems.

Indications for radiography of the spine are perhaps more numerous than for the dog or cat. Any rabbit showing signs of limb dysfunction, discomfort, abnormal or inappropriate behaviour or lack of grooming is a potential candidate for spinal radiography.

Physical examination

Prior to radiographic examination, attempts should be made to localize pathology to a specific site or sites. A general physical examination followed by a specific neurological examination should be performed on every patient presenting with non-specific illness or specific neurological signs. Given the rabbit's nervous nature and tendency to hide pain this is not always easy, or indeed possible, but should be attempted. Localization of pathology allows collimation of the X-ray beam, reducing scatter radiation and optimizing clarity of the image, which is essential in small patients.

Examination may proceed along similar lines to that of the dog or cat, but bearing in mind that the rabbit is a prey species and exhibits some significant differences:

- Systemic disease is common and often advanced at the time of presentation and can both cause and mimic neurological disease

- Conditions such as bilateral pododermatitis and cruciate ligament disease are common and may mimic spinal disease
- Certain tests may be inaccurate in some patients as a result of fear and stress and should be interpreted with caution, e.g. proprioceptive positioning and menace reflexes
- The pain response may be significantly inhibited or markedly exaggerated, depending on the individual patient, owing to stress.

The aim of the neurological examination is to localize any lesion to either the brain or one of four major spinal cord divisions. The spinal cord divisions are: cranial cervical (C1–C5); cervical enlargement (C6–T2); thoracolumbar (T3–L3); and lumbosacral (L4–Cd (caudal)). The spinal cord ends around the second sacral vertebra (S2), and cord segments do not correlate with vertebral number. It should also be noted that the cord segments may correlate with different vertebrae in different patients because the number of thoracic and lumbar vertebrae may vary.

Great care should always be taken to prevent the rabbit injuring itself during examination. Iatrogenic spinal fractures and/or luxation are unfortunately common but are completely avoidable with correct restraint. The spinal column of the rabbit has limited flexibility in the dorsoventral (DV) plane. If undue downward pressure is applied to the thoracic spinal column during restraint (e.g. when the rabbit is held by the scruff or across the shoulders), the resultant upward force exerted by the hindlimbs during attempts to escape can easily over-flex the vertebral column, resulting in injury. Similarly, if the rabbit escapes restraint and kicks out suddenly with the hindlimbs, over-extension of the spine may occur. Generally rabbits respond well to very calm and gentle restraint. Administration of a sedative is always preferable to, and safer than, excessively firm manual restraint.

Indications for radiography

The following are some of the common indications for radiography of the rabbit spine:

- Thoracic and pelvic limb paresis or paraparesis
- Mono-, para- or quadriplegia
- Suspected vertebral deformities
- Ataxia

- Stiffness, inactivity and/or reluctance to move
- Urine incontinence/scald
- Caecotroph accumulation
- Failure to groom, acariasis, myiasis
- Otitis externa (resulting from inability to groom the ears using the hindlimbs)
- Gastrointestinal stasis.

Positioning for radiography

Whole body survey radiographs are helpful to identify concomitant underlying conditions, e.g. lung metastases or urolithiasis, that might otherwise go undetected. However, they should not replace targeted, well collimated radiographs of specific areas of interest localized by a thorough and systematic physical and neurological examination.

General anaesthesia is usually required to obtain accurate, diagnostic radiographs of the spine and is mandatory for myelography. Manual restraint and immobilization techniques may not provide the accurate positioning required for diagnosis, could cause artefacts and may result in further injury and stress to the patient (see Chapter 3 and Appendix 4).

Lateral view

For the lateral view it is essential that the spine is parallel to the cassette; the patient is placed in right or left lateral recumbency with the hindlimbs and forelimbs extended. Full extension should be maintained only for the duration of exposure of the film, to avoid respiratory compromise. The limbs should be kept parallel to the cassette with the use of cotton wool or small foam wedges and should be secured to the X-ray table or cassette using tape; sandbags and rope ties are generally too bulky. For the cervical spine the skull should be positioned with the nares and pinnae in perfect vertical alignment; the nose may need to be elevated slightly with the use of a foam wedge. Foam supports may be positioned under the neck and lumbar spine to ensure that the spine does not kink, depending on the conformation of the rabbit. Gentle traction on the skull and spine may be utilized with care to reduce rotation and other positioning artefacts. Correctly positioned views should demonstrate superimposition of the osseous bullae, wings of the atlas, transverse processes, ribs and wings of the ilia (Figures 6.1 and 6.2).

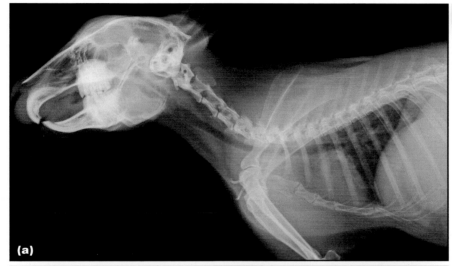

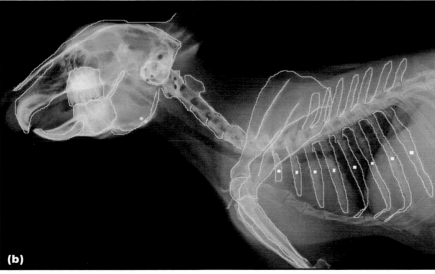

6.1 **(a,b)** Normal lateral view of the cervical and thoracic spine of a 3-year-old entire male dwarf rabbit. Early signs of dental disease were an incidental finding. The alignment of the tympanic bullae (black asterisks), ribs (white squares), wings of atlas (red circles) and mandibles (yellow circles) denote correct positioning. (continues) ▶

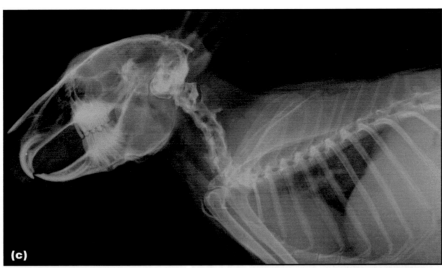

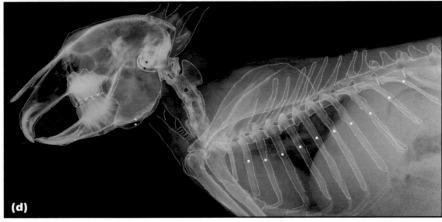

6.1 (continued) **(c,d)** Normal flexed-neck lateral view of the cervical and thoracic spine of a 3-year-old entire male dwarf rabbit. Early signs of dental disease were an incidental finding. The alignment of the tympanic bullae (black asterisks), ribs (white squares), wings of atlas (red circles) and mandibles (yellow circles) denote correct positioning.

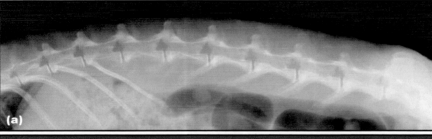

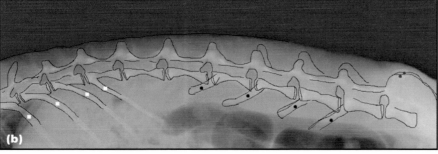

6.2 **(a)** Normal lateral view of the lumbar spine of a 2-year-old neutered male Dwarf Lop rabbit presented with gastrointestinal stasis. **(b)** The alignment of the lumbar transverse processes (black circles), ribs (white squares) and wings of the ilia (red circles) denote correct positioning.

Ventrodorsal view

For the ventrodorsal (VD) view the patient is placed in dorsal recumbency, preferably supported by radiolucent foam wedges or a plastic trough. The limbs may be held in a relaxed position or can be held with equal extension and slight inward rotation with the use of adhesive tape fixed to the cassette or X-ray table. As before, gentle traction on the skull and spine may be utilized with care to reduce rotation and other positioning artefacts. Correctly positioned views should be symmetrical, with centrally positioned spinous processes (Figure 6.3).

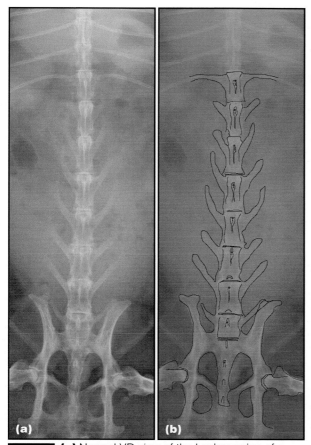

6.3 **(a)** Normal VD view of the lumbar spine of a 2-year-old neutered male Dwarf Lop rabbit presented with gastrointestinal stasis. **(b)** The symmetry and centrally positioned spinous processes (red circles) denote correct positioning.

Myelography

Myelography is generally used to determine whether a bone or disc lesion identified on plain radiographs is causing spinal cord compression, or to identify spinal lesions not identifiable on plain radiographs such as neoplasia, abscesses and degenerative disc disease. The procedure for myelography is described in Technique 3.1.

As with other techniques, familiarity with normal myelographic anatomy is essential in order to interpret a myelogram effectively. The three main locations for pathological abnormalities that may be identified on a myelogram are intramedullary, intradural–extramedullary and extradural. Additionally, contrast medium may enter the spinal cord parenchyma in cases of spinal cord malacia.

A number of significant side effects have been associated with myelography following injection of the contrast agent, including apnoea, seizures, hypotension and paresis/paralysis. In cats, ketamine has been shown to raise intracranial pressure and increase the risk of brain herniation following withdrawal of cerebrospinal fluid (CSF). This may not be the case in rabbits, but it may be wise to avoid ketamine in sedative/anaesthetic combinations during myelography in this species (Chitty, 2007). General anaesthesia is considered essential, and intubation and intravenous access are recommended to reduce and/or treat potential complications that might occur.

A number of different techniques have been described in detail by Whittington and Bennett (2011) and Chitty (2007) and are described further in Chapter 3. Capello et al. (2008) commented that, anecdotally, injection of contrast medium into the cerebellomedullary cistern has resulted in the death of rabbit patients and suggested that there may be an apparent anatomical and/or physical contraindication to this procedure in this species. However, other practitioners have successfully performed this procedure several times without complications (John Chitty, personal communication).

With more advanced imaging techniques such as computed tomography (CT) and magnetic resonance imaging (MRI) becoming more readily available, myelography may become less useful or indeed desirable given the potential side effects associated with the procedure. However, myelography is readily achievable with minimal equipment, expense and experience and still has merit, especially in cases where speed of diagnosis is required, finances are limited, or the owner is unable to travel but still desires a more accurate diagnosis, e.g. cases of suspected spinal cord compression causing hindlimb paresis. In such circumstances a decision on prognosis and treatment may be made promptly with minimal stress to the patient, without the need for extra travel and an additional anaesthetic.

Approach to the paralysed or paretic rabbit

Generally a holistic medical approach to the rabbit patient is advised. Unfortunately poor rabbit husbandry is still common. This, coupled with the rabbit's tendency to hide illness, means that many rabbits presented to the veterinary surgeon will have more than one significant condition requiring attention, e.g. dental disease and degenerative joint disease, spinal disease and urine scald. Furthermore, the stress and/or pain of many conditions often mean that gastrointestinal stasis and/or ulceration are common complications that need to be addressed if a successful outcome is to be expected.

The paralysed or paretic rabbit is typical of these cases. In the early stages of disease rabbits will have, or be at risk of, urine scald, gastrointestinal stasis and pododermatitis. With increasing severity and time, myiasis, urinary tract infections and progression of pododermatitis to osteomyelitis are increasingly common. Systemic diseases such as chronic renal failure, dental disease, malnutrition and hepatic lipidosis may be additional complications.

A suggested diagnostic approach to the paralysed/paretic rabbit is summarized in Figure 6.4. It

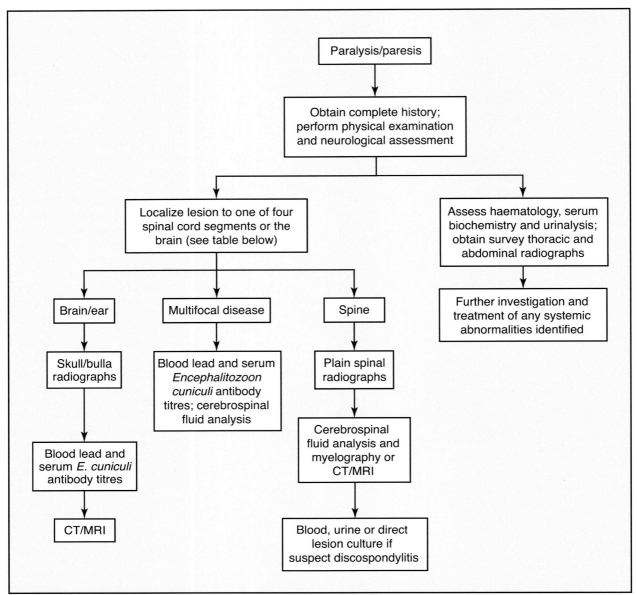

Brain	Spinal cord division			
	Cranial cervical (C1–C5)	*Cervical enlargement (C6–T2)*	*Thoracolumbar (T3–L3)*	*Lumbosacral (L4–Cd)*
UMN signs in all four limbs or fore- and hindlimb on single side; ± cranial nerve deficits; altered mental state; seizures	UMN signs in both forelimb(s) and hindlimb(s)	LMN signs in thoracic limb(s); UMN signs in pelvic limb(s); reduced or absent ipsilateral cutaneous trunci reflex if C8–T1 segment involved	Normal thoracic limbs; UMN signs in pelvic limb(s); reduced or absent cutaneous trunci reflex caudal to the level of the last intact dermatome	Normal thoracic limbs; LMN signs in pelvic limb(s); urinary incontinence; faecal incontinence

6.4 Suggested diagnostic approach to the paralysed/paretic rabbit. LMN = lower motor neuron signs; UMN = upper motor neuron signs.

is ideal to investigate the potential for underlying systemic diseases as thoroughly as possible. Standard nursing protocols should include the provision of warm dry bedding with access to hay *ad libitum*. Great attention should be paid to the removal of oculonasal discharges and soiled/matted fur. Administration of fluids, analgesics, prokinetics and antacids should be routine in most cases.

Normal radiographic anatomy

The vertebral formula of the rabbit is C7–T12–L7–S4–Cd15–Cd16, although variations are relatively common. In a study by Greenaway *et al.* (2001) that evaluated 64 New Zealand White rabbits, 43.8% had 12 thoracic and 7 lumbar vertebrae, 32.8% had 13 thoracic and 6 lumbar vertebrae, and 23.4% had 13 thoracic and 7 lumbar vertebrae.

The lumbar vertebrae of rabbits have several differences from those of other domestic mammals. The first three lumbar vertebrae have a ventral crest. All the lumbar vertebrae have a prominent mammillary process of the cranial articular process, where the powerful lumbar musculature attaches to the vertebral column. Unlike those of other domestic mammals, the dorsal aspect of the lumbar vertebral mammillary process is level with, or slightly ventral to, the spinous process. The first three vertebrae of the sacrum are fused, while the 4th sacral vertebra is fused variably.

Features that can be diagnosed using radiography

Vertebral deformities
Kyphosis (Figure 6.5), lordosis, scoliosis and hemivertebrae are common in pet rabbits. These deformities are often incidental findings but may also be associated with significant disease. Pain and/or reduced mobility secondary to these lesions may result in urine scald, perineal soiling with caecotrophs and reduced ability to groom, which in turn increases the risk of myiasis and acariasis.

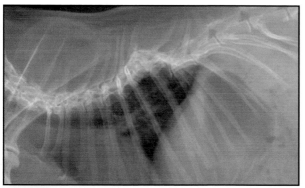

6.5 Kyphosis of the mid-thoracic spine in a 2-year-old neutered female Dwarf Lop rabbit with chronic perineal soiling. Reduced mobility resulting from the kyphosis resulted in caecotroph accumulation around the perineum. The problem was managed by regular shaving of the fur around the perineum, which reduced the accumulation of caecotrophs and allowed easier cleaning by the owner.

Deformities may be congenital but may also occur secondary to poor husbandry and diet. Diets that are low in calcium predispose the rabbit to reduced vertebral bone density. Breeding does kept in small cages that restrict normal movement have been shown to have an increased prevalence of spinal deformity (Drescher and Loeffler, 1996); the increased demand for calcium due to gestation and lactation results in reduced vertebral bone density. Similarly, young growing rabbits fed on cereal mixes may develop nutritional secondary hyperparathyroidism, resulting in generalized demineralization of the skeleton.

Spondylosis
Spondylosis (Figure 6.6) is common in middle-aged and older rabbits and may occur anywhere along

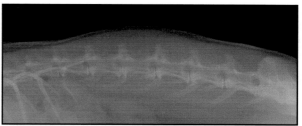

6.6 Lumbar vertebral spondylosis in a Dwarf Lop rabbit with a history of reluctance to exercise and obesity. There were no neurological deficits and there was no evidence of spinal pain. A calorie-controlled diet was advised, consisting of predominantly hay with an eggcupful of pellet diet daily. Free exercise and foraging were encouraged.

the length of the spinal column. Clinical signs, if present, result from reduced flexibility of the spine and/or discomfort and are similar to those described for vertebral abnormalities.

Discospondylitis
In dogs, discospondylitis is thought to occur most commonly secondary to haematogenous spread of bacteria or fungi; sources of infection include migrating foreign bodies (grass awns), bacterial endocarditis, and dental and urinary tract infections (LeCouteur and Grandy, 2000). Given the apparent relatively high incidence of dental and urinary tract infections in rabbits, and their access to hay which often contains awns, it is perhaps surprising that discospondylitis appears to be rare in rabbits. This may simply reflect under-diagnosis, again due to the rabbit's tendency to mask pain and the difficulty in obtaining a definitive diagnosis of the condition.

In dogs, typical radiographic signs are destruction of the bone endplates adjacent to an infected disc, collapse of the intervertebral disc and varying degrees of new bone formation; similar signs would be expected in affected rabbits (Figure 6.7). Supporting evidence for discospondylitis may include increases in CSF white cell counts and protein levels, and/or positive urine, blood or

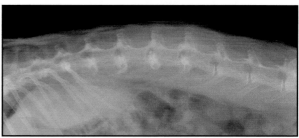

6.7 Discospondylitis in a 7-year-old neutered male rabbit with a recent history of sudden-onset severe depression, lethargy and anorexia. Physical examination revealed hindlimb paresis, lumbar pain and a doughy abdomen. Abnormalities on the radiograph include collapse of the intervertebral disc spaces and osteosclerosis of the vertebral endplates from T12–T13 through to L3–L4. Calcified disc material is visible in the L2–L3 intervertebral foramen. There is also gas dilation of the gastrointestinal tract. The owner declined further investigation and elected for euthanasia.

CSF cultures. The use of CT/MRI and surgical exploration to obtain samples for culture and cytology may be required in selected cases to obtain a definitive diagnosis.

Intervertebral disc disease

In the laboratory rabbit, intervertebral disc disease (IVDD) would appear to be relatively common; Green *et al.* (1984) performed post-mortem examinations of the spines of 35 laboratory rabbits ranging in age from 3 months to 8.5 years. They observed degenerative changes of the intervertebral disc (IVD) in individuals as young as 3 months and vertebral spondylosis in animals from 24 months of age, which suggests that at least subclinical disc disease may occur frequently in pet rabbits.

Clinical reports of IVDD are rare in the rabbit, though this may reflect under-diagnosis. Smith Baxter (1975) described two cases of disc protrusion and extrusion of nuclear material in pet rabbits, associated with posterior paralysis and urinary and faecal incontinence. Both cases appeared to result from hyperflexion of the spine and resulted in compression of the spinal cord. Both rabbits were euthanased after failing to respond to corticosteroids.

Clinically, IVDD may be demonstrated by radiopacity of the intervertebral disc space (IVDS) with or without the presence of mineral opacities in the intervertebral foramen and/or narrowing of the IVDS (see Figure 6.7). Spinal cord compression may be confirmed by myelography (Figure 6.8), CT or MRI.

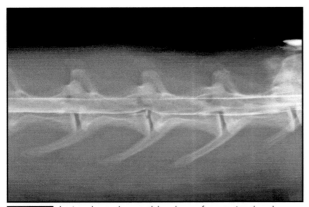

6.8 Lateral myelographic view of an extradural compression on the ventral aspect of the spinal cord at the L4–L5 intervertebral disc interspace of a rabbit that had sustained a fracture of the vertebral endplate of the 4th lumbar vertebra. (Courtesy of Frances Harcourt-Brown)

Forelimb neuropathy

Forelimb neuropathy in a rabbit was attributed to lateralized intervertebral disc protrusion (John Chitty, personal communication). The affected individual presented with an abducted forelimb and triceps muscle wastage associated with spondylitic lesions at T1–T2 and T3–T4 (Figure 6.9).

Muscle wastage and cutaneous sensitivity can be used to localize the lesion. It appears that the order of nerve emergence from the brachial and

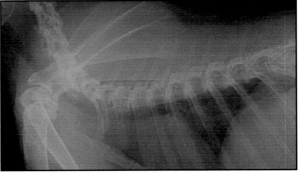

6.9 Radiograph of a 6-year-old giant-breed rabbit presenting with the right forelimb extended laterally at a 45-degree angle from the body. Wastage of the triceps musculature was noted; the left forelimb was also affected but to a much lesser extent. There is spondylosis evident at T1–T2 and T2–T3. (© John Chitty)

lumbosacral plexuses and the muscles innervated are similar to those in dogs. Survey spinal radiographs in such cases may demonstrate IVDD, enlarged intervertebral foramina in cases of peripheral nerve sheath tumours, or lytic changes indicative of other neoplasms or infection.

Fractures and luxations

The most common site of vertebral fracture or luxation is in the lumbosacral region (L6–L7). Injuries are most frequently caused by improper restraint (Figure 6.10). In some cases the injury may occur when a rabbit is not being handled but is attempting to flee a perceived or actual danger. Such cases may be presented having been found by the owner with acute hindlimb paresis or paralysis with no history of trauma or handling.

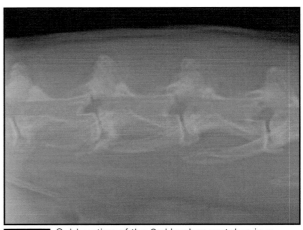

6.10 Subluxation of the 3rd lumbar vertebra in a 5-year-old crossbreed neutered female rabbit with a history of hindlimb paresis following a recent fall from its hutch. The clinical signs improved following treatment with oral meloxicam.

Spinal injuries resulting from dog (Figure 6.11) or fox bites, falls and entrapment under furniture, and/or being trodden on by owners, are also relatively common in pet rabbits, whilst gunshot injuries and road traffic collisions are common in wild or stray rabbits.

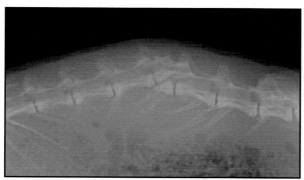

6.11 Vertebral body fracture (L4) in a 1-year-old entire female Dutch rabbit with a recent history of dog attack. The rabbit presented with acute-onset hindlimb paralysis with no deep pain sensation. The rabbit was euthanased.

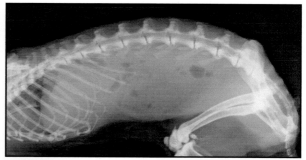

6.12 Marked generalized osteosclerosis of the axial and appendicular skeleton of a 6-year-old entire male Dwarf Lop rabbit with chronic renal failure. The rabbit was presented because of forelimb pain and polydipsia. Note also the calcified aorta, which is a common feature in chronic renal failure.

Injuries are usually readily identified on plain survey radiographs but some cases are subtle, and myelography or more advanced imaging such as CT/MRI may be required to identify lesions and, more importantly, to assess spinal cord trauma. Luxation may be transient following a traumatic event and radiographic signs may be subtle despite significant injury and spinal cord trauma.

Excess mineralization

Chronic renal failure in rabbits can lead to hypercalcaemia as a result of impaired excretion of calcium by the kidney in the face of continued calcium absorption from the intestine (Harcourt-Brown, 2007). Excess calcium may subsequently be deposited in the skeleton (osteosclerosis) and soft tissue, resulting in excess mineralization of these structures which is readily appreciable on radiographs (Figure 6.12). Nephroliths and aortic calcification may be identifiable on survey spinal radiographs. This is in contrast to dogs and cats, in which chronic renal failure is more likely to cause mineral loss from the axial skeleton as a result of renal secondary hyperparathyroidism. Hypervitaminosis D may cause identical lesions.

Owing to the generalized nature of the skeletal changes, and particularly in the early stages of disease, excess mineralization is easily overlooked. Reference to a normal rabbit radiograph is invaluable for comparison and, ideally, a prepared bone or bones may be placed alongside the patient during radiography for comparison. This helps to minimize the effect of inadequate exposure and/or faults in developing the film.

Neoplasia

Primary neoplasia of the spinal column appears to be rare; however, with the increasing age of the pet rabbit population and owners seeking more proactive veterinary investigations and treatment, it would seem likely that more cases of spinal neoplasia will be reported in the future. Published cases include osteosarcoma (Weiss and Müller, 2011) and lymphoma (Reed *et al.*, 2009). Metastatic neoplasia is possible and is most likely to be associated with uterine adenocarcinoma.

References and further reading

Capello V, Lennox AM and Widmer WR (2008) The basics of radiology (contrast radiography). In: *Clinical Radiology of Exotic Companion Mammals*, ed. WR Widmer, pp. 40–42. Wiley-Blackwell, Ames, IA

Chitty J (2007) Clinical techniques: the subarachnoid space, its clinical relevance in rabbits. *Journal of Exotic Pet Medicine* **16**, 179–182

Drescher B and Loeffler K (1996) Scoliosis, lordosis and kyphosis in breeding rabbits. *Tierärztliche Praxis* **24**, 292–300

Green PW, Fox RR and Sokoloff L (1984) Spontaneous degenerative spinal disease in the laboratory rabbit. *Journal of Orthopaedic Research* **2**, 161–168

Greenaway J, Partlow G, Gonsholt N *et al.* (2001) Anatomy of the lumbosacral spinal cord in rabbits. *Journal of the American Animal Hospital Association* **37**, 27–34

Harcourt-Brown FM (2007) Radiographic signs of renal disease in rabbits. *Veterinary Record* **160**, 787–794

LeCouteur RA and Grandy JL (2000) Diseases of the spinal cord. In: *Textbook of Veterinary Internal Medicine, 5th edn*, ed. SJ Ettinger, pp. 608–656. WB Saunders, Philadelphia

Reed SD, Shaw S and Evans DE (2009) Spinal lymphoma and pulmonary filariasis in a pet domestic rabbit (*Oryctolagus cuniculus domesticus*). *Journal of Veterinary Diagnostic Investigation* **21**, 253–256

Smith Baxter J (1975) Posterior paralysis in the rabbit. *Journal of Small Animal Practice* **16**, 267–271

Weiss ATA and Müller K (2011) Spinal osteolytic osteosarcoma in a pet rabbit. *Veterinary Record* **168**, 266

Whittington JK and Bennett RA (2011) Clinical technique: myelography in rabbits. *Journal of Exotic Pet Medicine* **20**, 217–221

7

Radiographic interpretation of the abdomen

Angela M. Lennox

Many indications for abdominal radiography in the rabbit are similar to those in other species, and can be inferred from history (e.g. straining to urinate, haematuria), physical examination findings (e.g. abdominal pain, palpable gas accumulation, abdominal masses) or other supportive laboratory diagnostics (e.g. biochemistry, urinalysis). Owing to the high incidence of gastrointestinal (GI) disease in rabbits, abdominal radiography is an important part of the initial diagnostic plan for any rabbit with decreased appetite or anorexia. In rabbits with GI disease, serial radiographs are critical for monitoring response to therapy. Radiographs of the normal abdomen are shown in Figure 7.1.

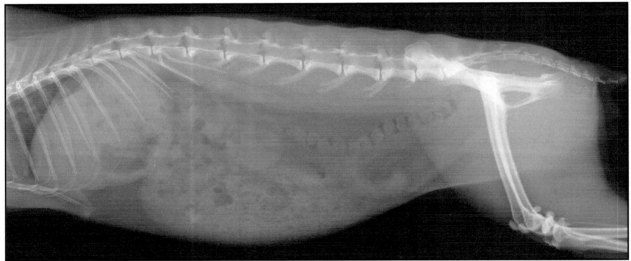

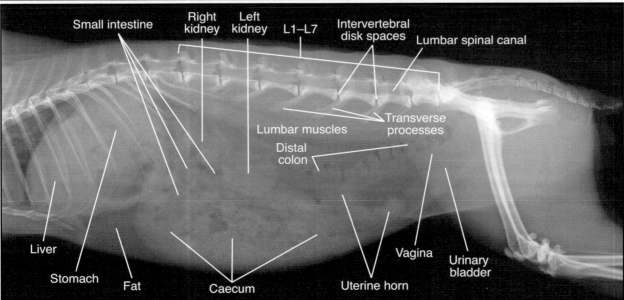

7.1 Lateral and VD views of the abdomen of a normal 1.4 kg intact female rabbit. (Reprinted from Capello and Lennox (2008) with permission of John Wiley & Sons) (continues) ▶

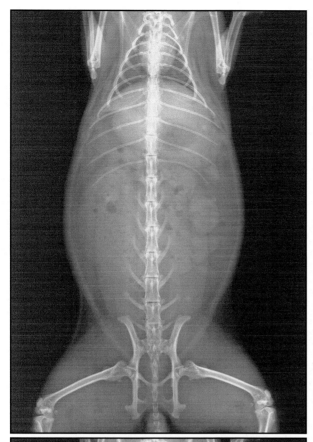

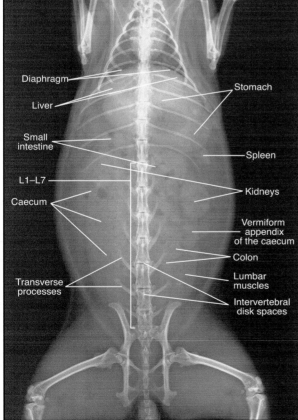

7.1 (continued) Lateral and VD views of the abdomen of a normal 1.4 kg intact female rabbit. (Reprinted from Capello and Lennox (2008) with permission of John Wiley & Sons)

Labels (VD view): Diaphragm; Liver; Small intestine; L1–L7; Caecum; Transverse processes; Stomach; Spleen; Kidneys; Vermiform appendix of the caecum; Colon; Lumbar muscles; Intervertebral disk spaces

Radiographic techniques

Techniques for radiography of the rabbit are reported in detail elsewhere (see Chapters 3 and 14 and Capello and Lennox, 2008). The increased interest in computed (digital) radiography (Figure 7.2) has implications for abdominal radiography. Traditional analogue radiographs must be optimal for proper diagnosis; both over- and underexposure carry risks of incomplete or inaccurate diagnosis. Similarly, errors of diagnosis can occur with digital radiography, in particular with improper scanner setting and adjustment of the greyscale (Figure 7.3).

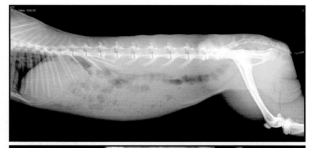

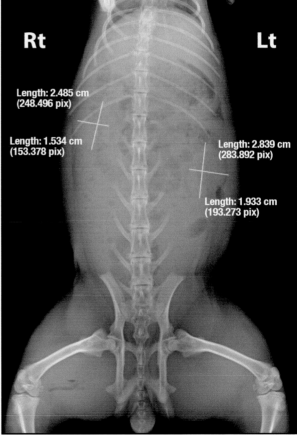

Rt   Lt

Length: 2.485 cm
(248.496 pix)

Length: 1.534 cm
(153.378 pix)

Length: 2.839 cm
(283.892 pix)

Length: 1.933 cm
(193.273 pix)

7.2 Computed (digital) radiography was used to produce lateral and VD views of the abdomen of a normal 1.4 kg intact male rabbit. Note the differences in contrast and greyscale compared with traditional film images. DICOM (digital imaging and communications in medicine) viewers allow measurement of organ size; in this rabbit the right kidney is 2.5 × 1.5 cm, and the left kidney is 2.8 × 1.9 cm. (Courtesy of Vittorio Capello)

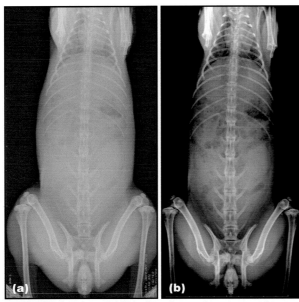

7.3 Computed (digital) radiography was used to obtain a DV radiograph of the rabbit shown in Figure 7.2. This position is suboptimal because the pelvic limbs are not extended as in the VD view. However, this technique is useful for monitoring changes in the GI tract. In this case, the rabbit is healthy. Note that **(a)** and **(b)** show the same radiograph, before and after adjustment of the greyscale. Correct computer processing of digital images is important and can greatly affect visualization and diagnosis. (Courtesy of Vittorio Capello)

Restraint

In most cases, sedation or general anaesthesia is required to reduce patient stress and to obtain ideal positioning for optimal radiographs. However, sedation or anaesthesia may be risky in debilitated patients, or for those undergoing multiple radiographic procedures. A useful technique for rabbits requiring repeated views of the GI tract is simple positioning on the radiographic plate without restraint. Lateral radiographs can be obtained by placing the rabbit in lateral recumbency with a sandbag across the neck (see Chapter 14). For a dorsoventral (DV) view, depending on the temperament of the patient, the pelvic limbs may be positioned normally or in a 'frog-leg' position (Figure 7.4). The disadvantage of this technique is superimposition of the limbs, and it is observed that this position produces a more narrow or compressed view of the abdomen; however, visualization of stomach size and gas patterns is not negatively affected.

For extremely debilitated animals for which sedation or general anaesthesia may be risky, manual restraint with the use of proper radiographic protection equipment may be indicated. Use of sedatives and anaesthetics must be selected with consideration of the temperament and overall condition of the patient (see Chapter 1).

Positioning and views

Proper positioning and symmetry are extremely important for most views, with the exception of oblique or other specialized positions, which are seldom indicated for radiography of the abdomen.

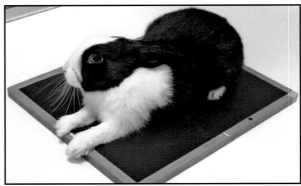

7.4 Depending on temperament or level of debilitation of the rabbit, dorsoventral radiographs of the abdomen may be obtained without restraint. While positioning is not ideal, evaluation of the GI tract is possible. (Courtesy of Vittorio Capello)

An indication for an oblique view of the abdomen is visualization of both ureters in the lateral view during contrast urography. In most cases, ideal positioning requires extension of the limbs to avoid superimposition over abdominal structures. Radiographs should always be taken in at least two views, lateral and standard ventrodorsal (VD), or, in situations where dorsal recumbency is considered risky, a DV projection may be considered. Other than organ position, the DV view does not significantly change the radiographic anatomy of the abdomen.

Care must be taken to include all of the targeted area in the radiographic view. The abdomen of the rabbit is relatively large when compared with the smaller thorax. Errors of omission occur when the entire abdomen is not imaged.

> **PRACTICAL TIP**
> The entire perineum should be included in abdominal radiographs of the rabbit. While this is not technically in the abdomen, distal urethral uroliths can be missed when the perineum is not included within the radiographic view.

Interpretation

Before beginning, it is important to ascertain whether the radiograph is of diagnostic quality in regard to radiographic technique (contrast, greyscale) and positioning. Each radiograph should be evaluated in a systematic manner, from cranial to caudal.

For the lateral radiograph, the following topographical areas should be observed:

- The hypochondrial area, including liver, diaphragm and stomach
- The dorsal and retroperitoneal area (kidneys and ureters)
- The middle/ventral abdominal area (small intestine, caecum)
- The caudal abdominal area, from dorsal to ventral (colon, vagina and uterus in the female, urinary bladder)
- The perineal area (distal urethra).

The VD projection is similarly evaluated, observing both single and paired structures:

- The liver and diaphragm
- The stomach on the left side, and the pylorus with the proximal duodenum on the right side
- The more cranial right kidney and more caudal left kidney
- The caecum on both sides of the abdomen, but mostly on the right
- The ureters and the urinary bladder; note that the vagina and uterus are not usually visible on the VD view unless they are enlarged
- The perineal area.

Owing to the variation in size of pet rabbits (800 g to >5 kg), production of reference ranges for organ size is not practical. Some generalizations can be made, however, and are included below.

Normal radiographic anatomy

The GI tract occupies the great majority of the abdominal cavity, and often obscures most other abdominal structures (see Figure 7.1). Unlike those of carnivorous species, the GI tract of the rabbit is never empty. Normal GI anatomy is extremely variable and depends upon the current phase of digestion and the amount of food in the stomach and in the caecum, which when full is the largest portion of the digestive tract (see Chapter 14). Food content in the normal rabbit has a mottled appearance on radiographs, with small interspersed pockets of gas.

The stomach is oval in both lateral and VD views, and is located caudal to the liver, mostly in the left quadrant, with the pylorus extending to the right quadrant. The stomach may appear more rounded after a large meal, and the caudal border may extend slightly beyond the costal arch. There are always at least some ingesta in the stomach, which may be mixed with small pockets of gas. On the VD view, the stomach is asymmetrical, with the largest curvature on the left side. Grooming results in normal ingestion of hair, and some hair is always found in the stomach of the rabbit. Normal hair in the stomach is not distinguishable from food contents. The stomach is relatively small compared to the rest of the GI tract.

The small intestine also contains digesta, and gas is usually evenly dispersed. The caecum may be partially or completely filled, and when full it occupies the majority of the abdomen. Larger pockets of gas may intermittently appear in the intestines of the normal rabbit.

The rectum may contain faecal material that takes on the characteristic shape of hard round faecal pellets.

The diaphragm can usually be viewed in its entirety, especially on the VD view; the stomach may obscure it on the lateral view. The liver is cranial to the stomach, and is mostly contained within the ribs in the normal animal (see Figure 7.1); the stomach is superimposed on the liver.

The kidneys are often visible, the right kidney just caudal to the last rib and the left more caudal

than the right, as in other mammalian species. In some cases a full caecum may make visualization difficult. The shape of the kidney is similar to that of dogs and cats. Its length is approximately 2–2.5 rib spaces, and the width is approximately 2 rib spaces. The left kidney is more ventral on the lateral view (see Figure 7.1).

The bladder may be visible, especially when it contains mineral-dense urine. In the intact female, reflux of urine from the bladder to the large vagina is normal; therefore, the vagina may appear as a second 'bladder' distinct from the actual urinary bladder. The ureters and urethra are generally not visible, but their location can be inferred from the presence of uroliths. The female reproductive tract is difficult to discern in the normal animal.

In extremely obese animals, abdominal and retroperitoneal fat may be seen displacing the kidneys and intestines cranially (Figure 7.5).

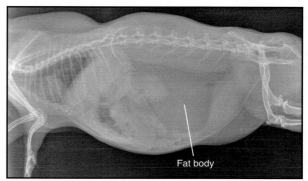

7.5 Lateral view of an obese rabbit, demonstrating cranial displacement of most of the GI tract by abdominal fat. (© John Chitty)

Specific conditions

Gastrointestinal tract

Contrast radiography is not commonly described in rabbits, but is discussed in Chapter 3. Its usefulness is limited because, in contrast to carnivores, it is impossible to achieve an empty or nearly empty GI tract in the rabbit. Potential benefits may include the identification of hernias, or space-occupying lesions displacing the contrast-filled GI tract.

Gastrointestinal stasis

Gastrointestinal stasis is defined as impaired flow of ingesta, and can include any portion of the GI tract. The term rabbit gastrointestinal syndrome (RGIS) has been proposed to define this complex group of signs and pathological conditions, which can include gastric and intestinal impaction, gas accumulation and obstruction. Other disease processes can have a direct impact on the GI tract, including pancreatitis, reproductive disease and hepatic disease (Lichtenberger and Lennox, 2010). GI stasis is discussed in more detail in Chapter 14.

Radiography is the single most important test for evaluation of the GI tract, and for monitoring the response to therapy. Serial radiography is important for patients with GI disease.

Identification of the true surgical patient is difficult. Some authors advocate early surgical intervention for any rabbit with evidence of obstruction, for example marked depression, extreme stomach dilation, hyperglycaemia and suggestive radiographic findings (Harcourt-Brown FM, 2007; Harcourt-Brown TR, 2007) while others note that many rabbits, including those with evidence of obstruction, respond well to aggressive supportive therapy. The outcome of treatment may depend on whether the patient has an intermittent obstruction or moving foreign body (see Chapter 14). When supportive therapy is chosen, overall patient condition is monitored carefully, along with repeated radiographs, taken every 2–3 hours initially. Both are key to assessing the progress of the condition. Radiographic evidence of deterioration includes increasing stomach size and gas accumulation, while evidence of improvement may include

decreasing stomach size and distribution of gas accumulation (Figures 7.6 and 7.7). Radiographs are taken less frequently, up to every 24 hours, in more stable patients.

Conditions of the stomach

While the stomach of the rabbit always contains at least some food, a filled or overfilled stomach in the presence of anorexia must be considered abnormal. Even in the anorexic patient, the stomach often continues to fill with fluid from gastric secretions and with gas. The abnormal stomach begins to take on a more filled or rounded shape as the contents accumulate. The completely distended stomach is round and very large, compressing the diaphragm (see Figure 7.6a). Other contents may include foreign material, which may appear as irregular radiopaque densities. Ingestion and accumulation of foreign

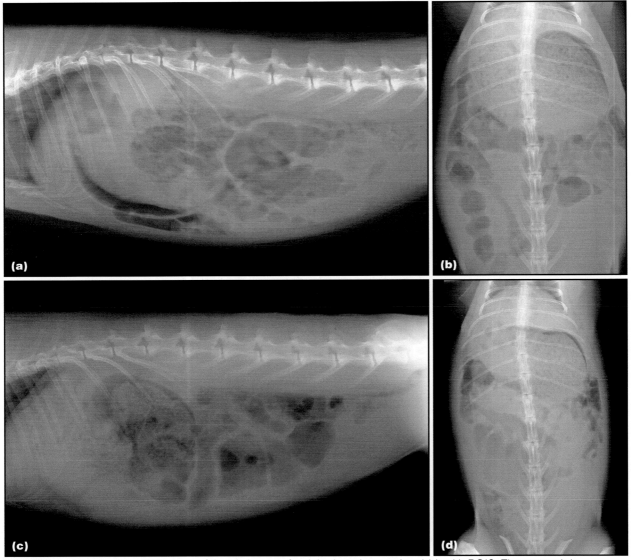

7.6 **(a,b)** Lateral and VD views of the abdomen of a dehydrated anorexic rabbit with RGIS. The stomach is enlarged, filled with ingesta and rounded in appearance. There is evidence of intestinal and caecal gas. **(c,d)** The same rabbit 2 hours after initiation of treatment, which included analgesics and intravenous fluid administration. The clinical condition had not deteriorated. A slight reduction in size of the stomach indicates that the condition is not worsening, and surgical intervention is probably not indicated. The rabbit went on to recover fully; the cause of the RGIS was unknown. (© Angela Lennox)

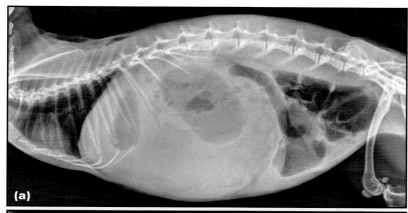

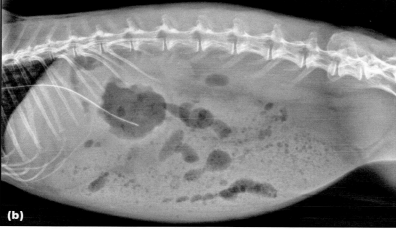

7.7 **(a)** Lateral view of the abdomen of a depressed, anorexic and dehydrated rabbit with severe gastric and caecal gas accumulation. The stomach is very large and round in appearance, and displaces the gas-filled caecum caudally. **(b)** Lateral radiograph of the same rabbit 8 hours after medical treatment, which included intravenous fluid administration, analgesia and administration of food via a nasogastric tube (visible in the radiograph). The severity of the initial condition suggested that surgical intervention might have been warranted, but this was declined by the owner. The rabbit went on to recover fully with medical therapy alone. (Reprinted from *Veterinary Clinics of North America: Exotic Pet Practice* **13**(3), 2010, with permission of Elsevier)

bodies in the stomach is relatively rare in the rabbit, but may include carpet fibres, paper, cat litter or other material (Harcourt-Brown, 2002a). Abnormal accumulations of hair in the stomach can occur, but these are impossible to identify radiographically.

Conditions of the intestines

The most common radiographic intestinal abnormality is gas accumulation, which eventually occurs in all cases of intestinal stasis. Gas may appear in large pockets in any part of the intestines, and in severe cases portions may be completely filled with gas (see Figures 7.6 and 7.7). Intestinal obstruction occurs most commonly at the proximal duodenum and, in the author's experience, less frequently at the ileocolic junction (Harcourt-Brown FM, 2007). Rabbits with partial to complete intestinal obstruction may demonstrate typical radiographic findings, including a rounded stomach filled with fluid and gas, with an intestinal gas pattern ending abruptly at the site of the obstruction. In some cases, gas may appear both proximal and distal to the site of obstruction, probably as a result of an obstructive accumulation of gas and of accumulation due to secondary functional ileus. Foreign material in the intestines may appear as radiopaque densities. Intestinal masses are more difficult to identify; some neoplasms may produce mineralization, which aids identification (Figure 7.8a,b).

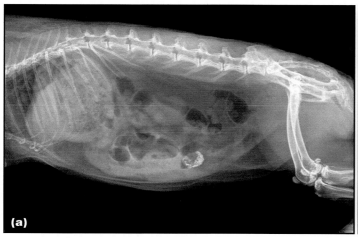

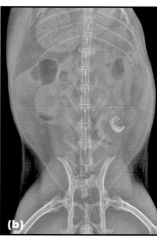

7.8

(a,b) Lateral and DV views of the abdomen, demonstrating a mineralized density that was identified as a calcified necrotic lipoma and was successfully removed at surgery. (a,b © John Chitty) (continues) ▶

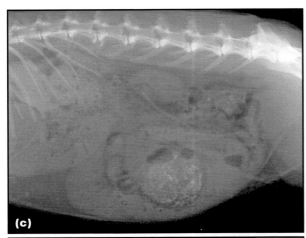

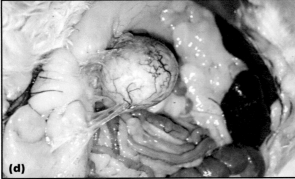

7.8 (continued) **(c)** Lateral view of the abdomen of a different rabbit, showing a larger mineralized mass. This was identified as an abscess and removed surgically **(d)**. (c,d courtesy of Frances Harcourt-Brown)

Conditions of the caecum

The caecum normally varies greatly in size, but when identified it contains mottled food material. Material resembling clumps or with irregular density is always abnormal. The abnormal caecum may become impacted (Figure 7.9), with irregular radiopaque densities, or contain larger abnormal pockets of gas. The gas-distended caecum is easily identified by the presence of clearly visible sacculations.

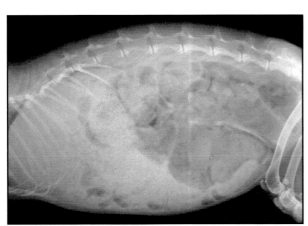

7.9 Lateral view of the abdomen of a rabbit with caecal impaction. Note the accumulation of round dense material of variable size in the enlarged caecum, which occupies most of the abdomen. (© Angela Lennox)

Conditions of the liver

Hepatic torsion has been described in the rabbit, but the radiographic findings are non-specific. In most cases, such rabbits present anorexic and depressed, and the radiographic findings suggest secondary RGIS (Starke *et al.*, 2011). Depending on its degree, hepatic enlargement can be identified radiographically and the liver may displace the stomach caudally. Some hepatic diseases may produce mineralization, for example some hepatic neoplasms or cysts (Figure 7.10).

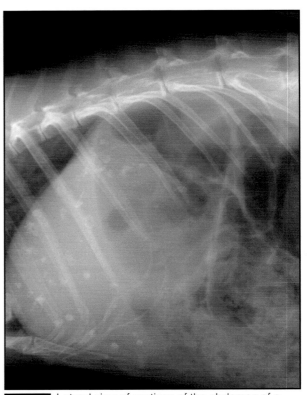

7.10 Lateral view of portions of the abdomen of a female rabbit. Note the multiple focal mineralized lesions associated with the liver. These lesions have been described in other rabbits following hepatic coccidiosis. They were an incidental finding. (Courtesy of Frances Harcourt-Brown)

Urinary tract

Urolithiasis

Urolithiasis is common in rabbits and uroliths can appear anywhere from the kidneys (unilateral or bilateral) to the distal urethra. Uroliths vary in number, density, size, shape and location (Figure 7.11). Uroliths can be located in the very distal urethra in both male and female rabbits, and can be missed if the radiographic view does not include the entire perineum of the patient. It is a common error to focus on large, easily identified uroliths in the bladder and to miss smaller, less obvious uroliths in the kidneys or ureters, which carry a more guarded prognosis. It should also be noted that mineral in the GI tract can obscure, or be mistaken for, urolithiasis; in this case, serial radiographs are used to identify repeatable lesions.

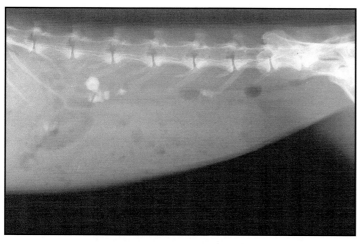
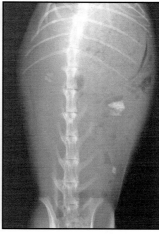

7.11

Bilateral nephrolithiasis and unilateral (left) ureterolithiasis in a dehydrated 5-year-old female rabbit. Both views are essential for localization of the uroliths. Further diagnostic imaging would include ultrasonography and contrast urography. (Courtesy of Vittorio Capello)

The presence of mineral in the bladder of male rabbits, and in the bladder (Figure 7.12) and possibly vagina of female rabbits, is common. Normal mineral accumulation can be mild to moderate, and it can appear and disappear with serial radiographs as the rabbit voids. Abnormal, dense mineral accumulation is often referred to as hypercalciuria, or 'sludge', and is thought to be a result of incomplete voiding (liquid urine is expelled leaving heavier mineral in the bladder) and gradual accumulation over time (see Chapter 15). Sludge can be very dense, persistent and often palpable. Rabbits with abnormal accumulations of sludge often present with clinical signs (frequent urination, dysuria, discomfort, urine scalding; Harcourt-Brown, 2002b). In some cases, chronic accumulation produces marked enlargement of the bladder (Figure 7.13); in others, mineral is so dense it can be difficult to distinguish from a solid urolith. Figure 7.14 shows a female rabbit with dense hypercalciuria and multiple uroliths in the bladder.

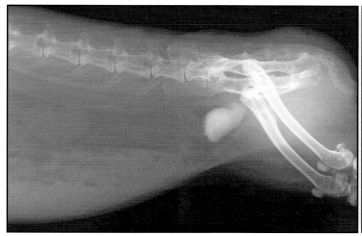
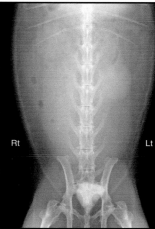

7.12

Lateral and VD views of the abdomen of a female rabbit with hypercalciuria. Note the accumulation of radiodense material in the bladder. (© Angela Lennox)

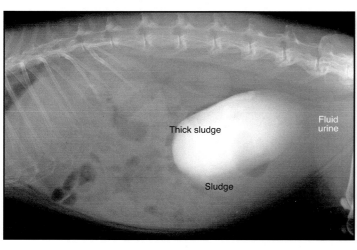
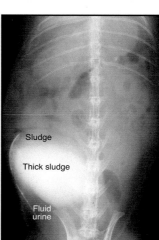

7.13

Lateral and VD views of a 9-year-old spayed female rabbit with chronic hypercalciuria. Note the abnormal dilation of the bladder, and accumulations of urine and sludge of varying densities. (© Angela Lennox)

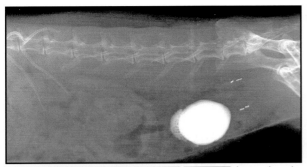

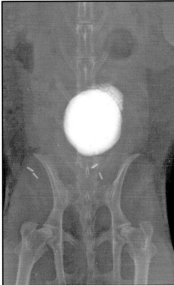

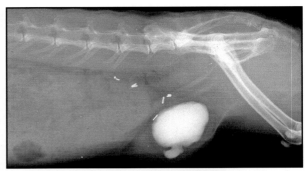

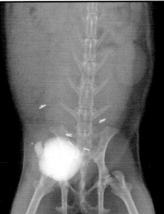

7.14 Lateral and VD views of the abdomen of a female rabbit with multiple cystoliths, including one very large and multiple small stones. The metal densities are haemostatic clips placed on the ovarian pedicles during ovariovaginectomy (OVV). In this animal, OVV was performed at a young age, before enlargement of the uterus; therefore, the haemoclips appear further caudally than expected. (© Angela Lennox)

7.15 Lateral and VD views of a 9-year-old female rabbit with hypercalciuria and inguinal herniation of the urinary bladder. The bladder was readily palpable under the skin in the inguinal region, and gentle palpation caused expression of urine. The presence of mineral helped to localize the urinary bladder outside the margin of the peritoneal cavity on the lateral view. (© Angela Lennox)

Bladder rupture

Herniation of the bladder has been described in both male and female rabbits. In all cases, the bladder was palpable subcutaneously in the inguinal region, and gentle palpation resulted in expression of urine. In some patients, the presence of mineral in the urine supports the diagnosis, because the bladder can be easily identified outside the peritoneal wall (Figure 7.15). In the author's case and a single published case, surgical repair was successful.

Abdominal masses

In rabbits with uterine disease, the uterus may appear as a space-occupying mass ventral to the colon and dorsal to the bladder (Figure 7.16). Depending on its size and shape, it may cause cranial displacement of the intestines, and/or dorsal displacement of the colon. Some uterine neoplasms contain areas of mineralization, producing easily identified radiodensities (Figure 7.17). Uterine neoplasia can undergo metastasis, especially to the lungs. Local abdominal metastasis may be more difficult to identify radiographically. In cases of uterine neoplasia without metastasis, ovariohysterectomy is the treatment of choice.

Pregnancy

Fetuses may not be identifiable in the abdomen of the rabbit until ossification appears between days 18 and 23. Diastasis of the ischiopubic symphysis does not occur in this species.

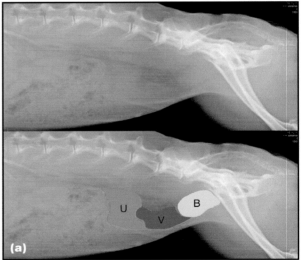

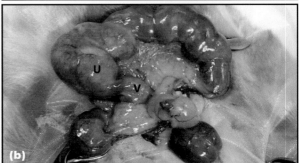

7.16 **(a)** Lateral view of the abdomen of an intact female rabbit. Note the bladder (B), vagina (V) and portions of an enlarged, abnormal uterus (U). **(b)** At surgery, the vagina (V) can be seen in relation to the uterus (U). The urinary bladder is not visible in this image. (Courtesy of Vittorio Capello)

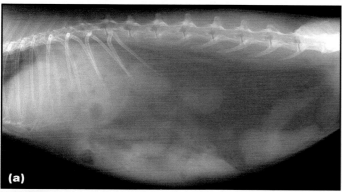

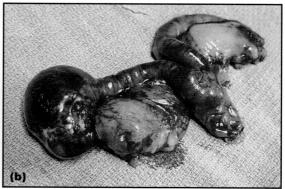

7.17 **(a)** Lateral view of the abdomen of an intact female rabbit with a palpable mass in the caudoventral abdomen, and vaginal bleeding. Note the presence of a soft tissue mass with fine mineralization correlating with the palpation findings, and consistent with a uterine mass. **(b)** Uterine mass excised at surgery. (© Angela Lennox)

References and further reading

Capello V and Lennox A (2008) *Clinical Radiology of Exotic Companion Mammals*. Wiley-Blackwell, Ames, IA

Harcourt-Brown F (2002a) Digestive disorders. In: *Textbook of Rabbit Medicine*, pp. 249–291. Butterworth Heinemann, Oxford

Harcourt-Brown F (2002b) Urogenital diseases. In: *Textbook of Rabbit Medicine*, pp. 335–351. Butterworth Heinemann, Oxford

Harcourt-Brown FM (2007) Gastric dilation and intestinal obstruction in 76 rabbits. *Veterinary Record* **161**(12), 409–41

Harcourt-Brown TR (2007) Management of acute gastric dilation in rabbits. *Journal of Exotic Pet Medicine* **16**, 168–174

Lichtenberger M and Lennox A (2010) Updates and advanced therapies for gastrointestinal stasis in rabbits. *Veterinary Clinics of North America: Exotic Pet Practice* **13**(3), 525–541

Silverman S and Tell LA (2005) *Radiology of Rodents, Rabbits, and Ferrets: An Atlas of Normal Anatomy and Positioning*. Elsevier, St. Louis

Starke NJ, Graham JE, Orcutt CJ *et al.* (2011) Successful outcome of hepatectomy as treatment for liver lobe torsion in four domestic rabbits. *Journal of the American Veterinary Medical Association* **238**, 1176–1183

8

Ultrasonography

Sharon Redrobe

The rabbit ultrasonographer is faced with a number of difficulties. There are few reference data regarding the normal and abnormal ultrasonographic anatomy of this species and also relatively few individuals who are familiar with both ultrasonography and the veterinary aspects of the rabbit patient. The basic terminology of ultrasonography needs to be grasped (Figure 8.1), and the differentiation of 'real' images from artefacts (Figure 8.2) needs to be understood in order to maximize the potential of this useful diagnostic technique. Artefacts can occur as a result of incorrect transducer positioning and machine settings, as well as for the reasons outlined in Figure 8.2; therefore good technique and an understanding of the workings of the ultrasound machine in use is essential. Artefacts and over-diagnosis are common in rabbit ultrasonography. It is vital therefore that the ultrasonographer is familiar with both the normal anatomy of the rabbit and the basic practice of ultrasonography. Interpretation of the ultrasound image requires knowledge of where the probe was placed on the animal; moving images are more easily interpreted than still images. This makes forming a second opinion of ultrasonographic findings difficult. Radiography is a much more familiar imaging technique to most clinicians and the images, once taken, can be read by others.

Term	Explanation
Anechoic	An anechoic structure does not produce any internal echoes and thus appears black
Attenuation	The ultrasound beam undergoes a progressive weakening as it penetrates the body, owing to absorption, scattering and beam spread. The amount of weakening is dependent on frequency, tissue density and the number and types of interfaces
B-mode	Brightness modulation: a two-dimensional display. The A-mode spikes are electronically converted into dots and displayed at the correct depth from the transducer
Complex	Refers to a mass that has both fluid-filled and solid areas within it
Enhancement (acoustic)	Sound is not weakened (attenuated) as it passes through a fluid-filled structure and therefore the structure behind appears to have more echoes than the same tissue beside it
Frequency	The number of complete cycles per second (Hertz)
Gain	The amount of amplification of the returning echoes
Homogeneous	Of uniform appearance and texture
Hyperechoic	A relative term used to describe a structure that has greater brightness relative to an adjacent structure
Hypoechoic	A relative term used to describe an area that has lower brightness relative to an adjacent structure
Interface	Strong echoes delineate the boundary of organs, caused by the difference between the acoustic impedance of the two adjacent structures. An interface is usually more pronounced when the transducer is perpendicular to it
M-mode	The motion mode, displaying moving structures along a single line in the ultrasound beam
Noise	An artefact that is usually caused by the gain control being too high
Shadowing	Failure of the sound beam to pass through an object, e.g. a bone does not allow any sound to pass through it and there is only shadowing seen behind it

8.1 Ultrasonography terminology.

Artefact	Cause
Enhancement	Increase in brightness caused by reflections behind a poorly attenuating structure, e.g. masses, cysts
Reverberation	Multiple reflections caused by a strong echo bouncing back and forth between transducer and tissue. Common in bladder and heart
Shadowing	Blocking of the sound wave by strong reflectors or attenuating material, e.g. gas, bone
Speckle	Interference caused by scattering within a tissue, causing a granular appearance

8.2 Common ultrasonography artefacts and their causes.

Equipment

A table or bench with an area cut out to allow access of the probe to the dependent side of the animal is useful. Equipment for shaving the rabbit is required, although a minimal area should be shaved to prevent chilling of the patient during the procedure and while the hair is regrowing. Rabbit fur is very thick, and good quality clippers are required for hair removal. However, their skin is quite fragile and care must be taken not to tear the skin or accidentally remove nipples.

Given that rabbits can range in size from 900 g to over 5 kg, a range of ultrasonography equipment is required to enable highly detailed images to be obtained from all rabbit patients:

- For the small rabbit breeds, a minimum requirement is a high-definition curvilinear transducer (7.5–10 MHz) with a footprint of <2 cm
- Larger rabbits may be scanned with a 5 MHz linear probe to equally good effect
- For structures such as the eye, a 10 MHz probe is preferable.

A useful additional piece of equipment is a stand-off for visualizing structures <2 cm from the body surface, which is the case for many rabbit organs. However, the difficulty of working with a stand-off may offset the useful gain in image quality; many small rabbits can be imaged adequately using a 7.5–10 MHz curvilinear probe without a stand-off.

Functions other than two-dimensional (2D) real-time imaging, e.g. colour Doppler, power Doppler, pulse wave and M-mode capabilities, are required to image blood flow and to perform echocardiography. An additional consideration for echocardiography of the rabbit is a machine with an update rate/frame rate sufficiently fast to cope with the rabbit's rapid heart rate.

Image capture capability, for both still and moving images, is ideal for review of the images at a later date, archiving, sending for a second opinion and explaining to the owner. Moving images are far superior to still images for understanding the structures and for later review, especially for the inexperienced ultrasonographer. Many ultrasound machines contain an image capture function but if not, attaching a handheld camcorder or other digital recording device can often be attempted with good results.

Indications for ultrasonography

There is much to be said for considering radiography and ultrasonography as complementary tools for investigation of the rabbit patient; one does not necessarily replace the other. The author usually considers survey radiography (skull, thorax, abdomen, including spine and limbs) together with ultrasonography of the abdominal structures and heart to form part of the minimum database in working up the rabbit case.

Ileus is a common presenting sign in rabbits and ultrasonography can be very useful in evaluating intestinal movement, searching for evidence of blockage and assessing for the presence of peritoneal fluid. Almost every rabbit patient presents with a history of anorexia; it is essential to establish whether the rabbit has developed potentially irreversible hepatic lipidosis before committing to prolonged or involved therapy. Rapid ultrasonography of the liver, in the conscious patient, can readily indicate whether a degree of lipidosis is present, as indicated by increased echogenicity when compared with normal. The degree of lipidosis may be accurately determined via liver biopsy; however, a rapid estimation of the extent of hepatic lipidosis can be readily achieved within seconds and will help to inform the clinical prognosis and management of the case.

Patient restraint and preparation

In all but the most tractable individuals, it is often preferable to sedate them or to perform general anaesthesia to prevent undue stress or even injury to the rabbit if it struggles.

It is rarely possible in rabbits to scan through the fur, even with plenty of gel to exclude air, because rabbit fur is so thick. Some hair removal is therefore required but should be minimized; large areas of hair loss can predispose the rabbit to (mild to moderate) hypothermia if they are later housed outside in cold weather. The rabbit is typically shaved from xiphisternum to pubis and laterally for half the width of the ribcage to the iliac crests. Acoustic coupling gel is applied liberally to the skin and transducer.

Abdominal ultrasonography

Ultrasonography of the abdominal organs may be hindered by the presence of the large hindgut found in rabbits. Ultrasound waves are blocked by gas, and therefore ultrasonography of the abdomen of the rabbit is greatly hampered by the pockets of gas present. Ultrasonography of the bladder, uterus, liver and spleen is possible percutaneously via the ventral abdomen in most species. Ultrasonography of the kidneys and ovaries is easier percutaneously via the flank. Rabbits possess an open inguinal canal and therefore the testes may ascend into the abdomen when palpated; ultrasonography can be used to trace and detect an abdominal testis in the case of undescended testis. Ultrasonography of the abdominal organs is summarized in Technique 8.1.

Knowledge of the general relative echogenicity of organs is helpful in differentiating normality from pathology. The order of normal relative echogenicity, starting with the least echogenic, is: kidney < liver < spleen < fat.

The liver
Probe positioning is illustrated in Technique 8.1.

Position and anatomy

The liver lies just behind the diaphragm, two thirds on the right and one third on the left of the median plane, and is positioned almost perpendicular to the longitudinal body axis. The rabbit liver is divided into four lobes:

- The right and left lobes are each divided into cranial and caudal lobules
- The quadrate lobe (attached to the right lobe) lies caudal to the gallbladder
- The small circular caudate lobe lies adjacent to the right kidney and has a narrow attachment.

The gallbladder is found deep within the right cranial lobule. The right cranial lobe is pushed forward from the gastric pylorus. The most developed liver lobes are the right cranial and left caudal lobes. The quadrate lobe lies behind the xiphoid cartilage.

Normal ultrasonographic appearance

The liver parenchyma has heterogeneous echogenicity, with the biliary tree and blood vessels easily detected (Figure 8.3). The rabbit liver is hypoechoic compared to the surrounding soft tissues. Its contours are regular and close to the hyperechoic diaphragm. The gallbladder is noted as an anechoic elongated oval shape. Its walls are hypoechoic. The cystic duct may be observed at the edge, where it joins the left hepatic duct. Both structures are elongated ovals, in contrast to the biliary ducts which are anechoic tubular structures without walls. The normal gallbladder has several areas noted on ultrasonography: the body is an oval structure, filled with anechoic content, its walls are hypoechoic, and the walls of the infundibulum and neck are hypoechoic. These two anatomical parts are elongated structures merging into the cystic duct. The portal vein has a wide lumen and hyperechoic, easily visualized walls. Parallel to the vein, the cystic duct is observed as a thin tubular structure.

The pancreas

Position and anatomy

The pancreas is diffuse and located in a pocket formed by the transverse colon, stomach and duodenum. It is very difficult to detect unless there is significant fibrosis, and therefore if it can be seen on the ultrasound scan it is abnormal. The pancreatic duct and the bile duct are separate structures.

The spleen

Probe positioning is illustrated in Technique 8.1.

Position and anatomy

The spleen is flat and elongated and lies on the dorsolateral surface of the greater curvature of the stomach. The rabbit spleen has an elongated to oval shape; its borders are parallel. Its dorsal end is situated at the level of the last rib. A portion is located cranial to the left kidney and the rest is caudal to the ribs. The spleen lies against the dorsal abdominal wall between the stomach, jejunum and caecum. Its hilus is elongated and separates the gastric surface from the intestines. The spleen is on the caudomedial surface of the stomach.

Normal ultrasonographic appearance

The rabbit spleen has a distinct acoustic structure and borders, when compared with the surrounding soft tissues (Figure 8.4). The spleen is hypoechoic and more homogeneous than the adjacent liver. The spleen has an elongated shape longitudinally. In the transverse ultrasonographic plane the shape is almost triangular. The capsule is often a distinct hyperechoic and heterogeneous striped area. The parenchyma is more hypoechoic towards the capsule. It is more homogeneous and uninterrupted towards the organ capsule. The parenchyma contains many small linear hyperechoic areas, among which small hypoechoic spaces are seen. The blood vessels appear as oval anechoic areas within the spleen parenchyma. The spleen parenchyma has low to medium echogenicity, compared with the higher echogenicity of the liver parenchyma.

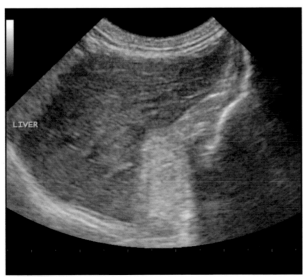

8.3 Ultrasonographic appearance of the normal liver of a rabbit, obtained using a 10 MHz curvilinear probe.

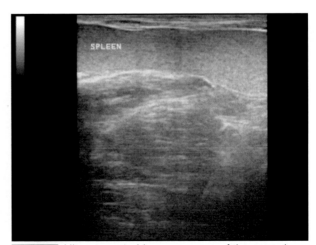

8.4 Ultrasonographic appearance of the normal spleen of a rabbit, obtained using a 10 MHz curvilinear probe.

The kidneys
Probe positioning is illustrated in Technique 8.1. It is important that a complete scan of both kidneys is performed in both transverse and longitudinal planes before making a diagnosis.

Position and anatomy
Rabbit kidneys are unilobular (unipyramidal) and are placed asymmetrically in the retroperitoneal space. The right kidney is found extending from the 11th or 12th rib to the 2nd lumbar vertebra. The cranial pole touches the liver beneath the last rib. The caudal pole of the right kidney approaches the descending part of the duodenum. The left kidney lies between the 2nd and 4th lumbar vertebrae and is caudal and ventral to the right kidney. The jejunal loops lie ventral to the left kidney, and the descending colon and the body of the pancreas lie cranially and ventral to it. The left kidney touches the left abdominal wall and can be scanned caudal to the rib cage, left of midline, using the spleen as an acoustic window.

Normal ultrasonographic appearance
The normal renal cortex is finely granulated, homogeneous and more hypoechoic than the parenchyma of the adjacent liver and spleen. The high echogenicity of the liver and spleen is an advantage in the evaluation of the ultrasonographic scans of the kidneys, and allows easy detection of the kidneys in the abdominal cavity. The renal cortex has low echogenicity, while the spleen has the highest echogenicity in this region. The renal medulla is hypoechoic.

The kidneys appear oval in both longitudinal (Figure 8.5) and transverse planes. The borders are well defined against the adjacent soft tissues. The fibrous capsule appears as a thin hyperechoic line over the cortex. The adipose capsule is relatively hyperechoic, with rough and irregular borders. The renal cortex has a rough granular appearance, heterogeneous echogenicity and multiple linear hyperechoic areas. The renal cortex is uniform in echogenicity, hyperechoic to the renal medulla, hypoechoic to the spleen, and isoechoic to the hepatic parenchyma. The kidney medulla has a lower echogenicity than the cortex and the pelvic structures. Pelvic septa are

situated among the parts of the renal pyramid, which are hyperechoic to the other two renal regions. The renal pelvis is a centrally located hyperechoic structure surrounded by the hyperechoic peripelvic adipose tissue.

The urinary bladder
Probe positioning is illustrated in Technique 8.1.

Position and anatomy
Ultrasonographic evaluation of the urinary bladder is typically performed with the rabbit in dorsal recumbency. This position allows optimal visualization of the urinary bladder. The bladder should be moderately distended with urine and the patient should have free access to water before examination.

Normal ultrasonographic appearance
Urine is the major route of excretion for calcium in rabbits; serum calcium levels are not maintained within a narrow range, but are dependent largely on dietary intake, with excess excreted via the kidney. Rabbit urine is often thick and creamy owing to the presence of calcium carbonate crystals. On ultrasonography the urine often contains hyperechoic flecks within the hypoechoic (fluid-filled) bladder. Normal bladder wall thickness as measured using ultrasonography varies from 1.70 to 2.50 mm in the New Zealand White rabbit.

The uterus and ovaries

Position and anatomy
The rabbit uterus has no uterine body but two separate uterine horns and two cervices that open into the vagina (see Chapter 12). It lies dorsal to the urinary bladder.

Normal ultrasonographic appearance
The vagina is large and flaccid and may contain some urine, forming an 'extra' hypoechoic (fluid-filled) structure next to the bladder that is sometimes mistaken for the bladder or a cystic structure. The mesometrium is a major site of fat deposition and is often readily identifiable during abdominal ultrasonography owing to its high echogenicity relative to the other soft tissues.

The ovary appears as a solid hyperechoic structure, typically adjacent to the left kidney (Figure 8.6).

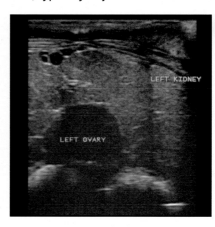

8.6 Ultrasonographic appearance of the normal kidney and ovary of a rabbit, obtained using a 10 MHz curvilinear probe.

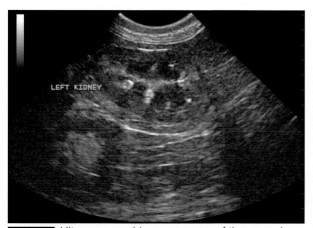

8.5 Ultrasonographic appearance of the normal kidney of a rabbit, obtained using a 10 MHz curvilinear probe.

The testes

Position and anatomy

The testes are easily visible in a sexually mature male rabbit; the age of maturity varies with breed. The testes typically descend on the 6th day of age and are fully in the scrotum at day 22. Despite this, much later ages are often quoted for testicular descent in the pet trade and in veterinary texts, e.g. 3–5 months; although this is physiologically inaccurate, it demonstrates the difficulty in detecting the small immature descended testes. Sexual maturity (production of sperm) occurs at around 20 weeks (4–5 months) of age; the testes are then quite large and externally visible. Adult sexually mature testes are approximately 33 mm × 11 mm in size.

Normal ultrasonographic appearance

Higher-frequency probes provide more detailed images, but reducing the frequency of the probe means that the entire image of the testis fits into a single frame, making it easier to compare the echogenicity of the testes on the same screen. Fixing the testis on a rubber pad with a central hole large enough to surround the funiculus spermaticus under a water sac not only improves the quality of the image, but also keeps the testis out of the inguinal canal (see Technique 8.1).

The testicular parenchyma is homogeneous and moderately echoic. The epididymis is identified as a homogeneous structure that is less echoic than the parenchyma. The scrotal skin and subscrotal layers are seen as a single hyperechoic band surrounding the scrotal contents. A centrally located hyperechoic mediastinum may be observed in sagittal plane images of approximately 70% of testes. The cauda of the epididymis is identified as a homogeneous, less echoic structure located next to the testicular parenchyma in sagittal plane images.

Thoracic ultrasonography

The lungs and thymus

Position and anatomy

The lungs have three lobes; the cranial lung lobes are small (left smaller than right). Large amounts of intrathoracic fat are often present.

The normal thymus remains large in the adult rabbit and lies ventral to the heart, extending into the thoracic inlet. It can therefore be imaged lying next to the heart by placing the probe in the intercostal spaces. The area of the thymus of a normal adult rabbit (at least 3 months old) is approximately 30–40 mm^2 (it is 50–60 mm^2 at 4 weeks of age).

Normal ultrasonographic appearance

Healthy lungs are rarely seen using ultrasonography because the air prevents formation of an image.

The appearance of the normal thymus is typical on ultrasound examination. It has low echogenicity with multiple echogenic lines and foci, representing cross-sections either of connective-tissue septa or of blood vessels within a septum.

Echocardiography

Patient preparation and probe positioning are described in Technique 8.2.

The heart rates of rabbits are much faster than those of humans (for which most machines are designed) and dogs. The rabbit heart rate varies between 150 and 300 beats/min, depending on the size of the rabbit and whether it is excited or calm. The ultrasound machine must have a frame rate or update rate fast enough to image these 'fast hearts' or the cardiac image will be merely a blur.

The ultrasonographer should note the sedative or anaesthetic drugs used to restrain the animal because many drugs affect myocardial contractility and other parameters. For example, myocardial contractility in rabbits is higher under isoflurane/nitrous oxide anaesthesia than under halothane/nitrous oxide anaesthesia. In addition, ultrasonography has been used to evaluate heart damage caused by general anaesthetics, for example myocardial fibrosis has been associated with ketamine/xylazine anaesthesia in rabbits.

Position and anatomy of the heart

The heart of the rabbit is situated close to the sternum, and its longitudinal axis is almost parallel to the thoracic base. The heart is relatively small and lies cranially in the thoracic cavity. The right atrioventricular (AV) valve has only two cusps. The rabbit aorta shows neurogenic rhythmic contractions.

The transthoracic ultrasonographic investigation of the rabbit heart is mainly performed via the intercostal windows of the 3rd, 4th and 5th left intercostal spaces, and the 3rd and 4th right intercostal spaces. The parasternal probe position is used for the sagittal and transverse 2D visualization of the heart cavities and valves. Three main positions of the transducer are used for 2D transthoracic echocardiographic study of the rabbit heart:

- Left parasternal on the longitudinal axis of the heart
- Right parasternal on the longitudinal axis
- Left parasternal on the short heart axis.

The following measurements may be the most useful and accurate in small mammals:

- Left ventricular systolic time intervals
- Right ventricular systolic time intervals
- Right ventricular end-diastolic dimension
- Left atrial internal dimension
- Left ventricular end-diastolic and end-systolic dimensions
- Systolic slope of the interventricular septum
- Mid-diastolic partial closure of the mitral valve (the EF slope)
- Systolic slope of the posterior aortic wall.

Normal ultrasonographic appearance of the heart

The walls of the heart cavities are hyperechoic compared with their lumens.

The left parasternal plane on the longitudinal axis of the heart allows visualization of both left heart chambers. The bicuspid valve is evident as a hyperechoic line moving between the left ventricle and atrium.

The right parasternal view shows the ascending aorta and aortic valve as hyperechoic areas in the centre of the heart image (Figure 8.7), surrounded by the hypoechoic left and right atria, parts of the right ventricle, pulmonary ostium, the beginning of the pulmonary trunk and the pulmonary valve. The pulmonary valve may be noted as a hyperechoic line moving at the beginning of the aorta.

The parasternal plane on the short axis of the heart gives a transverse image (Figure 8.8). The tricuspid and pulmonary valves may be identified.

M-mode

To perform M-mode echocardiography, the apical pulse is identified and the transducer placed at the same intercostal space. Images of the left AV valves are obtained first. Standard views are then obtained (Figure 8.9) at the apex, left AV valve, cranial left AV leaflet, aortic root, right AV valve and pulmonic valve.

Echocardiographic M-mode measurements reported for dogs vary proportionally with body size (weight) and therefore type or breed, whereas those reported for ferrets and chinchillas do not vary greatly, perhaps because these species are similar in size. In rabbit studies published so far, no significant associations between bodyweight and

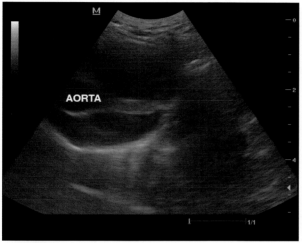

8.7 Parasternal view showing the hypoechoic lumen of the ascending aorta.

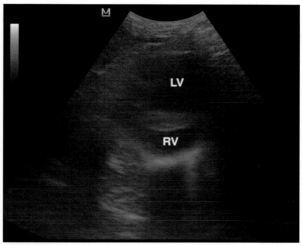

8.8 Parasternal short axis view showing right (RV) and left (LV) ventricles.

8.9

The four main positions for M-mode measurements. aml = anterior mitral leaflet; Ao = aorta; av = aortic valve; ECG = electrocardiogram; IS = interventricular septum; LA = left atrium; LV = left ventricle; mv = mitral valve; per = pericardium; PW = posterior wall; RV = right ventricle; TW = thoracic wall. (Reproduced with permission from Tello de Meneses *et al.*, 1989)

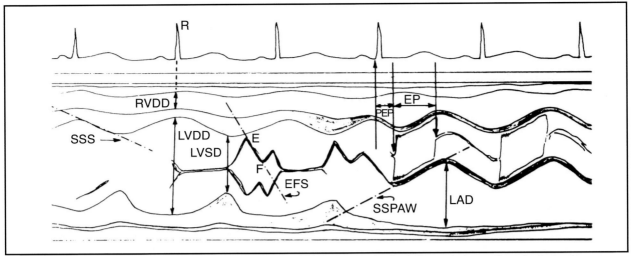

8.10 Diagram summarizing M-mode measurements. EF slope = early diastolic posterior motion of mitral valve; EP = ejection period; LAD; left atrial interval dimension; LVDD = left ventricular end-diastolic dimension; LVSD = left ventricular end-systolic dimension; PEP = pre-ejection period; RVDD = right ventricular end-diastolic dimension; SSPAW = systolic slope of the posterior aortic wall; SSS = systolic slope of the septum. (Reproduced with permission from Tello de Meneses *et al.*, 1989)

echocardiographic measurements have been reported. However, individual rabbits and breeds of rabbit do vary considerably in size, and perhaps there are yet too few studies to establish whether the measurements may be different in larger or smaller breeds.

The results from one M-mode examination in a rabbit (Figure 8.10; Tello de Meneses *et al.*, 1989) yielded the following results:

- Mean ± standard deviation (SD) heart rate = 155 ± 29 beats/min
- Mean ± SD measurements in diastole and systole for interventricular septum thickness, left ventricular internal diameter, and left ventricular free wall thickness were: 2.03 ± 0.37 mm and 3.05 ± 0.45 mm; 14.37 ± 1.49 mm and 10.25 ± 1.22 mm; and 2.16 ± 0.25 and 3.48 ± 0.55 mm, respectively
- Mean ± SD of the ratio of the left atrial to aortic diameter was 1.17 ± 0.14, and the mean ± SD mitral valve E-point to septal separation interval was 1.71 ± 0.29 mm

- Mean ± SD for fractional shortening and ejection fraction were 30.13 ± 2.98% and 61.29 ± 4.66%, respectively
- Mean ± SD maximal aortic and pulmonary artery outflow velocities were 0.85 ± 0.11 m/s and 0.59 ± 0.10 m/s, respectively. The peak E to peak A wave velocity ratio of the mitral valve was 2.19 ± 0.46.

Ultrasonography of the eye

Ultrasonography is a valuable technique for ophthalmic evaluation in the rabbit (Figure 8.11). The conscious rabbit will tolerate scanning of the globe following topical anaesthesia to the eye and sedation is rarely required. A high detail, high-frequency probe is required, typically a 10 MHz sector probe. Normal measurements of the various structures of the eye can be taken using ultrasonography (Figure 8.12).

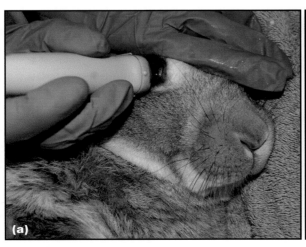

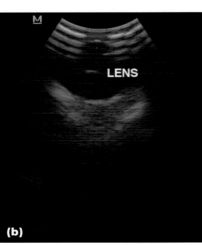

8.11 (a) Position of probe used to obtain an image of the globe. (b) Normal ultrasonographic appearance of the rabbit globe.

Dimension	Measurement (mm)
Cornea thickness	0.50 ± 0.12
Lens thickness	6.28 ± 0.23
Vitreous chamber depth	9.23 ± 0.61
Axial globe length	18.28 ± 0.17

8.12 Ocular measurements in the rabbit. Data based on 10 healthy adult rabbits (20 eyes). (Data from Adel, 2011)

Examples of conditions for which ultrasound examination can be diagnostic

Retrobulbar and intraocular lesions

Exophthalmos in the rabbit should be investigated using ultrasonography of both the eye and the surrounding tissues for masses, but the mediastinum should also be examined because thymoma often presents as intermittent or persistent exophthalmos (see Chapter 17). In the typical rabbit with a retrobulbar abscess, ultrasonography will reveal a mass ventromedial to the eye, with hyperechoic areas that cast an acoustic shadow and appear typically homogeneous (Figure 8.13). If osteomyelitis is also present the bony orbit may appear incomplete, the mass may extend laterally, and the contralateral globe may appear indented by the pressure of the adjacent mass. Tapeworm cysts will appear as large hypoechoic areas representing fluid-filled structures (see Chapter 29). Tumours will be seen as hyperechoic 'solid' masses, which are often heterogeneous in appearance.

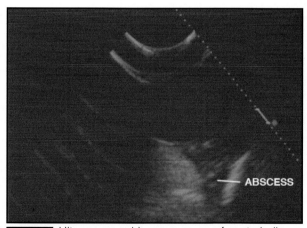

8.13 Ultrasonographic appearance of a retrobulbar abscess in a rabbit, obtained using a 10 MHz curvilinear probe.

Cardiovascular disease

Echocardiography is recommended for evaluation of the heart in rabbits presenting with exercise intolerance or dyspnoea. Pet rabbits can develop cardiovascular disease, and radiography, electrocardiography and echocardiography are useful non-invasive diagnostic procedures that can be used to provide a highly specific assessment of cardiac size, arrhythmias, and internal structure and function (dynamics), respectively.

The author has detected a ventricular septal defect in a rabbit presenting with chronic dyspnoea. Cardiomyopathy is a relatively common post-mortem finding in aged rabbits. As the lifespan of pet rabbits has increased, the incidence of heart failure and atherosclerosis has also been increasing. Confirmation is obtained by demonstrating reduced fractional shortening on ultrasonography. Bacterial endocarditis (associated in particular with severe osteomyelitis) and occasional cases of pericardial effusion have all been noted by the author in rabbits presenting with non-specific signs such as anorexia, weight loss or general 'illness'. It is likely that as this technique becomes more widely used in the rabbit patient, more conditions will be identified *in vivo*.

Rabbits are prone to arteriosclerosis, either as a result of a high-fat diet (which may be seen in overfed house rabbits) or associated with renal failure and soft tissue mineralization. The condition may be clinically silent in its early stages or present as lethargy and inappetence. Ultrasonography is much more sensitive than radiography for detecting the condition. Calcification of the aorta, reportedly associated with renal failure (and therefore lack of renal calcium clearance in the rabbit) can be detected on ultrasonography (Figure 8.14), even if the calcification is not yet detectable on radiography.

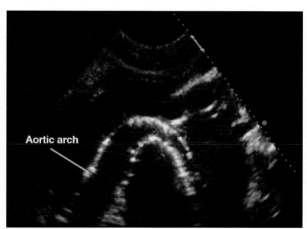

8.14 Ultrasonographic appearance of calcification of the aortic arch of a rabbit with 'early' arteriosclerosis, obtained using a 10 MHz curvilinear probe.

Thymoma

Rabbits with thymoma often show clinical signs of dyspnoea and bilateral exophthalmos. Cytology of samples collected by ultrasound-guided biopsy can be an accurate diagnostic tool for the identification of thymomas and differentiation of the type of neoplasia where present. Ultrasonography of the cranial mediastinum via an intercostal approach, with the rabbit in either sternal or lateral recumbency, is used. The thymoma will appear as a heterogeneous hypoechoic mass cranial to the heart, with hypoechoic (cystic) regions of varying size. As the thymoma is typically large and takes up most of the cranial mediastinum, lung artefacts do not tend to interfere with the image. Larger cystic lesions in the thymoma are sometimes detected (see Chapter 19), which may be aspirated under ultrasound guidance to relieve dyspnoea.

Lung masses

Normal lung fields do not lend themselves to ultrasonography because the air contained within them interferes with image formation. However, lung pathology related to chronic pneumonia is very common in the pet rabbit and an element of lung consolidation can sometimes be detectable using ultrasonography. In some cases known to the author, the condition has progressed to lung abscessation, the extent of which can also be traced using ultrasonography.

Liver disease

Liver lobe torsion in rabbits is well known as a cause of ileus, anorexia and depression. Ultrasonographic findings include an enlarged liver with heterogeneous liver parenchyma in the affected area (Figure 8.15) and free abdominal fluid. Ultrasound-guided fine-needle aspiration of the liver may reveal unremarkable liver cytology, or in some cases be suggestive of neoplasia – such is the extent of hepatocellular disruption. Free anechoic fluid may be found in the cranial abdomen. In some cases a heterogeneous area of liver-like tissue may be identified adjacent to the right kidney, so it is important to scan the whole liver when this condition is suspected. Owing to the presence of gas within the stomach and intestinal tract it will be difficult to connect this abnormal tissue to the liver. In other cases, the stomach and caecum appear to be distended with luminal gas, resulting in acoustic shadowing. There may be minimal bowel motility in the intestinal tract, consistent with ileus.

Contrast agents may be used to enhance the visualization of hepatic and splenic masses, and this technique has been reported to be successful in the rabbit experimentally. Detection on ultrasonography of dilation of the biliary tree has been associated with hepatic coccidiosis, which is common in pet rabbits though often undiagnosed in clinical practice.

Kidney disease

Early signs of renal failure, where mild renal calcinosis is present on histology but not yet visible on radiography, is easily detected by the hyperechoic appearance of the renal cortex using ultrasonography, a finding that can be easily noted by even an inexperienced rabbit ultrasonographer (Figures 8.16 and 8.17). Scarring associated with, for example, encephalitozoonosis may be detected as hyperechoic regions. An ultrasound-guided biopsy of the kidney may be used in order to perform histology and reach a definitive diagnosis.

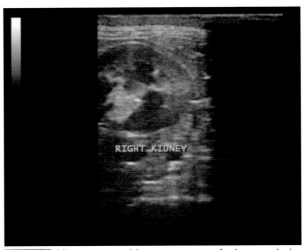

8.16 Ultrasonographic appearance of a hyperechoic area of the kidney suggestive of nephrocalcinosis in a rabbit, obtained using a 10 MHz curvilinear probe.

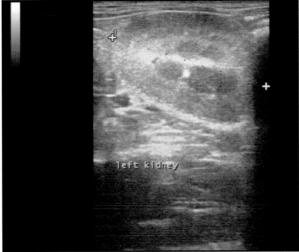

8.17 Ultrasonographic appearance of the kidney of a rabbit showing a marked hyperechoic cortex consistent with nephrocalcinosis and (early) renal failure. The nephrocalcinosis was not yet visible on plain radiography. This rabbit died 8 months later and renal failure was confirmed on post-mortem examination. Image obtained using a 10 MHz curvilinear probe.

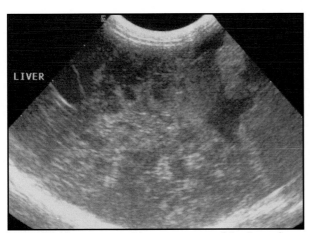

8.15 Ultrasonographic appearance of the liver of a rabbit with liver lobe torsion. The right side of the liver was enlarged and heterogeneous. Image obtained using a 10 MHz sector probe.

Urolithiasis and cystitis

The finding of 'sand' (hyperechoic flecks) in the urinary bladder is not unusual in the rabbit and may or may not be associated with disease, making a decision on whether this finding is of clinical relevance difficult. However in some cases the bladder wall is thickened and apparently irritated by this excessive 'sand'. In the author's opinion the finding of hyperechoic material in the bladder coupled with a thickened bladder wall is often associated with urine scalding in the rabbit, because flushing of the bladder contents under anaesthesia to remove the sandy material often results in clinical resolution of the urine scalding. Formed uroliths may be detected using ultrasonography, with which smaller stones may be more easily detected; radiography readily detects larger stones.

Pregnancy

Pregnancy diagnosis via ultrasonography is possible in female rabbits after the 7th day of pregnancy, when ultrasound images may reveal the blastocyst stage of the embryos; by day 8 the embryonic vesicles may be detected as round anechoic areas. Heartbeats of the fetuses are generally detectable between days 11 and 19 of gestation. The best time for counting the number of the fetuses using ultrasonography is suggested to be day 11.

Uterine pathology

Uterine adenocarcinoma and pyometra in the rabbit may be diagnosed and differentiated by ultrasonography; the solid, more hyperechoic appearance of the tumour contrasts with the hypoechoic appearance of pyometra. Uterine adenocarcinoma has a reportedly high incidence in rabbits and can be detected using ultrasonography often before it is readily palpable on abdominal examination. The hyperechoic homogeneous masses consistent with uterine adenocarcinoma are typically visualized against the contrast of the hypoechoic fluid-filled urinary bladder (Figure 8.18).

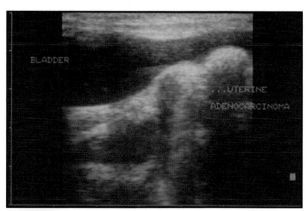

8.18 Ultrasonographic appearance of the bladder and uterine adenocarcinoma, obtained using a 7.5 MHz sector probe.

References and further reading

Adel A (2011) Two-dimensional sonography biometry evaluation of rabbits' eyes. *Global Veterinaria* 6, 220–222
Aksoy M, Erdem H, Hatipoğlu F *et al.* (2009) Ultrasonographic examination of the scrotal content in the rabbit. *Reproduction in Domestic Animals* 44(1), 156–160
Dimitrov R, Vladova D, Stamatova K, Kostov D and Stefanov M (2011) Transthoracal two-dimensional ultrasonographic anatomical study of the heart in the rabbit (*Oryctolagus cuniculus*). *Trakia Journal of Sciences* 9(3), 45–50
Dimitrov RS (2012) Ultrasound features of kidneys in the rabbit (*Oryctolagus cuniculus*). *Veterinary World* 5, 274–278
Du Boulay GH and Wilson OL (1988) Diagnosis of pregnancy and disease by ultrasound in exotic species. *Symposia of the Zoological Society of London* 60, 135–150
Fontes-Sousa APN, Brás-Silva C, Moura C *et al.* (2006) M mode and Doppler echocardiographic reference values for male New Zealand White rabbits. *American Journal of Veterinary Research* 67, 1725–1729
Kienle RD and Thomas WP (2002) Echocardiography. In: *Small Animal Diagnostic Ultrasound, 2nd edn*, ed. TG Nyland and JS Matton, pp. 354–423. WB Saunders, Philadelphia
Kunzel F, Hittmair KM, Hassan J *et al.* (2012) Thymomas in rabbits: clinical evaluation, diagnosis, and treatment. *Journal of the American Animal Hospital Association* 48, 97–104
Maurer JK, Gibbons BA and Bruce RD (1990) Morphometric assessment of thymic size variation in laboratory rabbits. *Toxicological Pathology* 18, 407
Moarabi A, Mosallanejad B, Ghadiri AR and Borujeni MP (2011) Ultrasonographic evaluation of the urinary system in New Zealand white rabbit and Tolai hare. *Veterinary Research Forum* 2(2), 113–120
Moïse NS and Fox PR (1999) Echocardiography and Doppler imaging. In: *Textbook of Canine and Feline Cardiology, 2nd edn*, ed. PR Fox *et al.*, pp. 130–171. WB Saunders, Philadelphia
Orcutt C (2000) Cardiac and respiratory disease in rabbits. *Proceedings of the British Veterinary Zoological Society, Autumn meeting 2000*, pp. 68–73
Pizzi R, Hagen RU and Meredith AL (2007) Intermittent colic and intussusception due to a cecal polyp in a rabbit. *Journal of Exotic Pet Medicine* 16(4), 113–117
Rajfer J (1982) Endocrinological study of testicular descent in the rabbit. *Journal of Surgical Research* 33, 158–163
Redrobe S (2001) Imaging techniques in small mammals. *Seminars in Avian and Exotic Pet Medicine* 10(4), 187–197
Soroori S, Dehghan MM and Molazem M (2008) Ultrasonographic assessment of gestational age in rabbits. *Proceedings of the 15th Congress of the Federation of Asian Veterinary Associations, 27–30 October 2008, FAVA–OIE Joint Symposium on Emerging Diseases. Bangkok, Thailand*, pp. 367–368
Stamatova-Yovcheva K, Dimitrov R, P. Yonkova *et al.* (2012) Comparative imaging anatomic study of domestic rabbit liver (*Oryctolagus cuniculus*). *Trakia Journal of Sciences* 10(1), 57–63
Tello de Meneses R, Mesa MD and Gonzalez V (1989) Echocardiographic assessment of cardiac function in the rabbit: a preliminary study. *Annales de Recherches Vétérinaires* 20, 175–185
Thomas WP, Gaber CE, Jacobs GJ *et al.* (1993) Recommendations for standards in transthoracic two-dimensional echocardiography in the dog and cat. Echocardiography Committee of the Specialty of Cardiology, American College of Veterinary Internal Medicine. *Journal of Veterinary Internal Medicine*, 7 247–252
Ward ML (2006) Diagnosis and management of a retrobulbar abscess of periapical origin in a domestic rabbit. *Veterinary Clinics of North America: Exotic Animal Practice* 9, 657–665

TECHNIQUES →

TECHNIQUE 8.1:
Ultrasound examination of the abdomen

Positioning

Dorsal recumbency (also lateral for the kidneys).

Assistant

Required for restraint of rabbit, even when sedated (as shown here).

> **WARNING**
> If the rabbit is difficult to restrain manually, use chemical sedation, e.g. intravenous midazolam 1 mg/kg. Attempting to restrain a fractious rabbit manually can result in spinal injuries leading to permanent paresis or paralysis.

Equipment extras

Warmed gel.

Patient preparation

1 Shave the abdominal area from sternum to pubis and wide enough to permit access to the left kidney.

2 Clean skin with surgical spirit to remove debris.

3 Apply sufficient amounts of acoustic gel.

> **PRACTICAL TIP**
> Use warm gel (place the tube in a jug of warm water prior to use) to prevent the rabbit jumping when cold gel is applied. Rub warm gel in before scanning starts, just after shaving; this ensures better contact and therefore a better image when scanning starts.

Technique

Apply a methodical approach to ensure that every organ listed is checked and each organ is scanned across its entire length and breadth.

Liver

The probe is positioned just caudal to the ribs, aiming cranially. The normal liver extends only a small distance outside the ribcage and is barely palpable. The whole width of the rabbit should be scanned to image every aspect of the liver, to ensure that focal as well as diffuse lesions are noted. The gallbladder is on the right.

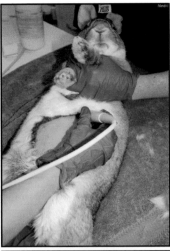

Alternative positions of probe used to obtain an image of the liver.

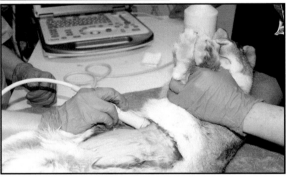

Spleen

Place the probe on the left side of the rabbit just caudal to the ribcage.

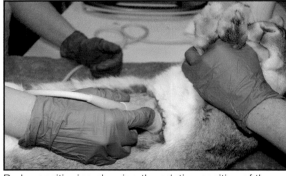

Probe positioning showing the relative position of the spleen in the cranial abdomen.

Right kidney

The probe is positioned on the right side just caudal to the liver. This kidney is often imaged accidentally when examining the liver lobes on the right.

→

TECHNIQUE 8.1 continued:
Ultrasound examination of the abdomen

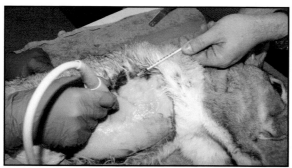

Position of probe used to obtain an image of the right and left kidneys.

Left kidney

There are two methods of imaging the left kidney:

- Palpate the abdomen and gently hold the left kidney in one hand whilst applying the probe with the other. The left kidney is more loosely attached than the right one and lies between the 2nd and 4th lumbar vertebrae.
- Image the right kidney, pull the probe gently directly caudally by 2–3 lengths of the right kidney and press a little more firmly; it is possible to image the left kidney via the right side of the rabbit.

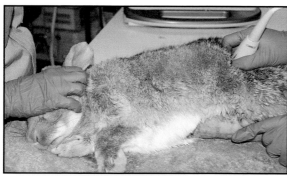

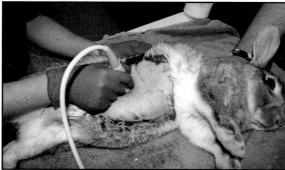

Alternative positions of probe used to obtain an image of the left kidney.

PRACTICAL TIP
Rather than shaving a large amount of hair from the rabbit's abdomen, and risking chilling of the outdoor rabbit until hair regrows, shave only an area three clipper widths centrally and when aiming to image the kidneys merely shave over these discrete areas.

Urinary bladder

Place probe in the region of the pubis to the umbilicus (depending on how full the bladder is).

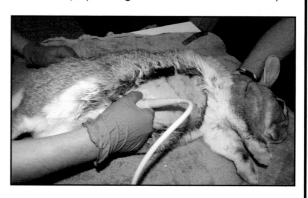

Uterus and ovaries

Lying dorsal to the urinary bladder, these can be imaged using the full urinary bladder as an acoustic window.

Testes

Apply probe directly over the testes via the thin scrotal sac.

PRACTICAL TIP
To prevent the rabbit retracting the testes during examination, restrain the testes using a rubber ring.

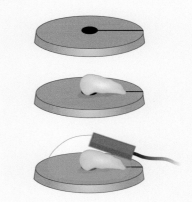

TECHNIQUE 8.2:
Echocardiography

Positioning

Lateral recumbency.

Assistant

Required for restraint of the rabbit, even when sedated.

> **WARNING**
> If the rabbit is difficult to restrain manually, use chemical sedation e.g. intravenous midazolam 1 mg/kg. Attempting to restrain a fractious rabbit manually can result in spinal injuries leading to permanent paresis or paralysis.

Equipment extras

Warmed gel.

Patient preparation

1 Shave the area from the ventral and lateral thoracic wall in the region from the manubrium (cranially) to the xiphoid process (caudally), and laterally to the right and left axillary region.

2 Clean skin with surgical spirit to remove debris.

3 Apply sufficient amounts of acoustic gel.

> **PRACTICAL TIP**
> Use warm gel (place the tube in a jug of warm water prior to use) to prevent the rabbit jumping when cold gel is applied. Rub the warm gel in before scanning starts, just after shaving. This ensures better contact and therefore a better image when scanning starts.

Probe positioning

- **Left parasternal plane on the longitudinal axis of the heart, showing the left ventricle and parts of the heart cavities:** Incline the transducer consecutively in the 3rd and 4th left intercostal spaces, laterally from the sternum.
- **Right parasternal plane on the longitudinal axis of the heart, demonstrating the four heart cavities:** Place the transducer consecutively in the 3rd and 4th right intercostal spaces laterally.
- **Left parasternal plane on the short axis of the heart, showing the aortic valve and the left and right ventricles:** Place the transducer consecutively in the 3rd and 4th left intercostal spaces, close to the sternum.
- **Apical plane, showing the heart cavities:** Place the transducer in the 5th intercostal spaces on the left and right sides.
- **Right subcostal plane on the longitudinal axis of the heart, demonstrating parts of the four cavities:** Place the transducer horizontally between the right costal arch and the xiphoid process.

9

CT and MRI scanning and interpretation

Stefanie Veraa and Nico Schoemaker

Diagnostic imaging modalities in veterinary medicine are becoming increasingly sophisticated, and the use of computed tomography (CT) and magnetic resonance imaging (MRI) has increased over the last decade. In the early years, limiting factors for implementation of CT and MRI in rabbit medicine were the long duration of the imaging procedures, length of anaesthesia, the small size of the animal and limited resolution of the images. In recent years, the modalities have evolved, resulting in decreased procedure times and high resolution images, and CT and MRI scanning in rabbit medicine have become routine imaging techniques in some clinics. However, equipment for CT and MRI is expensive, in terms of both acquisition and maintenance, and an extensive knowledge of the technique and the acquired images is a necessity. These requirements can be difficult to accomplish in small veterinary practices. Fortunately, CT and MRI are becoming increasingly available in diagnostic imaging departments at veterinary universities and referral clinics, so patients that are in need of CT or MRI can be referred to these centres.

Principles and equipment

CT and MRI are both tomographic techniques, *tomos* meaning 'slice' in Greek. In both techniques the object is displayed as multiple images or pictures, with every image representing one slice of the object. Every picture consists of pixels (picture elements) that have a thickness equal to the slice thickness. These three-dimensional (3D) 'pixels' are called voxels (volume elements) (Bushburg *et al.*, 2002a). Creating CT and MR images is a complex process and therefore only some of the technical aspects will be highlighted in this section.

Computed tomography

Computed tomography (CT), or computed axial tomography (CAT) as it was previously named, was introduced in 1972. In the early period it took about 5 minutes to create one slice that was 13 mm thick and had pixels of 3 mm × 3 mm. The images were of low resolution with many artefacts (Bushburg *et al.*, 2002a). Many developments, such as helical scanning and multi-slice techniques, have improved the imaging process such that, within milliseconds, high-resolution images can be created that have a

slice thickness of <1 mm. Helical scanning, consisting of continuous movement of the X-ray tube around the patient and simultaneous table movement, was introduced in 1989 and has improved scanning speed. The multi-slice technique, in which multiple slices are created in one rotation of the X-ray tube, was introduced in 1992 (Bushburg *et al.*, 2002a). The development and availability of advanced software programs has made image reconstruction and rendering possible and, as slice thickness decreases, high-resolution 3D image reconstruction or multi-planar reconstruction (MPR) become available. The 3D image reconstruction enables evaluation of the shape of anatomical structures such as the skull or blood vessels (CT angiogram). In MPR images, all views in the x-, y- and z-axes are available for reviewing, and all the structures in the reconstructed slice can be evaluated without superposition of other structures. The equipment available in veterinary medicine currently consists mostly of 1 to 64 multi-slice, helical scanners.

CT images are created by rotating an X-ray tube around the patient and computing the data (amount of X-rays) collected by a ring of X-ray detectors that is positioned around the gantry (the central opening in which the patient is located). The different anatomical tissues and fluids are projected in the image in varying grey values, which are named Hounsfield units (HU), according to the amount of X-ray attenuation by the tissues. Pure water has an HU value of zero, and therefore darker (hypoattenuating) areas in the image (e.g. air and fat) will have a negative HU value and lighter (hyperattenuating) areas (e.g. soft tissues, mineralized structures, contrast medium or metal) will have a positive HU value.

Intravenously injected contrast medium can be applied during CT imaging in rabbits using the same agents that are used in radiographic procedures (i.e. ionic or non-ionic iodinated). The contrast medium will cause hyperattenuation where it is present in the image (Dennis and Herrtage, 1989).

There are up to 4200 grey values in every image, but the human eye can only detect up to 256. To maximize the visibility of these varying grey values, images are displayed in certain ranges. The centre of the range is called the level (L), and the width of grey values above and below this centre is called the window (W). To optimize evaluation of, for example, soft tissues or bones, these parameters will be changed to HU values of, respectively, 350 (W) and 50 (L) or 3500 (W) and 500 (L). This is called windowing and levelling and allows the creation of soft tissue and bone settings. These images can be further improved by using filters that enhance various characteristics of the tissues, for example a soft tissue filter will smooth the image but a bone filter will enhance the bone borders by edge enhancement. All these improvements of the image quality for varying tissues are performed after image acquisition (Bushburg et al., 2002a).

Magnetic resonance imaging

Magnetic resonance imaging (MRI) was introduced in the mid-1980s as a sequel to spectroscopic studies in chemical and biochemical research (Bushberg et al., 2002b). MRI scanners have evolved during recent decades and are now available in veterinary medicine mostly as low-field 0.2–0.3 Tesla (open) systems or high-field 1–3 Tesla superconducting systems. The main difference between the low- and high-field systems is the fact that low-field systems are generally magnetized only temporarily. These systems only create a magnetic field as electric power is turned on and they can be switched off in an emergency (Bushberg et al., 2002c). The high-field systems use a superconducting wire kept in a cryogenic liquid such as liquid helium. A permanent current runs through the wire, creating a permanent magnetic field that can only be switched off by removing the cryogenic liquid (Bushberg et al., 2002c). As this is a very costly operation, precautions must be taken to minimize the risk of an emergency requiring the shutdown of the system. All MRI systems are placed in a shielded room (Faraday cage) to protect the environment from the extensive magnetic field but more importantly to protect the MRI system from environmental radio frequency (RF) pulses. RF pulses (e.g. FM broadcasts) interfere with the creation of the MR image because they are in the same range as the frequencies that the body emits during an imaging procedure (Bushberg et al., 2002c). All equipment and material inside the shielded room has to be MR-compatible, because all non-compatible objects can become lethal weapons when attracted by the magnet (e.g. pairs of scissors, needles, chairs, oxygen tanks, anaesthesia monitors and machines). Even very small magnetic objects in the patient, such as identification chips or staples, can create large susceptibility artefacts in the MR images and removal is advised when they would be in the scanning field of view.

Image acquisition for MRI is very different from CT image acquisition because there is only one method of creating an image in CT but several in MRI. The magnetic field created by the MRI system causes protons in the tissues to align accordingly, as if they were small magnets in a low-energy state. Images are created by stimulating these protons using RF pulses. Some of the protons take up energy from these RF pulses and will eventually return to their low-energy state, emitting some of the energy absorbed previously by sending a weak RF signal. This signal will be captured, processed and the MR image created, and every type of tissue or fluid will emit the RF pulses in a different time span. By differentiating the times of RF pulse stimulation (TR, time of repetition; TI, time of inversion) and readout (TE, time of echo), the MR characteristics of these tissues, namely the T1, T2 and proton density, will become visible. In this way, several MRI sequences can be created with different grey scales for the different tissues. For example, cerebrospinal fluid (CSF) will be dark (hypointense) on T1-weighted images and bright (hyperintense) on T2-weighted images.

The intravenous contrast medium used in MR image acquisition is in most cases a derivative of gadolinium and affects the relaxation times (time to reach the low-energy state) of the protons. This is best appreciated on T1-weighted images. The T1 characteristics of the tissues in which the contrast medium is present will be brighter in the image (hyperintense) because protons in the tissues retain the energy of the RF pulse for a shorter duration (Kuriashkin and Losonsky, 2000). Lesions are more evident if there is increased vascularization or stasis of blood within these lesions.

There are at least three ways of creating an MRI sequence; the most frequently used in veterinary medicine are called spin echo, gradient echo and inversion recovery. All these sequences have T1, T2 and proton density imaging characteristics but are created in different ways. The major advancement for gradient echo sequences is the fact that images with very thin slices can be created, and therefore 3D reconstruction and MPR of the scanned area can be made. The inversion recovery sequences used in veterinary MRI consist of the fluid-attenuated inversion recovery (FLAIR) sequence, in which the signal of aqueous liquids (such as CSF) will be dark, and the short tau inversion recovery (STIR) sequence, in which the signal of fat will be dark (fat suppression). The MRI sequences can be made in all desired planes (dorsal, transverse, sagittal), unlike CT where only the transverse plane is available (when the rabbit is positioned longitudinally on the table). All these sequences, or a combination of these sequences, will be acquired after each other and therefore an MRI study can be lengthy (Bushberg et al., 2002b).

Resolution and scanning times are improving in MRI scanning as more and more high-field systems are introduced in veterinary medicine and imaging protocols with specific high-resolution sequences are developed (e.g. gradient echo). Because MR imaging with low-field systems is still inferior in image acquisition times to the relatively fast CT image acquisition, its use has been lagging behind. The fragility and sensitivity to complications of rabbits during and after general anaesthesia requires use of the shortest scanning time possible. The increasing availability of high-field MRI systems in veterinary medicine is offering new possibilities for rabbit imaging, as it has done in research facilities. In these facilities, high-field MRI systems have been available for many years and rabbits have been used frequently as MRI or CT models. Therefore an extensive databank on MR and CT imaging in rabbits is available, and can be used as a guide and reference for imaging in veterinary medicine (Mavinkurve *et al.*, 2005; Yuan *et al.*, 2005; Casteleyn *et al.*, 2010; Qiuhang *et al.*, 2010; Van Caelenberg *et al.*, 2010, 2011; Zhao *et al.*, 2010; Zhang *et al.*, 2011; Wei *et al.*, 2012).

Indications for CT and MRI

Radiography and ultrasonography are the primary imaging techniques used in veterinary medicine; they are affordable and available for many veterinary practices and often provide sufficient information to enable diagnosis. However, given that medical CT and MRI systems offer high-resolution images in conjunction with excellent 3D and MPR possibilities, these techniques can be used as a clinical aid in diagnostics, to help in surgical planning and even in planning radiotherapy protocols (Mavinkurve *et al.*, 2005; Zotti *et al.*, 2009; Figure 9.1). Most rabbits require CT or MRI scanning because of the need to specify the differential diagnosis and treatment options. CT and MRI are indicated in areas where radiography and/or ultrasonography offer insufficient information owing to technical limitations or tissue characterization. This can be a result of the superimposition of multiple anatomical structures (e.g. in the head), the lack of soft tissue differentiation in radiographs, the lack of overview in ultrasound images or the limited acoustic penetration of ultrasound waves where bone or air (e.g. in the lungs) is present.

Currently, CT examination of the head is performed most frequently for clinical signs related to dental problems such as anorexia, soft tissue swellings, epiphora or exophthalmos. The lack of superimposition of multiple anatomical structures in the CT and MR images is a major benefit. Smaller structures can be identified and evaluated for their position, shape, structure and size related to the adjacent anatomical structures. The images acquired allow moderate to good soft tissue differentiation, overview and penetration into all anatomical structures. The use of intravenously applied contrast medium in both MRI and CT enhances tissue differentiation because of the differences in tissue vascularization. Necrotic areas will not be vascularized and will therefore lack contrast enhancement, but surrounding areas are often hypervascularized as a result of inflammation and will be enhanced strongly (ring enhancement). In the rabbit, this is most often seen in abscesses, where the centre will not be enhanced but the capsule surrounding the abscess will. The visibility of all these structures will assist in the diagnostic process and narrow the differential diagnosis list to the most plausible option. The images created can be used in planning of surgery (e.g. abscess drainage) or radiotherapy. The transverse images and possible 3D and MPR options are of great value at this stage (Figure 9.2). Note: All transverse CT and MR images in this chapter are displayed with the left lateral aspect of the rabbit on the right side of the image.

CT	MRI
General concept	
Mineralized structures (e.g. dental structures, bone); air-containing structures (e.g. ear canal and tympanic bulla); soft tissues; however, minimal differentiation possible without intravenous contrast medium; intravenous contrast medium is used to evaluate vascularization of tissues	Soft tissues (e.g. brain, vertebral canal and spinal cord, abdominal organs, muscles, tendons, intervertebral discs); soft tissue changes in bone (e.g. bone marrow, osteomyelitis, neoplasia); intravenous contrast medium is used to evaluate vascularization of tissues
Head	
Dental problems (e.g. malocclusion, apical infection, fractures); abscess (e.g. apical dental infection, foreign body); exophthalmos (e.g. dental problem, neoplasia); epiphora (e.g. dental problem, inflammatory plug, neoplasia); rhinitis (e.g. infection of nasal passages, apical dental infection, foreign body, neoplasia); ear problems (e.g. otitis externa, media and interna)	Epilepsy (primary or secondary); abnormal behaviour such as circling and neurological deficits such as paralysis or ataxia (e.g. meningoencephalitis, hydrocephalus, infarct, neoplasia)
Spine	
Paresis or paralysis (e.g. traumatic fracture, discospondylitis, neoplasia)	Paresis or paralysis (e.g. traumatic myelopathy, intervertebral disc herniation, haemorrhage, neoplasia)
Thorax	
Screening for metastases; dyspnoea (e.g. bronchopneumonia, neoplasia, foreign body); evaluation of size and position of mass lesions seen on radiographs (e.g. thymoma, pulmonary neoplasia)	(Functional imaging: cardiac)
Abdomen	
Evaluation of size, position, structure of mass lesions (e.g. abscess, neoplasia); screening for metastases; vasculature; intestinal problems (e.g. foreign body, neoplasia)	Evaluation of size, position and structure of mass lesions; screening for metastases (more sensitive than CT in soft tissues such as liver and spleen); vasculature
All areas	
Surgical planning; radiotherapy planning; screening for metastases	Surgical planning; screening for metastases

9.1 Comparison of indications for CT and MRI in the rabbit.

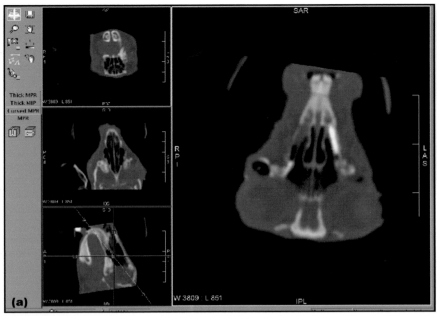
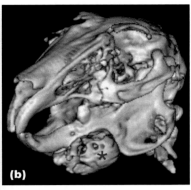

9.2 **(a)** MPR enables the creation of CT images in all planes. The right-hand image (with the yellow box lining) corresponds to the yellow line in the left lower image. **(b)** 3D bone reconstruction, showing the head of a rabbit with bilateral apical infection of the mandibular cheek teeth at the level of the premolars. This is visible as a bony expansive lesion (*) ventral to the mandible.

CT *versus* MRI

MR images are superior in soft tissue differentiation to CT images, but CT images are superior for bone imaging to MRI; therefore MRI is, for example, used most frequently for the brain or spinal cord and CT for the rest of the head or vertebrae. Soft tissues have a narrower range of attenuation (grey values) in CT images, making them harder to differentiate from each other, especially when positioned close together. Intravenous contrast can be of assistance in differentiating well vascularized and poorly vascularized tissues from each other, in both CT and MRI (MRI being more sensitive than CT for smaller changes). Cortical bone and mineralization is black on MRI and therefore small areas of mineralization are better visualized with CT. However, some bone pathologies (e.g. bone necrosis or oedema) can be appreciated with MRI at an early stage but not detected with CT at all.

Restraint and positioning

CT and MRI examinations in the rabbit are performed under general anaesthesia. Preparation and scanning time for a CT scan is short (usually less than 20 minutes). The patient is prepared for the anaesthesia in or near the scanning room to reduce the duration of anaesthesia. In most cases, pre-medication with an anxiolytic drug (e.g. midazolam) followed by an inhalant anaesthetic (e.g. isoflurane) is sufficient. An intravenous catheter is placed when a contrast study is deemed necessary and this is the most time-consuming procedure of the entire examination. MRI scanning takes considerably more time (up to an hour) than CT scanning. The anaesthetic equipment has to be MR-compatible, as do the monitors and positioning materials.

The rabbit is positioned in ventral recumbency and as symmetrically as possible, especially for the head, neck, thorax and pelvis. Although positioning the animal in dorsal recumbency creates a better spatial distribution of the abdominal organs, the pressure on the diaphragm, and therefore on the thorax, has to be kept in mind. Modern rendering and reconstruction software can recreate a symmetrical image, but anatomical structures are very small and therefore positioning is important in creating the best images. After positioning the patient, straps are placed around the table and the rabbit to keep it in exactly the same position during movement of the table and, if the animal should wake up during scanning, to prevent it jumping off the table. Electro-cardiography cables, catheters, infusions and anaesthetic equipment should be kept out of the CT and MRI (even when MR-compatible) gantry as much as possible, because they may cause artefacts which degrade the images.

Conditions in which CT or MRI scanning may be diagnostic

Given that imaging techniques are a sequel to clinical examination, the clinical findings are an important part of image interpretation. A preliminary differential diagnosis guides the CT or MRI technician and radiologist in creating the correct images (choosing the appropriate scanning protocols) and interpretation.

The head

CT examination of the dental structures with adjacent bony structures, nasal passages, nasolacrimal canal, ear canal (external ear canal, tympanic bullae and inner ear) and calvarium is the most common CT procedure performed. MRI of soft tissue structures and the brain can also be performed.

The teeth and nasal passages

The position, shape and attenuation (in HU) of the dental structures and the adjacent bony and soft tissue structures can be evaluated with CT (Van Caelenberg *et al.*, 2008). When interpreting the CT images, the position of the crown and root is evaluated in all dental structures, starting with the incisors and continuing caudally to the maxillary and mandibular cheek teeth. The crown and occlusal surface of the incisors can easily be evaluated clinically but, as the root is elongated and reaches to the nasal passages, this area is not visualized clinically. CT of this area allows evaluation of the tooth roots as well as the surrounding alveolar bone and nasal passages. Some of the cheek teeth are poorly visualized during clinical examination owing to their caudal position. With CT, the entire row of cheek teeth can be visualized, because there is no superimposition of cheek teeth as would be present on a radiograph.

- Malocclusion of the dental structures and secondary changes such as hooks or accumulation of cementum near the roots are all easily visualized with CT.
- The surrounding tissues such as the alveolar bone and nasal passages can be evaluated for possible secondary osteolysis or malformation due to periapical abnormalities (Figure 9.3a).
- Periapical abscesses that deform the alveolar bone are visible as widening of the alveolar space surrounding the roots. CT imaging is very sensitive for detection of minor changes in this area, and a hypoattenuating zone will be the first change visible.
- If inflammation has spread to the nasal passages to cause rhinitis or an abscess, the extent of deformation and destruction of the conchal structures, mucosal swelling and presence of purulent material can be evaluated with CT.
- The existence of an oronasal fistula due to destruction of the alveolar bone in an apical abscess is most often visible as osteolysis of the alveolar wall and concurrent changes (e.g. fluid accumulation) in the nasal passages.
- Abscess formation in conjunction with dental and bony abnormalities can be detected (Figure 9.3b) (Arzi and Sinclair, 2002; Van Caelenberg *et al.*, 2008).

Contrast studies: Intravenous contrast medium can further specify the soft tissue attenuating structures in the images and more clearly demarcate lesions on CT and MR images in fluid, necrotic areas or vascularized tissues. Contrast

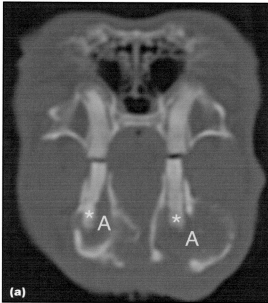

(a)

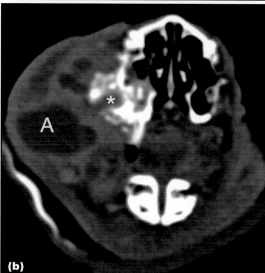

(b)

9.3 **(a)** Transverse CT image (bone setting) of the same rabbit as in Figure 9.2b. It shows bilateral severely deformed mandibles due to extensive apical abscessation (A) of the premolar cheek teeth (*). The roots of the involved cheek teeth are deformed and hypoattenuating. **(b)** Transverse CT image (soft tissue setting) of a different rabbit, showing a large lobular abscess (A) lateral to the right maxilla. Ring enhancement is present. The adjacent maxillary bone is irregular (*), and apical infection with minimal nasal mucosal swelling and fluid is visible.

enhancement patterns can differentiate abscesses and diffuse inflammation from neoplastic masses. Diffuse inflammation will be vaguely defined and cause an increase in attenuation of the fascial fat lines as these are most often involved in the process. Neoplastic masses are more often well defined and, although necrosis or bleeding can be present in the mass, it will cause a diffuse patchy enhancement in both CT and MRI (Figure 9.4). CT and MRI can assist in evaluating the extent of the lesion, detection of the possible origin and treatment planning (Wagner *et al.*, 2005; Ward, 2006).

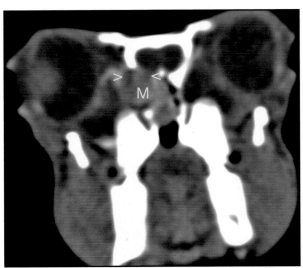

9.4 Transverse CT image (soft tissue setting after intravenous contrast injection) of the head at the level of the cribriform plate. A well defined space-occupying neoplastic mass (M) is visible in the nasopharynx, extending intracranially and in the retrobulbar area via osteolytic areas of the cribriform plate (<) and medial orbital wall (>). Minimal right-sided exophthalmos is present.

The nasolacrimal canal

Blockage of the nasolacrimal duct can be evaluated by performing a CT dacryocystography (Yoshikawa *et al.*, 1998; Nykamp *et al.*, 2004). The contrast medium is instilled directly into the nasolacrimal duct via the punctum lacrimale; if no abnormalities are present, the contrast medium will be visible in the entire canal and nasal passage. Given that CT offers a 3D and complete evaluation of the contrast material in the nasolacrimal canal, the exact location, extent, possible cause of the blockage and clinical or surgical options can be evaluated (Figure 9.5). The advanced software available can create images in three-dimensional planes (MPR) with no superposition, which are superior to radiographs. A virtual endoscopy session can be created. The wall and the lumen of the nasolacrimal duct and the surrounding structures can all be evaluated with CT

scanning. Abnormalities in the lumen can be differentiated from external pressure caused by abnormalities in the surroundings.

The ear canal

Head tilt, head shaking or other neurological deficits can indicate ear problems. Extensive evaluation of the ear is possible with CT scanning because the external ear canal, the tympanic bullae, the petrous bone and cochlea, and even the small ear ossicles may be seen (Stieve-Caldwell *et al.*, 2009). With MRI, the emerging nerves and cochlear fluid can be evaluated.

The external ear canal is normally filled with air and has a certain diameter. In otitis externa, the air will be replaced partially or completely by a soft tissue structure and the lumen becomes narrowed or completely obliterated. This may be due to sebaceous material or an increase in soft tissue, e.g. swelling or neoplasia of the wall of the external ear canal.

In the middle ear, the tympanic bulla is normally filled with air and delineated by a thin, smooth and well defined wall of bone (Figure 9.6a). Otitis media is visible as a partial or complete filling of the tympanic bulla by a mucous to soft tissue material that is visible on both CT and MRI (Figure 9.6b). Destruction of the tympanic bulla wall together with dystrophic mineralization can be present in chronic infections and the extent can be evaluated with CT (Figure 9.6c). Contrast CT and MRI offer further diagnostic possibilities when otitis interna is suspected but no bony abnormalities are visible. Evaluation of adjacent structures, such as the fluid in the cochlea and the cranial nerves, is possible.

The brain and meninges

Meningitis or meningoencephalitis due to an intracranial extension of inner ear infection will cause enhancement of inflamed and hypervascularized tissues, and treatment can be changed accordingly. Other intracranial conditions, such as pituitary adenomas, infarcts or haemorrhage, hydrocephalus or neoplastic lesions, can be detected with both CT and MRI (Figure 9.7) though they are not often encountered in the rabbit (Sikoski *et al.*, 2008; Qiuhang *et al.*, 2010; Wei *et al.*, 2012).

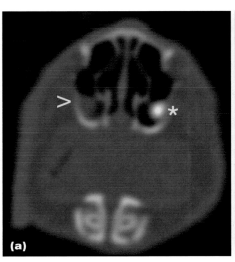

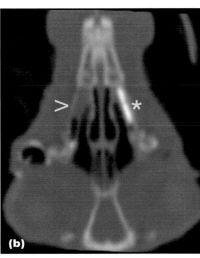

9.5 Dacryocystography. **(a)** Transverse CT image (bone setting) of the head at the level of the premolars. Contrast medium is visible in the left nasolacrimal duct (∗). Soft tissue attenuating material is present in the right nasolacrimal duct (>). **(b)** Dorsal MPR of the same rabbit. Contrast medium is present in the left nasolacrimal canal (∗). Only a minimal amount of contrast medium is visible, followed by air that is outlining a soft tissue attenuating structure blocking the right nasolacrimal canal (>). The large extent of the blockage is clearly visualized.

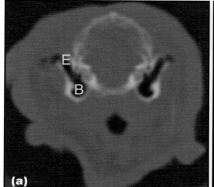
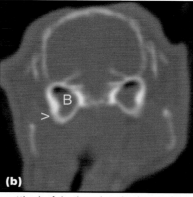
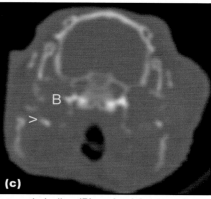

9.6 **(a)** Transverse CT image (bone setting) of the head at the level of the tympanic bullae (B) and axial external ear canal (E). Both are air-filled and the wall of the tympanic bulla is smooth and thin. **(b)** Transverse CT image (bone setting) of the head at the level of the tympanic bullae (B): the tympanic bullae are almost completely filled with a soft tissue attenuating material bilaterally. Note the minimal thickening of the tympanic bulla wall (>). **(c)** Transverse CT image (bone setting) of the head at the level of the tympanic bullae (B): note the bilateral extensive deformation and osteolysis of the tympanic bulla wall (>). The tympanic bullae are completely filled with a soft tissue attenuating material.

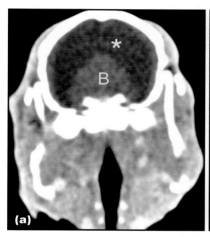
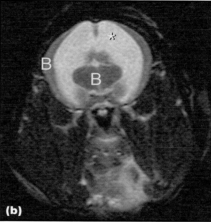

9.7 **(a)** Transverse CT image (soft tissue setting after intravenous contrast medium) of the head at the level of the cranium. The slightly hyperattenuating structure in the central and ventral part of the cranium, together with the very small hyperattenuating rim adjacent to the cranial bones, represents the brain tissue (B). The hypoattenuating area in between these two represents fluid in the lateral ventricles (*). The diagnosis was severe hydrocephalus. **(b)** Transverse T2-weighted MR image of the same rabbit. The fluid in the lateral ventricles is hyperintense (*) and the brain tissue (B) at the centre and near the cranial bones is slightly hypointense.

The thorax and abdomen

CT of the thorax and abdomen in rabbits is mainly performed to evaluate the lungs, lymph nodes and other structures for metastasis (Figure 9.8). A major advantage of radiography and ultrasonography of the thorax and abdomen is that these modalities can be used in rabbits that are in poor body condition where sedation is not possible. However, CT has a much higher sensitivity for the detection of lung changes and therefore metastases will be detected at an earlier stage. Thoracic CT in companion animals such as dogs, cats and birds has become more popular in recent years and is used to evaluate and characterize lung lesions such as lower airway disease, spontaneous pneumothorax, neoplastic lesions or air sac disease in birds. CT of the abdomen is used for the evaluation of the various organs and vasculature. MRI is being used more frequently for abdominal scanning and it seems likely that the use of CT and MRI in evaluation of the thorax and abdomen in rabbits will increase in the future. CT has already been used in radiotherapy for thymoma in rabbits for planning of radiation dose and treatment area (Morrisey and McEntee, 2005).

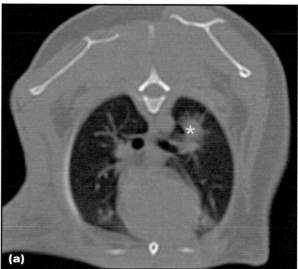

9.8 **(a)** Transverse CT image (bone setting) of the thorax at the level of the caudal main bronchi: a soft tissue attenuating nodule is visible dorsal to the left caudal main bronchus (*). Multiple soft tissue nodules of varying size were present in the lungs and were considered to be metastases of a previously diagnosed uterine carcinoma. (continues) ▶

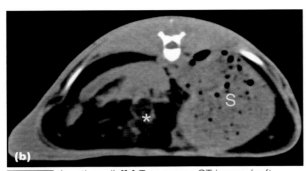

9.8 (continued) **(b)** Transverse CT image (soft tissue setting) of the abdomen at the level of the stomach (S) of the same rabbit. Irregular nodular changes (✳) are seen in the abdominal fat, consistent with carcinomatosis of the uterine carcinoma.

The vertebral column and extremities

CT or MR imaging of the neck and trunk of the rabbit, as well as of intramedullary lesions, has been described mainly for research purposes (Mavinkurve *et al.*, 2005; Zotti *et al.*, 2009). In rabbit medicine, the use of these advanced techniques for diagnosis or treatment planning has been limited but they would be an excellent alternative to myelography and radiographic studies. MRI has almost completely replaced myelography in dogs and cats, and CT has proven to be much more accurate in the detection of bony abnormalities such as vertebral fractures or medial coronoid dysplasia in the elbow.

References and further reading

Arzi B and Sinclair KM (2002) Diagnostic imaging in veterinary dental practice. *Journal of the American Veterinary Medical Association* **236**, 405–407

Bushburg JT, Seibert JA, Leidholdt EM Jr and Boone JM (2002a) Computed tomography. In: *The Essential Physics of Medical Imaging, 2nd edn*, pp. 327–372. Lippincott Williams & Wilkins, Philadelphia

Bushburg JT, Seibert JA, Leidholdt EM Jr and Boone JM (2002b) Nuclear magnetic resonance. In: *The Essential Physics of Medical Imaging, 2nd edn*, pp. 373–414. Lippincott Williams & Wilkins, Philadelphia

Bushburg JT, Seibert JA, Leidholdt EM Jr and Boone JM (2002c) Magnetic resonance imaging. In: *The Essential Physics of Medical Imaging, 2nd edn*, pp. 415–468 Lippincott Williams & Wilkins, Philadelphia

Casteleyn C, Cornillie P, Hermens A *et al.* (2010) Topography of the rabbit paranasal sinuses as a prerequisite to model human sinusitis. *Rhinology* **48**, 300–304

Dennis R and Herrtage ME (1989) Low osmolar contrast media: a review. *Veterinary Radiology* **30**, 2–12

Kuriashkin IV and Losonsky JM (2000) Contrast enhancement in magnetic resonance imaging using intravenous paramagnetic contrast media: a review. *Veterinary Radiology and Ultrasound* **41**, 4–7

Mavinkurve G, Pradilla G, Legnani FG *et al.* (2005) A novel intramedullary spinal cord tumor model: functional, radiological, and histopathological characterization. *Journal of Neurosurgery and Spine* **3**, 142–148

Morrisey JK and McEntee M (2005) Therapeutic options for thymoma in the rabbit. *Seminars in Avian and Exotic Pet Medicine* **14**, 175–181

Nykamp SG, Scrivani PV and Pease AP (2004) Computed tomography dacryocystography evaluation of the nasolacrimal apparatus. *Veterinary Radiology and Ultrasound* **45**, 23–28

Qiuhang Z, Zhenlin W, Yan Q *et al.* (2010) Lymphatic drainage of the skull base: comparative anatomic and advanced imaging studies in the rabbit and human with implications for spread of nasopharyngeal carcinoma. *Lymphology* **43**, 98–109

Sikoski P, Trybus J, Cline JM *et al.* (2008) Cystic mammary adenocarcinoma associated with a prolactin-secreting pituitary adenoma in a New Zealand White rabbit (*Oryctolagus cuniculus*). *Comparative Medicine* **58**, 297–300

Stieve-Caldwell EL, Morandi F, Souza M and Adams WH (2009) What is your diagnosis? *Journal of the American Veterinary Medical Association* **235**, 665–666

Van Caelenberg A, De Rycke L, Hermans K *et al.* (2008) Diagnosis of dental problems in pet rabbits (*Oryctolagus cuniculus*). *Vlaams Diergeneeskundig Tijdschrift* **77**, 386

Van Caelenberg AI, De Rycke LM, Hermans K *et al.* (2010) Computed tomography and cross-sectional anatomy of the head in healthy rabbits. *American Journal of Veterinary Research* **71**, 293–303

Van Caelenberg AI, De Rycke LM, Hermans K *et al.* (2011) Low-field magnetic resonance imaging and cross-sectional anatomy of the rabbit head. *Veterinary Journal* **188**, 83–91

Wagner F, Beinecke A, Fehr M *et al.* (2005) Recurrent bilateral exophthalmos associated with metastatic thymic carcinoma in a pet rabbit. *Journal of Small Animal Practice* **46**, 393–397

Ward ML (2006) Diagnosis and management of a retrobulbar abscess of periapical origin in a domestic rabbit. *Veterinary Clinics of North America: Exotic Animal Practice* **9**, 657–665

Wei XE, Zhang YZ, Li Y *et al.* (2012) Dynamics of rabbit brain edema in focal lesion and perilesion area after traumatic brain injury: a MRI study. *Journal of Neurotrauma* **29**, 2413–2420

Yoshikawa T, Hirota S, Ohno Y *et al.* (1998) Basic study of MR-dacryocystography. *Nihon Igaku Hoshasen Gakkai Zasshi* **58**, 758–760

Yuan YH, Xiao EH, He Z *et al.* (2005) MR diffusion-weighed imaging of rabbit liver. *World Journal of Gastroenterology* **11**, 5506–5511

Zhang LJ, Wang ZJ, Lu L *et al.* (2011) Dual energy CT ventilation imaging after aerosol inhalation of iodinated contrast medium in rabbits. *European Journal of Radiology* **78**, 266–271

Zhao C, Kurita H, Kurashina K *et al.* (2010) Temporomandibular joint response to mandibular deviation in rabbits detected by 3D micro-CT imaging. *Archives of Oral Biology* **55**, 929–937

Zotti A, Banzato T and Cozzi B (2009) Cross-sectional anatomy of the rabbit neck and trunk: comparison of computed tomography and cadaver anatomy. *Research in Veterinary Science* **87**, 171–176

10

Endoscopy

Alessandro Melillo

Endoscopy has been under-utilized in rabbits for many years, despite their popularity as pets. Recently, the usefulness of endoscopy has been recognized and a variety of papers concerning the applications of clinical endoscopy in the companion rabbit can be found.

Patient evaluation

Endoscopic procedures are usually performed under general anaesthesia, so careful attention to the clinical condition of the patient before performing anaesthesia is important. Stabilization may be necessary. Pre-anaesthetic assessment is described in Chapter 1. Given that rabbits hide signs of disease, a clinical profile, including complete blood count and routine urinalysis, may be useful to highlight possible metabolic problems. A chest radiograph may help to exclude subclinical cardiac or respiratory problems. Careful examination of the skull, including different radiographic views, is mandatory when endoscopic procedures are intended for exploration of the nose, mouth, throat or ear.

Anaesthetic considerations

Anaesthetic protocols for endoscopy are related to the nature of the disease that is under investigation, as well as to the clinical condition of the patient. In most cases, premedication with a benzodiazepine combined with an opioid is indicated, followed by induction with ketamine and medetomidine or with sevoflurane delivered by facemask.

When the patient is in an optimal state of relaxation, intubation can be performed and an appropriate plane of anaesthesia can be maintained using isoflurane in oxygen. Tracheal intubation should be performed for surgery and invasive procedures. A nasal mask may be sufficient for faster or less invasive procedures.

Instillation of lidocaine into the nasal cavity is helpful to reduce sensitivity during rhinoscopy. Some authors (Divers, 2010b) suggest the use of neuromuscular blockers (e.g. atracurine) that inhibit reflex movements. The use of these agents means that lower concentrations of inhalational anaesthetics are required, but careful monitoring and ventilation are necessary (see Chapter 1).

Equipment

Most endoscopic procedures can be performed with a basic set of instruments, a good source of light, a camera, a monitor and a rigid endoscope.

Rigid endoscopes

The most useful rigid endoscope is 2.7 mm x 18 cm with a 30 degree oblique view. This allows investigation of several organ systems and the body cavities of most companion rabbits, and a wide variety of tools can be used through its service channel. With its sheath, the diameter of a 2.7 mm endoscope increases to 4.8 mm, and this can be a problem with investigation of delicate structures in small rabbits, especially the nasal cavities. For this indication a 1.9 mm endoscope with a sheath built to give a total diameter of 3.3 mm is more appropriate for rabbits that weigh <1 kg, but this has the disadvantage of only being able to work with a reduced range of dedicated tools.

Flexible endoscopes

A 3 mm fibreoptic endoscope is appropriate for the majority of flexible endoscopic procedures in the rabbit. The most frequently used ancillary instruments are biopsy forceps and 'crocodile teeth' forceps. The applications of flexible endoscopy in rabbits are limited, partly because of their small size and partly because the primary indication for flexible endoscopy is gastroscopy and duodenoscopy in carnivores. These procedures are severely limited in rabbits because their stomach is never empty. There are descriptions of flexible tracheobronchoscopy procedures in rabbits and the endoscopic anatomy of the respiratory system has also been published, but such applications in daily practice are very rare.

Light sources

The endoscope is connected via a fibreoptic cable to a light source. A xenon source is recommended for its bright and intense light, even though cheaper halogen light sources may also provide acceptable results for most simple procedures and in animals <2 kg.

Cameras and monitors

Direct observation through the eyepiece of the lens is acceptable for short procedures and manipulation is easy, but the position does not allow the freedom of movement that is needed for minimally invasive surgery. The use of a camera and a monitor is considered essential for the surgical procedures described in this chapter, and optional for diagnostic procedures such as rhinoscopy or tracheoscopy. An additional advantage of video equipment is the ability to collect and store images, which are useful both for teaching and for communication with the owner.

Carbon dioxide

Insufflation is beneficial for the visualization of many structures through an endoscope. Laparoscopic procedures require CO_2 insufflation. A special (dedicated) pump can be used but compressed ambient air insufflated with an aquarium pump or a syringe is acceptable, although there is a small risk of introducing air. The gas is introduced through the valves of the operating sheath, and it is also possible to use this channel to introduce irrigation fluids, such as saline, to dilate orifices such as the nasal conchae or urethra.

Ancillary instruments

In order to work on the structures that can be visualized with endoscopy, it is necessary to use instruments that can pass through the operating sheath. The most frequently used devices in rabbit medicine are biopsy forceps and grasping forceps, which are useful for debridement and/or to retrieve foreign bodies from ears and nostrils. A flexible needle is useful to aspirate the contents of cystic structures and/or to irrigate cavities that are hard to reach.

Operator positioning

The best position in which to use the endoscope is determined, within certain limits, by the individual operator, who will develop working practices in accordance with his/her individual abilities and preferences. Secure control over the endoscope is essential because the equipment is expensive and fragile. Flexion of the endoscope easily breaks the cylindrical lenses inside the device.

In order to perform endoscopy, it is necessary to master the technique of maintaining the rigid endoscope with a single hand. For a right-handed operator the left hand holds the lens, placing it between the extended thumb and palm, and wrapping it with the other fingers; the right hand remains free to use the ancillary tools. At first, it may be useful to have the help of a second person, but to be efficient it is necessary to learn to do it alone. It should be stressed that even the most modern cameras have most of their weight at the upper end of the endoscope, so it is necessary to hold the equipment in two places. The camera is held with the whole hand, with the thumb and forefinger at the point of entry into the body of the patient.

Direct observation through the eyepiece of the lens can be used for fast procedures but does not allow a suitable ergonomic position to be maintained during prolonged observation. A camera and a monitor are necessary. It is essential that the monitor is directly in front of the operator's eyes and, ideally, the endoscope should be directed toward the monitor itself. This simple practice can help to maintain an ergonomic position and facilitates rapid mental association between hand movements and images on the monitor.

For minimally invasive surgery, when several sites of access on both sides of the patient are needed, the use of two monitors is preferred. Alternatively, an assistant can be instructed to move the monitor when the surgeon changes position, but effective collaboration of the surgical assistant with the procedure is then compromised.

Patient positioning

The rabbit can be placed in dorsal, sternal or lateral recumbency, according to the procedure that is to be performed. It is helpful to have the ability to tilt the patient's head upwards in order to gain good access to the liver during laparoscopy, or downwards to improve access to the caudal organs such as the bladder or intra-abdominal testes, or to facilitate the flow of irrigation fluid during rhinoscopy.

Endoscopic examination of the ear

The prevalence of subclinical otitis in rabbits, especially in lop-eared breeds (see Chapter 16), warrants special attention to endoscopy of the ear. It is always better to sedate the rabbit, in order to avoid sudden movements that may cause damage to the ear canal or the instrument. The patient may be maintained in sternal or lateral recumbency. The normal ear canal contains wax. Often there is a mild degree of inflammation, which produces a large amount of debris, so mechanical cleaning is required before introducing the endoscope. Irrigation with sterile saline is preferred because this will allow sample collection for bacteriology.

The endoscope is inserted along the length of the ear canal down to the eardrum; the examination may reveal generalized or localized inflammation (Figure 10.1), foreign bodies, mites or tumours. If the tympanic membrane is ruptured or perforated by infection, syringotomy to collect material for analysis, and to decrease pressure and relieve clinical signs, may be helpful.

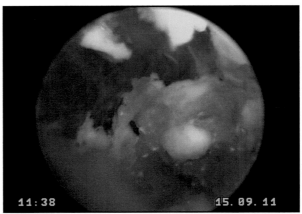

10.1 An endoscopic view of an inflamed ear canal containing a wax plug and pus.

Endoscopic evaluation of the pharynx and larynx

The larynx in rabbits is covered by the soft palate, which needs to be lifted in order to visualize the glottis, to insert an endotracheal tube or to obtain a tracheal swab sample. Foreign bodies may be visualized in the larynx.

Endoscope-guided endotracheal intubation

Unlike in dogs, cats and ferrets, in rabbits it is not possible to visualize the glottis directly simply by opening the mouth; endotracheal intubation is therefore more difficult. Although 'blind' intubation is possible, endoscopy-guided intubation is faster and safer. A small-gauge paediatric laryngoscope that is slightly curved is particularly useful because it provides a route for an oxygen supply, which reduces the risks associated with the procedure. It is recommended that lidocaine gel be applied to the endotracheal tube prior to intubation to reduce the risk of laryngeal spasm.

Alternatively, a 2.7 mm 0 degree straight probe may be employed, either by inserting it inside the tube or by placing it adjacent to the tube. Inserting the endoscope into the tube is usually only possible in rabbits large enough to be intubated with 3 mm tubes, unless a 1.9 mm endoscope is available that can be used in smaller rabbits. It may be necessary to shorten the endotracheal tubes: their length should not be greater than that of the endoscope, otherwise steam or saliva can accumulate in the tip, obstructing vision.

To insert an endotracheal tube alongside an endoscope, the anaesthetized rabbit is placed in sternal recumbency with its head and neck raised and extended. The head is supported dorsally to avoid compression of the trachea. It may be convenient to place the animal on a mobile dental platform or to use a dental gag. The tongue is pulled out to aid progression of the endoscope through the oral cavity, following the median groove to maintain the correct direction. If the endoscope is oriented ventrally to the larynx, the larynx will be visible through the transparent soft palate. At this point, the tube is advanced to the side of the endoscope until it enters the visual field. Progressing gently, the tip of the endoscope will lift the soft palate and release the larynx, so the tube can be inserted during inhalation (see Technique 1.2).

Proper placement of the tube is confirmed by direct observation, by the sight of vapour in the transparent tube or, if the 'scope in the tube' technique is used, by observation of the tracheal rings. The advantages of this technique are the ability to use endotracheal tubes of the widest calibre possible, the security of not introducing foreign material into the trachea and the ability to intubate a rabbit who is not breathing.

Rhinoscopy

Rhinitis is a common problem in rabbits, and has a varied and multifactorial aetiology. Treatment is often frustrating and an early aetiological diagnosis is important to guide appropriate therapy, otherwise the problem tends to become chronic. Rhinoscopy is an invaluable aid in making a diagnosis: it permits irrigation of the nasal cavities, which removes excess secretions; it is used to detect infection or neoplasia and to collect biopsy samples for bacteriology, cytology and histopathology; and can aid removal of foreign bodies. Some endoscopic views of the nose, throat, mouth and trachea are shown in Figure 10.2.

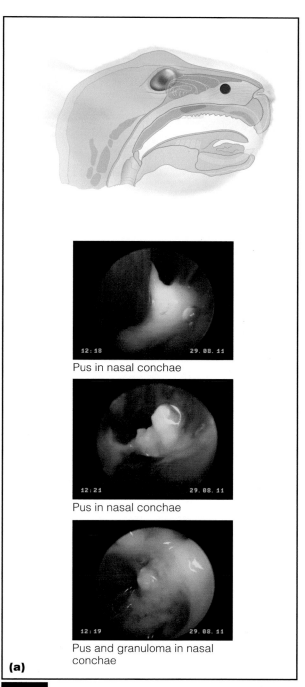

Pus in nasal conchae

Pus in nasal conchae

Pus and granuloma in nasal conchae

(a)

10.2 **(a)** Endoscopic views of the nose. (continues) ▶

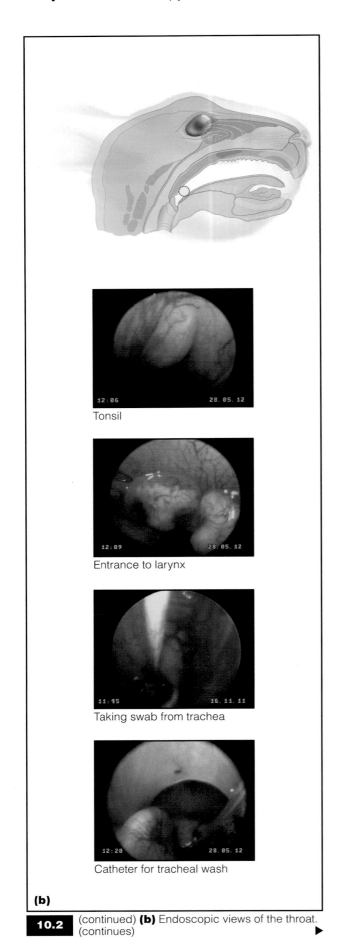

Tonsil

Entrance to larynx

Taking swab from trachea

Catheter for tracheal wash

(b)

10.2 (continued) **(b)** Endoscopic views of the throat. (continues) ▶

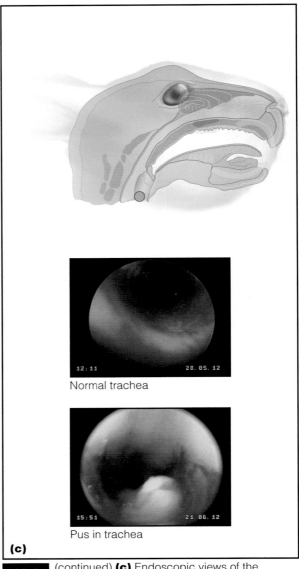

Normal trachea

Pus in trachea

(c)

10.2 (continued) **(c)** Endoscopic views of the trachea.

Given that the nasal mucous membranes are very sensitive, a deep plane of anaesthesia is required as well as local analgesia, such as a lidocaine spray. The intubated animal is placed in sternal recumbency with the head slightly lower than the body (10–20 degrees). As an uncuffed endotracheal tube is normally used, it is important to fill the mouth with soft gauze to absorb any liquid and prevent its inhalation. Placing a towel under the animal is also useful, because of the extensive irrigation that is required for this examination.

In rabbits <2 kg, a 2.7 mm endoscope with its sheath is too large to reach the deep nasal cavity. A 1.9 mm endoscope with a built-in sheath is preferable. Alternatively, a 2.7 mm endoscope can be used without the sheath, irrigating the nasal passages using a syringe intermittently, but the results are much less satisfactory.

After introduction of the endoscope, the lens is guided gently through the nasal passages (Figure 10.3). The endoscope needs to be placed medially

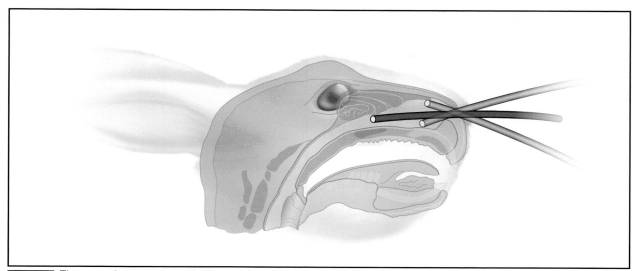

10.3 There are three meatuses in the nasal cavity: dorsal, middle and ventral. The endoscope needs to be directed into the middle meatus because the dorsal and ventral meatuses are blind-ended. In order to explore the delicate nose of smaller rabbits a fine scope (1.9 mm) with built-in sheath is advisable. Some bleeding is to be expected. Foreign bodies, chronic infections and complications from odontogenic abscesses are common findings in this region.

because the mucosa of the turbinates is fragile, especially if inflamed, and may bleed profusely. It is almost impossible not to cause minor bleeding, even if the procedure is conducted carefully.

It is also possible to access the nasal cavity and paranasal sinuses by rhinotomy or facial osteotomy to explore the cavity before a major surgical procedure (Figure 10.4). This application can be particularly useful in cases of odontogenic abscesses involving the nasal region (Divers, 2010c).

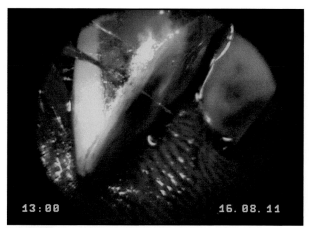

10.4 Tooth fragment in the maxillary sinus. The sinuses can be explored endoscopically after trephining a hole through the bone.

Tracheobronchoscopy

This is one of the few applications for flexible endoscopy in the rabbit, although a rigid endoscope will reach the tracheal bifurcation. For tracheobronchoscopy, the head and the neck must

be kept extended and aligned, to avoid any trauma to the sensitive tracheal mucosa. To avoid problems with gas exchange, only small diameter endoscopes should be used and only for short periods of time, or oxygen can be introduced through the instrument channel of the endoscope (Figure 10.5).

Tracheobronchoscopy is useful for removing foreign bodies and to obtain an aetiological diagnosis in cases of severe respiratory disease. Chronic inflammatory processes may be caused by mucosal injury and complicated by tracheal stenosis followed by severe respiratory failure.

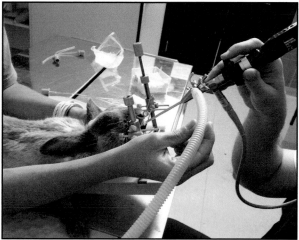

10.5 Tracheoscopy. Using a rigid endoscope of appropriate size, with some care and attention the rabbit trachea can be explored down to the bronchial bifurcation. The normal tracheal mucosa is a bright red colour, which can be confused with inflammation. Tracheal stenosis and obstruction cause severe respiratory distress and it is mandatory to provide extra oxygen to the rabbit during the whole procedure.

Vaginoscopy, urethroscopy and cystoscopy

Haematuria is a frequent clinical sign in rabbits and, although other diagnostic imaging techniques (radiology, ultrasonography) are commonly used to determine the cause, endoscopy is a valid aid for examination of the vagina (Figure 10.6), urethra (Figure 10.7), bladder and cervix. With a rigid endoscope, it is possible to manipulate urethral stones that would otherwise be unreachable because, for example, they are in the pelvic stretch of the urethra. Endoscopy can also be used to take biopsy samples and remove small papillomas. The patient is usually positioned in dorsal recumbency with the perineum at the edge of the table. Dilation of the urethra is facilitated by irrigation with warm saline. Some endoscopic views of the urogenital tract are shown in Figure 10.8.

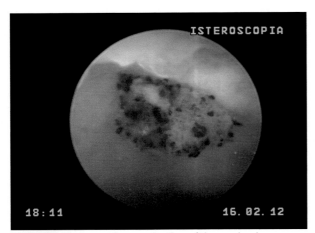

10.6 Endoscopic examination of the vagina is straightforward. The openings of the urethra separate the vaginal vestibulum and the long soft uterine vagina. In this image a mass can be seen in the vaginal wall. Although ultrasonography is more frequently used to diagnose uterine diseases in does, hysteroscopy allows the surgeon to obtain biopsy samples of pathological tissue before surgery and to obtain a more precise prognosis.

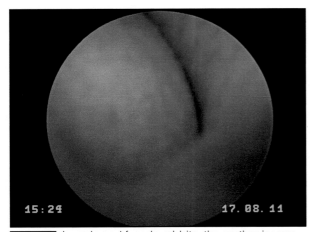

10.7 In male and female rabbits, the urethra is very elastic and easily allows the passage of the endoscope. This may be the only way to retrieve stones lodged in the pelvic stretch of the urethra. Biopsy samples of bladder mucosa can be taken in a relatively non-invasive way.

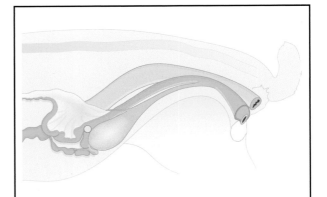

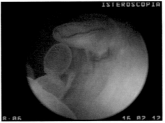

Carcinoma in left cervix

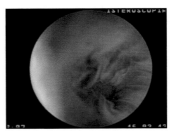

Opening of right cervix

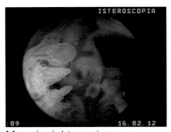

Mass in right cervix

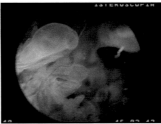

Mass in right cervix

(a)

10.8 **(a)** Endoscopic views of the cervix. (continues) ▶

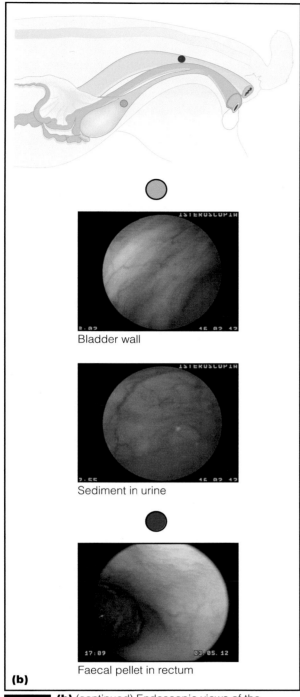

Bladder wall

Sediment in urine

Faecal pellet in rectum

(b)

10.8 **(b)** (continued) Endoscopic views of the bladder and rectum.

Endoscopy of the digestive tract

Although this is the most commonly used endoscopic technique in domestic carnivores, in rabbits gastroscopy is almost impossible because the stomach is never empty. It is possible to use the endoscope for colonoscopy and rectoscopy (see Figure 10.8b) and, in cases of papillomatosis, endoscopy can be used to rule out the presence of papillomas in areas not visible following simple protrusion of the rectal mucosa (Figure 10.9).

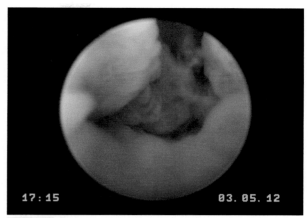

10.9 Rectal papillomatosis is quite common in rabbits and colonoscopy can help to locate masses not immediately evident on simple evagination of rectal mucosa. These masses can be excised using traditional surgery, cryosurgery or surgical laser (see Chapter 18).

Laparoscopy

Laparoscopic investigation (see also Chapter 13) and minimally invasive abdominal surgery are in their early days in the rabbit, but several authors have emphasized the advantages in terms of reduced tissue trauma, less pain and faster postoperative recovery. However, the owner must be informed that, in the case of complications, access by traditional open surgery may still be necessary.

Laparoscopic procedures in rabbits include ovariectomy (Divers, 2010a), liver and kidney biopsy, and endoscope-assisted cystotomy for removal of small uroliths. Laparoscopy requires additional care when compared with endoscopic examination of natural orifices. A pneumoperitoneum must be generated to visualize the abdominal organs and to move among them. This is usually achieved by insufflation with carbon dioxide, which is considered safer than ambient air because there is less risk of embolization or combustion if electrocautery is used. Creating a pneumoperitoneum increases the pressure in the abdominal compartment and hinders diaphragmatic excursion so it is essential to work only with intubated rabbits receiving mechanical ventilation. The increased intra-abdominal pressure also alters haemodynamics as a result of compression of the aorta and the vena cava. Although this problem is marginal in large rabbits, in patients <5 kg it is recommended not to exceed an intra-abdominal pressure of 8 mmHg.

For most procedures, the patient is placed in dorsal recumbency. The fur is shaved and the skin prepared as for conventional surgery. Insufflation of gas takes place through a special cannula with a trocar (Veress needle) that is inserted in the caudal midline. It is advisable to ensure that the rabbit has an empty bladder because it is possible to traumatize viscera with the Veress needle. Other causes of organomegaly (gastric dilatation, pregnancy, pyometra, abscess, neoplasm) should also be considered before proceeding to laparoscopy. Some authors consider it safer to make a small incision in the abdominal wall and raise the midline with a clamp or sutures before using a scalpel as in a traditional laparotomy incision. Subsequent introduction of a blunt cannula is less likely to cause organ damage. The incision is closed around the cannula with a haemostat or sutures.

Once gas has been introduced into the abdomen, insufflation must progress smoothly and with a gradual increase of pressure. A sudden rise in pressure is a sign that the gas is being introduced subcutaneously.

Once the abdomen is insufflated, an endoscope is inserted just caudal to the umbilicus, and the procedure begins with general visualization of the abdominal cavity. If there are no significant contra-indications to laparoscopy (adhesions, masses, important iatrogenic damage), access points are identified for an accessory trocar, which must always be visible from both inside and outside the abdomen (see Chapter 11). The light from the endoscope trans-illuminates the abdominal wall and shows the blood vessels, which helps to identify a site for incision and insertion of the accessory trocar. Instruments can be introduced through the accessory trocar for haemostasis, or probes for manipulation of the viscera.

When the laparoscopy is complete, the trocars are extracted and the valve of the insufflation cannula is opened. Once the air has been fully evacuated, the incisions are closed. In humans, residual gas in the abdomen is very painful; it is not known if this is the case in other species.

Thoracoscopy

Thoracoscopy is generally considered easier than laparoscopy because there are fewer organs to be displayed and because it is easier to maintain a pneumothorax than a pneumoperitoneum. Given that thoracic surgery is more difficult and delicate than abdominal surgery, one would expect a much greater use of thoracoscopy because it is minimally invasive, less painful and is associated with faster postoperative recovery.

In rabbits, however, there are difficulties associated with anaesthesia during thoracoscopy. Intermittent positive pressure ventilation is always required (see Chapter 1). The applications that have been described for thoracoscopy in the rabbit involve biopsy of mediastinal and lung masses, as well as the collection of fluid for cytology and culture. The approach can be parasternal (usually more suitable for small rabbits) or intercostal (in larger individuals). The small incisions through which the endoscope and trocars are inserted need to be sutured carefully and the insufflated air fully sucked out. The vital signs and blood oxygenation of these patients need to be closely monitored before, during and after the procedure.

References and further reading

Divers SJ (2010a) Clinical technique: endoscopic oophorectomy in the rabbit (*Oryctolagus cuniculus*), the future of preventative sterilization. *Journal of Exotic Pet Medicine* **19**, 231–239

Divers SJ (2010b) Endoscopy equipment and instrumentation for use in exotic animal veterinary medicine. *Veterinary Clinics of North America: Exotic Animal Practice* **13**(2), 171–185

Divers SJ (2010c) Exotic mammal diagnostic endoscopy and endosurgery. *Veterinary Clinics of North America: Exotic Animal Practice* **13**(2), 255–272

Divers SJ (2012) Exotic mammal diagnostic and surgical endoscopy. In: *Ferrets, Rabbits and Rodents, Clinical Medicine and Surgery*, ed. KE Quesenberry and JW Carpenter, pp. 485–501. Elsevier, St. Louis

Hernandez-Divers SJ (2004) Small mammal endoscopy. In: *Ferrets, Rabbits and Rodents, Clinical Medicine and Surgery*, ed. KE Quesenberry and JW Carpenter, pp. 392–394. Elsevier, St. Louis

Hernandez-Divers SJ (2005) Rabbit ear, nose and mouth endoscopy. In: *Proceedings of the North American Veterinary Congress, Jan 8–12, Orlando, Florida*, pp. 1330–1331

Melillo A and Grande D (2010) Pratica endoscopica nei piccoli mammiferi. In: *Exotic Files Endoscopia degli Animali Esotici*, ed. Dr Lorenzo Crosta, pp. 21–26. Editore SCIVAC, Palazzo Trecchi, Cremona [In Italian]

Selleri P (2011) Endoscopia negli animali esotici – piccoli mammiferi. In: *Endoscopia degli Animali d'Affezione (Cane, Gatto, Esotici) Testo Atlante*, ed. E Bottero and P Ruggiero, pp. 279–291. Poletto Editore srl Vermezzo, Milan [In Italian]

Basic principles of soft tissue surgery

Molly Varga

The general principles of soft tissue surgery are as applicable to rabbits as they are to cats and dogs. These include Halsted's basic principles of soft tissue surgery.

Halsted's principles
- Gentle tissue handling
- Accurate haemostasis
- Preservation of adequate blood supply
- Strict asepsis
- Avoidance of tension on wounds
- Careful tissue approximation
- Obliteration of dead space

The aim of this chapter is to highlight both the similarities and differences between rabbits and cats and dogs, so that veterinary practitioners can modify their existing surgical skills where necessary.

Rabbits as surgical candidates

Soft tissue broadly comprises skin, skeletal elements (muscles, tendons, ligaments), nervous tissue, cardiovascular tissue and viscera. Differences in the ways that these tissues respond to insult (surgical or pathological) affect the way they need to be handled clinically (Figure 11.1).

Dogs	Cats	Rabbits	Surgical consequences in the rabbit
Skin			
Stratum corneum 45 cells thick; collagenous bridges exist between dermis and deeper tissues; healing mainly by wound contraction; skin wound healing significantly faster than in cats and full tensile strength reached more rapidly	Stratum corneum 12 cells thick; collagenous bridges exist between dermis and deeper tissues; healing by epithelialization and central pull, takes significantly longer than in dogs	Stratum corneum 2–3 cells thick; no collagenous bridges between dermis and subcutaneous layer, creating a 'fracture plane'; very densely haired tissue, with lots of primary and secondary follicles per square millimetre; healing by epithelialization and fibrous tissue formation	It is relatively easy to create unwanted dead space adjacent to skin incisions if tissue is not handled carefully; this can be potentially difficult to deal with clinically, leading to seroma or abscess formation
Muscle			
Heals well, though muscle contraction occurs over time	Heals very easily with minimal contraction in many cases	Significant muscle contraction can occur rapidly, potentially making fracture fixation difficult; 'plasty' techniques to elongate muscle may be required	Surgical fixation of muscular damage needs to be addressed rapidly; healing by primary intention indicated
Gut			
Serosal surfaces need to be apposed to ensure rapid healing; generous omentum, allowing omentalization of gut wounds	Serosal surfaces need to be apposed to ensure rapid healing; generous omentum, allowing omentalization of gut wounds post repair	Direct apposition of edges required to minimize lumen diameter reduction; omentum is smaller and less flexible compared to cats and dogs, so is less useful for supporting gut wounds	Edges of rabbit gut must be apposed directly to prevent stenosis; single layer gut closure is indicated (unlike cats and dogs); omental support postsurgically cannot be relied upon
Urogenital tract			
Double layer of inverting sutures indicated for repair; sutures penetrating bladder wall and remaining for long periods can become a nidus for infection and urolith formation	Double layer of inverting sutures indicated for closure; penetration of bladder lumen with non-absorbable sutures can act as foci for infection and urolith formation	Double layer of inverting sutures indicated for closure; penetration of suture material into bladder lumen can form a nidus for infection or urolith formation; therefore sutures penetrating full wall thickness not recommended	Careful repair of bladder incisions required to avoid iatrogenic urolithiasis that can persist for as long as the suture material does

11.1 A comparison of species differences in tissues often requiring surgical intervention.

Skin

Rabbit skin is thinner and more fragile than the skin of cats and dogs and as such requires careful handling. The epidermis is thinner and there is no collagenous adherence between the dermis and deeper layers, creating a cleavage plane (Billingham and Medawar, 1951). This allows the skin to be detached from the underlying tissue easily, making rabbits good candidates for skin flap and grafting procedures. The disadvantage is that dead space can easily be created inadvertently, giving the potential for serous/serosanguineous fluid or pus to collect. The thinness of the skin can mean that the ends of knots from suture lines in tissues under the skin, e.g. the linea alba, can cause significant irritation to the rabbit, particularly if they are not covered by subcuticular suture lines.

Unless an individual rabbit is very overweight, there is much less subcutaneous tissue available compared to other species. One consequence of this is that subcuticular sutures, while desirable, are much more difficult to place. This is because of the thinness of rabbit skin compared with that of cats and dogs, which makes it very easy for sutures to go through instead of tunnelling within the skin, leaving a portal for entry of infection. In areas where there is more subcutaneous fat this is not so much of a problem, e.g. behind the elbow area in fatter individuals or in the dewlap region.

Rabbit skin heals rapidly but is easily traumatized. Due to the formation of very viscous sticky pus, a consequence of the enzyme content of the rabbit heterophil/neutrophil compared to the cat/dog neutrophil (Baggiolini et al., 1969, 1970), wound infection can be very difficult to manage, and abscessation is a common consequence. Rabbits are also prone to overproduction of granulation tissue during healing and are commonly used experimentally as models of wound healing for this reason (Gordon et al., 1974; Bayat et al., 2006; Abramov et al., 2007; Onderdonk et al., 2009). This in turn can lead to large fibrous scars, so that healing by primary intention is preferable, for better cosmetic and functional results.

Musculoskeletal elements

Damaged muscles heal by fibrosis. This fibrous tissue does not have the functional capability or strength of normal muscle. This, and the fact that significant contracture can occur prior to fixation of damaged bones, can cause functional problems in the longer term. Severe muscle contraction, for example in the quadriceps femoris when the femur is damaged, may necessitate surgical muscle lengthening 'plasty' techniques (Merck, 2011). Fibrous healing does not yield a highly functional tissue, compared with the healing achieved by prompt surgical repair. Formation of adhesions, particularly in tendon healing, can limit range of motion and therefore function (Shrive et al., 1995).

Abdominal viscera

Handling of the serosal surfaces of rabbit viscera can cause the formation of 'adhesions' or internal scars between organs, particularly affecting gut motility after abdominal surgery. They can, however, occur after any soft tissue trauma. Fat necrosis occurs readily, with the decomposition resulting in the formation of fatty acids and glycerol. The fatty acids combine with ions such as sodium and calcium to promote adhesion formation. Foreign material, such as talcum powder from gloves or fibres from swabs, can also elicit adhesion formation. The omentum is smaller and less flexible than in cats and dogs and therefore less useful for omentalizing viscera.

Wound healing and repair

Wound healing in the rabbit progresses in the same way as in other species. However, there are quantitative differences with regard to epidermal migration and connective tissue maturation (Srivastava and Lossin, 1976; Onderdonk et al., 1979; Bayat et al., 2006; Abramov, 2007; Aziz and Aziz, 2008; Hashemi et al., 2011).

There are four main phases.

1. **Haemostasis:** the coagulation cascade is activated by tissue damage, and a blood then fibrin clot is formed in the defect. The fibrin clot is the main support for the wound until cellular healing occurs.
2. **Inflammation:** soluble chemotactic factors attract various cell types to the wound. In rabbits, polymorphonuclear heterophils (PMHs) are the predominant cell type in the hours and days after injury. They kill and phagocytose bacteria, remove debris and secrete proteases to break down damaged tissue. Once the PMHs have completed this process they undergo apoptosis and are in turn phagocytosed by macrophages. Macrophages also remove any remaining cellular debris and bacteria, and continue the breakdown of damaged tissue by producing proteases. They replace PMHs as the predominant cell type within 48 hours of insult.
3. **Proliferation:** formation of granulation tissue. This is stimulated by chemotactic factors secreted by macrophages, which attract fibroblasts (cells involved in re-epithelialization and angiogenesis). This starts to occur 2–3 days post insult, although it can be delayed if the wound is severely contaminated. Granulation tissue contains a variety of cell types, including vascular tissue, white blood cells, fibroblasts and macrophages. It acts to protect the underlying tissue from infection and further trauma. Re-epithelialization occurs over the surface of the granulation tissue. Fibroblasts lay down collagen, which acts as a matrix within which all the other cell types can proliferate. Wound contraction also occurs at this stage; myofibroblasts contract, drawing the wound edges together. Rabbits are particularly prone to excessive production of granulation tissue.
4. **Remodelling:** collagen is remodelled from type 3 to type 1 (increasing in tensile strength) and realigned in response to tissue forces. The tensile strength of the wound increases until it approaches that of undamaged tissue.

- The ideal for wound healing is **primary intention healing**, allowing return to maximum function in minimum time. The criteria for this are: accurate apposition of tissue, usually achieved by suturing; and lack of infection. Surgical wounds most closely approximate this ideal; however, traumatic wounds can fall into this category as long as measures are taken to prevent infection and there are no significant tissue deficits. Measures to prevent infection include careful wound cleaning and debridement, sensitive apposition of tissue so that there is no excess tension on the wound, suitable choice of suture material and antibiosis.

- For grossly infected wounds, either **secondary or delayed primary intention healing** is more appropriate. In practice, infected wounds should be thoroughly debrided and cleaned and then consideration given to how best to maintain healthy granulation tissue.

- One consideration specific to rabbits is that of **subcutaneous abscesses**. They are one of the commonest presenting problems and can occur secondary to fighting, in particular, or to skin trauma of any kind. The confounding factor in the rabbit is the consistency of the pus, which is thick, sticky and tenacious. This means that the traditional approach of lancing, flushing and placing a drain does not work, and is indeed contraindicated. Ideally, subcutaneous abscesses would be removed intact without disturbing the fibrous abscess capsule, and the wound could then be allowed to heal by primary intention. However, this is not always possible and other solutions must be sought. The general approach is to resect as much of the abscess capsule as possible and to marsupialize the edges of the capsule to the skin surface and allow healing by secondary intention. This effectively allows the abscess to heal from the inside out (see also Chapter 29).

- For both grossly infected wounds and initial treatment of cutaneous abscesses, the author advocates the use of **collagen matrix dressings** sutured tightly on to the wound for at least the first 3–5 days after debridement. This allows granulation tissue to form in a protective moist environment while wicking away any purulent exudates. Essentially, the pus gets locked into the dressing away from the wound. Packing the wound tightly appears to enhance this process without causing additional discomfort to the rabbit. Once the dressing is removed, sufficient granulation tissue has formed to allow direct cleaning of the wound (see Operative Technique 11.1).

- An alternative option is the use of classical **wet-to-dry dressings** using swabs moistened with sterile saline that are applied to the wound and allowed to dry *in situ*. As the dried swabs are removed this provides gentle wound debridement. Once infection is controlled and the granulation bed has formed, the decision can be made as to whether healing should continue by secondary intention or whether delayed primary closure should be attempted.

- **Honey** has been advocated as a bactericidal wound dressing (there are several proprietary formulations, but unpasteurized Manuka honey is also suitable). While it has been shown to be less effective than some other compounds, the advantages of a non-toxic effective wound dressing are obvious. The mechanism of action is via production of hydrogen peroxide within the wound, which then kills the bacteria present (this is also cytotoxic) so healing relies on effective phagocytosis. This is well accepted by rabbits.

- Once a healthy bed of granulation tissue has formed, the **skin deficit can be left open**, allowing the owner to clean (and thereby gently debride) the area once or twice daily. As rabbit wounds heal primarily by wound contraction and epithelialization the skin deficit can reduce rapidly (often 10–14 days for a 3 cm x 2 cm deficit).

- **Decision making** is based on the amount of tissue deficit, whether flap or advancement procedures can be employed, how well infection is controlled, the requirement for full return to function, and the projected long-term effect on the patient.

- Rabbits are generally good candidates for **flap or skin advancement procedures** as their skin is very flexible and the lack of collagenous attachment between the dermis and deeper tissues means it is practically easy to accomplish. This can be a useful tool for large skin wounds once infection has been addressed.

11.2 A practical approach to wound management.

A practical approach to wound repair is outlined in Figure 11.2. Wound repair can be accomplished in various ways:

- **Primary intention:** wound edges are in good anatomical apposition and healing progresses rapidly with minimal scar formation, e.g. surgical repair. This minimizes scarring and maximizes chances of tissue functionality
- **Secondary intention:** wound edges are not in apposition and granulation tissue formation is allowed. This produces a broader scar and slower healing. Functionality may be compromised. Typically seen in large infected wounds. Ongoing wound cleaning and debridement may be required to allow granulation tissue to form
- **Delayed primary or secondary intention:** the wound is cleaned and debrided for several days prior to closure, or is left purposefully open (e.g. to receive a tissue graft).

The rate of healing can vary with tissue type, e.g. skin heals rapidly while tendons may take up to a year to be fully repaired.

Skin preparation
Rabbit skin is very fragile and the hair is dense, making it difficult to clip without causing skin damage. The best option is to use new/sharp clipper blades with small fine teeth. It is sensible to have 'rabbit only' clippers that are not blunted by dog and cat hair. Gentle tension should be placed on the skin and clipping should be done slowly and against the direction of hair growth, with the clipper blades as near parallel to the skin as possible. Even with careful clipping, iatrogenic damage can occur. This can cause skin irritation, leading to self-trauma.

Some authors have suggested plucking hair for smaller procedures; however, in the author's experience, this can cause significant skin irritation and can lead to tearing. Hair removal creams have also been advocated; however, these are not widely used at this time and appear to have fallen out of favour.

Once the hair has been removed, skin cleaning and disinfection needs to be undertaken. This includes scrubbing with antiseptics such as chlorhexidine or povidone–iodine, and final preparation with surgical spirit. Excessive scrubbing can cause postoperative irritation and increase the potential for discomfort and self-trauma. Single-application products should be considered, e.g. chlorhexidine or povidone–iodine in surgical spirit, as these may prove less irritant; however, in cases where there is gross skin contamination they may not be appropriate.

In small individuals it is sensible to try to reduce heat loss by removing the least amount of hair that is practical, and consistent with good surgical access, and minimizing the amount of skin that is wet (the hair at the edges of the prepared area should be slicked down away from the incision line).

Tissue handling

Rabbits have been used extensively as models for postsurgical adhesion formation, due to their propensity to form fibrous adhesions after any tissue damage, whether surgical or traumatic (Gordon *et al.*, 1974). In humans, as many as 80% of patients have clinical problems related to adhesion formation in the 2 years after abdominal surgery (Steinleitner *et al.*, 1989, 1990). It is likely that as many, if not more, rabbits suffer in a similar way. From a surgical perspective, postoperative adhesion formation is significantly increased by rough or traumatic tissue handling. While adhesion formation can cause significant functional problems for the rabbit patient, the important point is that they frequently cause discomfort, if not pain.

Adhesions are 'internal scars' that form between viscera. Trauma to the visceral surface (e.g. surgical intervention or handling) causes fibrin to be deposited on to the damaged tissues. This acts to seal the injured area (fibrinous adhesion). Normally fibrinolytic enzymes act to limit the extent of adhesion formation. If the availability of these enzymes is compromised (e.g. due to the disease process) then the adhesion matures. Fibrinolysin levels are lower in rabbits than in cats and dogs. Macrophages, fibroblasts and blood vessels penetrate the fibrinous tissue and lay down collagen, forming a permanent fibrous adhesion.

Fat necrosis can also lead to adhesion formation and this is often seen in the fat of the broad ligament after ovariohysterectomy (see Chapter 12).

In the author's experience, lack of appropriate intraoperative haemostasis can also contribute to adhesion formation; for example, failure to ligate or cauterize the vessels in the broad ligament so that blood clots are left within the abdomen, which may eventually become adhesions. Equally, the use of inappropriate ligatures (e.g. catgut) for haemostasis can also result in adhesion formation.

In practical terms, the use of instruments rather than manual manipulation of tissue is advocated. This is mainly because powder from gloves can encourage adhesion formation. Manipulation using instruments is also more precise, and the tips of surgical instruments are significantly smaller than fingertips, which means that a smaller area of tissue is damaged; this way of working is therefore far less likely to cause significant adhesions. Sterile cotton buds can be helpful for haemostasis, again because their small size means less tissue is contacted.

Tissue desiccation is also a factor in adhesion formation; the use of instruments (meaning more viscera are kept inside the body cavity) as well as frequent irrigation of tissue exposed to air for any length of time will mitigate this. The use of moistened swabs rather than dry ones also helps to reduce adhesion formation, by reducing the likelihood of lint from the swab remaining on the tissue surface and by helping to keep the tissue moist. Many rabbit surgeons also advocate flushing the surgical site prior to closure.

One possible consequence of laparoscopic surgery in rabbits is the creation of a pneumoperitoneum with attendant tissue drying; this is dependent on the length of time the procedure requires.

> **PRACTICAL TIP**
>
> Adhesions may be prevented by:
>
> - Minimizing tissue handling and using gentle surgical technique
> - Paying careful attention to haemostasis
> - Keeping tissues moist, irrigating frequently and using wet gloves and moistened swabs
> - Minimizing surgical time
> - Using the smallest suitable suture material, with swaged-on needles.

Risk of haemorrhage

The clotting time in rabbits is shorter than that in many other species (Perry-Clarke and Meunier, 1991); however, intraoperative haemorrhage may still present the surgeon with problems. The blood volume of the rabbit is approximately 57 ml/kg bodyweight (5.7% of total bodyweight; therefore significantly less than the 10% estimate for a dog and 8% estimate for a cat). Loss of 15–20% of this volume (around 30–40 ml in a 3.5 kg rabbit) can lead to significant tachycardia, arterial vasoconstriction and redistribution of blood away from less essential areas such as gut and skin. Loss of blood in excess of this amount can prove critical or fatal. In practice, rabbits can be seriously affected if they lose a volume of blood that would be tolerated by a cat or a dog. Venous access and fluid support throughout surgery can mitigate blood losses, and maintenance of blood pressure during surgery can make visualization of potential bleeds easier.

Good surgical technique will minimize blood loss, although haemorrhage is sometimes unavoidable. Traditionally, ligation of 'bleeders' using suture material has been the method of choice; however, the use of electrocautery or radiosurgical instrumentation can be very helpful. It is worth considering that the use of electrocautery causes inflammation within the surrounding tissues, but so does the swabbing-up of blood and placing ligatures. Vessel-sealing handpieces (e.g. Ligasure) may also be used. Good knowledge of blood vessel anatomy will allow the surgeon to be specific in sourcing and correcting the origin of a bleed. Ligatures of absorbable monofilament suture are least reactive and minimize inflammation and adhesion formation in the longer term (McFadden, 2011).

Instrumentation

Most rabbit surgery can easily be accomplished using normal surgical kits of suitable size. For most rabbits a cat-sized kit is appropriate, while for larger individuals (>7 kg) a dog-sized kit may be necessary. When surgery on very young or small individuals is contemplated, ophthalmic or microsurgical instrumentation may be helpful. Rabbit-specific surgical kits are available commercially. The smallest instruments that are practical should be selected.

A typical surgical kit should include:

- Small (iris) scissors
- Long (Metzenbaum) scissors
- A pair each of dressing forceps and atraumatic or rat-toothed forceps
- A scalpel handle
- 3x artery forceps
- 4x towel clamps
- A pair of needle-holders.

In all kits it is useful to have DeBakey atraumatic forceps; these have ridged ends without the points that are found on rat-toothed forceps, allowing very good grip with minimal tissue damage. Magnification loupes are helpful for smaller patients and radiosurgical units may also be useful, particularly where haemostasis may be an issue. Sterilized cotton buds are another helpful addition.

Non-powdered gloves are preferable as they can reduce the potential for adhesion formation (see above).

Suture materials and patterns

Selection of an appropriate suture material is critical to the success of any surgery. The general principles applied to cats and dogs are also true for rabbits. The role of a suture is to maintain surgically incised or injured tissue in apposition so that it can heal. The suture material needs to provide enough tensile strength and for long enough to allow healing to be completed (Figure 11.3). Different tissues heal at different rates, so sutures need to stay in position for varying amounts of time. Bladder and uterine tissue heal rapidly (normal tensile strength achieved in 14–21 days), whereas fascia can take in excess of 42 days to repair. Within the gut, small intestine heals significantly faster than large intestine (14 *versus* 28 days).

The ideal suture material exhibits knot security, resistance to infection, and no inflammatory, immunological, or carcinogenic reactions. Such material does not exist, so a compromise must be made based on knowledge of healing and suture material characteristics.

As rabbits are commonly used experimental animals, much information has been generated on the reaction to and persistence of various suture materials in this species. In general, non-absorbable sutures that remain in tissues cause a persistent inflammatory response. Biological absorbable materials (e.g. catgut/chromic catgut) cause a greater inflammatory response than synthetic ones. Biological sutures are broken down by phagocytosis whereas synthetic ones are broken down by hydrolysis to simple molecules which are then absorbed and metabolized by the body (McFadden, 2011).

Rabbits form excessive granulation tissue in response to foreign material such as sutures. Suture selection is therefore very important, as suture reactions are a common postoperative complication.

- Monofilament suture materials are more resistant to infection than multifilament ones, and tend to cause less tissue reaction. The use of monofilament absorbable suture material for internal sutures (e.g. polydioxanone (PDS)) is recommended.
- External sutures should be non-absorbable but preferably also monofilament (e.g. monofilament

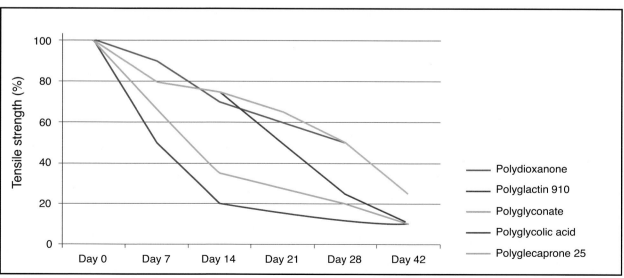

11.3 Deterioration in tensile strength (as a percentage of original strength) in a variety of commonly used sutures. (Data from McFadden, 2011)

nylon). Surgical steel staples are also suitable, but often less well tolerated from a comfort point of view, leading to self-trauma of the wound. In cases where exuberant granulation or fistulous tracts are formed secondary to suture placement, surgical excision may be necessary. Cyanoacrylate tissue glue may also be used for skin closure. However, a significant exothermic reaction occurs as it cures, which can cause skin necrosis in severe cases, so it should be used with caution.

- One possible use for catgut is in infected wounds, where the sutures can then be removed by phagocytosis along with any associated bacteria (Harcourt-Brown, 2002). This, however, can potentially prolong the inflammatory phase of wound healing and increase the potential for excessive formation of granulation tissue.

PRACTICAL TIP
The size of the suture material has more effect on adhesion formation than the suture material itself (McFadden, 2011); therefore, the finest practical suture material should be chosen.

For most wound closures it is desirable not to create any tension on the wound and the suture pattern chosen should reflect this.

- **For closure of the gut**, simple interrupted non-crushing suture patterns are advised. The submucosal layer of the gut is the most important for healing, as it contains the most collagen. It is important not to evert or invert the edges of rabbit intestine but to bring them into direct apposition without crushing the tissue. This is in contrast to similar surgery in dogs and cats, where serosal contact and inverting sutures are indicated. Single-layer closures are acceptable as double-layer closures will reduce gut lumen and functionality; however, the former are more prone to breakdown. The lack of a large, freely motile omentum means that intestinal wounds cannot be supported in this way. Inverting suture patterns will cause lumen stenosis and, particularly in the large intestine, can affect the function of the haustra. The most suitable suture material in this situation is a monofilament absorbable suture such as polydioxanone (PDS) 1 or 1.5 metric (5/0 or 4/0 USP).
- **For the uterus or bladder,** continuous inverting suture patterns such as Lembert or Cushing would be suitable. Penetration of the bladder lumen should be avoided, as it can cause calculus formation for the duration of the life of the suture. Therefore sutures that do not penetrate the wall fully are advocated, using 1 or 1.5 metric (5/0 or 4/0 USP) absorbable monofilament materials (e.g. PDS).
- **The abdominal wall** is closed in a single layer of either simple interrupted or simple continuous sutures (see Operative Technique 11.2). If a

continuous suture pattern is used, the knots at each end of the incision must be secure and several extra throws placed at each end. Absorbable monofilament or braided sutures are suitable (e.g. PDS or polyglactin 910 (e.g. Vicryl)). The size should be suitable for the size of patient, e.g. 1.5 metric (4/0 USP) for a 2 kg rabbit.

- **Subcuticular sutures** are ordinarily made in a simple continuous pattern; however, for wounds with a large skin deficit, it can be easier to place several interrupted subcuticular horizontal sutures to ensure the skin is where it is intended to be, prior to placing a full subcuticular suture. Ideally, the knot at the end of the subcuticular suture should be buried (Aberdeen knot, Figure 11.4). Either monofilament or braided absorbable sutures are suitable in this location (e.g. PDS, Vicryl); the size should be the smallest suitable for the patient, e.g. 1.5 metric (4/0 USP) for a 2 kg rabbit.
- **For skin,** the pattern chosen depends on the type of wound and the amount of subcuticular support already provided. Horizontal mattress, cruciate or simple interrupted suture patterns are all suitable. Stainless steel skin staples could also be used.

The Aberdeen knot is a buried knot suitable for the end of a subcuticular suture pattern. Its main advantage is that the knot is secure but small and the end is buried in a tunnel of tissue rather than cut off short, potentially allowing it to poke through the suture line.

1. At the end of the subcuticular suture, keep the last loop of suture material loose and place a final stitch.
2. Loop the end of the suture material nearest to your hand through the last suture.

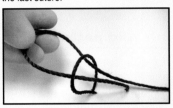

3. Pull the loop so that the last suture is tightened, then pull the end of the suture nearest you again through the remaining loop to make a third loop.

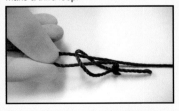

4. Place tension on the third loop so that the second loop is tightened.
5. Repeat this process for at least four to six throws and on the last throw pass the free end of the suture through the final loop and pull tight to secure the knot.
6. Tunnel the end of the suture material for a short way under the skin and up through the surface.
7. Pull it tight and cut off close to the skin surface, allowing the knot to pull back under the skin when released.

11.4 The Aberdeen knot. (Photos courtesy of Geraldine Hunt and reproduced from *BSAVA Manual of Canine and Feline Surgical Principles: a Foundation Manual*)

Potential complications and their prevention

Common presenting problems, their potential causes, and actions that should be taken to address them are summarized in Figure 11.5.

Wound breakdown
The correct placement and choice of suture are vital for the prevention of wound breakdown, as are the tension placed on the wound, the tightness of the suture and the sterility of the procedure. However, regardless of the care and planning undertaken, breakdown can still occur. Revision surgery is often necessary and consideration must be given to:

- The patient's comfort
- The immediate support the wound requires
- Addressing any infection
- Whether a second attempt at primary closure is warranted or whether delaying primary closure may be a more viable option.

Wound infection
Sterile technique and judicious use of antibiosis should reduce the likelihood of wound infections significantly. Equally, careful clipping, gentle tissue handling, and suitable suture selection with sutures that are not too tight will all reduce the likelihood of inflammation, tissue necrosis and self-trauma. Signs that a wound is infected include pain, swelling, redness, heat and the presence of purulent discharge.

Pus in rabbits is thick and sticky in consistency due to the mucolytic and proteolytic enzyme levels found in heterophils (a relative deficiency in myeloperoxidase means there is not enough of this enzyme to break down dead cells into thinner pus) (Baggiolini *et al.*, 1969, 1970). This presents a significant problem to the surgeon, as rabbit pus does not flow; so drain placement, a traditional way of dealing with infected wounds in other species, does not help and is even contraindicated as the drain itself can act as a nidus for further infection (Harkness *et al.*, 2010). Wounds that become infected may be dealt with by planning for healing either by delayed primary intention or by secondary intention. The area should be thoroughly and extensively debrided and cleaned repeatedly prior to considering delayed closure. Most rabbit surgeons advocate treating abscessed wounds as radically as one would a tumour (see Operative Technique 11.1).

Adhesions
Adhesions can be thought of as 'internal scars' that form between soft tissues after any tissue trauma (e.g. surgery). They are commonly recognized

Presenting problem	Possible causes	Actions
Wound red	Normal healing; inflammation; self-trauma; bleeding	Check wound. Assess antibiosis and pain relief. Check clotting ability if necessary
Wound swollen	Normal healing; inflammation; seroma formation; sutures too tight; infection; abscessation; suture reaction	Check wound. Consider drain placement if seroma formation. Consider culture and sensitivity testing (NB pus may be a poor sample for culture). Review antibiosis and pain relief. Revision surgery may need to be considered
Wound open	Self-trauma; lack of exercise restriction; suture failure	Review antibiosis and pain relief. Revision surgery may need to be considered
Purulent discharge	Wound infection or abscessation; secondary to suture reaction; secondary to self-trauma	Review antibiosis and pain relief. Revision surgery must be considered. Obtain sample from pyogenic membrane for culture. Consider delayed primary intention healing, addressing infection and causative factors prior to revision surgery and closure
Not eating or defecating after surgery	Wound infection or breakdown; inadequate pain relief; reduced mobility due to incisions; acquired dental disease secondary to a period of anorexia related to the surgery or the reasons for it; reasons unrelated to surgery	Perform a full clinical examination (including a dental examination). Examine external wounds. Review antibiosis and pain relief. For abdominal surgery, consider either abdominocentesis or ultrasonography to look for free peritoneal fluid and potential wound breakdown. Provide supportive care, including fluids and assisted feeding. Take a blood sample (blood glucose level may help to assess prognosis)
Abdomen swollen	Excess fluid or gas within gut; excess free fluid within peritoneal cavity; abnormal abdominal mass formation (abscess or tumour growth)	Perform a full clinical examination including auscultation for gut sounds. Use abdominocentesis or ultrasonography to look for free peritoneal fluid and abnormal mass formation. Review antibiosis and analgesia. Treat any abnormalities aggressively. Revision surgery is likely to be required
Lack of expected return to function (of area operated on)	Continued pain; adhesion formation; wound contracture affecting mobility of area in question; continued wound infection affecting healing	Perform full physical examination and compare current function with normal. Review antibiosis and pain relief. Revision surgery may be indicated. Consider physical therapy to aid in adhesion breakdown. Consider medical therapy for prevention of adhesion re-formation

11.5 Trouble-shooting guide for potential complications associated with wound healing.

Chapter 11 Basic principles of soft tissue surgery

between the viscera after abdominal surgery. In some cases they can significantly affect gut motility in the rabbit and may cause problems months or even years after surgery. In severe cases the gut can become obstructed. Adhesions are uncomfortable at best, and may cause significant pain. The surgeon should be aware of the causes of adhesions, and utilize techniques to reduce them, including gentle tissue handling, wet gloves/swabs, minimal handling of viscera except with instruments, and careful haemostasis. In cases where extensive tissue handling is unavoidable, or where there has perhaps been significant bleeding (and therefore haemostatic attempts), consideration should be given to the use of drugs to minimize adhesion formation, e.g. verapamil and pentoxifylline. Verapamil can be used at 200 µg/kg q8h for nine doses (Steinleitner et al., 1989) and pentoxifylline at 2.5 mg/kg q12h for six doses (Steinleitner et al., 1990).

Recombinant tissue plasminogen activator (Dorr et al., 1990) has been proven to act synergistically with verapamil and to reduce adhesion formation even further. In severe cases, revision surgery may need to be considered. The point of this is to go back into the body cavity and resect the adhesions manually, while striving to prevent further adhesion formation. This should be undertaken in parallel to aggressive drug therapy, as detailed above.

Pentoxifylline has also been shown to reduce re-formation of adhesions after surgical breakdown (Steinleitner et al., 1990). Other medical therapies being postulated for reduction of adhesion formation include: diltiazem (another calcium-channel blocker; Golan et al., 1989); nimesulide (an anti-inflammatory; Guvenal et al., 2001); non-selective non-steroidal anti-inflammatory drugs (NSAIDs) such as ibuprofen (Green et al., 2005); melatonin (Ozcelik et al., 2003); surfactant compounds (phospholipids); hydrolytic enzyme complexes; and anti-adhesive polypeptide complexes (Binda and Koninckx., 2009; Anilkumar et al., 2011). In the longer term, some of these may well be very useful to the rabbit surgeon. Currently, topical intra-abdominal treatments are not commonly used after surgery in rabbits, and of the medications previously advocated, only NSAIDs at therapeutic doses can be advised clinically.

Self-trauma
In most cases, rabbits are unlikely to chew or damage skin sutures. However, if the sutures are tight, there is tension on the wound, or the wound is swollen due to infection or suture reaction, then they certainly will. It is preferable to address the underlying cause of the discomfort, and make certain that pain relief is comprehensive. If self-trauma continues then local anaesthetic blocks, transdermal local anaesthetic cream or bitter sprays may be helpful. Dressings can be more difficult to maintain and they may not stop attempts to damage the area in question. In the author's opinion Elizabethan collars (Figure 11.6a) are not suitable for use in rabbits as they prevent prehension of caecotrophs, can inhibit eating, and often damage the backs of the pinnae. Soft collars that are tied around the neck and flap

down over the shoulders (Figure 11.6b) may be used for wounds in some positions and these appear to be well tolerated. Body-stockings/'onesies' are now available commercially for use in rabbits and can provide a comfortable and secure way of preventing self-trauma.

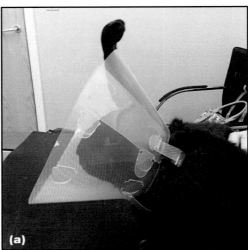

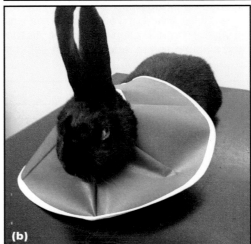

11.6 **(a)** A rabbit in a normal rigid Elizabethan collar. Note that this restricts the rabbit's ability to groom, to eat and to prehend caecotrophs. The edge of the collar can rub against the external side of the pinnae, causing skin erosion and pain. **(b)** A soft collar that can be folded down over the shoulders is better accepted and less restrictive. This type of collar works well for wounds around the shoulder and chest, and does not restrict access to the perineal area, so caecotrophy can occur. It is, however, not useful for wounds that are located more caudally. (© Molly Varga)

Endosurgery (minimally invasive surgery)

Endoscopy is a familiar and well recognized tool in many aspects of veterinary medicine. 'Keyhole' or minimally invasive surgery, the natural extension of this, is increasingly available to veterinary surgeons and is of particular use in rabbits because the minimally invasive nature of the procedure allows a rapid return to normal function. A rigid endoscope can be used to visualize body cavity contents, while certain surgical procedures can be performed endoscopically, such as exploratory laparoscopy, thoracoscopy, harvesting of thoracic or abdominal organ biopsy samples, neutering (see Operative Technique 11.3), cystotomy and foreign body retrieval.

The advantage of endoscopic surgery is that it allows access to internal organs through much smaller incisions compared to traditional surgical techniques. This results in a reduced risk of postoperative wound breakdown, as smaller wounds are less likely to be disturbed by excessive exercise, less likely to herniate, and less likely to get infected. There is also a shorter, less painful recovery period. However, potential complications can include iatrogenic damage to organs, desiccation of viscera due to insufflation with gas, infection or abscessation of the portal entry sites and seeding of tumours (Mehler, 2011). The advantages and disadvantages of endosurgery *versus* traditional surgery are summarized in Figure 11.7.

Traditional surgery	Endoscopic surgery
Large entry incision	Several small entry incisions
Good visibility and access	Visibility and access more restricted
10–14 days minimum recovery period	Recovery period shorter as wounds less vulnerable
Anecdotally more painful recovery	Anecdotally less painful recovery
Possibility of wound rupture and infection	Possibility of wound rupture and infection
Iatrogenic damage to organs unlikely	Iatrogenic damage to organs a potential complication
Iatrogenic tissue drying likely	Iatrogenic tissue drying a possibility

11.7 Advantages and disadvantages of endosurgery *versus* traditional surgery.

For most endoscopic surgical procedures the patient is placed in dorsal recumbency (Figure 11.8); however, this can vary depending on the site of interest. Where a head-down position is indicated (e.g. for laparoscopic access to the bladder) it is wise to consider mechanical ventilation, as significant respiratory impairment may occur due to pressure build-up within the abdomen and the additional weight of the viscera on the diaphragm. In all cases patients should be clipped and aseptically prepared in the same way as for any other surgical intervention.

Basic equipment needs are discussed in Chapter 10. The trocars/cannulas allow entry into the body cavity (Mehler, 2011). They are usually inserted in three positions depending on where/what the organ of interest is, oriented either in a triangle with its base facing away from the area of interest and the tip being the tissue of interest (Figure 11.9), or in a straight line, usually along the midline. These ports allow for insufflation, and act as portals for

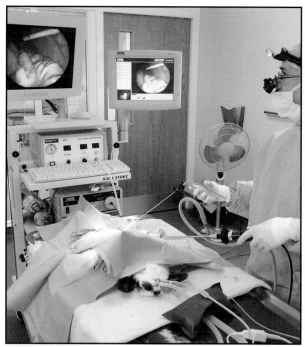

11.8 A rabbit undergoing a laparoscopic procedure. Note the positioning in dorsal recumbency, with two ports in use, one for the endoscope and one for the forceps. (© Romain Pizzi, Zoological Medicine Ltd)

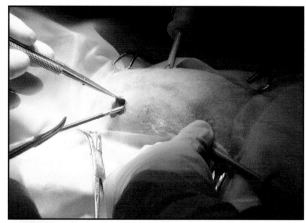

11.9 A rabbit undergoing laparoscopic surgery with three entry portals, illustrating the triangulation technique for port placement. (© Romain Pizzi, Zoological Medicine Ltd)

insertion of the endoscope and accessory instruments. The surgeon then uses the endoscope for visualization while manipulating one or two instruments, using a triangulation process. It is vital that there is enough room for the surgeon to manipulate the instruments inside the body, so the trocars should be placed far enough apart that the instruments will not be too close to the area of interest. This means there will be a wider field available within which the surgeon can manoeuvre.

Once entrance into the body cavity has been achieved, the tissues must be moved away from the end of the endoscope to create a space in which the surgeon can work. The medium used needs to be transparent. Either water/fluid or gas may be used and in modern endoscopy carbon dioxide (CO_2) is infused into the body cavity to expand its volume (Figure 11.10), allowing the viscera to separate and the operator to see around the organs. Insufflation of gas requires an airtight seal between the body cavity and the environment. This is achieved using closed trocar–cannula units. Closed trocar–cannula units contain valves that stop gas leakage, while open ones do not. Open trocar–cannula units can be used, but it takes longer for the CO_2 to insufflate the body cavity adequately as the gas is not stopped from flowing out. Most CO_2 delivery systems deliver the gas at a variable flow rate to produce a constant pressure in the body cavity. In rabbits, producing a high intra-abdominal pressure can significantly impair respiration, so the lowest pressure that allows the procedure to be performed should be used.

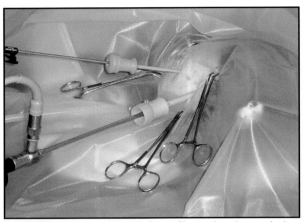

11.10 A two-portal technique, illustrating the sealed ports. Note the degree to which the abdomen has been distended by the gas insufflation. (© Romain Pizzi, Zoological Medicine Ltd)

Instruments can be inserted through the trocars in order to perform endoscopic procedures. A blunt probe is used to move or palpate organs. These are often engraved with measuring rulers to allow the estimation of organ or mass size. Biopsy cups or forceps are used for tissue collection, as are core biopsy needles. Grasping forceps, scissors, retractors, clip applicators and heat ligation cutting tools are also used.

References and further reading

Abramov Y, Golden B, Sullivan M et al. (2007) Histologic characterization of vaginal vs. abdominal surgical wound healing in a rabbit model. Wound Repair Regeneration 15(1), 80–86
Anilkumar TV, Jaseer M, Anumol J et al. (2011) Advantages of hyaluronic acid as a component of fibrin sheet for care of acute wound. Biologicals 39, 81–88
Aziz N and Aziz NR (2008) A gross anatomical and histological inspection of the mammalian integument post treatment with aluminium nitrate. Annals of Microscopy 8, 4–13
Baggiolini M, De Duve C, Masson PL and Heremans JF (1969) Association of lactoferrin with specific granules in rabbit heterophil leukocytes. Journal of Cell Biology 45, 559–571
Baggiolini M, Hirsch JD and De Duve C (1970) Further biochemical and morphological studies of granule fractions from rabbit heterophil leukocytes. Journal of Cell Biology 45, 586–596
Bayat M, Asgari-Moghadam Z, Maroufi M et al. (2006) Experimental wound healing using microamperage electrostimulation in rabbits. Journal of Rehabilitation Research and Development 43, 219–226
Billingham RE and Medawar PB (1951) The technique of free skin grafting in mammals. Journal of Experimental Biology 28, 385–407
Binda MM and Koninckx PR (2009) Prevention of adhesion formation in a laparoscopic mouse model should combine local treatment with peritoneal cavity conditioning. Human Reproduction 24, 1473–1479
Divers SJ (2010) Exotic mammal diagnostic endoscopy and endosurgery. Veterinary Clinics of North America: Exotic Animal Practice 13(2), 255–272
Dorr PJ, Vemer HM, Brommer EJP et al. (1990) Prevention of post-operative adhesions by tissue-type plasminogen activator (1-PA) in the rabbit. European Journal of Obstetrics and Gynaecology and Reproductive Biology 37, 287–291
Golan A, Wexler S, Lotan G et al. (1989). Calcium antagonist effect on adhesion formation. Acta Obstetrica et Gynecologica Scandinavica 68, 529–532
Gordon S, Todd J and Cohn ZA (1974) In vitro synthesis and secretion of lysozyme by mononuclear macrophages. Journal of Experimental Medicine 139, 1228–1248
Green AK, Alwayn IPJ, Nose V et al. (2005) Prevention of intra-abdominal adhesions using antiangiogenic COX-2 inhibitor celecoxib. Annals of Surgery 242, 140–146
Guvenal T, Cetin A, Ozdemir H et al. (2001) Prevention of post operative adhesion formation in a rat uterine horn model by nimesulide; a selective COX-2 inhibitor. Human Reproduction 16(8), 1732–1735
Harcourt-Brown FM (2002) Textbook of Rabbit Medicine. Butterworth Heinemann, Oxford
Harkness JE, Turner PV, Van de Woude S and Wheler CL (2010) Harkness and Wagner's Biology and Medicine of Rabbits and Rodents, 5th edn. Wiley-Blackwell, Ames, IA
Hashemi B, Bayat A, Kazemei T and Azarpira N (2011) Comparison between topical honey and mafenide acetate in treatment of auricular burn. American Journal of Otolaryngology 32, 28–31
Lhermette P and Sobel D (2008) BSAVA Manual of Canine and Feline Endoscopy and Endosurgery. BSAVA Publications, Gloucester
McFadden MS (2011) Suture materials and suture selection for use in exotic pet surgical procedures. Journal of Exotic Pet Medicine 20, 173–181
Mehler SJ (2011) Minimally invasive surgery techniques in exotic animals. Journal of Exotic Pet Medicine 20, 188–205
Merck (2011) Myopathies in small animals. In: The Merck Veterinary Manual. www.merckvetmanual.com. Merck and Co, New Jersey
Nilsson T (1981) Closure of the abdominal wound with single layer and double layer technique. Acta Chirurgica Scandinavica 147, 399–403
Onderdonk AB, Kasper DL, Mansheim BJ et al. (1979) Experimental animal models for anaerobic infections. Reviews of Infectious Diseases 1, 291–301
Ozcelik B, Serin LS, Basburg M et al. (2003) Effect of melatonin in the prevention of post-operative adhesion formation in a rat uterine horn adhesion model. Human Reproduction 18(8), 1703–1706
Oznurlu Y, Celik I, Sur E, Telatar T and Ozparlak H (2009) Comparative skin histology of the white New Zealand and Angora rabbits: histometrical and immunohistochemical evaluations. Journal of Animal and Veterinary Advances 8, 1694–1701
Perry-Clark LM and Meunier LD (1991) Vascular access ports for chronic serial infusion and blood sampling in New Zealand White rabbits. Laboratory Animal Science 41, 495–497
Ruggiero SL, Bertolami CN, Bronson RE and Damiani PJ (1987) Hyaluronidase activity of rabbit skin wound granulation tissue fibroblasts. Journal of Dental Research 66, 1283–1287
Shrive N, Chimich D, Marchuk L et al. (1995) Soft-tissue 'flaws' are associated with the material properties of the healing rabbit medial collateral ligament. Journal of Orthopaedic Research 13, 923–929
Srivastava CM and Lossin C (1976) A comparative study of the healing of wounds made by scalpel and electrosurgery in rabbits. Australian Dental Journal 21, 252–257
Steinleitner A, Kazensky C and Lambert H (1989) Calcium channel blockade prevents postsurgical reformation of adnexal adhesions in rabbits. Obstetrics and Gynecology 74, 796–798
Steinleitner A, Lambert H, Kazensky C, Danks P and Roy S (1990) Pentoxifylline, a methylxanthine derivative, prevents postsurgical adhesion reformation in rabbits. Obstetrics and Gynecology 75, 926–928
Williams J and Niles J (2005) BSAVA Manual of Canine and Feline Abdominal Surgery. BSAVA Publications, Gloucester
Xie JL, Bian HN, Qi SH, et al. (2008) Basic fibroblast growth factor (bFGF) alleviates the scar of the rabbit ear model in wound healing. Wound Repair and Regeneration 16, 576–581

OPERATIVE TECHNIQUE 11.1:
Removal of subcutaneous abscesses
(Adapted from Harkness *et al.*, 2010, and the author's experience)

The aim of treatment of subcutaneous abscesses is to remove the abscess in its entirety without breaching the pyogenic membrane and fibrous capsule. This needs to be achieved while maintaining the functional and structural integrity of the underlying soft tissues.

Positioning

The area of interest must be easily accessible to the surgeon.

Assistant

An assistant is not usually required.

Equipment

A normal surgical kit is acceptable in most cases. For very extensive abscesses, a retractor (e.g. a Lone Star retractor) and intraoperative radiography, using contrast material to outline the extent of the abscess, may be helpful.

Approach

1 The rabbit should be anaesthetized and positioned so that the area of interest is easily accessible to the surgeon.

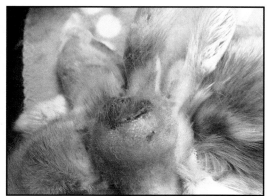

A large abscess located near to but not connected to the base of the ear. (© Molly Varga)

2 The area of interest should be clipped with a wide margin around to allow for aggressive abscess removal.

3 The area should be aseptically prepared.

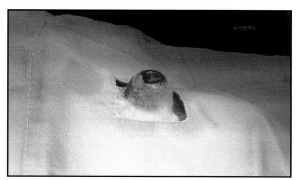

The abscess has been clipped, aseptically prepared and draped for surgery. (© Molly Varga)

4 If the skin does not appear to be attached to the fibrous abscess capsule, then the skin can be carefully excised to expose the abscess underneath. Care needs to be taken at this stage to handle the skin and subcutaneous tissues gently as the skin may adhere to the abscess capsule at certain points and rough handling would then cause the capsule to tear.

5 Blunt dissection is used to remove the skin from the abscess, using moistened cotton buds, wet swabs, artery forceps or, cautiously, blunt-tipped scissors. Any prominent vessels should be either ligated or coagulated using an electrocautery or radiosurgical unit (e.g. Ellman Surgitronic).

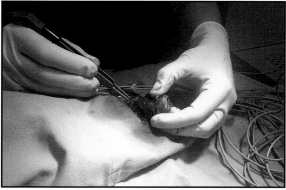

The abscess capsule is dissected out in an attempt to remove as much of the abscess as possible intact. Bipolar radiosurgery forceps are being used to provide haemostasis. (© Molly Varga)

OPERATIVE TECHNIQUE 11.1 continued:
Removal of subcutaneous abscesses

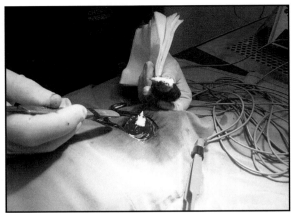

Most of the abscess has been removed, leaving only that portion that is so intimately attached to the underlying tissue that removal would cause unacceptable damage. All remaining pus is scooped out and the abscess capsule curetted using a Volkmann's scoop. (© Molly Varga)

6 Ideally, the whole abscess should be removed in this manner and the skin closed routinely.

7 If the abscess is deeply attached to subcutaneous structures that cannot be removed, as may occur with abscesses around the perineum or near the base of the ear, then another strategy should be used. Infiltration with radiographic contrast medium and radiography may be indicated in order to delineate the exact extent of the abscess. Marsupialization may be the preferred option (see Chapter 29).

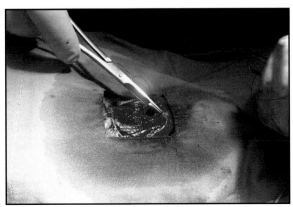

The abscess capsule is sutured to the surrounding skin or 'marsupialized'. (© Molly Varga)

8 The remains of the fibrous capsule can then be left open, to allow daily cleaning (e.g. using chlorhexidine scrub) and application of topical treatment (e.g. Manuka honey, F10 barrier ointment or other antibacterial preparations (see Chapter 29), as long as the active ingredients are not potentially harmful if the rabbit licks them). An alternative strategy is to cover the open area with a hydrocolloid-based absorbent dressing (e.g. Covidien, Smith and Nephew or Granuflex, ConvaTec). The easiest option is to suture the dressing directly around the wound. The absorbance of the dressing draws the pus away from the surface of the wound, maintains moisture in the granulation tissue and physically protects it, making the open surface less uncomfortable for the patient. After 3–5 days the dressing can be removed and the open wound cleaned and treated topically as described above.

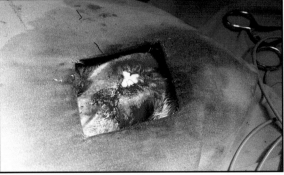

A small pad of foam dressing is sutured into the wound. This draws any discharge away from the wound surface and provides protection to allow a bed of granulation tissue to form. The foam dressing can be soaked in injectable antibiotics prior to placement in order to hold antibiotics in contact with the pyogenic membrane. The dressing may be left *in situ* for 3–5 days after surgery; it is then removed and direct cleaning of the abscess void can commence. (© Molly Varga)

9 Regular cleaning and topical medication should continue for as long as possible and the wound should be encouraged to stay open until it heals from the inside out.

10 The surgical and topical treatment should continue in parallel with oral or parenteral antibiosis and analgesia until the wound is completely resolved.

OPERATIVE TECHNIQUE 11.2:
Abdominal closure

(Adapted from *BSAVA Manual of Canine and Feline Abdominal Surgery*)

Positioning

Dorsal recumbency.

Assistant

An assistant is not usually necessary.

Equipment

A normal surgical kit is sufficient.

Approach

1 With the rabbit in dorsal recumbency, the abdominal cavity is checked for haemorrhage and potential damage prior to closure. If problems are noted, these must be addressed prior to closure.

2 The linea alba should be repaired in a single layer (it has been shown there is no advantage to more layers; Nilsson, 1981). Try to include the peritoneum in each stitch. Simple interrupted sutures of monofilament absorbable suture material are ideal; however, continuous patterns may be used as long as secure knots are placed at each end of the suture line. Care should be taken not to make the sutures too tight as ischaemic necrosis can occur, causing adhesions internally as well as pain at the incision site.

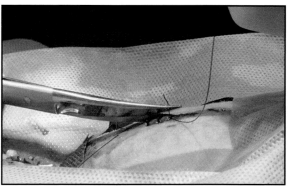

Sutures being placed in the abdominal wall (linea alba). Note the small size of the suture material. Care must be taken not to tie these sutures too tightly, or necrosis of the edge of the abdominal wall and discomfort and self-trauma may occur. (© Molly Varga)

3 Subcuticular sutures can then be placed in a continuous pattern, preferably ending in a buried (Aberdeen) knot (see Figure 11.4). Some individuals have very little subcutaneous tissue to work with. Rabbit skin is very thin and fragile and care must be taken that these sutures really are subcuticular and do not penetrate the surface of the skin, as this can cause a point of entry for infection.

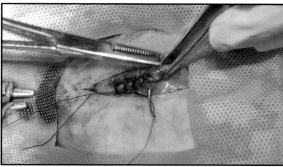

Subcuticular sutures being placed. These sutures appose the skin edges, and cover the underlying suture line. Care must be taken to bury the ends of the final knot (Aberdeen knot) so they do not protrude through the skin, allowing entry of infection. (© Molly Varga)

4 If needed, skin sutures (either simple interrupted, cruciate or horizontal mattress) can be placed using a non-absorbable suture material. Staples or skin glue are also appropriate (NB cyanoacrylate glue can cause a significant exothermic reaction and skin necrosis in some individuals).

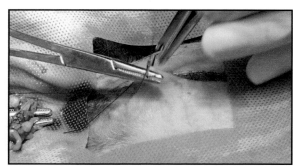

The first suture being placed in the skin. Again, care must be taken not to tie these sutures too tightly; otherwise, discomfort and self-trauma may occur. (© Molly Varga)

5 The use of spray-on wound sealants, local anaesthetic blocks or local anaesthetic creams can all help reduce the incidence of interference with the wound.

OPERATIVE TECHNIQUE 11.3:
Laparoscopic ovariectomy

(Adapted from: Divers, 2010; P Cornwell, personal communication; *BSAVA Manual of Canine and Feline Endoscopy and Endoscopic Surgery*)

This procedure should only be undertaken by surgeons familiar with endosurgical techniques. It requires airway support, and mechanical ventilation is an advantage. The small size (≤800 g) of many prepubertal rabbits limits its use in this group, although individuals of 500–1000 g can be operated on satisfactorily using 3–5 mm equipment. In many small individuals, the length of the laparoscopic incisions is similar to the length of a routine spay incision.

The author (MV) and Roman Pizzi (provider of the images) do not recommend this procedure currently unless undertaken in prepubertal individuals, as there is a potential risk for uterine changes to have already occurred prior to surgery. Any older females neutered in this way should be carefully followed postsurgically for uterine changes. In one series of cases where rabbits were ovariectomized between 6 and 9 months of age and followed ultrasonographically for 3 years, no uterine changes were noted, and in the USA, where even very small specimens are being ovariectomized, this has become the technique of choice (P Cornwell, personal communication; Divers, 2010).

Dr Thomas Goebels reports that in a series of 700 rabbits under 9 months of age undergoing ovariectomy, none subsequently showed signs of uterine disease. In rabbits of 9–18 months, visualization of the uterus determined whether ovariectomy or ovariohysterectomy was performed, and in 50% of cases a full ovariohysterectomy was performed. Uterine disease was noted in one rabbit, 3 years after ovariectomy. (Dr Thomas Goebels, personal communication)

Positioning

Dorsal recumbency.

Assistant

An assistant is an advantage, although this technique can be accomplished by a single surgeon.

Equipment

A normal surgical kit and laparoscopic equipment (cannulas, rigid endoscope, bipolar cutting forceps, Babcock forceps) are required.

Approach

1 The rabbit is anaesthetized, intubated, placed in dorsal recumbency and clipped as for a normal spay procedure, so that if something unexpected is encountered during the procedure the incision line can be extended to allow a full surgical laparotomy.

2 The surgical site is aseptically prepared.

3 The first port can be placed either surgically (this may be preferable as there is less risk of damaging underlying viscera) or using a Verres needle. If surgical placement is undertaken, the abdomen is opened as normal, the port placed and the entrance incision tightened around the port using a suture. The port should be placed at the umbilicus on the midline. This port accommodates the rigid endoscope. In dogs, the initial incision is made just off the umbilicus in order to avoid the falciform fat; however, this is not advocated in rabbits.

4 The abdomen is insufflated to a suitable pressure (see Chapter 10). Care must be taken not to compromise breathing at this time, and manual or mechanical ventilation may be required.

5 The second port is placed 2–5 cm cranial to the umbilicus, depending on the size of the patient. This port is generally placed with direct visualization through the first port. The Babcock or locking forceps are introduced through this portal.

6 The third port is placed in the same way, 2–5 cm caudal to the umbilicus depending on the size of the patient. This port allows introduction of the cutting device. This port placement allows access to both ovaries.

7 The patient is then rotated from dorsal recumbency towards the surgeon into semi-lateral recumbency. The abdominal contents fall towards the dependent side of the abdomen, creating a space dorsally. The ovary in the dorsal-most side is located and grasped with Babcock or locking forceps introduced through the cranial portal.

OPERATIVE TECHNIQUE 11.3 continued:
Laparoscopic ovariectomy

8 The ovary is held up against the abdominal wall and a bipolar cutting device (e.g. Ligasure or Hotblade) is sited across the ovarian ligament, pedicle and uterine attachments. These are then transected.

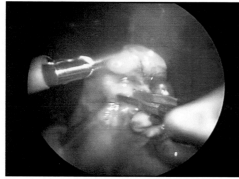

The ovarian artery is grasped using bipolar forceps. (© Romain Pizzi, Zoological Medicine Ltd)

9 The ovary is grasped and removed through the lumen of the cannula or, if it is too large, by removal of the cannula and direct traction through the body wall.

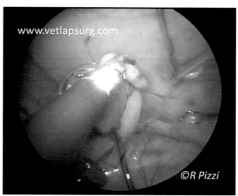

Grasping the ovary. (© Romain Pizzi, Zoological Medicine Ltd)

10 The rabbit is then rotated on to its other side and the procedure repeated on the opposite side.

11 The ports can then be removed and the surgical wounds sutured as normal (see Operative Technique 11.2).

Postoperative care

Postoperative care should include monitoring carefully for return to normal feeding, provision of analgesia and routine surgical wound care.

12

Neutering

Frances Harcourt-Brown

Neutering rabbits is becoming an everyday procedure in small animal practice.

Considerations prior to neutering

Reasons to neuter rabbits

Reasons to neuter female rabbits
- To prevent unwanted litters.
- To reduce hormonal territorial behaviour and aggression
- To prevent false pregnancies.
- To prevent reproductive disease, which is very common and often silent in mature entire females. Uterine adenocarcinoma is life-threatening and extremely common. It has been reported that 60% of entire females will have adenocarcinoma by the time they are 4 years old and 75% will have it by the time they are 7 years old (Greene, 1941).

Reasons to neuter male rabbits
- To prevent breeding.
- To prevent fighting with other rabbits. Neutered male rabbits can live together companionably.
- To prevent undesirable behaviour such as urine spraying or 'inappropriate' copulatory actions.
- To reduce sexual frustration and obsessive compulsive behaviour displayed by entire males that live on their own or in proximity with others.
- To reduce sexual behaviour towards a companion rabbit (or guinea pig, although this is not recommended as a good arrangement for either species).
- To treat male reproductive disease such as inguinal hernia, cryptorchidism, testicular neoplasia or testicular torsion.

Elective neutering is recommended for all female rabbits that are not intended for breeding. However, no real health benefits are gained from neutering young male rabbits and so, if the rabbit is kept as a sole house rabbit, many owners prefer to leave them entire. Entire male rabbits tend to have a stronger personality than neutered ones and not all of them show undesirable male behaviour. Entire males that have a lot of interaction and companionship can become very closely bonded with their owners. There is no medical reason to neuter these rabbits. Most reproductive problems develop later in life and are obvious to the owner. By this time, the rabbit's personality and behaviour is well established and castration is unlikely to alter it.

Suitable ages for neutering

Females
Does can be neutered at any age, although the procedure is more difficult in immature females because the uterine horns are tiny, threadlike, difficult to locate and may break if any pressure is applied (Figure 12.1). For this reason, it is preferable to leave females until they are hormonally active, usually at about 5 months of age. The easiest time to neuter females is between 6 and 9 months, before large amounts of fat are laid down in the mesometrium.

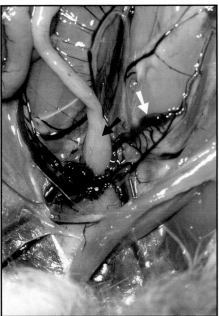

12.1 The post-mortem appearance of the uterus of a 14-week-old female rabbit. The caecum, proximal colon and small intestine have been removed. The small size of the vestigial uterus (white arrow) can be compared with the rectum (black arrow) that lies adjacent. At this age the uterus is difficult to locate, friable and easily broken as it is exteriorized, which makes ovariohysterectomy difficult.

Ovariohysterectomy can be performed at any time during pregnancy or pseudopregnancy but after a doe has given birth it is preferable to delay surgery until the babies are weaned at 4–5 weeks old.

Males
Males can be neutered as soon as testicles are evident within the scrotal sacs, which can be as early as 10 weeks. Rabbits with absent testicles should be left until they are at least 6 months old to give time for the testicles to descend. There is no upper age limit for castration.

Female reproductive anatomy and physiology

Anatomy of the reproductive tract
A diagram of the female reproductive tract and its relationship with neighbouring organs is shown in Figure 12.2. Both ovaries lie in the dorsal abdomen, close to the kidneys. They are elongated elliptical structures that, in a sexually mature female, contain multiple follicles at varying stages of development (Figure 12.3). The cranial end of the ovary is attached to the fimbriae, which open into the infundibulum. This is attached to the ampulla tubae uterinae, which forms a semicircle that encloses the ovary. These structures are enclosed in a discrete body of fat, the mesovarium, which is part of the mesometrium.

The caudal end of the ovary is attached to the mesovarium by a short ligament. The fallopian (uterine) tube is long and red in colour and can resemble a blood vessel. It opens into a long convoluted

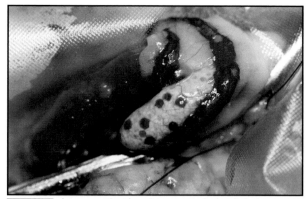

12.3 An ovary that has been exteriorized during ovariohysterectomy. It contains follicles in various stages of development. The ovary is encompassed by the ampulla tubae uterinae, which is a deep red colour and resembles a blood vessel.

uterine horn, which ends in a cervix. The right and left uterine horns are completely separate so that the two cervices are attached to form a single structure (bicornuate cervix) that separates the uterus from the vagina. There is no uterine body. The vagina is a long flaccid but muscular structure that fills with urine during micturition. Contractions of the vagina occur readily and may be seen during ovariohysterectomy. The urethra lies ventral to the vagina and opens into it about half way along its length, beneath the pubic bone. The part of the vagina that is distal to the urethral opening (vestibulum vaginae) is attached to supporting musculature, which can constrict and move the vagina and vulva during urination, mating and parturition.

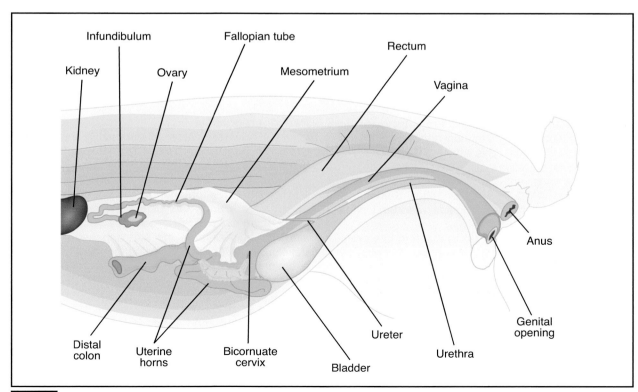

12.2 Anatomy of the female reproductive tract and its relationship with neighbouring organs.

Reproductive physiology

Rabbits are well known for their ability to reproduce quickly. As babies, they can be difficult to sex (Figure 12.4) but this becomes easier once they reach puberty at 4–9 months of age. Smaller breeds mature earlier than larger breeds.

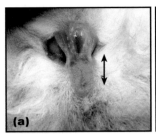
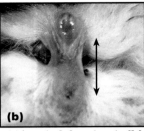

12.4 Genitalia of 6-week-old female **(a)** and male **(b)** siblings. At this age, the testicles are not descended and it is easy to sex the rabbits incorrectly. The genital orifice needs to be retracted to expose (a) the cone-shaped vulva with a slit-shaped opening or (b) a small tubular penis. The distance between the genital opening and the anus is greater in the male than in the female.

Rabbits are induced ovulators with no defined oestrous cycle, although a cyclic rhythm in sexual receptivity exists. Follicular development occurs in waves, with 5–10 follicles on each ovary at any one time (see Figure 12.3). When the follicles reach maturity they produce oestrogens for about 12–14 days; if ovulation has not occurred during this period the follicles then degenerate with a corresponding reduction in oestrogen level and sexual receptivity. After about 4 days a new wave of follicles develops and the doe becomes receptive again. Mating stimulates ovulation approximately 10 hours after coitus.

The average litter size is 5–8 and females are able to conceive within hours of giving birth. Rabbits can be lactating while they are pregnant, and it is possible for a single female to give birth to over 40 offspring each year.

Pregnancy

Gestation lasts for 30–32 days. Pregnancy can be detected by abdominal palpation and the best time for diagnosis is 10–14 days after mating, when the fetal units can be felt as olive-sized masses. Fetal resorption is relatively common in rabbits and can take place up to 20 days post coitus. Sometimes viable fetuses are found alongside resorbing ones (Figure 12.5).

Mammary development takes place in late pregnancy when the doe starts to prepare her nest by filling it with hay or other material before lining it with fur pulled from the hip, dewlap and mammary glands. After parturition, the doe pulls even more fur from her body to cover the litter in the nest. It is advisable to remove other rabbits from the hutch during late pregnancy.

Parturition

Parturition usually takes place in the morning and lasts less than 30 minutes. The babies are born blind, without hair and helpless. After giving birth,

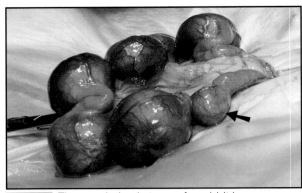

12.5 The exteriorized uterus of a rabbit in mid-pregnancy undergoing ovariohysterectomy. Viable fetal units and a resorbing one can be seen. The resorbing fetal unit is much smaller than the rest (arrow); dissection of the uterus showed that this unit contained a mass of amorphous tissue. The other units contained fetuses.

maternal behaviour is minimal and the babies are left alone in the nest for most of the time. The doe only returns to the nest for less than 10 minutes once or occasionally twice a day to feed them. The entrance to the nest is stopped up with leaves, earth or bedding material and hidden between visits, so owners may be unaware of the existence of the babies or, if they find them, may think they have been deserted. Owners may need reassurance that it is normal for their rabbit to be out of the nest when she has a litter and that she may be particularly aggressive and protective during this period. Lactation takes place for approximately 5 weeks after parturition.

During lactation, the mother stays close to the nest and may attack potential intruders, including human owners. She is particularly susceptible to disturbance in the first few days after parturition and may cannibalize or mutilate the young if she is upset. The legs or ears may be bitten, or even removed, or the skin stripped from over the neck, thorax or abdomen.

Pseudopregnancy

Ovulation can take place without mating and result in pseudopregnancy. Ovulation can be stimulated by the proximity of other rabbits or by the act of being mounted by another female. Pseudopregnancy is shorter than true pregnancy, lasting approximately 16–18 days. During this period the doe may show many of the signs of late pregnancy, such as aggression, pulling hair from the stomach and mammary development. Abdominal palpation and ultrasound examination are the best ways of differentiating the two conditions.

Female aggression

Female rabbits show many behavioural characteristics that are related to their hormonal status. Sexual receptivity, pregnancy, pseudopregnancy and nursing a litter of babies can radically affect the temperament and behaviour of a female pet. In the wild, the choice of nesting site has a strong influence on the survival of the young, and competition for a good site is strong. Females will dig out a nesting chamber before they are pregnant and defend it from predators and other rabbits. Some female pet rabbits display this behaviour towards their owners and other rabbits or pets that come close to their chosen nesting site, which is often their hutch or sleeping area because they have no other choice. To the owner, the transformation from an endearing baby rabbit to an adolescent one that strikes, growls or even bites when it is approached in its cage can be upsetting. Neutering can make a difference by removing the hormonal triggers for this behaviour.

Diseases of the female reproductive system

There are many diseases that can affect the female reproductive tract. The clinical signs that might alert the owner and practitioner to these problems are listed below. Diagnosis is confirmed by abdominal palpation, ultrasonography (see Chapter 8), abdominal radiography (see Chapter 7) and exploratory laparotomy.

Diseases of the female reproductive tract are more likely to be encountered as age increases. Many of the disorders show few obvious clinical signs until the condition is advanced. The clinical signs include:

- Palpable abdominal masses
- Abdominal distension
- Bleeding from vulva (may be sudden and severe)
- Haematuria. Blood from the uterus mixes with urine in the vagina so they are voided together. Close observation shows more blood at the end of urination. Blood clots are suggestive of uterine disease
- Regenerative anaemia
- Serosanguineous or purulent vaginal discharge
- Urinary incontinence due to an enlarged uterus pressing on the bladder
- Behavioural changes, such as aggression or increased sexual behaviour
- Mammary development, tumours or cysts
- Abnormal appearance of vulva due to vaginal prolapse or bladder eversion
- Anorexia and weight loss in advanced stages of some conditions.

Radiography and ultrasonography are useful to gain more information and can help to differentiate between the various conditions but laparotomy is always necessary to treat the disorders.

Endometrial hyperplasia
Endometrial hyperplasia results from prolonged oestrogenic stimulation. It is characterized by thickening of the endometrium, development of mucus-filled glands and accumulation of mucus in the lumen of the uterus. It is common in entire female rabbits (Saito *et al.*, 2002) and usually occurs in rabbits over 3 years of age, although it has been reported in rabbits under a year old (Walter *et al.*,

2010). The condition has few clinical signs and is usually discovered during elective ovariohysterectomy. A serosanguineous discharge may be noticed by observant owners. It is not clear whether endometrial hyperplasia progresses to uterine neoplasia or whether both conditions are hormonally stimulated and therefore have the same predisposing factor (Walter *et al.*, 2010).

Uterine tumours
Adenocarcinoma of the uterine endometrium is the most common neoplasm encountered in rabbits. The incidence increases with age and has been reported to reach 60% in females over 4 years of age and 75% by 7 years (Greene, 1941). Uterine adenocarcinomas are often multicentric and involve both horns of the uterus, appearing as globular polypoid structures that project into the uterus (Figure 12.6). As the condition advances, the tumours enlarge and coalesce so that large portions of the uterus are affected and they become progressively more palpable. They may contain large areas of haemorrhage, necrosis or calcification. Metastasis is slow and occurs via local spread into the peritoneum and other abdominal organs, such as the liver, or by haematogenous spread to distant sites, such as the lung, brain, skin or bones.

Not all uterine tumours are adenocarcinomas. Carcinosarcoma, adenoma, metastasis from ovarian tumours, leiomyoma and leiomyosarcomas have also been reported (Saito *et al.*, 2002; Walter *et al.*, 2010).

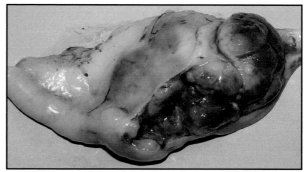

12.6 A section of the uterus of a 5-year-old Dutch rabbit that had a palpable abdominal mass. The uterus was removed. The polypoid mass extended into the lumen and into the underlying muscle layers. This is the typical gross appearance of a uterine adenocarcinoma. The diagnosis was confirmed histologically.

Pyometra
Pyometra is manifested by lethargy, inappetence, a purulent vaginal discharge, abdominal distension and a palpable abdominal mass. *Pasteurella multocida* is often present and pyometra has been cited as a manifestation of pasteurellosis (Johnson and Wolf, 1993). As in other species, pyometra is a life-threatening disease but is complicated in rabbits by the ready formation of adhesions between the infected uterus and other structures and the friability of the tissue. Rupture of the uterus can occur during surgery but surgery is the only option for treatment and can be successful.

Developmental abnormalities

Developmental disorders, such as absent uterine horns, are sometimes encountered during ovariohysterectomy in rabbits. Other abnormalities, such as a rudimentary vagina or an absent cervix, have been reported. Some abnormalities occur concurrently with other problems, such as absent kidneys (Thode and Johnston, 2009).

Endometrial venous aneurysms

Aneurysms of the uterine and myometrial venous plexuses can develop in some females, causing episodic bleeding, which can be dramatic and fatal. Intermittent haematuria may be evident.

Hydrometra

The clinical signs of hydrometra are loss of body fat and muscle and abdominal distension. There may be no change in bodyweight. The uterus is grossly enlarged (Figure 12.7) and filled with clear fluid. The condition occurs in mature females and can be diagnosed by ultrasound examination. Ovariohysterectomy is curative.

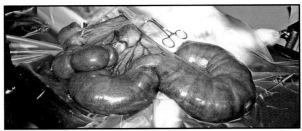

12.7 The uterus of a French Lop rabbit that was presented for neutering. The uterus was filled with fluid (hydrometra). Prior to surgery the rabbit weighed 4.5 kg; following surgery she weighed 3.4 kg. The rabbit was thin with a distended abdomen and no body fat despite eating well. She made a full recovery following ovariohysterectomy.

Extrauterine pregnancy

Extrauterine pregnancy is relatively common in domestic rabbits (Bergdall and Dysko, 1994). It is due to the escape of a fertilized ovum into the abdominal cavity or the rupture of a pregnant uterus (Harper and Ensley, 1982). Implantation usually occurs on the parietal peritoneum. The fetus becomes mummified and is palpated as an abdominal mass. Radiology or ultrasonography can be used in the differential diagnosis of this condition or it may be discovered during ovariohysterectomy (Figure 12.8).

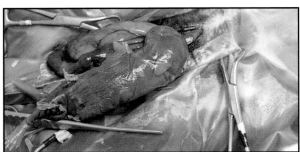

12.8 This ectopic fetus was found in the abdominal cavity during routine ovariohysterectomy.

Vaginal prolapse and bladder eversion

Prolapse of the vagina or eversion of the bladder occasionally occurs in rabbits that have recently given birth. Affected does are presented with a mass protruding from the vagina. They may be straining and unable to urinate. Replacing the prolapsed organ and putting in a purse string suture around the vulva can be successful.

Infection of the perineum and vulvar skin folds

Infection in the skin folds around the genitalia is common in mature rabbits that are overweight or loose-skinned. The hairless pouches that contain the scent glands, on either side of the genital opening, can also become infected. Affected rabbits have soiled fur under the tail and around the genitalia, which may smell strongly. There may be purulent material within the skin folds that can be mistaken for a vaginal discharge. The most effective treatment is to remove the skin folds, which is described in Chapter 21.

Behavioural changes, such as aggression

Rabbits that are pregnant, pseudopregnant or have adrenal disease (see Chapter 20) can become increasingly aggressive towards their owners or other rabbits.

Mammary development, cysts or neoplasia

Abnormalities of the mammary tissue often co-exist with uterine disease. Mammary development is a feature of pregnancy, pseudopregnancy or ovarian disease. Marked mammary development can also be associated with neoplasia and may be a sign of pituitary adenoma (Sikoski *et al.*, 2008). Malignant mammary tumours, notably adenocarcinomas, can occur. Metastasis to the lung may take place.

Surgical technique for neutering female rabbits

The technique for ovariohysterectomy is described in Operative Technique 12.1.

Considerations for ovariohysterectomy

- Rabbits are prone to uterine tumours, so it is advisable to remove the uterus, especially in animals over a year old. However, the risk of uterine disease is greatly diminished by removing the ovaries, so ovariectomy may be sufficient to prevent uterine disease if the procedure is performed before the rabbit is old enough (<1 year) to develop reproductive tract problems.
- Spaying sexually immature females is more difficult than spaying mature females because the immature uterus is small, thin and friable (see Figure 12.1).
- Rabbit blood clots quickly but the blood vessels that supply the ovaries and uterus are so large that they need to be tied off in the mesovarium and mesometrium.

- Rabbits have two uterine horns and two adjoined cervices. As in other species, the cervix acts as a seal and a barrier against infection and/or urine entering the uterus.
- The vagina is a long, friable, flaccid structure, which fills with urine during urination.
- In rabbits, if the cervices are removed, there is a risk of urine leaking into the abdomen unless the vaginal stump is effectively repaired or ligated. There is pressure on the ligature or vaginal suture line during urination.
- Ligating the vagina without leaving an area of devitalized tissue is difficult. If excess tissue is removed, the vagina easily slips out of the ligature unless a transfixing suture is used.
- The uterine artery is closely attached to the wall of the cervices and vagina. A transfixing suture can easily penetrate the uterine artery.
- The friable nature of the vaginal tissue can make oversewing difficult as the suture material can tear through the tissue.
- Rabbits are prone to fat necrosis in areas of the mesometrium that have been devitalized by ligation.
- Adhesions and granulomas form readily around any area of devitalized or traumatized tissue. These can cause problems, especially around the cervical or vaginal stump, which are anatomically close to the ureters, the rectum and the bladder (see Figure 12.2).
- Many of the problems associated with ovariohysterectomy can be avoided by ligating the cervices rather than the vagina. Each horn is ligated separately before encompassing and ligating the double cervix (see Operative Technique 12.1). The advantages of this technique are:
  - It is quick and simple
  - The ligature sits securely in the cervical tissue, which is much firmer than the flaccid vaginal tissue
  - The residual cervical tissue is an effective seal against infection or urine entering the abdomen from the vaginal stump
  - No transfixing suture is required so there is no risk of haemorrhage
  - The ligature is not close to the ureters, bladder, rectum or blood supply to the bladder.
- The only disadvantage of ligating the cervices is that a tiny amount of uterine tissue is left behind, but this is not significant unless the tissue is neoplastic or abnormal.
- Wound interference can be a postoperative complication after ovariohysterectomy. Subcuticular sutures and a comfortable wound repair help to prevent it (see Chapter 11). Other measures to prevent wound interference are described in Chapter 2.
- Rabbits are prone to gut stasis following any stressful event. Surgery and pain are stressful and ovariohysterectomy can trigger gut stasis. Good postoperative care, effective analgesia and careful observation by owners are essential (see Chapter 2).

Potential complications of ovariohysterectomy

Haemorrhage
Transfixing the cervices can result in haemorrhage into the abdomen and/or vagina from the uterine artery, which is closely attached to the wall of the cervices. Rabbit blood clots quickly so the haemorrhage is seldom a problem but can be avoided by tying off the uterine horns (see Operative Technique 12.1) rather than using a transfixing suture that can easily penetrate the uterine artery.

Transection of the vagina, resulting in urine leakage into the abdomen
The vagina is a flaccid structure that fills with urine during urination. If it is transected below the cervices and ligated or oversewn, pressure is applied to the ligature or suture line during urination and there is a risk of leakage. If this occurs, a local peritonitis can result, which may be life-threatening or may cause adhesions and tissue reactions involving the ureters, bladder or rectum, all of which are anatomically close to the vagina (see Chapter 13). These complications can be avoided by tying off the uterine horns at the cervix rather than transecting the vagina (see Operative Technique 12.1). The ligature is secure and the cervical stump is sealed.

Granulomas and adhesion formation
Any area of devitalized tissue can become necrotic. These areas can cause problems around the cervical or vaginal stump if they are close enough to occlude a ureter. Hydronephrosis can be the result. Granulomas can cause urinary incontinence from pressure on the bladder, especially if the vaginal stump is adherent to it. They can also adhere to the rectum and cause stricture. These complications can be reduced by ligating the mesometrium around the cervices rather than around the vagina.

Fat necrosis
Some fat necrosis is unavoidable around ligatures in the mesometrium of obese rabbits. The fat decomposes into fatty acids and glycerol. With time, these areas of fat necrosis can calcify as calcium binds with the fatty acids. Areas of fat necrosis in the mesometrial remnants seldom cause problems but may be obvious on abdominal radiographs (Figure 12.9). If infection is present, these areas can become abscesses that spread along the lymphatics or into the omentum. The risk of fat necrosis is reduced by using fine suture material (1.5 metric, 4/0 USP) and avoiding catgut.

Wound interference
The occasional rabbit will interfere with its abdominal wound, no matter how comfortably repaired it was or how much analgesia is used. Thin, healthy, lively young rabbits (especially wild rabbits) are most likely to remove their sutures. Elizabethan collars are not recommended as they are stressful and can therefore cause anorexia and gut stasis. An effective, temporary method of preventing a rabbit

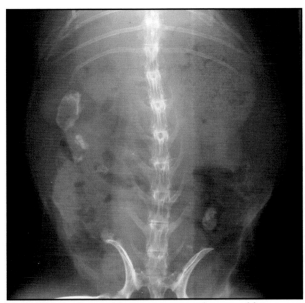

12.9 Radiographic appearance of areas of fat necrosis in the mesometrium. This is a dorsoventral view of a 7-year-old female rabbit that was neutered 6 years previously. The radiopaque areas were an incidental finding. Post-mortem examination confirmed that these lesions were solid calcified areas in the remnants of the mesometrium.

removing its skin sutures is to blunt its incisors by grinding off the tips (<1 mm). The effect lasts for 3–4 days (see Chapter 2).

Postoperative gut stasis
Like all abdominal surgery, ovariohysterectomy has the potential to trigger gut stasis. Good postopera-

tive care and effective analgesia are essential (see Chapter 2). After the rabbit has returned home, owners must be aware of the risk of gut stasis and the importance of knowing whether their rabbit is eating and defecating. Occasionally, female rabbits may not eat for 24–36 hours after surgery and will require analgesia, prokinetic therapy and syringe feeding during this period.

Ovariectomy *versus* ovariohysterectomy
In younger rabbits there is some debate about whether to perform ovariohysterectomy or ovariectomy, which can be performed endoscopically (Divers, 2010). Ovariectomy is quick and requires only a small incision. It also avoids suture and ligature placement close to the bladder, rectum or ureters. A concern about the procedure is that the uterine tissue that is left *in situ* can become cystic, neoplastic or infected. At the time of writing there are no published studies or case reports of this occurring but most veterinary surgeons prefer to perform an ovariohysterectomy. In rabbits over 1 year old, ovariohysterectomy is indicated because of the risk of uterine pathology.

Male reproductive anatomy and physiology

Anatomy of the male reproductive tract

External anatomy
The external anatomy of the male reproductive tract is shown in Figure 12.10. The sexually mature male has two external testicles that lie on either

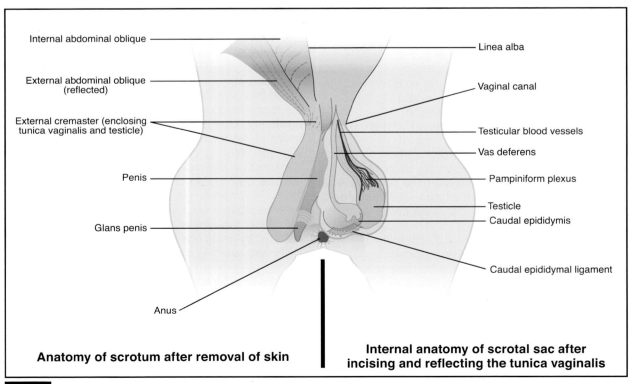

Anatomy of scrotum after removal of skin

Internal anatomy of scrotal sac after incising and reflecting the tunica vaginalis

Internal abdominal oblique

External abdominal oblique (reflected)

External cremaster (enclosing tunica vaginalis and testicle)

Penis

Glans penis

Anus

Linea alba

Vaginal canal

Testicular blood vessels

Vas deferens

Pampiniform plexus

Testicle

Caudal epididymis

Caudal epididymal ligament

12.10 Anatomy of external male genitalia.

side of the penis in two hairless scrotal sacs. The inguinal ring remains open throughout life and, during periods of food deprivation or illness, the testicles may be withdrawn into the inguinal canal by the well developed external cremaster muscle. Each testicle is enclosed in the tunica vaginalis, which has a long (2 cm) tubular section between the inguinal ring and the cranial end of the testicle. This section encloses the testicular blood vessels and the vas deferens. The caudal section of the epididymis is a prominent structure that can be seen through the thin scrotal skin at the caudal end of the scrotal sac where it is attached to the inner layer of the tunica vaginalis.

Internal anatomy

The external cremaster muscle is a section of the internal oblique abdominal muscle that passes through the inguinal canal and attaches to the tunica vaginalis; it is well developed in rabbits. In the abdomen, the vas deferens enters a seminal vesicle that opens into the urethra as it runs through the prostate gland. There is a vesicular gland in the dorsal wall of the seminal vesicle and a small pair of bulbourethral glands immediately posterior to the prostate. Disease of the male accessory glands has not been described in the rabbit.

Normal male behaviour and secondary sexual characteristics

In rabbits the testicles descend at approximately 10–12 weeks and remain small for a further 6–8 weeks. During this period, sexual behaviour is minimal and the rabbit is unlikely to be fertile. At about 5 months of age, sexual behaviour increases and the testicles become larger. Aggression towards male siblings can become serious and severe fight wounds may be inflicted by individuals that previously lived together with no problems. Wounds on the back, ears, eyelids and scrotum are common.

As maturity continues, the scent glands on the chin and anus develop and the rabbit starts to scent mark objects and accepted members of his social group (including owners) by rubbing his chin against them. He may start to deposit faeces and urine at the boundaries of his perceived territory. Sexual behaviour increases and the rabbit may start to make copulatory actions in response to being handled by the owner or attempt to mate with objects such as cuddly toys, cushions or the owner's feet. Courtship behaviour involves running past a prospective mate (including the owner's feet) and squirting a jet of urine over them.

As entire males get older, their head shape changes. The cheeks become wider, and the skin can become thickened along the dorsum from the neck to the rump. Histologically, the skin shows prominent, thick, dermal collagen similar to the cheek skin from entire male cats. In old age, the testicles tend to atrophy. The scrotal skin becomes thin and stretched. Skin debris and exudate become trapped beneath the scrotum and secondary dermatitis is common. Affected rabbits are prone to fly strike.

Diseases of the male reproductive tract

Retracted testicles

Stressed, immature or debilitated rabbits can retract their testicles into the inguinal canal where they are just palpable. In most cases, they can be pushed into the scrotum by applying gentle pressure to the inguinal region. If the rabbit is to be castrated, an incision at the cranial end of the scrotal sac, close to the inguinal ring, will reveal the end of the tunica vaginalis just beneath the incision. The tunic can be opened over the epididymis, which can be grasped to draw the testicle out of the inguinal canal. Once the testicle is exteriorized, it can be removed in the same way as in routine castration.

Absent testicles

In some mature rabbits, one or both testicles cannot be palpated in the scrotum or inguinal canal. This may be due to previous surgical removal, fighting or cryptorchidism. If the behaviour and general appearance of the rabbit suggests that it is an entire male, examination of the penis can be helpful. The penis of an entire male is long, pointed and slightly curved. It readily becomes erect and looks completely different from the penis of a castrated male, which is short, flaccid, and difficult to evert from the genital orifice. If the penis suggests the rabbit is entire, the rabbit is probably cryptorchid, or possibly an aged rabbit with an adrenal tumour (see Chapter 20).

Close examination of the inguinal area of rabbits with absent testicles is helpful but requires the fur to be clipped. The inguinal skin of a cryptorchid is smooth on the side of the absent testicle because a scrotal sac has never developed. If the testicle is retracted or has been removed, the empty scrotum persists, either as a wrinkled empty structure (retracted testicle) or as a fold of skin (after castration). Scars may suggest that the testicle has been damaged or removed as a result of a fight. The scrotum is often damaged during fights between males, and part or all of a testicle can be bitten off. In these cases surgical exploration may show remnants of a testicle or its surrounding structures.

Herniated bladder

Inguinal hernias containing part, or all, of the bladder are occasionally encountered in aged entire male rabbits (Thas and Harcourt-Brown, 2013; Figure 12.11a) and one case has been reported in a female (Grunkemeyer et al., 2010). In the early stages, a palpable swelling in the inguinal region is often detected by the owner. In the later stages, dysuria may be the presenting sign because, once part of or the entire bladder has passed through the inguinal canal, sediment accumulates in the herniated part of the bladder, which cannot empty properly. In severe cases, partial or complete ureteral obstruction can occur (Grunkemeyer et al., 2010).

Surgical repair is usually straightforward. After clipping the fur, examination of the swelling shows a herniated sac that, in males, is separate from the testicle and associated structures (Figure 12.11b).

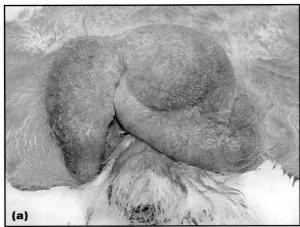

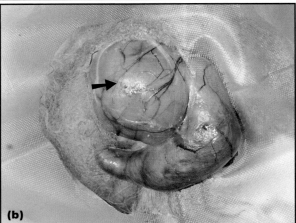

12.11 An inguinal hernia in a 6-year-old entire male Dwarf Lop. **(a)** A fluctuating swelling in the left inguinal region was revealed after the fur was clipped and some blue chlorhexidine solution applied to the area. **(b)** Surgical exploration revealed that the bladder had prolapsed through the inguinal musculature (arrowed). The rabbit made a full recovery following castration, re-placement of the bladder and closure of the inguinal canal and musculature.

After opening the skin of the swelling, the contents of the hernia can be identified by carefully opening the sac and examining the contents.

The bladder can be emptied by gently expressing it or by aspirating the urine. Cystotomy, with or without laparotomy, may be required in cases where a lot of sediment is present in the bladder. Once the bladder is empty, it can be re-placed into the abdomen. The hernial ring is identified and closed in the same way as for an inguinal hernia repair in a dog or cat, taking care not to compromise the nerves and blood vessels that lie close to it. The testicle also needs to be removed, ensuring that the inguinal canal is closed.

Neoplasia

Tumours of the testicle can occur in aged entire males. Sometimes they are very large before they are noticed by the owner. Benign interstitial cell tumours are the most common type and may be associated with other changes, such as mammary development (Maratea *et al.*, 2007).

Gonadoblastoma has also been described (Suzuki *et al.*, 2011). Urine scalding and dysuria may be the presenting signs if the tumour is so large that it distorts the external genitalia and diverts the stream of urine during urination (Figure 12.12). These rabbits often present with urine scalding on the inside of the contralateral leg.

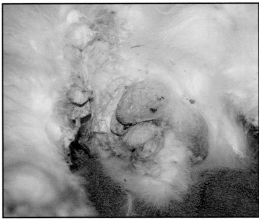

12.12 The external genitalia of an aged entire male rabbit that was presented for treatment because he was urinating down the inside of the right hindleg. Clinical examination revealed an enlarged right testicle, the size of a plum. It had expanded into the inguinal region and was distorting the scrotum so the penis was rotated. The rabbit urinated normally after he was neutered.

The author has encountered three cases of melanoma, with varying degrees of malignancy, all involving the scrotal skin, which was deeply pigmented, thickened and exfoliating dark pigmented scales, which were sometimes haemorrhagic.

Testicular torsion

Torsion of a testicle can occur. The condition may be seen in entire males of any age. It is a painful condition and sudden-onset depression and anorexia may be the presenting signs. The affected testicle is sore and tense. Its position in the scrotal sac is abnormal (Figure 12.13). Immediate removal of the twisted testicle is indicated.

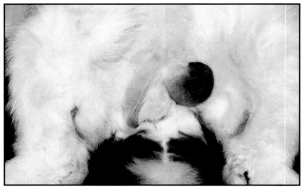

12.13 The external genitalia of a 1-year-old entire male Dwarf Lop that was suddenly depressed and anorexic. The left hemiscrotum was painful and distorted. The black coloration is pigmented skin. Exploratory surgery revealed a 180 degree torsion of the testicle. The rabbit was neutered and made a full recovery.

Persistent penile erection

Persistent penile erection can be a complication of sedation or anaesthesia in entire male rabbits that are easily aroused by handling. Some sedatives, especially opioids, do not dampen this response and the rabbit may have an erect penis throughout a surgical procedure, usually castration. Blood clots quickly in rabbits and it is probable that a blood clot prevents the corpus cavernosum from emptying. The erection may be maintained after the rabbit recovers from anaesthesia and can persist for hours or days. The exposed penis eventually becomes desiccated and inflamed. Mild cases are self-limiting and resolve with time, although lubrication of the penis, antibiotics and analgesia are required. In persistent cases, the penis becomes swollen, purple and gangrenous, and amputation may be necessary, which is usually successful.

In view of the risk of this complication, it is sensible to avoid potent opioids such as fentanyl for premedication or sedation of entire male rabbits.

Preputial adhesions

In some castrated male rabbits, especially obese ones, the penis can become adherent to the prepuce. In most cases, this is an incidental finding during eversion of the genital orifice as part of clinical examination when the penis everts to expose the distal urethra. If these rabbits develop urinary incontinence, the genital orifice and prepuce easily become inflamed and sore, which can exacerbate the adhesions and scarring so that urine is directed down the inside of one thigh.

Occasionally, the preputial opening becomes so stenotic that the rabbit can only dribble urine rather than direct a jet of urine away from the inside of the legs or under the tail. These cases may require surgery. In all cases, it is very important to clip all the urine-soaked fur from the skin on the inside of the legs and around the genitalia and tail before examining the prepuce and deciding how to improve the situation. Each case is different and treatment requires common sense. Tail amputation may be necessary (see Chapter 21); this procedure is as straightforward in rabbits as in other species.

Surgical techniques for neutering male rabbits

Routine castration

Several techniques for castration have been described and everyone has their own preference. The main consideration is to close the inguinal canal to prevent herniation of abdominal contents postoperatively. Some authors describe an open castration where the testicles are removed through a scrotal, prescrotal or even abdominal incision (Millis and Walshaw, 1992). These techniques require buried and skin sutures and carry a risk of herniation postoperatively.

A closed castration, either prescrotally or via the scrotum, is often recommended (Redrobe, 2000; Richardson and Flecknell, 2006). In these techniques, the tunica vaginalis is not opened but is dissected away from the interior of the scrotal skin. This can be difficult and time-consuming because the tunica vaginalis may be strongly connected to the scrotal skin, especially at the caudal end of the scrotum and in older males. The author prefers a mixed open and closed technique (see Operative Technique 12.2), which is quick and easy with no complications apart from the risk of mild skin trauma during preoperative clipping.

Neutering cryptorchid rabbits

In cryptorchid rabbits, one or both testicles fail to descend into the scrotum. They may be in the inguinal canal or the abdomen. Even if they are abdominal, it is often possible to remove them without a laparotomy by finding the caudal end of the tunica vaginalis in the inguinal canal, opening it and gently pulling on the ligament that attaches it to the testicle. The inguinal canal of rabbits is wide and retained testicles are elliptical and narrower than normal testicles so they can slide out of the abdomen and be removed (Figure 12.14).

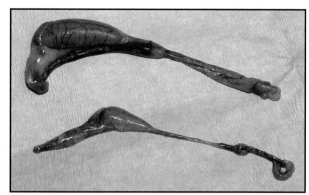

12.14 Comparative sizes of retained testicles. Both testicles were removed from a 9-month-old English rabbit. The testicle shown at the top of the picture was removed from the scrotum. The testicle shown below was removed from the abdomen, where it was lying close to the inguinal canal.

If abdominal exploration is necessary, a useful technique is to identify and exteriorize the bladder and reflect it to expose the ureters. The path of the ureter on the side of the missing testicle is followed to the point where the vas deferens loops over it. The vas deferens can then be followed until it ends in the retained testicle. Some abdominal testicles are very small and could be mistaken for a piece of abdominal fat.

Scrotal ablation

There are situations where it is advantageous to remove both scrotal sacs and the testicles, as well as all their attachments. The main indication is in elderly male rabbits, where the scrotal skin has stretched and deep folds have formed between the scrotum and genitalia. These rabbits cannot clean the folds, so skin debris collects and secondary infection develops. Testicular or scrotal skin tumours are another indication for scrotal ablation (see Chapter 21).

Scrotal ablation is a simple, effective procedure but is more time-consuming than routine castration. Sufficient skin must be left to repair the deficit with no tension on the wound, which might alter the direction of urine flow. Removal of the scrotal sacs gives good access to the inguinal canals so the tunica vaginalis can be identified and ligated securely. The skin is repaired with either buried subcuticular sutures or simple interrupted skin sutures (or both). The author's preferred suture material is 1.5 metric (4/0 USP) polyglactin 910 (e.g. Vicryl Rapide), because the material is soft and comfortable for the rabbit and the sutures will 'wipe off' after 10–14 days.

Potential complications of castration

Trauma to scrotal skin during clipping
The scrotal skin is very thin. It is not under tension and is easily nicked with clipper blades. Care is required to prevent such injuries but they are usually of little consequence and heal readily.

Postoperative complications
Complications following castration are extremely rare using the procedure described in Operative Technique 12.2.

> **Postoperative advice for owners**
> The postoperative advice after castration is the same as for any surgical procedure, although most rabbits eat straight away and continue to do so. Postoperative gut stasis is rare.
> After castration, the male can be considered sterile after a period of 4 weeks.

Postoperative swelling and oedema of the scrotal sacs
This follows closed castration, either via the scrotum or pre-scrotally, when the skin has been sutured so fluid can collect under it. Postoperative swelling is most common if it has been difficult to free the tunica vaginalis from the skin and the tissue has been traumatized. Fluid collects in the scrotal sac, which can become large and uncomfortable for the rabbit. Analgesia and time usually resolve the situation. The condition may resolve more quickly if the owner is willing to massage the hemiscrotal sacs delicately (Capello, 2005).

Postoperative infection
Postoperative infection is rare unless an inappropriate buried suture material is used or the surgical site was already infected or contaminated. Catgut should be avoided to ligate the spermatic cord as it can cause a tissue reaction in rabbits and act as a nidus for infection. In cases where the surgical site is already contaminated or infected, the author's preferred antibiotic is trimethoprim/sulphonamide.

Postoperative infection can be manifested by an inflamed, sore suture line that the rabbit chews at, or an inguinal swelling that may develop days or weeks after surgery. Surgical exploration and removal of all infected necrotic material, including residual suture material, is necessary. The wound is left open to drain like any other abscess.

Herniation of abdominal contents
If the inguinal ring is not closed effectively during castration, it is possible for abdominal viscera to herniate through it. The most likely organ to fit through the ring is a section of small intestine. The owner may see the prolapsed section of intestine if the scrotal wound was left open or the skin sutures were not adequate. If the scrotal skin is intact, they may see a swelling in the inguinal region or they may not notice anything at all. If the condition is not recognized and treated promptly, strangulation of the prolapsed section of small intestine can cause an intestinal obstruction so the rabbit develops gastric dilation and shock (see Chapter 14), usually within 72 hours of surgery. Treatment depends on the condition of the rabbit and the section of intestine that has prolapsed. If the condition is recognized early and the prolapsed contents are viable, they can be flushed copiously with warm saline and replaced through the inguinal canal before identifying and closing the tunica vaginalis and inguinal ring. If the intestine is not viable enterectomy or euthanasia may be necessary.

Male behaviour in castrated rabbits
Some aged castrated rabbits can develop male behavioural characteristics such as aggression towards other rabbits or humans and attempt to mate animate and inanimate objects. Pituitary or adrenal neoplasia is suspected in these cases. This subject is covered in Chapter 20.

References and further reading

Barone R, Pavaux C, Blin PC and Cuq P (1973) *Atlas d'anatomie du lapin.* Masson et Cie, Paris

Bergdall V and Dysko RC (1994) Metabolic, traumatic, mycotic and miscellaneous diseases. In: *The Biology of the Laboratory Rabbit, 2nd edn*, eds PJ Manning, DH Ringler and CE Newcomer, pp. 336–355. Academic Press, San Diego

Capello V (2005) Surgical techniques for orchiectomy of the pet rabbit. *Exotic DVM* **7**, 23–32

Divers SJ (2010) Clinical technique: Endoscopic oophorectomy in the rabbit (*Oryctolagus cuniculus*): The future of preventive sterilizations. *Journal of Exotic Pet Medicine* **19**, 231–239

Greene HSN (1941) Uterine adenomata in the rabbit. *Journal of Experimental Medicine* **73**, 273–292

Grunkemeyer VL, Sura PA, Baron ML and Souza MJ (2010) Surgical repair of an inguinal herniation of the urinary bladder in an intact female domestic rabbit (*Oryctolagus cuniculus*). *Journal of Exotic Pet Medicine* **19**, 249–254

Johnson JH and Wolf AM (1993) Ovarian abscesses and pyometra in a domestic rabbit. *Journal of the American Veterinary Medical Association* **203**, 667–669

Maratea KA, Ramos-Vara JA, Corriveau LA and Miller MA (2007) Testicular interstitial cell tumor and gynecomastia in a rabbit. *Veterinary Pathology* **44**, 513–517

Millis DL and Walshaw R (1992) Elective castrations and ovariohysterectomies in pet rabbits. *Journal of the American Animal Hospital Association* **28**, 491–497

Redrobe S (2000) Surgical procedures and dental disorders. In: *BSAVA Manual of Rabbit Medicine and Surgery*, ed. P Flecknell, pp. 117–134. BSAVA Publications, Gloucester

Richardson C and Flecknell P (2006) Routine neutering of rabbits and rodents. *In Practice* **28**, 70–79

Saito K, Nakanishi M and Hasegawa A (2002) Uterine disorders diagnosed by ventrotomy in 47 rabbits. *Journal of Veterinary Medical Science* **64**, 495–497

Sikoski P, Trybus J, Cline JM et al. (2008) Cystic mammary adenocarcinoma associated with a prolactin-secreting pituitary adenoma in a New Zealand White rabbit (*Oryctolagus cuniculus*). *Comparative Medicine* **58**, 297–300

Suzuki M, Ozaki M, Ano A, et al. (2011) Testicular gonadoblastoma in two pet domestic rabbits (*Oryctolagus cuniculus domesticus*). *Journal of Veterinary Diagnostic Investigation* **23**, 1026–1032

Thas I and Harcourt-Brown F (2013) Six cases of inguinal urinary bladder herniation in entire male domestic rabbits. *Journal of Small Animal Practice* [available online August 2013. DOI: 10.111/jsap.12120]

Thode HP and Johnston MS (2009) Probable congenital uterine developmental abnormalities in two domestic rabbits. *Veterinary Record* **164**, 242–244

Walter B, Poth T, Böhmer E, Braun J and Matis U (2010) Uterine disorders in 59 rabbits. *Veterinary Record* **166**, 230–233

OPERATIVE TECHNIQUES ➜

OPERATIVE TECHNIQUE 12.1:
Ovariohysterectomy

Positioning

The procedure is carried out under general anaesthesia (see Chapter 1.) The rabbit is placed in dorsal recumbency.

Equipment

Small instruments are required. The author's surgical kit for rabbits comprises:

- 5" Crile (two pairs) and Halsted (6 pairs) straight and curved artery forceps
- Martin splinter forceps
- 2 mm Debakey dissecting forceps
- 5" Adson dissecting forceps
- 5" Olsen Hegar scissor/needle-holder
- 5" straight sharp/blunt scissors
- 4.5" straight strabismus forceps
- 6" Metzenbaum scissors
- No. 9 scalpel handle
- No. 15 scalpel blade.

The author's preference for intra-abdominal suture material is 1.5 metric (4/0 USP) polyglactin 910 (e.g. Vicryl) and 1.5 metric (4/0 USP) poliglecaprone (e.g. Monocryl) to repair the abdominal incision.

Surgical technique

1 Make a 2 cm ventral midline incision approximately midway between the umbilicus and the pubic symphysis. In rabbits, the ovarian attachments are short but the vagina is long and the cervix is freely mobile, which makes a midline

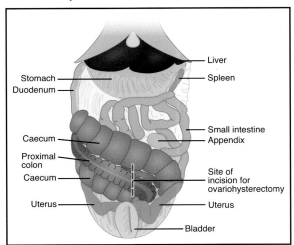

incision preferable to a lateral approach. The proximal colon or caecum is usually found immediately under the incision. A uterine horn or fallopian tube can be located under the ventral extremity of the incision in rabbits.

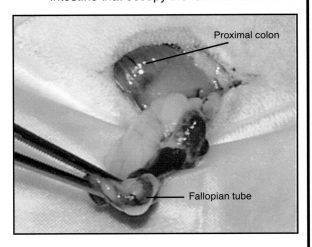

2 Exteriorize the uterine horn or fallopian tube with the attached mesometrium and follow it along to the ovary. The right ovary lies beneath the large ileocaecocolic complex, which occupies most of the right caudoventral abdomen. The left ovary is situated beneath the loops of small intestine that occupy the left mid-abdomen.

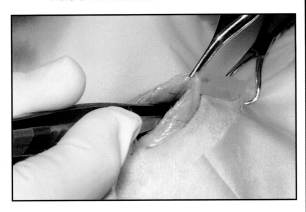

3 Exteriorize the ovary and its suspensory ligament, which contains a spherical body of fat. One end of the ovary is attached to the mesovarium by a small ovarian ligament, which can be safely torn, either deliberately or incidentally, during exteriorization of the ovary.

→

OPERATIVE TECHNIQUE 12.1 continued:
Ovariohysterectomy

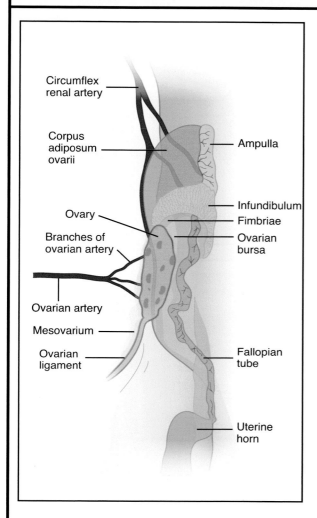

4 Locate the artery that lies within the body of fat around the ovary. This is a branch of the circumflex renal artery and supplies the ampulla, infundibulum and fimbriae. Clamp this artery and tie it off.

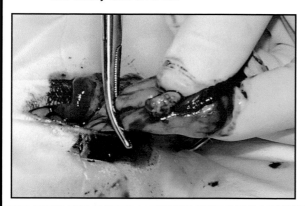

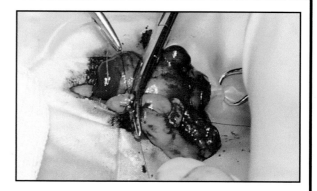

5 Separate the mesovarium to release the ovary.

6 Exteriorize the uterine horn and cervix that is attached to the ovary and locate the ovarian and uterine arteries within the mesometrium. At its cranial end, the uterine artery anastomoses with the ovarian artery in an arcuate arrangement to supply the uterine horn with numerous branches. At the cervical end, the large uterine artery curves round and attaches to the bicornuate cervix and runs along the vaginal wall.

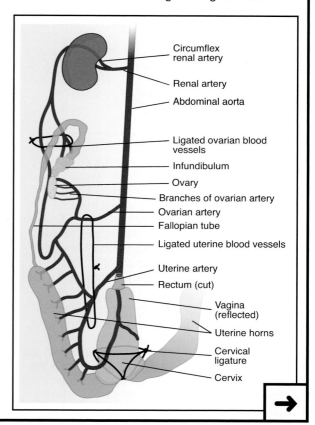

OPERATIVE TECHNIQUE 12.1 continued:
Ovariohysterectomy

7 Puncture the mesometrium within the curve of the uterine artery and apply a ligature that encompasses both the ovarian and uterine artery within the mesometrium (see also diagram opposite).

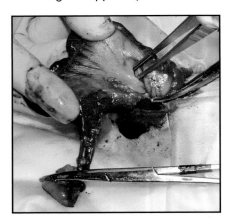

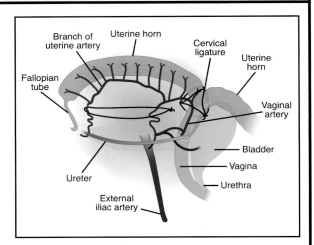

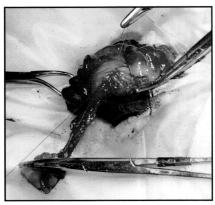

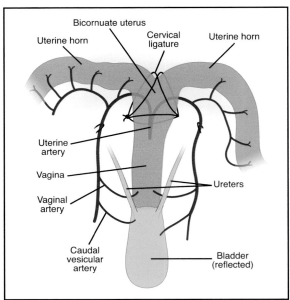

8 Locate the contralateral ovary and repeat the process on the other side.

9 After both ovaries and uterine horns have been exteriorized, the cervix must be securely ligated. Placement of this ligature is important because it needs to be away from the ureters or the blood vessels that supply the vagina and bladder. The anatomy and ligature placement are shown in the diagrams.

10 Ligate the cervix by applying a length of suture material around each uterine horn before encompassing the cervix. Once tightened, the ligature sits securely across the cervix without the need to transfix the vagina, which carries a risk of haemorrhage if the uterine artery is punctured. The cervical ligature prevents the risk of urine

leakage from the flaccid vagina, which fills with urine during micturition. It also reduces the likelihood of infection from the vagina entering the abdomen as the cervix is a natural barrier.

In order to place the ligature, first individually encompass and tie off each horn at the bifurcation by passing a length of suture material through the puncture in the mesometrium that was made to tie off the ovarian and uterine blood vessels. The ligature is then passed between the uterine horns so that it encircles only one of them. The ligature is tied but not cut.

→

OPERATIVE TECHNIQUE 12.1 continued:
Ovariohysterectomy

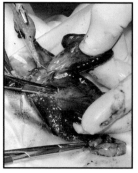

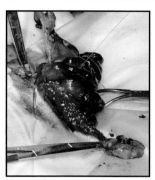

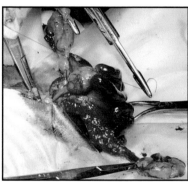

11 The same ligature is then taken through the puncture in the mesometrium on the contralateral side to encircle the other uterine horn. Again the ligature is tied but not cut. Once both horns are securely ligated, the ligature is taken around the cervical body and knotted to tighten it. The suture material is then cut.

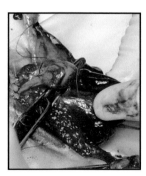

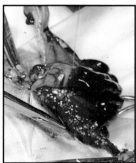

12 After placing the cervical ligature, section and remove the uterine horns and cut through the mesometrium.

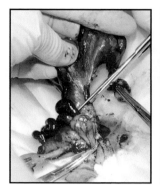

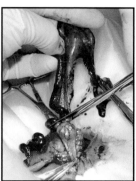

13 Inspect the cervical stump for haemorrhage.

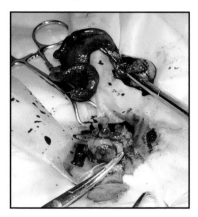

14 Then replace it into the abdomen and repair the incision.

Postoperative management

The use of antibiotics depends on the practice policy. Non-steroidal analgesia, such as meloxicam is always indicated and will need to be continued until the rabbit is eating well. Opioid analgesia, e.g. buprenorphine, tramadol or premedication with fentanyl/fluanisone, is also indicated (see Chapter 2).

Recovery from ovariohysterectomy is usually straightforward, although some rabbits may not eat properly for up to 48 hours

→

OPERATIVE TECHNIQUE 12.1 continued:
Ovariohysterectomy

after surgery and will need syringe feeding and prokinetic therapy. Hospitalization overnight following surgery can be beneficial to ensure the rabbit is eating, defecating and leaving the wound alone. If the rabbit goes home, the owners should be aware of the risk of gut stasis and should check the wound and make sure that the rabbit is eating and defecating postoperatively.

Possible complications

Haemorrhage, fat necrosis, adhesions, infection, wound interference and postoperative anorexia are possible complications of ovariohysterectomy although the risks are low if the above technique is used. These complications are discussed in more detail in the text.

OPERATIVE TECHNIQUE 12.2:
Castration

Positioning

The procedure is carried out under general anaesthesia (see Chapter 1.) Position the rabbit on its back. A trough is useful to keep the rabbit supported in dorsal recumbency. The testicles are found in hairless scrotal sacs on either side of the penis. The external cremaster muscle easily draws the testicle into the inguinal canal, even in response to handling prior to surgery. If this occurs, pressure on the inguinal canal will extrude the testicle back into the scrotum.

Equipment

The surgical kit that is used for ovariohysterectomy (see Operative Technique 12.1) is also suitable for castration.

Surgical technique

1 Clip the fur from the cranial end of the scrotal sacs and prepare the skin.

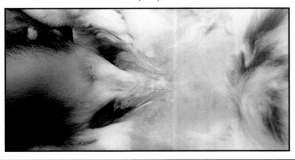

2 After draping the operation site, pick up and grasp a testicle between finger and thumb.

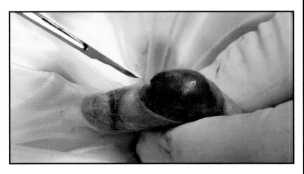

3 Make a 1 cm incision over the cranial end of the testicle to expose the tunica vaginalis.

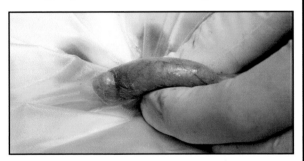

4 Incise through the tunica vaginalis to expose the testicle.

OPERATIVE TECHNIQUE 12.2 continued:
Castration

5 Squeeze the testicle out of the incision.

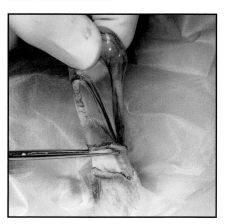

6 Grasp the testicle gently to exteriorize it and hold the testicle out of the scrotum to stretch the tunica vaginalis and the connective tissue between it and the scrotal skin (arrow).

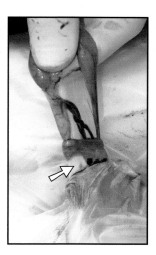

7 Section the attachment between the caudal end of the tunica vaginalis and the scrotal skin with scissors.

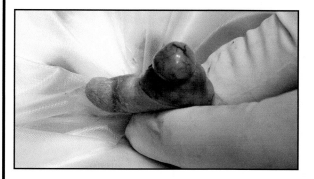

8 Use blunt dissection to free the length of the tunic (enclosing the vas deferens and blood vessels) to the inguinal ring. Clamp the testicular blood vessels.

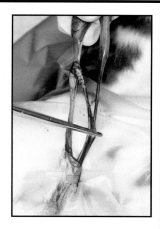

9 Ligate the blood vessels before sectioning and releasing them; they will then retract into the tubular section of the tunica vaginalis, which is about to be ligated at the site marked by the arrow.

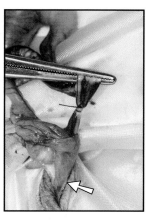

10 Close the inguinal canal by placing a ligature around the tunica vaginalis, after ensuring that the ligatures around blood vessels are contained within the residual tubular section of tunica vaginalis. They are visible through the thin tissue of the tunica vaginalis, especially if coloured suture material is used (arrow).

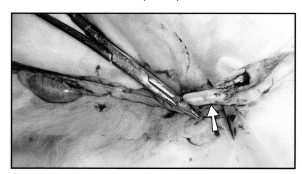

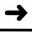

OPERATIVE TECHNIQUE 12.2 continued:
Castration

11 After the remnant of the tunica vaginalis is replaced under the skin, align the edges of the incision together with your fingertips. No sutures are required as there is no tension on the skin and the ligated tunica vaginalis prevents herniation of abdominal contents. The wound is comfortable so the rabbit will leave it alone.

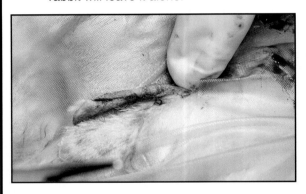

12 If the initial incision has been made in the prescrotal skin, e.g. over the inguinal canal to remove a retained or retracted testicle, skin sutures are often required to close the incision as there is less skin and the wound will gape. The author's preference is two simple interrupted sutures using an absorbable material.

13 Repeat the procedure for the other testis.

Postoperative management

Recovery from castration is usually straightforward, although some rabbits might be stressed by the disruption of their daily routine and having an operation. The owners should be aware of the risk of gut stasis and should make sure that the rabbit is eating and defecating after he goes home. The use of antibiotics depends on the practice policy. An injection of a non-steroidal analgesic such as meloxicam is indicated.

Possible complications

Haemorrhage, infection, wound interference and postoperative anorexia are possible complications of castration although the risks are negligible if the above technique is used. Complications of other techniques for castration are discussed in the text.

13

Exploratory laparotomy

Richard Saunders

Exploratory laparotomy involves a surgical approach to the abdominal cavity, to diagnose and potentially treat abdominal disease. In some cases, exploratory laparoscopy (see Chapter 11) may be performed in place of laparotomy.

Technically, the term 'laparotomy' describes a flank approach to the abdomen, and 'coeliotomy' describes a ventral midline approach. However, the term laparotomy is widely accepted to refer to any approach.

Patient assessment and preparation

Ideally, full haematology, serum biochemistry and blood gas analysis should be performed in rabbits prior to exploratory laparotomy. Abdominocentesis or diagnostic peritoneal lavage may also be employed. Imaging may have already been used to localize a lesion. However, where time or funds do not permit, a suggested minimum database should include packed cell volume (PCV), total protein, blood glucose and electrolytes. Prior collection of blood from a donor rabbit may be performed if expected to be required.

The only absolute contraindication to exploratory laparotomy is a patient unable to withstand the required anaesthetic. Unless the procedure is carried out as a life-threatening emergency, the patient should be stabilized as necessary before anaesthesia and laparotomy are performed. Where laparotomy is required to stabilize the patient (e.g. uncontrolled intra-abdominal blood loss), anaesthesia and surgery are performed without delay, although establishing vascular access (intravenous or intraosseous) facilitates blood replacement or other circulatory support and should be carried out first.

Blood transfusion in the rabbit

Where available, haemoglobin-based oxygen carriers (HBOCs) may be preferable to whole blood; their smaller molecules allow for much more effective (up to 10 times) tissue perfusion and efficacy in haemorrhagic shock. There are no concerns regarding donor welfare, cross-matching, clot prevention, disease transmission and short storage times, in contrast to blood. However, their expense and lack of commercial availability at this time makes blood an appropriate alternative.

Any of the following are indications for transfusion:

- A rapid decrease in PCV (to <15%)
- A loss of >30% (i.e. 30 ml/kg) of the circulating blood volume
- Blood loss associated with collapse
- Ongoing haemorrhage likely to lead to any of the above
- Lack of effective response to crystalloid and colloid treatment.

Donor concerns

Donors should be mature animals, no older than middle-aged (this varies by breed, but generally no older than 4 years for giant breeds and 6 years for small breeds), and in excellent health. Use of larger individuals is more practical and collection of greater volumes is safer from larger individuals. Donors should be disease-free, with negative *Encephalitozoon cuniculi* IgG and IgM antibody titres, or 4-week paired IgG titres. The donor's PCV should be measured prior to collection of blood, as a low PCV (<35%) may preclude safe blood collection or modify the collection volume required to achieve effective blood replacement in the recipient. Whilst the ethical arguments for blood donation in other species have been accepted, undue stress is a welfare concern for rabbits and so placid individuals should be used. The use of a companion rabbit as donor is ideal, as it is unlikely that new pathogens will be introduced to the recipient, and there is a benefit to the donor rabbit in increasing the likelihood of survival of a bonded companion animal. A maximum volume of 10 ml/kg may be taken safely from a healthy donor.

Blood collection

The jugular vein is the most appropriate site for collection. Butterfly or hypodermic needles may be used, connected to a 10–20 ml syringe. Syringes, needles and butterfly needle lines should be pre-prepared with anticoagulant. Anticoagulants commonly used for canine and feline blood collection may be employed, and the choice will depend on the required duration of storage of blood. ▶

Blood administration

Blood must be given at body temperature to avoid hypothermia. An in-line filter is used as part of the administration set, to prevent small clots entering the bloodstream. Blood may be given extremely rapidly (over a few minutes) in cases of severe acute haemorrhage, or otherwise over a period up to 4 hours, as required. If there are concerns about circulatory overload, and administration is deemed to be needed at a slower rate, the total volume of fresh blood should not be held at body temperature for >4 hours to avoid bacterial growth, and should instead be refrigerated at 5°C and rewarmed as needed. Blood may be given into the jugular vein or a large diameter peripheral vein, or via the intra-osseous route if no veins are available, which can be cannulated with a 22 G or larger bore catheter (to avoid lysis of red cells).

Donor monitoring

Baseline monitoring of temperature, pulse (rate and quality), respiration, mucous membrane colour and capillary refill time, PCV and general clinical appearance should be performed, and repeated at least every 30 minutes during and immediately after transfusion. The patient should be monitored continuously for the first 15 minutes, during which the administration rate should be no greater than 0.5 ml/kg/h, unless urgent trans-fusion is needed. Transfusion reactions are rare and cannot be prevented or minimized by prior administration of steroids or antihistamines. The PCV should be measured 1 hour after administra-tion to determine the response, and thus the need for further transfusions.

Cross-matching

Blood groups have been studied in the rabbit. However, their full significance is unclear, and some form of cross-matching should always be performed. One-off transfusions are generally considered safe. Related rabbits are likely to be more compatible (Joysey, 1955). Haemolysis is the most common transfusion reaction but is impossible to predict without sampling large volumes (2 ml). If this is not practical, then aggluti-nation testing is performed: two drops of plasma from one rabbit are mixed with one drop of blood from the other rabbit on a room temperature microscope slide, and left for 1 minute. The pres-ence of visible agglutination suggests incompati-bility (Lichtenberger, 2004a,b).

Volume required

The volume of blood required will depend on the degree of blood loss, the pre-transfusion PCV, the size of the rabbit, and any ongoing losses, as well as the donor PCV. Ideally, a post-transfusion PCV of >30% should be aimed for, in order to correct acute haemorrhagic blood loss. As a general rule of thumb, 2 ml/kg of whole blood will increase the recipient PCV by 1%. The formula below (Platt and Garosi, 2012) may also be used:

Blood required (ml) = bodyweight of recipient (kg) × circulating blood volume (66 ml/kg) × (desired recipient PCV – pre-transfusion PCV)/donor PCV

Autotransfusion

Autotransfusion may be employed following intra-operative blood loss, e.g. following vena cava perf-oration during liver lobectomy. It is important to filter and anticoagulate blood in these situations. The ease of collection, avoidance of disease risk and lack of detrimental effects on a donor are advantages. The main disadvantage is the low thrombocyte count in autotransfused blood, and subsequent effects on clotting (Silva *et al.*, 1984).

Anatomy

The normal anatomy of the abdomen is illustrated radiographically in Chapter 7, ultrasonographically in Chapter 8 and diagrammatically in Figure 13.1.

Indications for laparotomy

Abdominal trauma (including iatrogenic)

Exploratory laparotomy is the standard of care in cases with a history of significant abdominal trauma, where there is a reasonable suspicion of internal organ damage (e.g. road traffic accident; attack by a medium-sized to large dog; blunt force trauma such as being trodden on or kicked by a human or large animal; recent intra-abdominal surgery, such as ovariohysterectomy, recent laparoscopy). Any case where there is evidence of intra-abdominal bleeding, bladder or gastrointestinal tract rupture should be investigated by exploratory laparotomy. This includes any laparoscopic procedure where there is a reasonable suspicion of iatrogenic organ damage, which may require conversion to laparotomy.

Exploratory laparotomy should be carried out without delay in haemodynamically unstable trauma patients suffering from haemoperitoneum. These ani-mals are likely to have intraperitoneal bleeding from the liver, uterus, spleen or mesentery.

Exploratory laparotomy should be carried out following immediate patient stabilization in trauma patients with suspected urogenital or gastrointesti-nal tract rupture.

Acute-onset abdominal pain or discomfort

Any acute-onset abdominal pain or discomfort with clinical findings suggestive of intra-abdominal pathology should be evaluated promptly following immediate patient stabilization and a minimum data-base and, depending on the findings, exploratory laparotomy may be indicated. Causes may include ruptured abdominal organ, peritonitis, gastrointest-inal obstruction, ureteral blockage, liver lobe torsion, uterine torsion and bladder rupture, which are discussed in the relevant chapters.

A full clinical history should be taken, including reproductive status and expected parturition date if

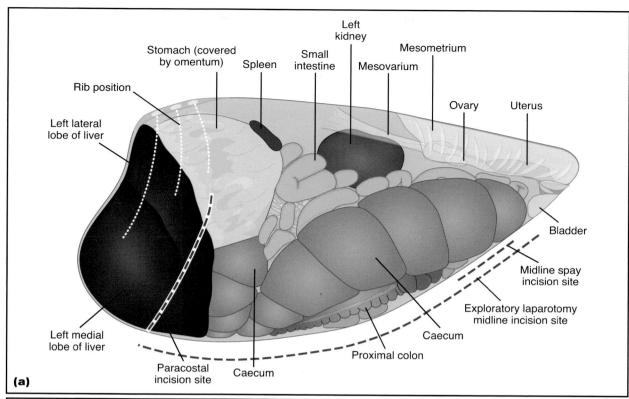

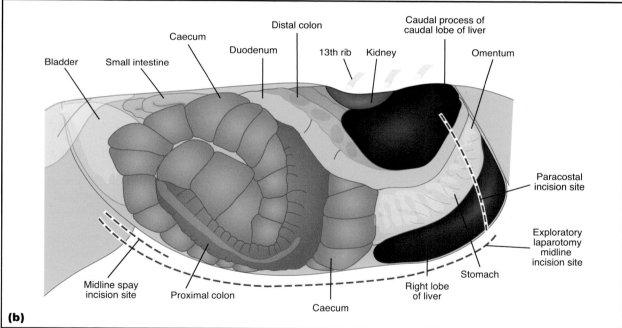

13.1 The normal anatomy of the abdomen: **(a)** left lateral view; **(b)** right lateral view.

pregnant, breed type, recent exertion, dental health status, food and treats offered, potential foreign body ingestion (e.g. fur mats, carpet fibres, clay-based cat litter, locust bean pods) and a prior history of gastrointestinal stasis. Appetite, passage of faeces, caecotrophs and urine should be noted. Impending parturition, especially in an obese doe, may be associated with pregnancy toxaemia and elective caesarean or ovariohysterectomy may be necessary.

Deep-chested large breeds such as French Lops and some Dwarf Lops appear over-represented as liver lobe torsion cases, as do rabbits that have had recent exertions, e.g. 'night fright' due to predators. Rabbits with dental disease and a poor state of grooming are predisposed to fur mat ingestion. Rabbits with a prior history of gastrointestinal stasis may have had intermittent partial obstructions previously, increasing the index of suspicion of current total obstruction. Recent oliguria may indicate bladder rupture or outflow obstruction.

Abdominal radiography and ultrasonography are extremely helpful in making the decision whether and when to perform an exploratory laparotomy. In cases of suspected intra-abdominal bleeding or liver lobe torsion, serial PCV measurement may provide an assessment of haemodynamic stability. In cases of suspected gastrointestinal foreign body, serial radiography and serum glucose measurement provide indicators of the presence or lack of successful progression of a foreign body through the gastrointestinal tract, and help determine the need for exploratory laparotomy. The presence of a PCV below 25%, and raised liver enzymes in an acutely anorexic and collapsed or lethargic rabbit is strongly indicative of liver lobe torsion (Saunders *et al.*, 2009; Wenger *et al.*, 2009). The presence of serum glucose measurements above 20 mmol/l in an acutely anorexic and collapsed or lethargic rabbit is strongly indicative of small intestinal obstruction (Harcourt-Brown and Harcourt-Brown, 2012).

Peritonitis (± ruptured viscus)
Peritonitis may be suggested by a history of recent trauma, surgery, gastrointestinal foreign body, urinary tract blockage or internal abscessation. There may be radiographic evidence of peritonitis (ground glass appearance and/or pneumoperitoneum), or ultrasound evidence (free fluid and/or gas), although these are not definitively diagnostic. Abdominal tap or diagnostic peritoneal lavage evidence of ruptured viscus is strongly indicative, but false negatives (insufficient or inaccessible fluid present) and false positives (iatrogenic viscus penetration) are both possible.

Abdominocentesis is potentially complicated in the rabbit by the high risk of perforation of the gut or bladder. This risk is greater in an animal with gas distension of the stomach or caecum, or a distended urinary bladder, and is therefore ideally carried out in dorsal recumbency, allowing the abdominal viscera to fall away from the site of needle entry. However, in this position, free fluid is also displaced away from the ventrum, so sample recovery is extremely poor. The voluminous gastrointestinal tract may block or enfold the needle or catheter, giving a negative finding, especially if the volume of fluid is small. In practice, ultrasound-guided abdominocentesis is a more precise, effective and potentially safer tool. An appropriately sized needle (typically 23 G, 1 inch) or catheter is introduced through an aseptically prepared site at right angles

to the body wall, just lateral to the ventral midline, and caudal to the umbilicus. A syringe may be used to withdraw a sample, or fluid may be allowed to drip from the needle hub (Fox, 2011).

Diagnostic peritoneal lavage is more likely to obtain meaningful results than blind abdominocentesis. The technique is as described for abdominocentesis, using an over-the-needle catheter. After introduction of the catheter, the stylet is removed, aspiration is attempted and, if no fluid is present, 20 ml/kg of warm sterile 0.9% saline is introduced slowly. Alternatively, a small midline skin incision may be made, and a larger bore catheter inserted, which is more invasive but less liable to produce false-negative results. A bung or three-way tap is placed on the catheter, and the rabbit is then gently rolled from side to side to disperse the fluid evenly throughout the abdominal cavity. A syringe may be used to withdraw a sample, or fluid may be allowed to drip from the catheter hub. Only a small proportion of the total instilled fluid is expected to be retrievable by this method (Fox, 2011).

Sedation or anaesthesia may be employed as required. In the collapsed animal it may not be necessary or appropriate to use chemical restraint. Local anaesthetic infiltration of the sampling site may also be performed.

Samples may be evaluated in a number of ways:

- Gross examination for the visual appearance of blood or gut contents or olfactory evidence of urine or gut content
- Biochemical analyses, such as:
  - Dipstick tests (e.g. Multi-Stix, Bayer) for the presence of blood
  - pH measurement
  - Serum biochemistry analysis for the presence of urea
  - Refractometry to quantify specific gravity in undiluted samples more accurately
- Cytological examination is helpful in diagnosing gastrointestinal rupture, bladder rupture, exfoliative neoplasia, and inflammatory or infectious conditions
- Bacterial culture and sensitivity, including anaerobic culture, may be performed in cases of bacterial peritonitis.

Samples may then be defined as transudate, modified transudate or exudate. The presence of urea is strongly indicative of bladder rupture, and an acidic pH is indicative of stomach rupture.

Treatment of organ rupture/secondary bacterial and sterile chemical peritonitis
Gastrointestinal, urogenital or other administration of barium-based positive contrast medium is absolutely contraindicated in suspected cases of hollow organ rupture, as it may provoke a severe chemical peritonitis.

Exploratory laparotomy is performed as described to examine the extent of the lesion(s) visually. Fluid is removed by suction to allow

visualization of the abdomen systematically. Even if a lesion is detected, a full examination should be carried out, in case other lesions are present. If possible, the affected area is isolated to prevent further contamination.

Hollow organ ruptures should be closed at this point. This may be achieved via a simple closure (e.g. gastrointestinal tract, bladder). If the site is

▶

not sufficiently viable to allow this (e.g. necrotic gastrointestinal tract), resection (enterectomy) is appropriate. The prognosis in such a case is significantly worse than for a more recent breach of an internal organ, with a lower degree and/or duration of contamination, and less risk of repeated contamination due to organ wound breakdown.

Bladder wall rupture repair should involve debridement of any tissue of questionable viability, taking care to avoid damage to the ureters. The bladder is closed in a single or double layer (McGrotty and Doust, 2004).

In ruptures of internal abdominal abscesses or abscessated structures, e.g. ovaries, complete removal of the infected area and associated organ, where possible, is ideal.

Samples of any abdominal contamination are obtained and submitted for cytology and aerobic and anaerobic bacterial culture and sensitivity. Broad spectrum antibiosis (as discussed in Chapter 29) is initiated, ideally via the intravenous route, pending results.

Urine, even if sterile, provokes a chemical peritonitis, particularly in the rabbit, due to its high sediment content. Bile is also capable of provoking a severe inflammatory response.

Chronic abdominal discomfort and gastrointestinal stasis

Chronic continuous or intermittent abdominal pain or gastrointestinal stasis may indicate a number of pathological conditions such as neoplasia, internal abscessation, uterine pathology, or abdominal adhesion formation. Whilst many of these will be diagnosed on imaging modalities such as ultrasonography or radiography, a full visual examination of the abdomen may be required for definitive diagnosis by examination and biopsy as necessary, and treatment, if possible.

Investigation of urogenital tract haemorrhage

Urogenital tract haemorrhage, in either sex, may be associated with neoplasia, infection, or adhesion formation anywhere along the urinary (Figure 13.2) and genital tracts. In the entire doe, endometrial venous aneurysm is an additional

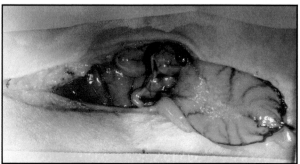

13.2 Mass adherent to bladder wall, causing persistent haematuria.

Any foreign, necrotic or fibrinous material is debrided and removed. The abdomen is thoroughly but gently lavaged with large volumes of warmed isotonic fluids (lactated Ringer's or isotonic saline, 200–300 ml/kg or sufficient to lavage until the fluid removed is clear, whichever is the greater).

Suture material used to close organs and the abdominal wall should be monofilament, to reduce the risk of bacterial infiltration in the fibres, and materials that provide support for a longer duration may be selected due to prolonged healing in peritonitis cases (e.g. polydioxanone II). Catgut is contraindicated due to its rapid degradation in the presence of inflammation (McGrotty and Doust, 2004).

Open peritoneal drainage (OPD) may also be employed. However, whilst the survival rates in domestic carnivores are similar (Staatz et al., 2002), animals undergoing OPD require much longer periods of hospitalization, and greater medical intervention, including blood transfusion and enteral feeding, and this author favours primary closure.

Heparin treatment via lavage fluid to reduce fibrin formation is controversial. It has been shown to improve survival in dogs with experimental peritonitis, but may lead to reduced tissue perfusion due to red cell aggregation.

differential. In the neutered doe, cervical or vaginal vestibular stump pathology may be present. In the male rabbit, prostatic pathology is a rare but reported condition. Abdominal and thoracic radiography, and abdominal ultrasound examination are indicated to assist in localizing the lesion and assessing organ architecture to complement and precede exploratory laparotomy. Contrast studies may be required, including excretory urography (see Chapter 3).

Investigation of ovarian remnant

Ovarian remnant syndrome may be noted in neutered female rabbits. The friability of the ovary and oviduct, especially in sexually immature rabbits, allows incomplete gonadectomy to occur (see Chapter 12). Ovarian tissue may also attach and revascularize to any intra-abdominal surface, effectively autotransplanting itself. In cases of suspected ovarian remnant, a full and complete examination of the abdominal cavity is required to ensure that all remnants are found and removed. An ovarian remnant may be suspected on history of hypersexuality and continuing oestrus behaviour in a neutered female rabbit, and confirmed on dynamic hormonal testing (progesterone–human chorionic gonadotropin stimulation test; Kellie et al., 2007; Varga, 2011; see also Chapter 20).

Adrenal gland disease

Adrenal gland disease has been reported in neutered male rabbits, and may potentially occur in neutered female rabbits and entire animals (see Chapter 20).

Organ biopsy

Exploratory laparotomy may be required for visual examination and biopsy of one or more organs within the abdominal cavity. The liver is the most commonly investigated organ (see Operative Technique 13.2), but the bladder, kidneys, pancreas, adrenal glands, gastrointestinal tract, visually abnormal intra-abdominal fat and any abdominal mass (abscess, neoplasia, etc.) may require exploration.

Myiasis

Myiasis, where there is entry or suspected entry into the abdominal cavity, is an indication for exploratory laparotomy to diagnose and treat any resultant peritonitis and foreign body reaction. Prior imaging may be helpful.

Retroperitoneal bleeding

Retroperitoneal bleeding is extremely uncommon given the low incidence of road traffic accidents involving domestic pet rabbits, but may be seen rarely, e.g. in conjunction with vertebral fracture.

Investigation of suspected adhesion formation

Adhesions may be suspected in cases of chronic continuous or intermittent gastrointestinal motility disorders, urine scalding or urinary incontinence, repeated urinary tract infections or episodic abdominal pain. Radiography and ultrasonography may be unrewarding and non-specific given the relatively small size of some adhesions, and the difficulty in differentiating them from solid masses in larger ones (Figure 13.3). Bladder or bowel malpositioning may be visible. Pockets of gas diffusely positioned through the gastrointestinal tract may be the only

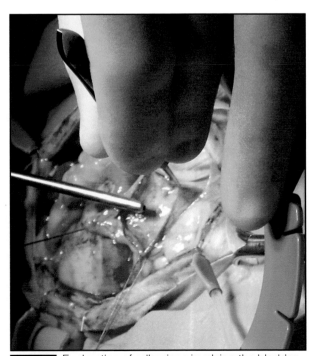

13.3 Exploration of adhesions involving the bladder. Note the use of suction to avoid abdominal contamination with urine.

signs on radiography. Where there has been urine leakage from the vaginal vestibulum, cystic fluid accumulations may be seen filling a space created by adhesions and fibrous tissue. Where adhesions have obstructed the ureters, ureteral dilatation proximal to the lesion, and hydronephrosis, may be seen (see Chapters 11 and 12).

Hernia and dehiscence repair

Revision surgery, following significant suture reaction, postoperative infection, partial or complete breakdown of the midline incision, eventration, herniation or dehiscence, is not an uncommon requirement in the rabbit. In the majority of cases the repair will be superficial only, but any suspicion of gut or other viscera herniation or entrapment, adhesion formation or peritonitis will necessitate an exploratory laparotomy.

Site and length of incision

Singular approaches

Whilst theoretically there are a number of approaches to the abdomen, in the vast majority of cases the ventral midline approach is favoured (see Figure 13.1 and Operative Technique 13.1). The main advantage of this approach is the excellent bilateral exposure to almost any area within the abdomen, depending on the length and position of incision, which may be easily extended as necessary either cranially to the xiphisternum and/or caudally to the pelvic symphysis. An incision through the linea alba is less painful postoperatively than incision through muscle, easier to repair, and produces less perioperative bruising and seroma formation.

The length and position of incision depends on the site of interest, with the approach to the liver or stomach only necessitating an approach from the umbilicus extending cranially to the xiphisternum, and the approach to the bladder or uterus from the umbilicus extending caudally or just cranial to the pelvic brim. These may need to be extended appropriately to view the remainder of the abdominal contents, or to gain better exposure, especially in deep-chested rabbits. It may be quicker and simpler in many cases to make a full-length incision at the outset, if this is anticipated to be necessary, although the shortest incision allowing adequate visualization is advised. Visual examination of the abdominal viscera, particularly the gastrointestinal tract, (with minimal handling and displacement) is preferable in the rabbit, and so a larger incision and less exteriorization of internal organs is advisable compared with the cat or dog.

The paramedian incision is less often used as it does not permit easy access to the contralateral side, and the muscle incision is more painful to make, more difficult to close, and has a greater incidence of complications. The key advantage in dogs, that it avoids dissection underneath the prepuce, is not a concern in the male rabbit due to the more caudally positioned penis. A flank approach is generally not employed, for the same reasons.

The paracostal approach, parallel and caudal to the last rib, is rarely employed in the rabbit. Gastropexy, although often required in domestic carnivores, is rarely performed in the rabbit, and more complete access to the stomach and gastrointestinal tract is required in this species.

Gridiron dissection is generally recommended for incisions through muscle layers, to avoid trauma through muscle fibres. However, this limits the possible size of the incision, making it generally impractical (Anderson, 2005).

Combined approaches

A combined approach is rarely required. A combined ventral midline and paracostal approach may be employed for improved access to deeper liver lobe lesions, but is more painful, with a greater incidence of postoperative wound complications.

Organ handling

The organs, particularly the gastrointestinal tract, should be handled as little and as gently as possible. Where possible the gastrointestinal tract should be examined for lesions *in situ*, avoiding unnecessary organ handling due to the risks of temperature loss, adhesion formation and ileus (see Chapter 11). However, when fully examining the gastrointestinal tract, it will be necessary to remove it from the abdomen, in which case it should be kept warm and moistened whilst exteriorized (Figure 13.4). It should be replaced so as to avoid undue folding of gas-filled sections, especially the caecum, to avoid causing pain and inhibiting the passage of gas and ingesta.

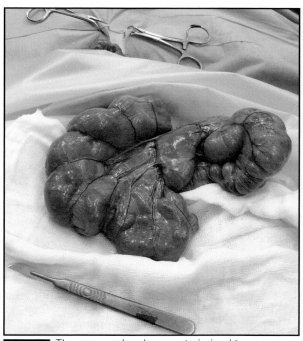

13.4 The caecum has been exteriorized to investigate chronic distension and avoid contamination of the abdomen, but must be kept warm and moist and re-placed carefully.

Potential problems and how to avoid them

Adhesion formation

Adhesion formation (see also Chapter 11) is the main potential postoperative complication of any laparotomy (Ray *et al.*, 1998). Rabbits are extremely prone to adhesion formation, and are used as a laboratory model (McDonald *et al.*, 1988). Adhesions may develop in response to any source of trauma, irritation or inflammation of any tissue (in this case, within the abdomen). The peritoneum, bladder, uterus or uterine stump, and intestines are the most common sites of adhesion formation. Both laparotomy and laparoscopy result in a similar incidence of adhesions, where the surgical procedure is otherwise the same (Becker and Stucchi, 2004).

Initiating causes are primarily associated with handling and exposure of tissues. Minor abrasions to the serosal or subserosal surfaces of any internal organ result in fibrin deposition, potentially allowing two areas of tissue to become adherent. This process starts within hours of the original insult.

Risk factors for adhesion formation
- Any handling of tissue that causes even the most minor trauma (e.g. use of rat-toothed forceps on tissues, the use of dry swabs to clean a surface of blood causing minor abrasions, the use of dry gloved hands).
- Excessive dryness of tissues (e.g. drying out under hot operating lights), or thermal damage from cautery or electrosurgery equipment.
- Chemical irritants (e.g. powder from gloves, excessive suture material remnants, or urine contamination of the abdomen).
- The presence of infection.
- Any devitalized or necrotic tissue or exposed serosal surfaces (e.g. the cervical stump/ vaginal vestibulum following ovariohysterectomy).

Surgery is not the only potential cause of adhesions. Any abdominal contamination (e.g. following bladder or intestinal content leakage, or intra-abdominal abscessation rupture) may lead to adhesion formation and should be rapidly addressed by exploratory laparotomy, closure of the organ, and thorough lavage of the abdomen (Figure 13.5).

Progression to permanent adhesions is not inevitable, but is more likely if tissues are compromised by drying and/or poor handling. Collagen is laid down in the fibrinous adhesions to produce fibrous adhesions, which may remain clinically silent or may cause chronic health issues. Depending on the organ systems involved, adhesions may cause problems in gut motility by preventing the free movement of gut within the abdomen, or constricting it to the point where gut content cannot pass freely (Figure 13.6).

Adhesions may affect bladder position or mobility, constrict bladder emptying, or may partially or completely obstruct the ureters to cause proximal

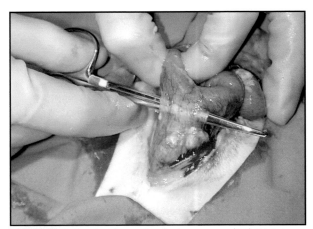

13.5 Adhesion formation between cervical stump and gastrointestinal tract. (Courtesy of Ron Rees Davies)

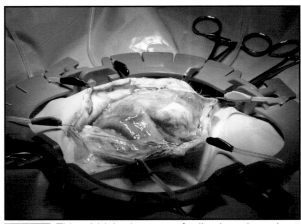

13.6 This rabbit had a mass of adhesions throughout the abdomen, involving the gastrointestinal tract and urogenital tract in particular.

ureteral dilatation and hydronephrosis. They may simply cause discomfort and pain within the abdomen, affecting the animal's demeanour, appetite, activity levels, behaviour and mobility. Pain may be due to prevention of free movement of intestinal content or urine, or caused by applying tension to sensitive structures, by entrapment of nerves, or by innervation with substance P-containing sensory neurons (Sulaiman *et al.*, 2001).

Treatment of adhesions is complex (see Chapter 11). Many rabbits may die without the benefit of the exploratory laparotomy required to diagnose and treat them. If they are identified, they may be too severe to attempt resection, as it is not possible in many cases to differentiate the margins of adhesion and normal tissue, and the blood supply, to the gastrointestinal tract in particular, may be compromised. Even if it is possible to remove adhesions cleanly and separate adhered tissues, the chance of recurrence is high. The remnants of adhesions may themselves form the basis on which further adhesions form (Fevang *et al.*, 2004).

The key to adhesion management is prevention, using the least abrasive swab material possible,

handling tissues carefully and no more than necessary, not exposing tissue to extremes of heat or cold, not allowing them to become desiccated, and not exposing them to chemical irritants such as hypertonic solutions, oil-based therapeutic agents or powder from gloves. Suture material used should be monofilament and unlikely to provoke tissue reaction (e.g. polydioxanone) rather than braided material with a greater surface area and a texture which, when pulled through tissue, causes microscopic trauma.

Catgut is particularly to be avoided, as it is broken down by phagocytosis, which is less reliable in the rabbit, and therefore it may persist for longer than hydrolysed materials. Pre-wetting surgical swabs and gloved hands, using normal saline or Hartman's solution at body temperature, to increase lubrication on handling tissues and avoid microtraumatic abrasion, is advised.

Closing the peritoneum is controversial in terms of adhesion formation, with some studies showing that it reduces adhesion development, and some showing that it increases it. The most recent work in rabbit models favours closure of the peritoneum under laparotomy incisions.

Inadvertent viscus penetration

The caecum lies directly dorsal to the peritoneum, and may be variably distended with gas, especially in the rabbit with gastrointestinal stasis. The stomach may also be hugely distended with gas in cases of outflow obstruction. Inadvertent penetration of either structure, or of a distended urine-filled bladder, is a potential complication, best avoided by the approach detailed below. Penetration of internal abscesses is also possible when dissecting them free. In re-operations, extreme care is necessary because the underlying gastrointestinal tract may be adherent to the parietal peritoneum, and it is even more likely that it may be inadvertently penetrated. In these cases, the peritoneum should be opened at a fresh point, preferably by extending the incision appropriately at either end.

Should the viscera be perforated, they should be packed off with moistened swabs or laparotomy packs, the lesion closed, and the abdomen lavaged gently with physiological saline (0.9%) or Hartmann's solution until no trace of contamination is seen. Appropriate antibiosis should start immediately, and should cover aerobic and anaerobic organisms. This author favours a combination of enrofloxacin (20 mg/kg q24h) with metronidazole (15 mg/kg q12h). A sample of contaminant should be submitted for aerobic and anaerobic bacterial culture and sensitivity testing against selected antibiotics.

Wound infection

Superficial wound infection may occur in rabbit exploratory laparotomy incisions, usually due to wound interference. This is best prevented by gentle surgical site preparation, atraumatic tissue edge handling, and avoiding toothed forceps where at all possible. Wound closure should be done carefully, apposing edges correctly, with no tension on wounds, and using the minimum quantity of minimally reactive suture material, on the finest, least traumatic swaged-on needles (see Chapter 11). Preoperative local anaesthetic infiltration may help minimize wound interference.

Seroma development may occur, providing a focus for interference and postoperative infection. It is prevented by good surgical technique, particularly haemostasis and avoidance of dead space. In most cases, this fluid is absorbed over time, but drainage may be necessary in some cases. It is important to distinguish between seroma formation and abdominal incision breakdown and herniation; careful palpation, ultrasonographic examination and exploratory surgery may be necessary where there is uncertainty.

External dressings are rarely required, but may be applied if necessary, particularly if drains are present. Rabbits are perfectly capable of removing dressings, and continuous observation, stockinette or other body bandages and Elizabethan collars may all be necessary in extreme cases, though collars are ideally avoided due to the stress they cause the rabbit, as well as making it difficult to drink water, eat food and prehend caecotrophs (see Chapter 11).

Ileus

Ileus is a common complication postoperatively. It may be secondary to inappetence due to perioperative pain, or primarily due to gut interference. Avoidance centres on excellent perioperative pain relief and minimal gut interference (see Chapter 2). Gut handling should only take place where necessary (e.g. foreign body removal or on moving aside to gain access to other structures). Handling should be gentle, using wetted gloved hands and atraumatic forceps where necessary. The gut should not be allowed to dry out or cool down, and should be covered with warm moistened swabs whenever it is exposed longer than momentarily (Figure 13.7).

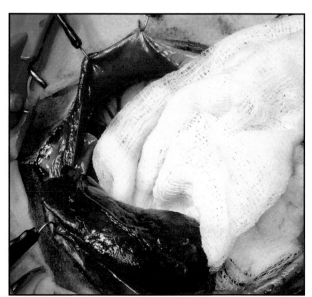

13.7 The abdominal viscera are covered in warm moist swabs when exposed during surgery.

Prophylactic use of gastrointestinal motility enhancers should be considered in any case of prolonged gut exposure or more than minimal handling. Cisapride, domperidone, ranitidine and metoclopramide have all been used. Lidocaine is used perioperatively in horses undergoing colic surgery (Nieto *et al.*, 2000) but is less well described in the rabbit (Taniguchi *et al.*, 2000).

Peritonitis/abscessation

Internal infection may result from the inadvertent penetration of non-sterile viscera, e.g. gut or abscess (although even sterile urine may provoke a chemical peritonitis). This may become walled off as an abscess (Figure 13.8) or generalized as peritonitis. Extreme care in entering the abdomen helps avoid this where the gut is closely underlying the linea alba. Surgical suction is helpful in emptying liquid content. When removing the uterus, the rabbit should not have its bladder compressed to empty it when positioned in dorsal recumbency, as this will reflux urine into the vaginal vestibulum, increasing the risk of leakage into the abdomen. With thick-walled cervical stumps, oversewing may be advisable to create a watertight seal and also reduce the risk of adhesions. Omentalization is not easily possible in the rabbit due to the minimal nature of the omentum. Suture patterns should be chosen to avoid leakage of material into the abdomen (see Chapter 11).

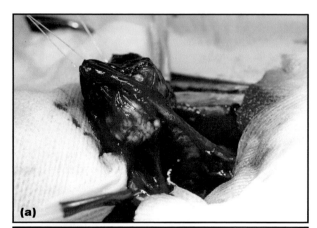

(a)

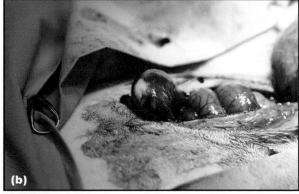

(b)

13.8 **(a)** This abscess followed scrotal castration and postoperative infection. On a thorough examination of the abdominal cavity, further abscesses were found **(b)**, but not generalized peritonitis.

Abdominal wall dehiscence and delayed abdominal herniation

Potential causes of abdominal wall dehiscence and delayed abdominal herniation are summarized in Figure 13.9.

Cause of failure	Examples
Technical error	Suture pull out due to incorrect placement Suture pull through (especially muscle sutures in flank incisions) Poor knot security Incomplete closure (especially at either end of a ventral midline incision) Fat trapped between sutured edges Inappropriate suture material Introduction of infection
Concurrent therapy	Corticosteroids
Concurrent disease	Cachexia/hypoalbuminaemia Obesity
Postoperative management	Failure to restrict activity Failure to prevent interference with sutures Postoperative pain resulting in abdominal tensing

13.9 Potential causes of abdominal wall dehiscence and delayed abdominal herniation.

The weight of viscera in the rabbit is proportionately greater than that in the dog or cat. Particularly with larger ventral midline incisions, this may lead to a greater strain on the suture line. Suture material may need to be slightly thicker than that for an equally sized carnivore, although excessive foreign material may provoke a reaction. Idiosyncratic reactions to suture material are not infrequent, resulting in abdominal muscle wound breakdown. Wound interference and excessive exercise, e.g. running up stairs in the house or double-decker hutch, should be avoided for about 7 days. Continuous sutures are quicker to place, but excellent knot security is vital to avoid dehiscence along the entire suture line. Extension of the linea alba incision below the skin edges, and subsequent incomplete closure at either end, should be avoided.

Heat loss

Heat loss occurs more rapidly on opening the abdominal cavity, and even more rapidly still if organs are exteriorized due to increased radiant and evaporative heat loss. Supplementary heating and covering exposed viscera help to avoid this (see Chapter 11).

References and further reading

Ahmad G, Duffy JMN, Farquhar C *et al.* (2008) Barrier agents for adhesion prevention after gynaecological surgery. *Cochrane Database of Systematic Reviews 2008*, Issue 2. Art. No.: CD000475. DOI: 10.1002/14651858.CD000475.pub2
Anderson DM (2005) The body wall. In: *The BSAVA Manual of Canine and Feline Abdominal Surgery*, ed. J Williams and J Niles, pp. 37–51. BSAVA Publications, Gloucester
Becker JM and Stucchi AF (2004) Intra-abdominal adhesion prevention: are we getting any closer? *Annals of Surgery* **240**, 202–204
Bourne D (2011a) Laparotomy in rabbits (Disease investigation and management. Treatment and care). [available at http://wildpro.twycrosszoo.org]
Bourne D (2011b) Liver biopsy in rabbits (Disease investigation and management. Treatment and care). [available at http://wildpro.twycrosszoo.org]
Browning A (2005) Diagnosis and management of peritonitis in horses. *In Practice* **27**, 70–75
De Iaco PA, Muzzupapa G, Bigon E *et al.* (2001) Efficacy of a hyaluronan derivative gel in postsurgical adhesion prevention in the presence of inadequate hemostasis. *Surgery* **130**, 60–64
Fevang B-TS, Fevang J, Lie SA *et al.* (2004) Long-term prognosis after operation for adhesive small bowel obstruction. *Annals of Surgery* **240**, 193–201
Fox N (2011) Abdominocentesis and diagnostic peritoneal lavage in rabbits (Disease investigation and management. Treatment and care). [available at http://wildpro.twycrosszoo.org]
Hailer NP, Blaheta RA, Harder S *et al.* (1994) Modulation of adhesion molecule expression on endothelial cells by verapamil and other Ca++ channel blockers. *Immunobiology* **191**, 38–51
Harcourt-Brown FM (2002) General surgical procedures and neutering. In: *Textbook of Rabbit Medicine*, pp. 352–360. Butterworth-Heinemann, Oxford
Harcourt-Brown FM and Harcourt-Brown SF (2012) Clinical value of blood glucose measurement in pet rabbits. *Veterinary Record* **170**, 674
Hellebrekers BW, Trimbos-Kemper TC, Trimbos JB, Emeis JJ and Kooistra T (2000) Use of fibrinolytic agents in the prevention of postoperative adhesion formation. *Fertility and Sterility* **74**, 203–212
Joysey J (1955) A study of the blood groups of the rabbit, with reference to the inheritance of three antigens and the agglutinability of the red cells carrying them. *Journal of Experimental Biology* **32**, 440–450
Kellie A, Fecteau BJ, Deeb JM *et al.* (2007) Diagnostic endocrinology: blood steroid concentrations in neutered male and female rabbits. *Journal of Exotic Pet Medicine* **16**(4), 256–259
Lichtenberger M (2004a) Transfusion medicine in exotic pets. *Clinical Techniques in Small Animal Practice* **19**, 88–95
Lichtenberger M (2004b) Principles of shock and fluid therapy in special species. *Seminars in Avian and Exotic Pet Medicine* **13**, 142–153
McDonald MN, Elkins TE, Wortham GF *et al.* (1988) Adhesion formation and prevention after peritoneal injury and repair in the rabbit. *Journal of Reproductive Medicine* **33**, 436–439
McGrotty Y and Doust R (2004) Management of peritonitis in dogs and cats. *In Practice* **26**, 358–367
Meredith A and Rayment L (2000) Liver disease in rabbits. *Seminars in Avian and Exotic Pet Medicine* **9**, 146–152
Nieto JE, Rakestraw PC, Snyder JR and Vatistas NJ (2000) In vitro effects of erythromycin, lidocaine, and metoclopramide on smooth muscle from the pyloric antrum, proximal portion of the duodenum, and middle portion of the jejunum of horses. *American Journal of Veterinary Research* **61**, 413–419
Niles J (2005) The liver and biliary tract. In: *BSAVA Manual of Canine and Feline Abdominal Surgery*, ed. J Williams and J Niles, pp. 168–194. BSAVA Publications, Gloucester
Platt S and Garosi L (2012) *Small Animal Neurological Emergencies*, p. 588. Manson, UK
Ray NF, Denton WG, Thamer M *et al.* (1998) Abdominal adhesiolysis: inpatient care and expenditures in the United States in 1994. *Journal of the American College of Surgery* **186**, 1–9
Redrobe S (2002) Soft tissue surgery of rabbits and rodents. *Seminars in Avian and Exotic Pet Medicine* **11**, 231–245
Saunders RA, Redrobe S, Barr F, Hotston Moore A and Elliott SC (2009) Liver lobe torsion in rabbits. *Journal of Small Animal Practice* **50**(10), 562
Silva R, Moore EE, Bar-Or D, Galloway WB and Wright ED (1984) The risk:benefit of autotransfusion – comparison to banked blood in a canine model. *Journal of Trauma* **24**(7), 557–564
Staatz AJ, Monnet E and Seim HB III (2002) Open peritoneal drainage versus primary closure for the treatment of septic peritonitis in dogs and cats: 42 cases (1993–1999). *Veterinary Surgery* **31**, 174–180
Steinleitner A, Lambert H, Kazensky C, Sanchez I and Sueldo C (1990) Reduction of primary postoperative adhesion formation under calcium channel blockade in the rabbit. *Journal of Surgical Research* **48**, 42–45
Steinleitner A, Lambert H, Montoro L *et al.* (1988) The use of calcium channel blockade for the prevention of postoperative adhesion formation. *Fertility and Sterility* **50**, 818–821
Sulaiman H, Gabella G, Davis MSC *et al.* (2001) Presence and distribution of sensory nerve fibers in human peritoneal adhesions. *Annals of Surgery* **234**, 256–261
Taniguchi T, Shibata K, Yamamoto K, Mizukoshi Y and Kobayashi T (2000) Effects of lidocaine administration on hemodynamics and cytokine responses to endotoxaemia in rabbits. *Critical Care Medicine* **28**, 755–759
Varga M (2011) Hypersexuality in a castrated rabbit (*Oryctolagus cuniculus*). *Companion Animal* **16**, 48–51
Wenger S, Barrett EL, Pearson GR *et al.* (2009) Liver lobe torsion in three adult rabbits. *Journal of Small Animal Practice* **50**, 301–305
Whitfield RR, Stills HF, Huls HR, Crouch JM and Hurd WW (2007) Effects of peritoneal closure and suture material on adhesion formation in a rabbit model. *American Journal of Obstetrics and Gynecology*, **197**, 644.e1–644.e5

OPERATIVE TECHNIQUE 13.1:
Exploratory laparotomy (coeliotomy) utilizing a ventral midline incision

Indications

Visual examination of abdominal cavity and organs within it in order to perform procedures such as biopsy, mass removal, adhesion investigation, exploration for gastrointestinal foreign body or other obstruction, and investigation for ovarian remnant or retained testis. It is the standard approach to the liver, urinary tract, female reproductive tract and other structures (Bourne, 2011a).

Positioning and preparation

The rabbit should be positioned in dorsal recumbency, in a 10–15 degree reverse-Trendelenburg position, allowing the liver and stomach to fall slightly away from the diaphragm and aid ventilation, but not so much that viscera exit the incision under their own weight. Positioning aids may be used, but must not prevent intraoperative warming equipment from being effective.

The largest possible incision should be prepared for. The fur should be clipped carefully and the skin aseptically prepared, from halfway up the costal arch to just caudal to the pelvic brim, and from just lateral to the nipples. Clipping and skin preparation should be as gentle and atraumatic as possible, to reduce skin tearing and irritation which could encourage wound interference after surgery.

The patient is draped and a right-handed surgeon is typically positioned on the rabbit's right side.

Equipment extras

The careful and gentle use of retractors can significantly improve exposure to the abdomen, especially to deeper abdominal organs, and can reduce the need for manual handling of the abdominal skin and muscle edges and internal organs. The Lone Star or Ring retractor system (Veterinary Instrumentation) are particularly useful in this regard, and tension and position of the retaining hooks can be varied as needed.

Assistant

An assistant may be helpful, especially to the less experienced surgeon, in retracting, positioning and ligating structures, and in operating suction equipment. Unnecessary handling of the viscera is to be avoided, however (see Chapter 11).

Surgical technique

A standard ventral midline incision is made, from the xiphisternum to the umbilicus or as far caudally as the pelvic symphysis, as required, through the skin, subcutis and linea alba.

The skin is extremely fine on the ventral abdomen, and there is often little or no subcutaneous fat present, necessitating a careful incision to expose the linea alba, which should then be carefully lifted with fine-toothed forceps to tent it away from the abdominal viscera. Metzenbaum scissors or an upturned No. 15 scalpel blade may be used to make a small incision in the linea alba.

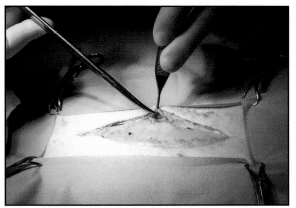
The linea alba is tented away from the viscera and carefully incised.

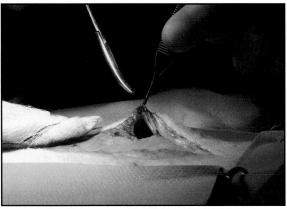
The incision is carefully extended with Metzenbaum scissors.

OPERATIVE TECHNIQUE 13.1 continued:
Exploratory laparotomy (coeliotomy) utilizing a ventral midline incision

At this point the release of the partial vacuum inside the abdomen usually allows the caecum to fall dorsally, but for added safety once an incision is made, forceps or a finger may be placed through the incision, parallel to the linea alba, lifting it away from and protecting the viscera, before extending the incision with scissors. The incision is continued cranially (pictured) and caudally as required.

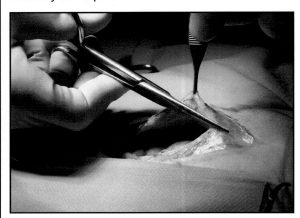

Any exposed viscera, particularly the gastro-intestinal tract, should be covered with surgical swabs soaked in warmed physiological saline (0.9%) or Hartmann's solution.

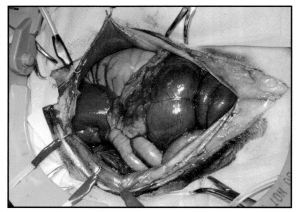

Whilst present in the rabbit, the falciform ligament does not generally obscure access to the abdomen, as it does in the carnivore, but it may be ligated and transected if necessary, to gain better access to the cranial abdomen.

Closure
For most rabbits 1 metric (4/0 USP) monofilament absorbable suture material is preferred for the linea alba closure, e.g. poliglecaprone 25 (e.g. Monocryl), glycolide/dioxanone/trimethylene carbonate (e.g. Biosyn), polyglytone 6211 (e.g. Caprosyn) or poly-dioxanone (e.g. PDS II). Larger sizes (2 metric, 3/0 USP) may be used for larger rabbits.

Continuous patterns may be used to minimize surgical time and the amount of suture material present. However, the risks of wound breakdown are greater and the potential consequences more severe, so single interrupted patterns may be preferred.

This incision was made from just below the xiphisternum to midway between the umbilicus and the pubis, and is sufficient for most abdominal surgery. The Lone Star retractor is used to further improve access and visibility. However, smaller incisions are advised, where possible, to minimize surgical time, adhesion risk and postoperative pain, and to minimize the risks and severity of wound breakdown subsequently.

OPERATIVE TECHNIQUE 13.2:
Liver biopsy and lobectomy

Indications

Liver biopsy is indicated for diagnosis and assessment of pathological abnormalities of the liver, e.g. neoplasia, hepatitis, vacuolar hepatopathy/lipidosis, as well as assessing the response to treatment or analyzing liver toxins (Meredith and Rayment, 2000). Liver lobectomy is indicated for lesions localized to one lobe (e.g. neoplasia, abscess, torsion) as a diagnostic and therapeutic procedure (Niles, 2005; Bourne, 2011b).

Patient preparation

Prior to performing a liver biopsy in a rabbit with suspected liver function compromise, blood clotting parameters and liver damage and function testing (serum biochemistry to include aspartate aminotransaminase, alanine aminotransferase, alkaline phosphatase, gamma-glutamyl transpeptidase, glucose dehydrogenase, bile acids, total protein, urea, albumin and globulin) should be carried out. Prophylactic antibiosis effective against aerobes and anaerobes is recommended prior to liver surgery (e.g. enrofloxacin and metronidazole).

After a standard ventral midline incision, as detailed above, from xiphisternum to umbilicus or further caudally as required, the liver should be approached carefully, gently reflecting the mesentery, omentum and stomach as necessary. The whole liver should be inspected. Note that accessory liver tissue may be positioned dorsally, some distance caudal to the main body of the liver, and apparently separated from it.

The area of interest in the liver should be identified and isolated. Where diffuse liver disease is present, the most accessible marginal area should be sampled from.

Biopsy punch

This is a useful technique for small samples, and is the most appropriate where multiple samples are required, e.g. in diffuse liver disease. An unused skin biopsy punch is applied to the required area(s) of liver. The punch is rotated in one direction until the metal end is completely within liver tissue. The punch is removed from the liver, with the specimen either remaining in place in the liver, or within the punch. If retained in the liver, it is detached using a No. 11 scalpel blade. If in the punch it may be removed carefully with forceps or a needle, avoiding tissue damage. Bleeding is usually minimal, and the application of foreign haemostatic material is to be avoided where possible.

Guillotine suture biopsy

This is a useful technique for peripheral lesions or samples. A loop is made in a piece of absorbable suture material. The first throw of a square knot is made and a peripheral piece of liver pulled through the loop. The loop is carefully tightened, crushing the liver tissue and ligating blood vessels.

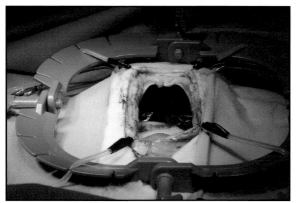

A Lone Star retractor used to improve exposure in a cranial laparotomy incision, giving good access to all but the deeper organs. Extension of the incision caudally would improve exposure further, but in deep-chested breeds, access to the dorsal viscera can be challenging.

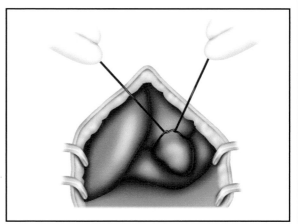

A loop of absorbable suture material is placed around the tip of a liver lobe.

OPERATIVE TECHNIQUE 13.2 continued:
Liver biopsy and lobectomy

Avoid excessive tightness, as this will 'cheesewire' through the blood vessels as well. The remaining throws are placed on the knot. The piece of liver is removed by sharp dissection or electrosurgery. (Note that with small samples, radio- or electrosurgery creates a proportionally larger area of thermally damaged tissue, rendering the sample less useful.) Bleeding is usually minimal, and the application of foreign haemostatic material is to be avoided where possible.

A suture packet may be placed below the sample, to provide a flat firm surface to cut down on to with a scalpel. The packet and sample may then be handed to an assistant for fresh frozen or formalin-preserved histopathology, avoiding the need to handle and damage the sample with forceps.

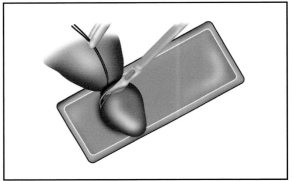

The suture is tied tightly and an empty suture packet is placed below the tip of the liver to act as a 'cutting board'. The hepatic tissue is cut approximately 5 mm from the ligature.

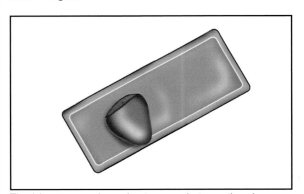

The biopsy sample and suture packet can then be handed to a non-sterile assistant to be frozen or put into formalin.

Excisional wedge biopsy: overlapping guillotine sutures

A row of slightly overlapping interrupted mattress sutures is placed through the full thickness of the liver parenchyma in a 'V', extending from the edge into the lobe, or taking a semicircular 'bite' from the edge. These should be tight enough, as above, to achieve haemostasis but not cut completely through the liver tissue. It is important to ensure they travel the full thickness through the liver parenchyma. The wedge of liver created by the sutures can be removed by sharp dissection or electrosurgery. (Note that with small samples, radio- or electrosurgery creates a proportionally larger area of thermally damaged tissue, rendering the sample less useful.) Bleeding is usually minimal, and the application of foreign haemostatic material is to be avoided where possible.

Lobectomy

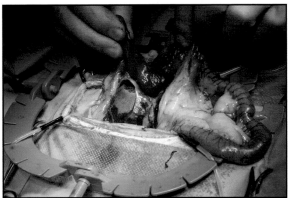

A diseased liver lobe (in this case an accessory lobe) is identified and exteriorized.

Partial lobectomy may be carried out by the two methods described above. In addition, the distal part of a liver lobe may be removed by incising superficially through the parenchyma just proximal to the demarcation between healthy and unhealthy tissue, and then bluntly fracturing the liver using fingers. As parenchymal vessels are exposed, they may be ligated or closed using radiosurgery or pressure/energy sealing systems.

Total lobectomy methods depend on the thickness of the attachment of the lobe to the liver.

OPERATIVE TECHNIQUE 13.2 continued:
Liver biopsy and lobectomy

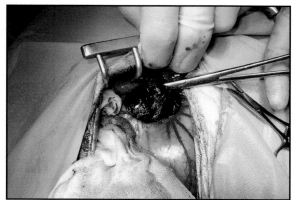

The required section (in this case an entire diseased lobe) is isolated with haemostats. Note the retractors used to improve access in this deep-chested breed.

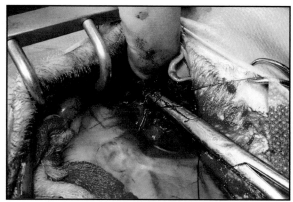

A suture is preplaced through the parenchyma and over the haemostats after removal of the tissue.

Surgical stapling devices of appropriate size may be used to crush and ligate the lobe at its base. Pressure/energy sealing systems (e.g. LigaSure) may be used, achieving haemostasis and tissue sealing in one. Extreme care should be taken when ligating the stalk of a liver lobe, as the vessels may be broad and short. Double ligation or stapling is advised. The removal of a torsed liver is usually more straightforward, as this tends to occur in lobes with a narrow attachment. These may be ligated with preplaced sutures before transecting, or isolated with haemostats as pictured below.

Postoperative care

Following surgery, it is suggested that the rabbit is placed in sternal recumbency to allow the liver's own weight to compress the biopsy site against the body wall and reduce haemorrhage.

The rabbit should be monitored for signs of haemorrhage (mucous membrane colour, pulse, capillary refill time, with PCV and blood pressure monitoring if there is cause for concern) for 24–48 hours, whichever technique has been used.

14

Gastric dilation and intestinal obstruction

Frances Harcourt-Brown

Gastric dilation is a common clinical syndrome in rabbits (Harcourt-Brown, 2007) and is often confused with ileus, gastrointestinal hypomotility or gut stasis. Some of the confusion originates in the terminology used, so the terms used in this chapter are defined in Figure 14.1. There is overlap between many of the conditions. Some authors use the term rabbit gastrointestinal syndrome (RGIS) to encompass them all (Lichtenberger and Lennox, 2010).

In order to understand and diagnose the clinical syndromes that can cause gastric dilation, knowledge of the anatomy and physiology of the rabbit's digestive system is required.

Anatomy and physiology of the gastrointestinal tract

Anatomy
The stomach of rabbits is a large, distensible organ that comprises about 15% of the volume of the gastrointestinal tract. The gastric fluid is very acidic. Saliva is continuously produced and swallowed, and water is secreted into the stomach so that the contents have a liquid consistency that varies with the time and texture of the last meal. The cardiac and pyloric sphincters are well developed and the stomach is never empty, even if the rabbit has not eaten for several days. The duodenum starts with a slight enlargement, approximately 1 cm from the pylorus, before the diameter suddenly narrows (Harcourt-Brown, 2001). After this point, the diameter of the small intestine remains the same until, at the distal end, the ileum opens into a spherical thick-walled enlargement known as the sacculus rotundus, which forms a T-junction between the ileum, caecum and colon. At the entrance to the sacculus rotundus is the ileocolic valve, which is another point at which the diameter of the small intestine narrows.

The caecum is a large, thin-walled organ, which forms a coiled spiral. It has mesenteric attachments with parts of the ileum and the colon, which follow its spiral pattern to form an ileocaecocolic complex (Figure 14.2) that occupies most of the caudoventral abdomen. The caecum has three sections:

- The bulbous ampulla caecalis coli from which the colon emerges
- The body of the caecum
- A finger-like appendix which forms the terminal portion of the caecum.

Term	Definition
Bloat	Abdominal distension due to gastric or caecal tympany
Dysautonomia	Dysfunction of the autonomic nervous system. In rabbits, dysautonomia is a cause of mucoid enteropathy, which is a syndrome that results in slow hindgut motility. The caecum fails to expel its contents, which become impacted and dry. The colon fills with mucus. Gastric dilation occurs in the later stages
Gastric or intestinal dilation	Distension of the stomach or intestines beyond their normal dimensions
Gastrointestinal hypomotility	Reduced peristalsis and diminution of flow of ingesta through the digestive tract triggered by adrenergic stimulation from a painful or stressful incident
Gut stasis	Cessation of flow of ingesta through the digestive tract due to gastrointestinal hypomotility
Ileus	Failure of peristalsis, which can be adynamic (i.e. gastrointestinal hypomotility and gut stasis), mechanical (caused by intestinal obstruction) or paralytic
Intestinal obstruction	Occlusion of the intestine by a foreign body or stricture
Paralytic ileus	Loss of all intestinal tone and motility as a result of reflex inhibition in acute peritonitis, from excessive handling during bowel surgery or prolonged or severe distension due to intestinal obstruction or dysautonomia
Rabbit gastrointestinal syndrome (RGIS)	A complex group of gastrointestinal signs, symptoms and pathological conditions. It includes gastric and intestinal impaction, gas accumulation, and obstruction (Lichtenberger and Lennox, 2010)
Trichobezoar	A ball of felted hair that is found in the digestive tract. In rabbits, trichobezoars can take one of two forms: 1. A satsuma-sized ball of stomach contents and fur found in the pylorus in rabbits with gut stasis 2. A small hard pellet composed of dry, compacted, felted hair that can cause an intestinal obstruction
Tympany	Distension of an organ (stomach, intestines, caecum) with gas

14.1 Definitions of terms.

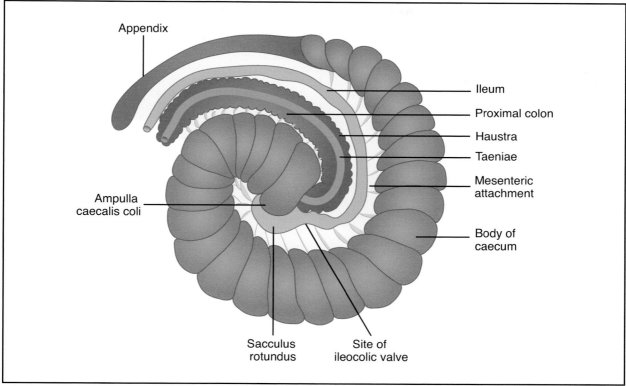

14.2 The ileocaecolic complex is a coiled spiral that contains the caecum, the proximal colon and the terminal ileum, which are attached to each other. It occupies most of the caudoventral abdomen.

The ampulla caecalis coli opens into the ascending colon, which has four anatomically distinct sections:

- A section with three bands of taeniae separating rows of haustra or sacculations
- A section with a single taenia and fewer, smaller haustra
- The fusus coli, a muscular area about 4 cm long
- A section that is histologically indistinguishable from the transverse and descending colon.

The fusus coli forms a natural division between two morphologically and functionally distinct sections of the colon. For this reason, the terms 'proximal' and 'distal' colon are often used, with the fusus coli as the dividing point. The diameter of the colon narrows at the entrance to the fusus coli.

Digestive physiology

The digestion and absorption of nutrients from the stomach and small intestine is similar to that in other animals, but digestion in the hindgut is different from other species, even other hindgut fermenters. Undigested food (i.e. mainly fibre) passes from the small intestine into the ampulla caecalis coli and the proximal colon where it is mixed and separated into small and large particles, which are simultaneously sent in opposite directions. The large particles are moved distally and compressed, to be expelled in hard faecal pellets. This occurs during the 'hard faeces phase' of digestion (Figure 14.3). During this phase, fluid and the small fibre particles are moved

proximally into the caecum to be degraded by the caecal microflora into nutrients such as amino acids, volatile fatty acids and vitamins. The caecum gently contracts rhythmically to mix in nutrients and fluid that enter from the ampulla caecalis coli. Periodically, the caecum and proximal colon stop moving and the caecum expels its contents into the colon to be passed through the anus as caecotrophs, which are immediately ingested by the rabbit as an additional source of nutrients. This is the 'soft faeces phase' of digestion (Figure 14.4).

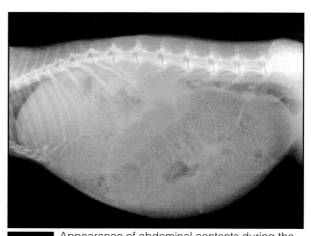

14.3 Appearance of abdominal contents during the hard faeces phase of digestion. The lateral view of the abdomen was taken at about 9 am, after the rabbit had been eating hay. The stomach and ileocaecocolic complex are full of full of ingesta, which is mottled due to its fibre content.

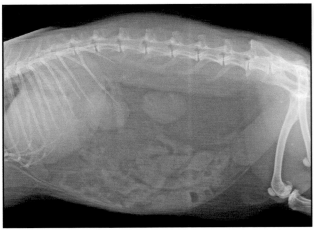

14.4 Appearance of abdominal contents during the soft faeces phase of digestion. This lateral view of the abdomen of a healthy rabbit with a normal appetite was taken in the late morning when the rabbit had been resting for a few hours. It shows a small stomach and ileocaecocolic complex containing ingesta with a homogenous appearance because it is composed of small particles. Some pockets of gas are visible. Soft faeces can be seen in the rectum. Other abdominal organs, such as the kidneys, can easily be identified because the abdomen is empty.

Predisposition to gastric dilation

In rabbits, the stomach often contains caecotrophs as well as ingested food. Caecotrophs are composed of the contents of the caecum that have been ingested from the anus and are rich in bacteria, many of which are gas producing. The cardiac sphincter is strong and effectively seals the cardia, which prevents stomach contents, including gas, from entering the oesophagus. Rabbits cannot vomit or burp. The only route for food and gas to leave the stomach is through the pylorus into the small intestine. If this exit route is obstructed, the stomach cannot empty and becomes increasingly filled with gas and fluid (Figure 14.5). It becomes dilated and eventually tympanitic (Figures 14.6 and 14.7). If the obstruction to the exit is not relieved in some way, the stomach, or intestine can eventually rupture and release ingesta into the abdominal cavity so the rabbit develops peritonitis and dies (Figures 14.8 and 14.9). All rabbits with an intestinal obstruction develop gastric dilation, but not all rabbits with a gastric dilation have an intestinal obstruction (see later).

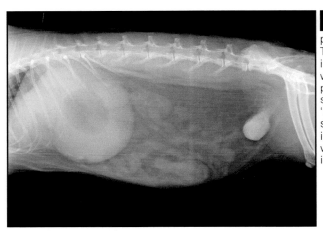

14.5 Gastric dilation. This lateral radiographic view of the abdomen shows a dilated stomach that was palpable behind the ribs on the left side of the abdomen. The stomach extends well beyond the costal arch and is just in contact with the ventral abdominal floor. The radiograph was taken with the rabbit lying on its right side and the pocket of gas that has collected in the pyloric area of the stomach can be seen as a dark circle in the stomach. This 'fried egg' appearance is typical of gastric dilation. There is some radiodense sediment in the urine, which is an incidental finding. On exploratory laparotomy, a foreign body was found in the small intestine and milked through to the ileocolic junction. The rabbit made a full recovery.

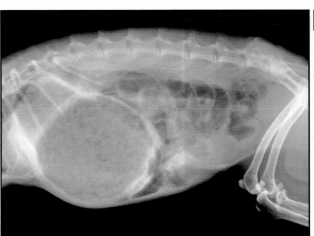

14.6 Gastric tympany. This lateral radiographic view of the abdomen was taken with the rabbit lying on its left side. The rabbit had been totally inappetent for 24 hours despite treatment by the owner with simethicone and pineapple juice. The stomach is grossly distended. It occupies half the abdomen and is in contact with the ventral abdominal floor. Loops of distended small intestine can be seen proximal to the site of the obstruction, which was due to marked thickening of the intestinal wall and narrowing of the lumen, causing a chronic partial obstruction. A large amount of hair was located at this site during post-mortem examination.

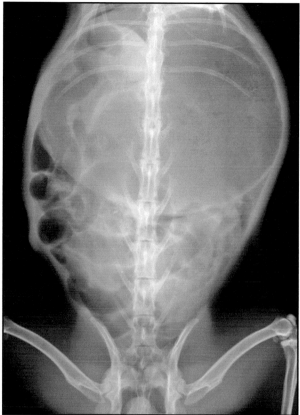

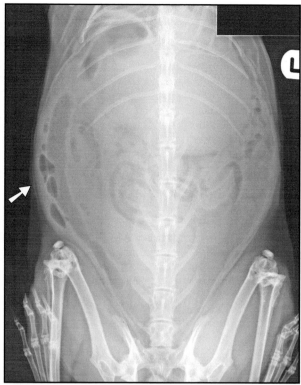

14.9 Ruptured intestine. This ventrodorsal view of the abdomen of a moribund rabbit was taken shortly after admission. It shows free gas in the abdominal cavity (arrow). The rabbit died after the radiograph was taken and post-mortem examination confirmed intestinal rupture. A pellet of hair was found in the ingesta that was released into the abdomen.

14.7 Ventrodorsal view of rabbit with gastric tympany. The radiograph shows the ventrodorsal view of the abdomen in the same rabbit as in Figure 14.6. A dilated section of small intestine can be seen leaving the pylorus and extending to the left side of the abdomen. Despite intravenous fluid therapy and passing a stomach tube, which released a large volume of gas and partially decompressed the stomach, the rabbit died shortly after induction of anaesthesia for exploratory laparotomy.

Intestinal obstruction

Intestinal obstruction is an easily missed but common cause of sudden death in rabbits. The sequence of events that follows obstruction of the intestine can be so rapid that the rabbit is eating and behaving normally one minute and dead 6–8 hours later. In other cases, the rabbit may show a transient episode of anorexia and abdominal discomfort before recovering spontaneously. The sequence of events depends on the cause, size and site of the obstruction and whether or not it passes through the ileocolic valve into the hindgut.

Sequence of events following occlusion of the intestine

1. **Accumulation of gas and fluid proximal to the site of obstruction.** Once the intestine is obstructed, the stomach and intestine proximal to the site of the obstruction start to fill with gas, fluid and ingesta. The more proximal the obstruction, the greater the speed and severity of the distension. At this point, differentiation between intestinal obstruction and other diseases is most difficult and affected rabbits need to be monitored closely.
2. **Pain and anorexia.** Abdominal pain associated with distension of the stomach and intestine

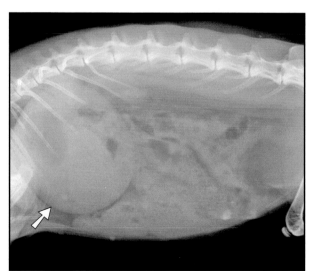

14.8 Free gas in the abdomen. This lateral radiograph of a moribund rabbit was taken prior to exploratory surgery. A duodenal foreign body was found and there was a small perforation in the stomach. Free gas in the abdomen can be seen outlining the ventral border of the stomach (arrow). The rabbit was euthanased.

175

causes anorexia. This may be intermittent if a moving foreign body is the cause of the obstruction. If the foreign body moves through the ileocolic valve, the gas and fluid can escape into the hindgut and distension of the stomach and intestines is relieved. The abdominal pain resolves and the rabbit may start to eat again.

3. **Gastric dilation.** If the intestinal lumen remains occluded, distension of the stomach and intestine changes to dilation, causing further abdominal pain, which may be severe (see Figure 14.5). Inflammation of the intestinal wall at the site of the obstruction is also painful.

4. **Gastric tympany.** If the intestinal obstruction does not resolve, the stomach becomes larger and larger until it is tympanitic and the rabbit quickly becomes shocked (see Figures 14.6 and 14.7). A number of secondary life-threatening events can occur, such as shock, hypovolaemia, and electrolyte and acid–base abnormalities. The dilated stomach compromises the venous return to the heart.

5. **Inflammation, ulceration, intestinal necrosis and peritonitis.** As the stomach becomes tympanitic, areas of inflammation develop, in some cases leading to areas of gastric ulceration. At the site of the intestinal obstruction, intestinal necrosis may occur, especially in cases of obstruction in the proximal duodenum. Peritonitis can also develop (see later).

6. **Gastric or intestinal rupture.** Gastric or intestinal rupture can occur, either as a result of intestinal necrosis or as a result of extreme tympany (see Figures 14.8 and 14.9). By this time, affected rabbits are shocked and moribund and usually die within an hour of examination.

Possible outcomes for rabbits with intestinal obstruction

- **Spontaneous resolution and recovery in rabbits with a moving foreign body.** In rabbits with moving foreign bodies, the intestinal and gastric distension can suddenly resolve as the foreign body moves through the ileocolic junction into the hindgut and releases the gas and fluid into the proximal colon and caecum (Figure 14.10). The rabbit then often starts to feel better and become more responsive. This recovery can be dramatic and may occur with or without treatment. It can be misinterpreted as a positive response to remedies such as fluid therapy, pineapple juice, simethicone or stomach massage.
- **Death.** This can be the result of shock, peritonitis, circulatory failure, acute renal failure or rupture of the stomach or intestine.
- **Partial improvement initially, but death within a few days.** An intestinal obstruction is a painful experience, even if a foreign body passes into the hindgut. The episode can trigger paralytic ileus (Figure 14.11) or acute renal failure, which may be fatal, especially if left untreated.

- **Recovery after surgical intervention.** Surgery to relieve the intestinal obstruction can be successful, especially if it is performed promptly.
- **Death during or after surgical intervention.** There are many reasons why a rabbit might die during or after surgery to relieve an obstruction. The rabbit will be shocked, with disturbed electrolyte and acid–base status and compromised cardiorespiratory function due to the dilated stomach. Complications associated with enterotomy or enterectomy can easily occur because of the narrow gut, and thin, friable tissue. Gastrointestinal hypomotility, gut stasis, paralytic ileus or acute renal failure may be triggered by the episode.

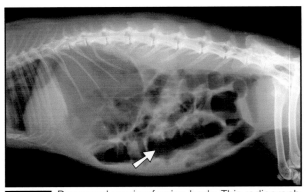

14.10 Presumed moving foreign body. This radiograph shows the lateral abdomen of a rabbit that had been totally anorexic for a number of hours. The stomach was palpably distended. The radiograph shows a dilated stomach and gas in the hindgut. The diameter of the section of intestine suggests that the gas was in the ileocaecocolic complex and colon (arrow). The gas shadow extends to the rectum. This radiograph suggests that an intestinal obstruction has moved through the ileocolic junction and allowed gas from the stomach and small intestine to escape into the hindgut. The rabbit was treated with analgesics and prokinetic therapy. He started to eat voluntarily within 2 hours of radiography.

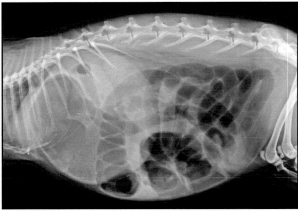

14.11 Paralytic ileus. This radiograph shows the lateral view of the abdomen of a rabbit that had been anorexic for 36 hours before undergoing surgery. It was shocked, hypothermic and collapsed. A pellet of hair was found obstructing the small intestine and was milked through to the colon. The rabbit died despite treatment with fluids, prokinetic therapy and analgesics. There is gas in the stomach, small intestine and ileocaecocolic complex.

Diagnosis of intestinal obstruction

Intestinal obstruction is more difficult to diagnose in rabbits than in other domestic species because they hide their pain. A dog or a cat with an intestinal obstruction would be vomiting, trembling and showing signs of illness and distress that are obvious to its owner. Horses show signs of colic and sweat, roll, kick and tremble. It is important to remember that rabbits that are dying with a serious abdominal condition may not look particularly unwell on cursory examination. The course of the disease depends on the cause and site of the obstruction. Clinical history and examination, blood sampling and abdominal radiography are the main diagnostic tools. Gastrointestinal hypomotility is a major differential diagnosis, especially in the early stages of intestinal obstruction. Other differential diagnoses include liver lobe torsion, ureteral obstruction, enterotoxaemia, peritonitis, pancreatitis and any other painful condition that can cause anorexia.

Clinical history

The owner's clinical history is often highly suggestive of an intestinal obstruction. Typical features include:

- **Rapid speed of onset.** Most owners say something like '*he was fine last night*' or '*she ate all her food this morning*'
- **Total anorexia.** Rabbits with intestinal obstruction are completely inappetent and this is usually the reason that owners seek veterinary treatment
- **Change in demeanour.** Rabbits with intestinal obstruction suddenly become very quiet and unresponsive (Figure 14.12)
- **Unusual behaviour.** The owners may have had to search for their rabbit before finding it hiding in an unusual place away from view
- **Signs of pain.** Overt signs of abdominal pain are rare, although some owners say they have noticed their rabbit changing its position suddenly or periodically pressing its abdomen to the ground
- **Bloated appearance.** In the later stages, many owners notice that their rabbit looks bloated. In the terminal stages, when the rabbit becomes shocked and moribund, it is obvious to the owner that it is seriously ill.

Clinical examination

Even in the early stages of intestinal obstruction, the stomach may be palpated as an enlarged structure behind the ribs on the left-hand side. This is a sign that should be checked for in any inappetent rabbit. A dilated stomach can be felt as a tense, balloon-like structure and is easily palpable unless the rabbit is obese. Further clinical examination is also necessary. It can reveal concurrent diseases, such as dental disease, grooming difficulties or upper respiratory problems, which may affect any decision to go for surgery. An assessment of the degree of dehydration, shock and pain is helpful. Shocked rabbits are hypothermic and ataxic with pale mucous membranes and poor capillary refill time.

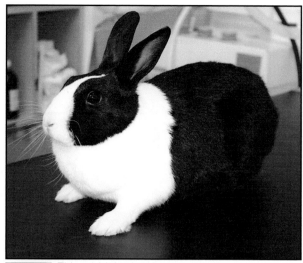

14.12 This rabbit had an inoperable obstruction in the duodenum. His stomach was tympanitic and the intestine was about to rupture at the site of the obstruction. The owner found him hiding in a corner when she returned from work. He had been eating well and behaving normally when she left for work 6 hours previously.

Heart rate is a measurable parameter that is useful in other species to assess shock and pain, but in rabbits the normal heart rate is 150–300 beats per minute (Meredith, 2006), which is too fast to count accurately, and a high rate can be normal. Blood glucose measurement can be more useful (Harcourt-Brown and Harcourt-Brown, 2012).

Blood biochemistry

A complete blood profile, including haematology, renal and liver function, calcium, phosphorus, electrolytes and acid–base parameters, with immediate results, is ideal for rabbits with suspected intestinal obstruction. For practices without the facilities to perform these tests immediately, a good compromise is a quick, informative, in-house profile that is easy to perform and only requires 3–4 drops of blood. It can help to differentiate between gut stasis and abdominal catastrophes with a poor prognosis, such as intestinal obstruction.

A glucose meter, centrifuge and spectrometer are required, to measure blood glucose, packed cell volume (PCV) and total protein, while the serum should be visually examined. Glucose is particularly important; it provides information that can help to decide whether a case of acute onset anorexia is surgical or medical. Blood glucose is easily measured with an inexpensive glucose meter that is available from pharmacists. These are hand-held, battery-powered devices that are used with individual test strips fitted with electrodes that measure glucose electrochemically (as glucose dehydrogenase) from 0.6 μl of blood. Results are displayed in 5 seconds and data is transferred from the strip via an infrared sensor.

In rabbits with serious abdominal conditions, such as intestinal obstruction, blood glucose levels rise rapidly to high levels of up to 30 mmol/l

(Harcourt-Brown and Harcourt-Brown, 2012). Conversely, rabbits with gut stasis rarely have blood glucose values above 15 mmol/l. In cases where decision making is difficult, blood glucose measurement can easily be repeated. Rising blood glucose levels signify a condition with a poor prognosis, in which surgery may be the only hope of saving the rabbit. Normal or slightly elevated glucose levels are indicative that immediate surgery is not necessary (Figure 14.13).

PCV is another useful parameter. It can easily be measured by collecting blood in a heparinized

Value	Significance	Possible reasons	Comments
Blood glucose (mmol/l)			
<2	Severely hypoglycaemic	Insulinoma; paraneoplastic syndrome; artefact; metabolic disease	
2–4.1	Moderately hypoglycaemic	Lack of food	Needs syringe feeding
4.2–8.2	Within laboratory reference range		Reassuring
8.2–12	Within normal range for pet rabbits in unfamiliar surroundings	Mild stress	Reassuring but indicative that the rabbit is stressed
12.1–15	Slightly hyperglycaemic	Stress	Probably stress-induced but could be start of serious disease; re-sample if necessary
15.1–20	Significantly hyperglycaemic	Stress/pain	Possibly but not definitely surgical; re-sample after 30–60 minutes; take radiographs
20.1–25	Severely hyperglycaemic	Pain/deranged glucose metabolism	Serious disease present; needs diagnosis and surgery is likely
>25	Critically hyperglycaemic	Pain/deranged glucose metabolism	Surgical or terminal
PCV			
<20%	Severely anaemic	Liver lobe torsion; autoimmune haemolytic anaemia; blood loss; chronic heavy metal poisoning	Further investigations are necessary
20–30%	Moderately anaemic	Chronic disease (e.g. dental disease); chronic or intermittent blood loss	
30–33%	Low end or less than laboratory reference ranges; apparently normal for pet rabbits		Reassuring
33–45%	Within normal laboratory reference range		Top end of range is unusual in pet rabbits, suggesting dehydration
>45%	High	Dehydration; polycythaemia (rare)	
Total protein (g/l)			
<54	Low	Protein-losing kidney or intestinal disease; liver disease; haemorrhage; malnutrition; excessive exudation, e.g. flystrike.	
54–75g	Normal		
>75g	High	Dehydration	
Visual examination of serum			
Abnormality	**Possible reasons**		**Comments**
Lipaemia	Obesity; hepatic lipidosis		Poor prognostic sign
Jaundice	Liver disease; haemolytic disease		Rare but significant

14.13   Interpretation of mini-laboratory profile that can be used to differentiate between medical and surgical emergencies.

capillary tube and spinning it in a centrifuge. Acute anaemia is a sign of liver lobe torsion, which is another cause of sudden onset anorexia. After the PCV is measured, the serum is visually inspected for lipaemia or jaundice before the tube is snapped so a drop of plasma can be placed in a spectrometer to measure total protein, which can indicate the hydration status of the rabbit. An interpretation of the results of this quick blood screen is summarized in Figure 14.13.

Abdominal radiography

Interpretation of abdominal radiographs is covered in Chapter 7. In rabbits with a suspected intestinal obstruction, the stomach, small intestine, ileocaecocolic complex and rectum are special areas of interest. The normal appearance of these areas changes throughout the day because of the two phases of digestion (see Figures 14.3 and 14.4).

Excessive amounts of liquid and gas in the gastrointestinal tract are the radiological features that are most easily identified on radiographs. Gas is an excellent contrast medium, which facilitates radiographic interpretation. In rabbits with intestinal obstruction and early gastric dilation, a pocket of gas often collects in the pylorus. If the rabbit is radiographed lying on its right side, this pocket of gas can be seen on radiographs as a 'fried egg' shape in the stomach (see Figure 14.5). As gastric dilation progresses, the stomach becomes large and tympanitic (see Figures 14.6 and 14.7). The small intestine proximal to the site of the obstruction also becomes dilated and tympanitic, which can be seen if the obstruction is in the distal small intestine but may not be obvious if it is in the descending duodenum.

Once a moving foreign body has moved through the ileocolic valve, the gas and fluid that was trapped in the stomach and small intestine is released into the ileocaecocolic complex and can be seen on radiographs. This is a good prognostic sign (see Figure 14.10).

Rabbits with intestinal obstruction have both gastric dilation and excessive amounts of fluid and/or gas in the stomach. However, there are other causes of either gastric dilation or gas in the stomach. These are summarized in Figure 14.14 and shown in Figures 14.15 to 14.17).

Radiographic sign	Cause
Gastric dilation and gas in stomach	Intestinal obstruction Mucoid enteropathy (Figure 14.15) Pyloric obstruction (rare) Paralytic ileus (Figure 14.11)
Gastric dilation	Intestinal obstruction Engorgement (Figure 14.16)
Gas in stomach but no gastric dilation	Early intestinal obstruction Aerophagia: dyspnoea (Figure 14.17) Oesophageal foreign body Stress Gut stasis

14.14 Causes of dilation or gas in the stomach of rabbits.

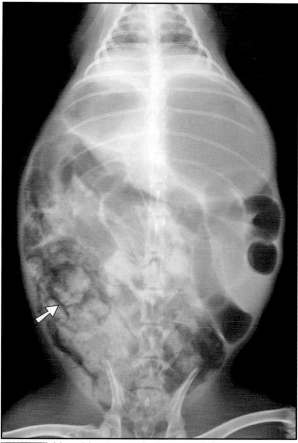

14.15 Mucoid enteropathy is a non-inflammatory condition that mainly affects the hindgut. The aetiology is not clear and dysautonomia has been confirmed in some outbreaks. The motility of the hindgut is affected so the caecum becomes impacted with hard dry ingesta (arrow) and the colon fills with mucus. Gastric dilation occurs in the late stages, as in this case. The ventrodorsal abdominal radiograph is of a 14-week-old rabbit that was one of number that had died at the same breeding establishment.

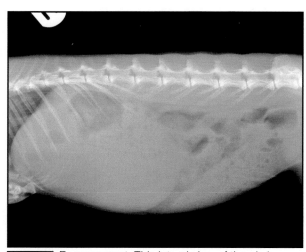

14.16 Engorgement. This lateral view of the abdomen was taken because an enlarged stomach was palpated during clinical examination of a rabbit presented for vaccination. The rabbit had just eaten a large bowl of dried food, which it did not normally have access to. She showed no other clinical abnormalities and was not ill.

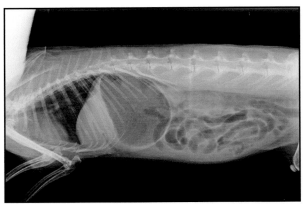

14.17 Aerophagia. This lateral view of the chest and abdomen shows hyperinflated lungs and a stomach full of gas. There is gas in the small intestine and rectum. The rabbit was presented for veterinary treatment because of a nasal foreign body, which was subsequently sneezed out.

Site of obstruction

Descending duodenum

The diameter suddenly narrows approximately 1–2 cm from the pylorus and this is a common site for obstruction. Affected rabbits carry a grave prognosis. The course of the disease is rapid and severe. Intestinal necrosis at the site of obstruction is common (Figure 14.18).

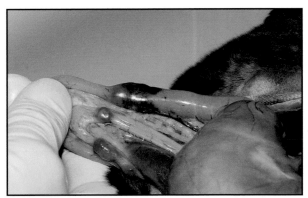

14.18 Duodenal obstruction. This image taken during post-mortem examination shows an inflamed, necrotic section of proximal duodenum containing a pellet of compacted hair (see Figure 14.19). The patient was a 6-year-old male neutered Rex house rabbit that was reluctant to eat at 11 pm the previous evening. By 6 am he was moribund and tympanitic. He died shortly after admission.

Small intestine

The small intestine can be obstructed anywhere along its length. The clinical signs and course of the disease depend on whether it is a foreign body that is causing a complete obstruction or moving and periodically obstructing. Tumours or other chronic abnormalities, such as strictures or diverticula, which partially occlude the intestinal lumen, may show more intermittent clinical signs, but gastric dilation is still a feature.

Ileocolic valve

The ileocolic valve is another common site of obstruction. In these cases, abdominal radiographs show lots of gas-filled intestine. The course of the disease is more protracted and the clinical signs less dramatic than in rabbits with a duodenal obstruction.

Hindgut

Obstruction of the hindgut is seldom due to an ingested foreign body. It is more likely to be due to a tumour, intussusception or a large piece of impacted caecal content that has moved into the colon. The fusus coli is the most likely site for obstruction of the colon by a caecolith or accumulation of foreign material. The diameter of the colon narrows at its entrance and strands of indigestible material, such as synthetic carpet fibre, can collect at this point and cause an obstruction.

Causes of intestinal obstruction

Pellets of impacted fur

A pellet of impacted fur is the most common cause of intestinal obstruction. The pellet is similar in size and appearance to a hard faecal pellet but is composed of tightly matted hair rather than plant material (Figure 14.19). The origin of these pellets has not been proven, although various suggestions have been put forward. For example, it has been postulated that the pellets are felts of matted hair that

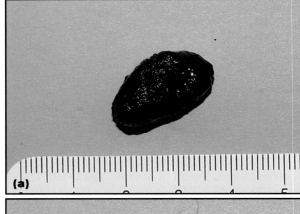

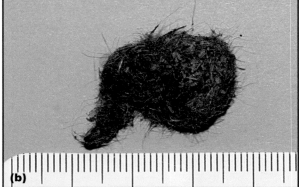

14.19 Typical pellet of hair that obstructs the small intestine. **(a)** The hard pellet that was obstructing the duodenum of the rabbit shown in Figure 14.18. **(b)** The same pellet after it was washed, dried and teased out.

have been removed from the coat and ingested during grooming, or that they are pieces of impacted stomach content that have broken off and passed into the small intestine. Current evidence indicates that neither of these explanations is correct. Although the pellets are more common during moulting and in long-haired rabbits, they also occur in short-coated breeds, such as Rexes. They have even been found in captive wild rabbits.

The most plausible explanation is that the pellets are formed by compression of ingested hair during its passage through the large intestine, especially when large quantities pass through the digestive tract during moulting. Fur is not broken down by digestive enzymes as it passes through the gastrointestinal tract so is compressed into pellets during its passage through the colon. These are sometimes seen as chains of faeces attached by strands of hair. Although rabbits are known to eat their caecotrophs, they are also coprophagic, and some rabbits will ingest hard faecal pellets as well as caecotrophs (Ebino *et al.*, 1993). This is not a problem if the pellet is small enough to pass through the small intestine, but if it is slightly larger it may periodically obstruct the small intestine on its way through. If the pellet is too large to pass through the small intestine then it will obstruct completely. Large amounts of hair (during moulting), large faeces (from a large companion), long fine mattable hair (angoras), intestinal abnormalities (adhesions, intestinal hypertrophy, diverticulitis) or slow gut motility (insufficient indigestible fibre) may be contributory factors.

Ingested foreign bodies
Occasionally, rabbits will swallow an object or material that can obstruct the intestine. At one time in the UK, locust bean seeds were a common cause of small intestinal obstruction but the incidence has reduced because locust beans are now excluded from most muesli mix diets. Other hard spherical objects, such as dried sweetcorn kernels, can also obstruct the small intestine.

Ingestion of large amounts of synthetic fibres (e.g. carpet) may obstruct the small intestine or they can pass, undigested, into the hindgut where they are separated from the rest of the ingesta and pass through the colon as large clumps. Occasionally obstruction can occur at the fusus coli.

Neoplasia
Intestinal neoplasia, especially lymphoma, is not unusual in rabbits. Affected rabbits may have a history of weight loss and inappetence before an acute episode of gastric dilation because the intestinal lumen is narrowed and eventually obstructed by the tumour. Other parts of the digestive tract, such as the caecum or rectum, can be involved and the clinical signs vary with the site of the lesion. Abdominal masses may or may not be palpable prior to surgery. Intestinal lymphomas are often aggressive and in many instances there is metastatic spread throughout the lymph nodes. There may be several tumours in the gut wall at the time of surgery.

Adhesions and other intestinal abnormalities
Adhesions with neighbouring structures can cause functional obstructions by creating bends or strictures in the intestine that impede the passage of a foreign object or pellet of fur through the intestinal tract. The adhesions may be chronic and long-standing, or acute. Long-standing adhesions may be the result of previous surgery or infection, or due to inflammation of a neighbouring structure, such as an abscess or a uterus full of pus. In acute cases, the adhesions may have formed because of peritonitis, which may be due to a perforated gut or from peracute enteritis or enterotoxaemia.

The author has encountered some other intestinal abnormalities that have caused intermittent bouts of obstruction. These include diverticulosis, and intestinal hypertrophy. These conditions were diagnosed during exploratory surgery or at post-mortem examination.

Torsions and strangulations
Gastric torsion in rabbits is not reported in the literature and has not been encountered by the author. Torsion of the intestine also appears to be very rare. Strangulations are more common and can be the result of adhesions or surgery, such as castration or laparotomy, where the abdominal repair has failed (Figure 14.20).

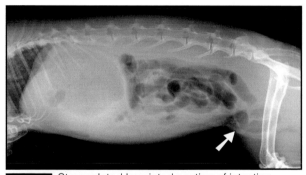

14.20 Strangulated herniated section of intestine. A lateral view of the abdomen of a rabbit that was presented ill 36 hours after castration. A section of small intestine had herniated through the inguinal canal and strangulated (arrow). The stomach was dilated and filled with gas and fluid.

Caecoliths
Occasionally, a large piece of impacted ingesta from the caecum (caecolith) may obstruct the colon, usually at the fusus coli, where the diameter of the colon suddenly decreases. This is a secondary problem. The primary cause is caecal impaction, which can be caused by intestinal hypomotility, mucoid enteropathy, inflammatory conditions, ingestion of small undegradable particles (e.g. chalk, barium, finely ground lignified material, clay cat litter) or chronic dehydration due to chronic renal failure. Ingestion of indigestible fine particulate material causes problems when it reaches the hindgut because, as the small particles are not degraded by bacteria, when they move into the caecum, they compress and can impact the caecum.

Tapeworm cysts

The author has seen a single case of obstruction of the colon that was caused by large numbers of tapeworm cysts in the mesentery. There were so many that they were occluding the transverse colon.

Moving foreign bodies

Although it is impossible to quantify the incidence, the ingestion of pellets of impacted hair seems to be a common occurrence and, in most cases, the pellet is small enough to pass through the small intestine without causing problems. Larger pellets can still pass through but periodically obstruct the small intestine on their way. Affected rabbits suffer from periodic bouts of abdominal pain over a few hours as the pellet obstructs and moves on. Evidence of this can be seen during surgery or at post-mortem examination, where a series of inflamed sections of small intestine are found where the foreign body has transiently lodged. In many cases, no definitive diagnosis is made because the rabbit makes a spontaneous dramatic recovery when the foreign body moves through the ileocolic junction and all the gas and fluid that was trapped in the stomach and small intestine is suddenly released into the colon (see Figure 14.10).

It is easy to confuse these cases with gut stasis because treatment with a variety of remedies that might help in cases of reduced gut motility (e.g. prokinetics, fluid therapy, analgesia, pineapple juice, simethicone, massaging the stomach, making the rabbit run round) may be misinterpreted as the reason the rabbit has recovered. The possibility that an obstruction could pass through without surgery complicates the decision-making process regarding how to treat a rabbit with gastric dilation.

Gastrointestinal hypomotility

Gastrointestinal hypomotility is the condition most often confused with intestinal obstruction. It is the result of stimulation of the sympathetic nervous system by stress. Discomfort or pain is stressful, so almost any disease can reduce gut motility and trigger a sequence of events that may be fatal if left untreated. This is summarized in Figure 14.21. Gastric dilation is not part of this sequence of events, which can be seen clinically and radiologically.

Stage 1: Onset

At the onset of gastrointestinal hypomotility, the rabbit may be quieter than usual and faecal output is diminished or absent. Any hard faecal pellets tend to be small and dry. Appetite is reduced, although the rabbit may pick at some favourite foods. There may be a history of a stressful event, e.g. surgery or loss of a companion. Clinical examination may reveal a condition that has triggered the gut stasis, e.g. dental spurs, urine scalding, painful hocks, etc. In some cases the initiating cause is not obvious. The abdomen feels empty and the stomach is not palpable.

Clinical findings	Radiographic findings
Initial (0–24 hours)	
Reduced appetite, often with a history of surgery, dental spurs or other painful or stressful incident, may be picking at food; reduced or absent faecal output, perhaps with small hard faecal pellets; empty abdomen; quiet demeanour; hypoglycaemia, normoglycaemia or mild hyperglycaemia (<15 mmol/l)	Reduced amount of ingesta in the stomach and ileocaecocolic complex; pockets of gas may be seen throughout the gastrointestinal tract and large amounts of faeces may be seen in the rectum
Intermediate (after 1–3 days)	
No appetite; absent faeces; depression; empty feeling abdomen; palpable firm small stomach; normoglycaemia or mild hyperglycaemia (<15 mmol/l); dehydration (± azotaemia)	Reduced amounts of ingesta in gastrointestinal tract; small stomach; increased amounts of gas in gastrointestinal tract, especially in the hindgut (there may be a gas halo surrounding the impacted stomach contents)
Late (after <4 days)	
Weight loss; depression; absent faeces; no appetite	Gas in stomach; impacted stomach contents; large amounts of gas in the caecum and colon
Terminal	
Hypothermia (<38°C); complete anorexia; collapsed and/or ataxic; ketosis; lipaemia; bizarre blood results; evidence of liver and kidney damage, acidosis, ketosis etc.; acidic urine with ketones	Same radiographic changes as in late stages; ultrasonography, especially of the liver, may be more useful than abdominal radiography

14.21 Clinical and radiographic signs of gastrointestinal hypomotility (gut stasis).

Radiography confirms that there is a reduced amount of food in the gastrointestinal tract. It may also show other conditions, e.g. nephroliths, that have triggered the episode of slow gut motility. Sometimes hard faeces can be seen accumulating in the rectum. A blood sample shows normal or slightly elevated blood glucose (>15 mmol/l), with PCV and total protein within the normal range. These rabbits often start to eat on their own, especially if they are offered grass, dandelions and other tempting foods. Syringe feeding, prokinetics and analgesia are never a bad idea. Any underlying problem also needs to be treated.

Stage 2: After 24–48 hours with treatment

Slow gastric emptying results in dehydration and impaction of the stomach contents and the formation of an impacted ball of hair, which may be seen on abdominal radiographs, often with a halo of gas around it. Pockets of gas are often seen throughout the intestines and hindgut. Clinically, the rabbit is quiet and less responsive with no faecal output. The stomach may be palpable in the empty abdomen as a solid, doughy structure behind the ribs on the left-hand side. At this stage, blood samples may or may not show mild dehydration and mild hypoglycaemia.

If urea and creatinine are measured, these may also be raised. Gastric ulceration can develop, which is impossible to diagnose with certainty in the live rabbit. Anti-ulcer medication, such as ranitidine, is a good idea as it also has a mild prokinetic effect. Tempting food, prokinetics such as domperidone, syringe feeding and analgesia are also indicated.

Stage 3: After 2–4 days without treatment
At this stage, the demeanour of the rabbit with gut stasis deteriorates. By this time it is totally anorexic and obviously unwell. There is no faecal output. This is often the time that an unobservant or inexperienced owner notices a problem and brings the rabbit for treatment. Large amounts of gas may be seen in the ileocaecocolic complex on abdominal radiographs. Blood samples may show signs of dehydration, i.e. raised PCV and total protein. If urea and creatinine are measured, these can be alarmingly high and it is easy to believe the rabbit is in renal failure, but the values will drop back to normal if treatment is successful. Blood glucose may be high but is unlikely to be higher than 15 mmol/l. At this stage, treatment is still usually successful unless the rabbit dies from a ruptured gastric ulcer.

Stage 4: Hepatic lipidosis
This develops after 4–7 days of untreated gut stasis. This is the endstage of gut stasis. Volatile fatty acids absorbed from the gastrointestinal tract are the major energy source for rabbits and, as the amounts decline due to reduction in caecal fermentation and ingestion of caecotrophs, free fatty acids are mobilized from adipose tissue instead. Fatty degeneration of the liver and β-oxidation of free fatty acids ensues, which causes ketone body production and metabolic acidosis. This is usually a terminal event. Clinically, these rabbits are depressed, cold and ataxic. There are no particular diagnostic radiographic features of hepatic lipidosis, although the change in liver consistency may be detected on ultrasound examination. All the signs of gut stasis may be seen on abdominal radiographs. Blood samples show lipaemia and a range of bizarre blood results including raised liver enzymes and kidney parameters. Marked hyperglycaemia is present in many cases. In the author's experience, hepatic lipidosis is a terminal event.

Gastrointestinal hypomotility *versus* intestinal obstruction

In the literature, there is considerable confusion between gut stasis and intestinal obstruction. Sometimes they are classed as features of the same syndrome when they are really two distinct clinical conditions with some common features, such as anorexia and gas in the digestive tract. The situation is further complicated by the rabbit's potential to develop secondary ileus in response to pain, so they can have both gut stasis and intestinal obstruction. Another source of confusion is that gut stasis and intestinal obstruction both involve balls of impacted hair, even though the balls are different in size and texture.

Hair ingested during grooming is not broken down by the stomach acid or digestive enzymes. In rabbits with gut stasis, the stomach contents become dry and impacted and form a large ball of hair mixed with food in the pylorus. The ball can be the size of a satsuma. In rabbits with intestinal obstruction, it is often a ball of fur that is causing the problem even though the 'hairball' is completely different. In this case, the hair is felted and tightly compacted and the ball is the size of a small bean (see Figure 14.19) rather than a satsuma.

The distinction between gut stasis and intestinal obstruction is an important one because prompt surgery may be necessary to save the life of a rabbit with an intestinal obstruction whereas gut stasis is always a medical condition and surgery is contraindicated. Clinical history, clinical examination, abdominal radiography and blood samples are useful to distinguish between the two. Figure 14.22 summarizes the differences between gut stasis, a moving foreign body and complete intestinal obstruction.

Feature	Intestinal obstruction	Moving foreign body	Gut stasis
Speed of onset	Rapid: owner often says rabbit was 'fine' a few hours before	Rapid	Slow: owners often can't say when signs began
Demeanour of rabbit at outset	Depressed, immobile, may hide in corners, may show signs of colic	Variable	Progressively quieter; becomes more depressed when anorexia has been present for 2–3 days (unless another condition is making rabbit ill)
Palpation of stomach	Large, balloon-like structure behind ribs on left-hand side	Dilated stomach is often palpable	Stomach is not palpable or can be felt as small, hard mass
Abdominal radiology	Gastric dilation; may or may not be distended loops of intestine (depending on site of obstruction); no gas in ileocaecocolic complex	Gastric dilation; distended loops of intestine usually visible, unless they are filled with fluid; large amount of gas in ileocaecocolic complex once foreign body passes through	Small stomach with or without impacted contents and halo of gas, depending on stage of gut stasis; gas in caecum is common; may be large amounts of caecal gas in later stages
Blood glucose	High >20 mmol/l	Raised 15–25 mmol/l	Low, normal or slightly raised (>15 mmol/l); low or within normal range in early stages

14.22 A summary of the differences between gut stasis, a moving foreign body and complete intestinal obstruction.

Protocol for rabbits with gastric dilation

Rabbits with a history of sudden onset complete anorexia and depression alongside a palpably distended stomach always require prompt investigation and treatment (Harcourt-Brown, 2007a). The following protocol can be life-saving and help with the decision-making process about whether a case is surgical, medical or hopeless.

- **Clinical assessment.** A rabbit that can still move around and show some interest in its surroundings carries a much better prognosis than one that is cold, ataxic and unresponsive. A palpably dilated stomach is a definite indication that the case is serious and requires immediate investigation and treatment.
- **Avoid massaging the stomach.** It is important to palpate the abdomen gently because a dilated stomach and small intestine are painful and can easily rupture. Stomach massage is contraindicated.
- **Provide immediate analgesia with opioids** if gastric dilation is present. The author's preference is fentanyl/fluanisone (e.g. Hypnorm 0.2– 0.25 ml/kg s.c.) as it is a potent analgesic and a mild sedative, which can be beneficial. Other analgesic protocols are given in Chapter 2.
- **Take radiographs.** A lateral view of the abdomen is easy to take in a conscious rabbit or after sedation. Although the positioning might not be perfect, in many cases the radiographic findings are diagnostic. The pattern of intestinal dilation can help to localize the site of an obstruction. Ideally, a dorsoventral or ventrodorsal view should be taken as well, as this will provide further information (see Chapter 7). Radiographs should be examined closely for evidence of other diseases (e.g. kidney stones) that may influence a decision to proceed with surgery. Gas in the caecum of rabbits with gastric dilation is a good prognostic sign as it indicates that a foreign body has passed through the ileocolic junction so gas has escaped into the hindgut (see Figure 14.10). Surgery is not indicated in these cases.
- **Attempt to decompress the stomach.** After taking radiographs, decompression of the stomach will reduce pressure, relieve pain, reduce the likelihood of perforation and improve venous return. It is worth attempting in all but the mildest cases of gastric dilation. Passing a stomach tube is effective in releasing gas and fluid in some cases and most rabbits will tolerate the procedure well (see Technique 14.1). Although decompression can also be accomplished by inserting a needle into the distended fundus of the stomach, it is preferable to perform this procedure when the stomach can be visualized during laparotomy so any leakage from the puncture site can be minimized, using a purse-string suture if necessary. Again, decompression is only successful if the needle does not block with food or hair.

Conscious radiography of the abdomen

Abdominal radiography can be performed on some rabbits without the need for sedation or anaesthesia, so the owner can wait rather than leave their rabbit at the practice. Non-manual restraint can be used in the conscious patient to allow the radiographer to move out of the designated area when the exposure is taken (see also Appendix 4 and Chapters 3 and 7). Note: Conscious radiography is not suitable for fractious or lively individuals, such as wild rabbits: these cases will require general anaesthesia/sedation.

In order to position the rabbit to take a lateral view of the abdomen, the author quietly lays the rabbit in dorsal recumbency until it relaxes (see Appendix 4 on Dorsal immobility response), then rolls it on to its side and positions it on the X-ray cassette. A sandbag is placed over the rabbit's neck and a towel over its head. The rabbit will remain still and can be positioned with the hindlimbs gently drawn back. Restraining the hindlimbs with sandbags or ties is counterproductive because it stimulates the rabbit to struggle. The rabbit will remain in this position as long as there are no loud or sudden noises or movements. Once the radiographs have been taken, the towel and sandbag can be removed so the rabbit can return to its normal position.

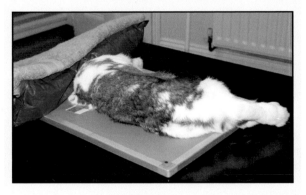

Dorsoventral views are more difficult to obtain without sedation because ideally the hindlimbs need to be extended, which is usually resisted. However, it is possible to gain some information without extending the hindlimbs and taking the radiograph with the rabbit sitting on the cassette (see Chapter 7). A ventrodorsal view can be obtained in some docile rabbits by leaving them in dorsal recumbency; wedges or sandbags can be used to aid positioning by supporting the rabbit on either side.

- **Provide supportive care,** i.e. intravenous fluid therapy and warmth (see Chapter 1).
- **Decide whether the case is surgical or medical.** A rabbit with gastric dilation always poses a dilemma. The rabbit might recover without surgery if the foreign body is small enough to pass through the intestine. If the pellet is large enough to cause a complete obstruction,

however, or the intestine is obstructed by a tumour, stricture, adhesion or strangulation, the only hope of saving the rabbit is by surgical intervention. If a tumour is present, laparotomy is the quickest way of finding it and provides an opportunity to remove it if it looks surgical or euthanase the rabbit if the tumour is inoperable. In the author's opinion, if there is a dilemma, prompt surgery is the best option. Surgery is quick, easy and, if performed correctly, well tolerated by rabbits. It is diagnostic and resolves the situation. It is preferable to perform surgery on a moving foreign body that could have moved through than to perform a post-mortem examination on a rabbit that you wish you had operated on.

Surgical treatment of intestinal obstruction

Exploratory laparotomy (see Chapter 13) is required to find and relieve an intestinal obstruction. Once the abdomen is opened, and the site of obstruction has been identified and examined, the situation can be re-appraised. Euthanasia may be necessary if the obstruction is caused by an inoperable tumour or if the intestinal tissue is so devitalized that surgery is difficult or impossible. If a foreign body is found, it can either be removed by enterotomy or milked carefully along the intestine until it can be squeezed through the ileocolic valve into the hindgut. Milking the obstruction along is usually preferable to an enterotomy or enterectomy as there is no risk of leakage or stricture postoperatively, but it can slow down recovery, presumably because much of the intestinal tract has been exteriorized so the abdominal contents need to rearrange themselves in the abdomen postoperatively. The technique for milking the obstruction through the intestine is described in Operative Technique 14.2.

If an enterotomy is performed, only the obstructed section of small intestine needs to be exteriorized and, if there are no complications, postoperative recovery can be rapid. However, enterotomy is more difficult in rabbits than in dogs and cats. The intestinal wall is so thin and friable that it can be difficult to make a leak-proof repair without causing a stricture. If enterotomy is performed, it is a good idea to move the foreign body into a healthy section of gut beforehand. It is also preferable to occlude the intestine by having an assistant to hold the intestine closed on either side of the incision rather than applying bowel clamps. It is important to maintain the blood supply to the affected area of intestine and to ensure the mesentery is not torn away from the gut. To remove the foreign body, the antimesenteric border is incised sufficiently to allow removal of the foreign body without tearing the intestinal wall. The incision is repaired with 4/0 or 5/0 monofilament absorbable suture material on a round-bodied needle. A simple interrupted pattern is often the only option as the intestinal wall is so thin and friable. Magnification is beneficial. After the enterotomy incision has been repaired, it must be tested for leakage by gently occluding the intestine proximal and distal to the intestinal repair and injecting saline into the lumen near to the suture line to gently dilate it. If the repair is satisfactory, omentalization can be attempted although the omentum is small in rabbits so it is often impossible. The abdomen is then closed. The postoperative care is the same as for milking an obstruction through the intestine.

References and further reading

Blood DC, Studdert VP and Gay CC (2007) *Saunders Comprehensive Veterinary Dictionary, 3rd edn*. Saunders Elsevier, Edinburgh

Ebino KY, Shutoh Y and Takahashi KW (1993) Coprophagy in rabbits: autoingestion of hard faeces. *Jikken Dobutsu* **42**, 611–613

Harcourt-Brown FM (2001) *Textbook of Rabbit Medicine*. Butterworth Heinemann, Oxford

Harcourt-Brown FM (2007a) Gastric dilation and intestinal obstruction in 76 rabbits. *Veterinary Record* **161**, 409–414

Harcourt-Brown FM and Harcourt-Brown SF (2012) Clinical value of blood glucose measurement in pet rabbits. *Veterinary Record* **170**, 674 [Epub 2012 Jun 1]

Harcourt-Brown TR (2007b) Management of acute gastric dilation in rabbits. *Journal of Exotic Pet Medicine* **16**, 168–174

Lichtenberger M and Lennox A (2010) Updates and advanced therapies for gastrointestinal stasis in rabbits. *Veterinary Clinics of North America: Exotic Pet Practice* **13**(3), 525–541

Meredith A (2006) General biology and husbandry. In: *BSAVA Manual of Rabbit Medicine and Surgery, 2nd edn*, ed. A Meredith and P Flecknell, pp. 1–17. BSAVA Publications, Gloucester

TECHNIQUES →

TECHNIQUE 14.1:
Passing a stomach tube to decompress the stomach

Positioning

The rabbit is placed in sternal recumbency with its head held in extension. The rabbit may be wrapped in a towel or sedated if necessary. Some rabbits with gastric dilation are so ill that the procedure can be carried out immediately and without sedation. If the rabbit is conscious, the procedure can be carried out with the rabbit in sternal recumbency. If the rabbit is anaesthetized or moribund, the procedure can be carried out with the rabbit in lateral recumbency. It is preferable to have an assistant to restrain the rabbit.

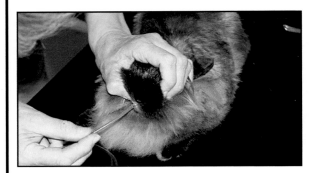

Equipment

A section of soft flexible tubing that will fit a luer fitting on a syringe is required. A feeding tube can be used or a section of giving-set (not paediatric) tubing cut to a length of 20–30 cm.

Procedure

1 Prior to insertion, the tube is measured against the body and the distance from the nose to the last rib is marked on the tube.

2 The tube is then passed through the mouth into the oesophagus to the stomach. This can be accomplished without a gag if the mouth is gently held closed so the rabbit cannot chew through the tube. Passing the tube through the larynx into the trachea is unlikely and is easily detected by:

- A change in breathing pattern
- The presence of breath sounds
- Condensation in the tube
- An inability to pass the tube past the level of the bronchi.

3 Once the tube is in the oesophagus it can be passed into the stomach. Minimal force should be used on the stomach tube, but slight resistance may be met as it passes through the cardia.

4 Once the tip of the tube is in the stomach, gas or fluid may be forced out of the tube as the stomach decompresses. Gently massaging the stomach can help this process. Attaching a syringe to the tube and sucking out fluid can also be successful. It is impossible to empty the stomach; the aim is to reduce its size by allowing gas and fluid to escape. Frequently, the tube clogs with hair and ingesta, in which case the procedure may have to be abandoned.

5 If the case is surgical, a stomach tube may or may not be left in place during surgery, depending on the size of the rabbit and whether or not it is providing an escape route for gas and fluid. In small rabbits, there may not be sufficient space in the pharynx for both the endotracheal tube and stomach tube without compromising the airway.

OPERATIVE TECHNIQUE 14.2:
Milking a foreign body through the small intestine

Positioning and equipment

The rabbit is positioned on its back. Restraining it in a trough will keep the midline straight.

Assistant

The procedure can be performed without an assistant.

Equipment

A standard surgical kit is required. The author's surgical kit for rabbits comprises:

- 5" Crile and Halsted straight and curved artery forceps (6 pairs)
- Martin splinter forceps
- 2 mm Debakey dissecting forceps
- 5" Adson dissecting forceps
- 5" Olsen Hegar scissors/needle-holder
- 5" straight sharp/blunt scissors
- 4.5" straight strabismus forceps
- 6" Metzenbaum scissors
- No. 9 scalpel handle.

Surgical technique

1 Laparotomy starts with a 2 cm midline incision at the umbilicus, which can be extended if necessary.

The presence of free ingesta in the abdomen indicates that gastric or intestinal rupture has already occurred and euthanasia is indicated. If it is not present, the small intestine can be located, exteriorized and followed to the site of the obstruction.

Inspection of abdominal radiographs can help to locate the obstruction. If the radiographs suggest that the obstruction is in the duodenum, it can be identified by finding the pylorus on the left side of the cranial abdomen and exteriorizing the descending section of intestine.

If the radiographs suggest the obstruction is more proximal, a loop of small intestine can be found and followed to the site of the obstruction. The intestine that is proximal to the obstruction is dilated in comparison with the intestine that is distal to the obstruction.

2 Once identified, the obstruction can be gently 'milked' along the small intestine. It is possible to push the foreign body along the whole length of the small intestine to the ileocolic valve at the entrance to the sacculus rotundus.

PRACTICAL TIP
It is important to be patient and gentle during this procedure. It is vital to handle the exteriorized intestine gently and to keep it moist by periodically dropping warm saline on to it to keep the tissue moist and lubricated.

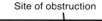
Site of obstruction
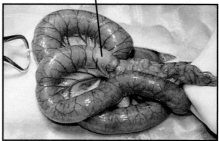
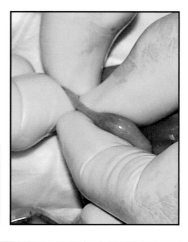

OPERATIVE TECHNIQUE 14.2 continued:
Milking a foreign body through the small intestine

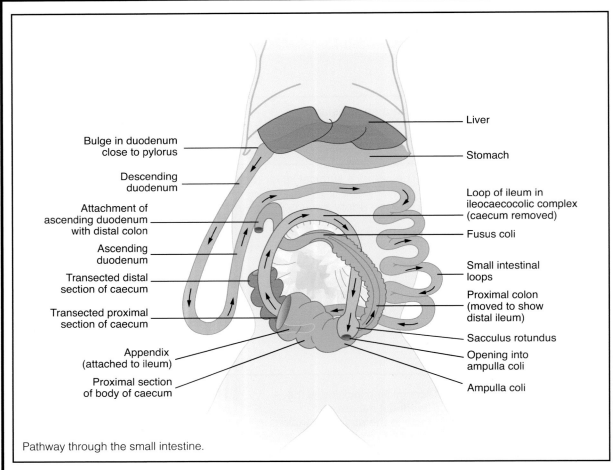

Pathway through the small intestine.

3 Distally, the small intestine is attached to other structures in the ileocaecocolic complex (see Figure 14.2)

When an intestinal foreign body is milked through the small intestine, the appendix is the first structure to be encountered.

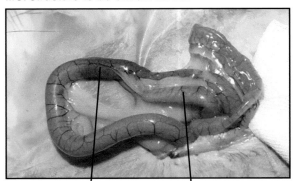

Small intestine containing foreign body   Appendix

At this point, the caecum and the proximal colon need to be exteriorized.

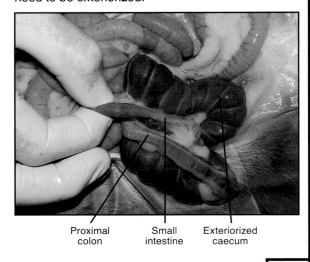

Proximal colon   Small intestine   Exteriorized caecum

OPERATIVE TECHNIQUE 14.2 continued:
Milking a foreign body through the small intestine

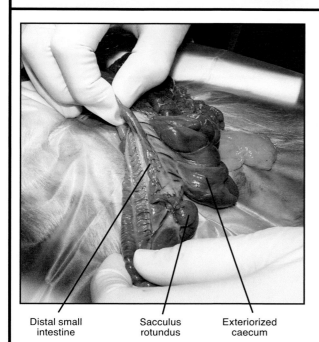

Distal small   Sacculus   Exteriorized
intestine   rotundus   caecum

4 The foreign body is gently moved along the distal part of the small intestine and squeezed through the ileocolic junction into the sacculus rotundus and then the ampulla coli. Once the foreign body is in the colon it will pass through without causing further problems.

5 The viscera can be replaced into the abdomen and the abdominal incision repaired.

Postoperative care

When surgery has been completed, the rabbit requires attentive management in a warm, quiet environment. Antibiotic cover is recommended. Fluid therapy should be maintained, taking care not to over-perfuse the patient. Aggressive prokinetic therapy is important. A prokinetic agent, such as cisapride or domperidone, can be given alongside metoclopramide to prevent paralytic ileus, which is a real risk after this procedure.

Syringe feeding immediately postoperatively poses a dilemma. Although food is necessary to prevent hepatic lipidosis, it also ferments in rabbits with paralytic ileus. The author's approach is to withhold syringe feeding immediately postoperatively and start a few hours after surgery, when the rabbit is starting to recover and the prokinetic and analgesic treatment is working. Syringe feeding may be necessary for a few days postoperatively.

Repeated doses of analgesia are very important and the rabbit should be offered food, particularly long fibre-containing food such as grass and dandelions, as soon as it recovers from anaesthesia.

15

Urinary tract surgery

Emma Keeble and Livia Benato

Urinary tract surgery can be technically demanding in rabbits due to their relatively small size and unique anatomy. Some techniques, however, such as cystotomy, are relatively common and fairly straightforward procedures. Thorough knowledge of rabbit anatomy, especially compared with that of more commonly seen species such as cats and dogs, is essential to avoid potential complications and achieve a successful outcome. This chapter will outline rabbit urinary tract anatomy, general surgical principles of urinary tract surgery and patient evaluation, and will detail surgical techniques and approaches to the urinary tract in the rabbit.

Anatomy of the urinary tract

Although the urinary tract of the rabbit (Figure 15.1) is similar to that of other small mammals, it has several unique features which need to be taken into consideration when undertaking urinary tract surgery.

The kidneys

Rabbit kidneys are bean-shaped with a smooth surface and are dark red in colour (Figure 15.2). They are found in the dorsal thoracolumbar area of the abdominal cavity on each side of the vertebral column, with the right kidney placed more cranially than the left. They are retroperitoneal and slightly mobile. The right kidney is slightly larger than the left kidney (Eken *et al.*, 2009).

The right kidney is positioned at the level of the 1st lumbar vertebra (Hristov *et al.*, 2006). The cranial pole of the right kidney is adjacent to the liver, while the caudal pole is adjacent to the right ovary and the duodenum. The right adrenal gland, the vena cava and the abdominal aorta are positioned on the medial aspect of the right kidney (Figure 15.3). The ventral surface of the kidney is adjacent to intestinal loops and the caecum. The left kidney is positioned between the 2nd and the 4th lumbar vertebrae (Hristov *et al.*, 2006). The cranial pole of the left kidney is adjacent to the stomach and spleen, while the caudal pole is adjacent to the left ovary. The left adrenal gland, the vena cava and the abdominal aorta are positioned on the medial aspect of the left kidney. The ventral surface of the kidney is adjacent to the pancreas, jejunum and colon.

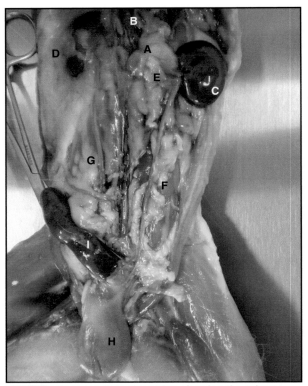

15.1 Post-mortem dissection showing the urinary tract of a rabbit. Notice the left kidney is free of its peritoneal attachment. A = left adrenal gland; B = right adrenal gland; C = left kidney; D = right kidney; E = left renal vessels; F = left ureter; G = right ureter; H = bladder; I = distal colon.

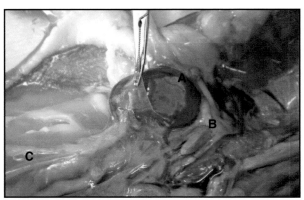

15.2 Post-mortem dissection showing the retroperitoneal attachment of the kidney (A). It also shows the anatomical position of the kidney in relation to the adrenal gland (B) and ureter (C).

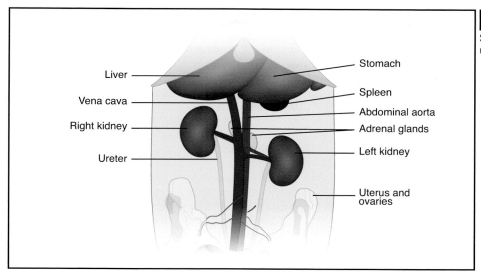

Schematic diagram of the upper urinary tract.

The kidneys are covered by a fibrous capsule that continues into the renal pelvis. On the medial border there is a mild depression called the hilum, where the vessels and ureter enter the kidney. The hilum then leads to the renal pelvis, inside the kidney. Rabbits have unipapillate kidneys (Figure 15.4). Renal parenchyma is divided into the cortex and medulla. The cortex is darker red in colour and contains the renal corpuscles, while the medulla is divided into outer and inner layers. The inner medulla projects inside the renal pelvis or calyx with only one papilla at the vertex of the renal pyramid. The renal artery, a branch of the abdominal aorta, enters the renal pelvis. The renal vein and ureter leave the renal pelvis and the renal vein then enters the caudal vena cava.

runs either side of the vertebral column and ends in the neck of the urinary bladder. Ureters are intimately attached to the lumbar muscles and covered and protected by the parietal peritoneum. The caudal ureteral artery, a branch of the vesicular artery, and the cranial ureteral artery, a branch of the renal artery, supply the distal and proximal ureter, respectively. The middle portion of the ureter has no external blood supply (Douglas and Hossler, 1995). Urine is moved from the kidney to the bladder by ureteral peristaltic contractions. Peristalsis starts

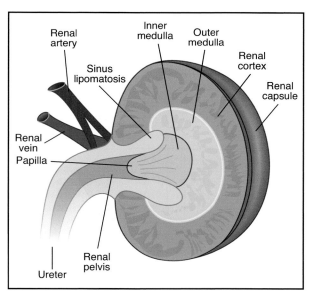

15.4 Diagrammatic representation of a cross-section through the rabbit unipapillate kidney.

The ureters

Ureters are smooth muscular tubes that convey urine from each kidney to the bladder (Figure 15.5). The ureter is a continuation of the renal pelvis that

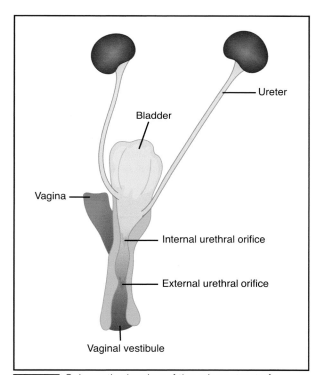

15.5 Schematic drawing of the urinary tract of a female rabbit (ventral view); the bladder and urethra have been opened to show the internal structure. The ureters run over the dorsal surface of the bladder and open level with each other into the neck of the bladder. The distal urethra opens into the vagina, approximately half way along the latter at the external urethral orifice.

in the renal pelvis, with the pacemaker being in the kidney, between the cortex and medulla (Dwyer and Schmidt-Nielsen, 2003).

The bladder
The urinary bladder (see Figures 15.1 and 15.5) is a muscular sac that stores urine. It is situated midline in the ventral caudal aspect of the abdominal cavity, ventral to the distal colon, and also the genital tract in the female rabbit. The wall is thin, elastic and easily distensible. Bladder capacity in a 4 kg rabbit is up to 60 ml of urine. The rabbit urinary bladder is divided into three parts: the apex, the body and the neck. The neck then continues as the urethra. The median ligament of the bladder runs along the ventral aspect of the body. Left and right vesicular branches of the internal and external iliac arteries and veins supply blood to the urinary bladder (Hossler and Monson, 1995). Contractions of the detrusor muscle empty the bladder.

The urethra
The urethra is a tubular smooth muscle structure that is the anatomical continuation of the neck of the bladder. The bladder and the urethra are divided by the internal urethral orifice, a smooth muscle sphincter. Urethral anatomy differs between the two sexes. In the male, the urethra starts from the internal urethral orifice of the bladder, runs along the pelvic floor and ends with the external urethral orifice at the tip of the penis (penile urethra); pudendal vessels and nerves supply the penile urethra. In the female rabbit the urethra is very short: it starts from the internal urethral orifice of the bladder and ends at the external urethral orifice in the floor of the vaginal vestibule, at the proximal end of the vagina (see Figure 15.5).

Patient assessment and decision-making

Urinary tract disease is common in rabbits. It may present acutely as a surgical emergency, or as a chronic condition.

Fluid therapy and preoperative care
Initial therapy, consisting of fluid replacement, analgesia, gastrointestinal motility drugs and provision of a high-fibre diet (see Chapter 1), and patient stabilization are paramount, prior to further diagnostic tests. It is essential to hospitalize the sick rabbit in a quiet area away from barking dogs and the smell of cats, to reduce external stressors and allow the rabbit to express normal behaviour.

Rabbits in acute renal failure should receive fluid therapy, aimed at correcting dehydration and increasing perfusion and diuresis to correct azotaemia and electrolyte and acid–base imbalances. Tubular regeneration can occur within 3 days with appropriate case management. In mild cases rehydration with 0.9% saline solution or Hartmann's solution is effective to correct mild metabolic acidosis or hyperkalaemia. Hartmann's, however, is contraindicated in cases with severe renal failure.

Urine production should be monitored carefully, and ideally measured, to assess the effects of fluid therapy. Creatinine clearance rate should be recorded so that the glomerular filtration rate can be estimated. Once hydration has been achieved and the rabbit is producing a good volume of urine, biochemistry should be repeated. At this stage fluids should be changed to those with a lower sodium content. Once biochemistry values are normal, fluid therapy should be reduced by 50% each day in order to avoid medullary washout. The authors usually administer fluids subcutaneously or intravenously prior to ultrasonography to ensure that the bladder is filled with urine and therefore easier to image.

History-taking and examination
A complete clinical history should be obtained and physical examination carried out. On physical examination the kidneys and bladder are generally easy to palpate, although in obese rabbits the kidneys may be difficult to evaluate due to the excessive amount of perirenal fat. Clinical signs and differential diagnoses for urinary tract disease in rabbits are outlined in Figure 15.6.

Disease process	Clinical signs	Differential diagnoses	Diagnostic tests and findings
Acute renal failure; pre-renal – dehydration, shock; renal – glomerular nephritis, tubular damage, interstitial renal disease, e.g. *Encephalitozoon cuniculi*; post-renal obstruction	Anorexia; lethargy; dehydration; bruxism; intestinal ileus	Dental disease; systemic disease; hepatic lipidosis; intestinal disorders; pyometra	Increased BUN (<35.7 mmol/l in pre-renal azotaemia); increased creatinine; no polydipsia/polyuria, weight loss or anaemia; isosthenuria, oliguria; metabolic acidosis; hyperkalaemia; radiography and ultrasonography to assess kidney size (enlarged and swollen)
Chronic renal failure; renal calculi; *E. cuniculi*; renal fibrosis; amyloidosis; pyelonephritis	Weight loss; polydipsia; polyuria; poor body condition; anaemia; occasional haematuria; reduced appetite; intestinal ileus	Any chronic systemic disease process; dental disease	BUN/creatinine elevated in severe disease; hypercalcaemia, hyperphosphataemia and osteosclorosis; increased UPC ratio; non-regenerative anaemia; isosthenuria (specific gravity 1.010–1.015); small irregular kidneys on palpation/ultrasonography/radiography; *E. cuniculi* serology; systemic hypertension

15.6 Clinical signs, differential diagnoses and diagnostic findings associated with urinary tract disease in the rabbit. BUN = blood urea nitrogen; UPC = urine protein:creatinine ratio. (continues)

Disease process	Clinical signs	Differential diagnoses	Diagnostic tests and findings
Urolithiasis/hypercalciuria	Hunched posture; teeth grinding; urine scald perineum; urinary incontinence; haematuria; dysuria; intestinal ileus	Severe intestinal ileus	BUN/creatinine may be elevated; radiography/ultrasonography to diagnose; bladder may be small and painful on palpation, or large with doughy material palpable in the lumen; urinalysis and culture – crystalluria, haematuria, proteinuria, bacteria may be present
Renal calculi	Teeth grinding; weight loss; polyuria; polydipsia; intestinal ileus	Any chronic systemic disease process; dental disease; chronic renal failure	BUN/creatinine usually elevated; radiography/ultrasonography to diagnose
Cystitis (bacterial, fungal, calculi, hypercalciuria)	Urinary scalding of perineum; urinary incontinence; dysuria; haematuria; hunched posture; vocalization on urination	Uterine adenocarcinoma; prostatic disease	Urinalysis – culture and cytology; ultrasonography and radiography
Calculi, bladder polyps, neoplasia (bladder/urethra), urethral stricture urethritis	Urinary incontinence (partial outflow obstruction) – dysuria, stranguria, urine dribbling, haematuria	*E. cuniculi* infection; uterine adenocarcinoma; uterine stump neoplasia/abscess	Radiography to assess bladder size and position; ultrasonography to look for polyps/neoplasia; *E. cuniculi* serology

15.6 (continued) Clinical signs, differential diagnoses and diagnostic findings associated with urinary tract disease in the rabbit. BUN = blood urea nitrogen; UPC = urine protein:creatinine ratio.

Laboratory tests

A serum chemistry profile, full haematology, urinalysis and culture, and urine protein:creatinine ratio (UPC) determination constitute a minimum database for each patient (Figure 15.7). Further specific diagnostic tests that may be performed on a case-by-case basis are outlined in Figure 15.8.

Full serum biochemistry and haematology are required to assess renal function prior to surgery (Figure 15.9; Harcourt-Brown, 2013). In the authors' experience, serum creatinine and blood urea nitrogen (BUN) values may be normal in mild cases, despite renal disease, and elevated UPC values are more useful for assessing renal function. A normal reference range of 0.11–0.40 has been reported for UPC in the rabbit (Reusch et al., 2009). In some cases UPC values are normal but an intravenous urogram (IVU) may reveal a reduced glomerular filtration rate of the contrast material, indicating reduced renal function. Renal biopsy for histopathological examination may be indicated in these cases if other causes have been ruled out.

Parameter	Normal findings	Comments
Urine volume	130 ml/kg per day	Urination usually sporadic in large volumes
Specific gravity	1.003–1.036	Ability to concentrate urine is useful in assessing renal function
Average pH	8.2	Sample must be freshly tested as bacteria can alter pH; can drop to 6 in anorexic rabbits
Crystals	Ammonium magnesium phosphate; calcium carbonate; calcium oxalate	Presence of large amounts of crystals in rabbit urine is not indicative of urinary tract disease
Casts, epithelial cells or bacteria	Absent to rare	If negative for bacteria does not rule out an infection; *Staphylococcus*, *Klebsiella* and *Pseudomonas* most common isolates; casts are rare in rabbits due to dissolution in alkaline urine
Leucocytes or erythrocytes	Occasionally present	Leucocytes indicate inflammation of the urinary tract; erythrocytes indicate inflammation or haemorrhage of the urogenital tract
Albumin	Occasionally present (especially in young rabbits)	If elevated may indicate renal damage, particularly if urine is dilute; check protein:creatinine ratio (UPC) and sediment analysis; can be renal or post-renal in origin
Glucose	Trace may be present	Increased if stressed
Ketones	Negative	May be found in anorexic rabbits

15.7 Reference ranges for routine urinalysis in the rabbit.

Diagnostic test	Comments
Plain radiography	Dorsoventral and lateral abdominal views useful for identification of uroliths and hypercalciuria, assessment of renal size and shape, position and shape of urinary bladder, soft tissue mineralization, osteosclerosis
Contrast radiography	Intravenous urogram; positive-, double- and negative-contrast cystogram; retrograde urethrocystogram
Ultrasonographic examination (see also Chapter 8)	Useful for assessment of kidneys, ureters, bladder and proximal urethra; uroliths, renal architecture, hydronephrosis, hydroureter, bladder wall thickening/masses, and hypercalciuria may all be assessed
Cystoscopy	Assessment of the bladder and urethra for disease in the female rabbit (e.g. small polyps); bladder wall mucosal biopsy possible with this technique
Computed tomography	Useful as an adjunct to other imaging modalities for complete assessment of the urinary tract, in particular bladder/uterine stump masses; intravenous contrast material may be used to assess renal filtration rates and ureteral obstruction

15.8 Further diagnostic tests for urinary tract disease evaluation in the rabbit.

Parameter	Reference range	Comments
Blood urea nitrogen (BUN)	10.1–17.1 mmol/l	Serum values affected by hydration status, dietary protein levels, liver function and intestinal absorption of nitrogen. Pre-renal elevation: may only be mildly elevated; secondary to cardiac disease, shock, dehydration, gastrointestinal haemorrhage; concurrent increased urine specific gravity. Renal elevation: usually greatly elevated; indicates damage to renal parenchyma and glomeruli; urine isosthenuric or dilute; indicates >75% loss of renal function if elevated. Post-renal elevation: urinary tract obstruction
Creatinine	74–171 μmol/l	Excreted by glomerular filtration; elevations can be pre-renal, renal or post-renal in origin; indicates >75% loss of renal function if elevated due to renal disease; measure urine specific gravity
Inorganic phosphate	1.0–2.2 mmol/l	Indirect glomerular filtration rate measurement as undergoes glomerular filtration and tubular reabsorption; elevated indicates reduced renal clearance, increased intestinal absorption, haemolysis, dehydration, increased vitamin D, nutritional secondary hyperparathyroidism
Total calcium	2.2–3.9 mmol/l	May be reduced in acute renal failure; variable with chronic renal failure, although in advanced chronic cases both calcium and phosphorus levels are typically elevated and this is a poor prognostic indicator
Ionized calcium	1.57–1.83 mmol/l	May be elevated in chronic renal failure associated with impaired calcium excretion
Potassium	3.3–5.7 mmol/l	May be elevated (acute renal failure, post-renal obstruction) or decreased with renal disease
Red blood cell count	$5.1–7.6 \times 10^{12}$/l	Chronic renal disease is associated with non-regenerative anaemia in rabbits

15.9 Biochemical and haematological assessment of renal disease in the rabbit.

Imaging

Radiographic and ultrasonographic examinations are the diagnostic methods of choice for evaluation of the urinary tract. The kidneys and bladder are generally easy to visualize radiographically. The ureters and urethra are more challenging, unless obvious pathology is present, such as hypercalciuria, urinary calculi or pathological enlargement. On ultrasound examination, both the upper and lower urinary tract are easy to follow and evaluate, unless a large amount of gas or ingesta in the gastrointestinal tract impedes visualization.

Radiography

Radiography is a useful tool for diagnosis of urinary tract disease (Harcourt-Brown, 2007; see also Chapter 7). Kidney size, shape and position can be assessed easily, with an average kidney size being 1.4–2.2 times the length of the second lumbar vertebra. Renal calculi are easily seen and are relatively common in the authors' experience. Calculi involving the ureters, bladder and urethra may also be seen radiographically.

Bladder position, size and content should also be assessed. Small amounts of radiodense material are normal findings in the bladder in rabbits and are associated with the presence of calcium carbonate crystals. The distinction between a bladder calculus and hypercalciuria may not always be obvious radiographically. In this case, ultrasound examination of the bladder will reveal an acoustic shadow if a calculus is present, whereas points of echogenic reflections, a 'snow storm' effect, will be seen if crystals only are present. Alternatively, gentle palpation of the bladder should alter the shape and formation of the bladder content on repeat radiography of the abdomen if crystals are present.

Contrast studies: Meglumine may be used for positive-contrast retrograde bladder cystography following placement of a urinary catheter. Negative-contrast studies (using air to create a pneumocystogram) of the bladder are performed following sedation and urinary catheterization. Midazolam may be used to help relax the urethralis muscle before 5–8 ml/kg of air is introduced via the catheter into the bladder.

Contrast studies are useful to help identify soft tissue structures within the bladder or urethral lumen and determine bladder wall thickness. Double-contrast studies can also be performed by administering 2 ml/kg iodinated contrast agent via the urinary catheter after air placement (Figure 15.10). Double-contrast studies are particularly useful to delineate the bladder wall if irregular or ulcerative lesions are suspected, e.g. in cases of bladder neoplasia.

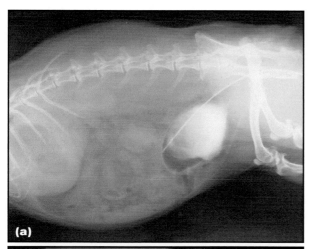

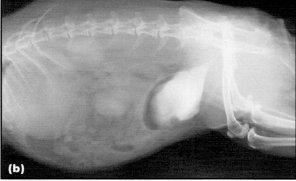

15.10 **(a)** Right lateral abdominal retrograde double-contrast cystogram in a 5-year-old male rabbit with hypercalciuria (16 ml air instilled via urinary catheter plus 2 ml Omnipaque). **(b)** Right lateral abdominal radiograph of the same rabbit using intravenous urography (4 ml Omnipaque), which revealed no obvious abnormalities of the kidneys or ureters. Contrast material can be clearly seen delineating both ureters 15 minutes after injection.

Further evaluation of the urinary tract is possible using excretory urography. An iodinated contrast medium is injected intravenously or intraosseously during radiographic examination (Porzio *et al.*, 2001); within minutes this enhances and defines the subgross anatomy of the urinary tract, from the renal pelvis to the urinary bladder. The size, shape and position of the kidneys and ureters can be determined, and the technique can also be used to help evaluate renal function. Excretory urography is also useful for examining the upper urinary tract for masses, obstructions or calculi, although ultrasonography is a less invasive imaging technique that can be used in these cases. Excretory urography

is particularly useful in cases of suspected ureteral, bladder or urethral rupture. The procedure is described in Chapter 3.

Ultrasonography
Ultrasonography of the urinary tract is an extremely useful diagnostic tool in rabbits; the technique is similar to that used in cats and dogs. Care should be taken that the rabbit does not become hypothermic if sedation is used or large areas are clipped. A 5 or 7.5 MHz sector scanner may be used. Animals that are used to being handled should tolerate this technique for short periods without sedation. More fractious animals or more invasive diagnostic ultrasound-guided sampling techniques (e.g. ultrasound-guided cystocentesis) may require sedation.

Diagnosis of hydronephrosis, hydroureter, renal cysts, renal calculi and differentiation between cystic calculi and hypercalciuria, are possible using ultrasonography. Renal size and shape can be assessed as well as the relative ratio of cortex to medulla (see also Chapter 8). The average kidney size in dwarf rabbits <2 kg is: length 22–36 mm, width 10.5–17 mm and height 12–20 mm. The size of renal papillae can also be assessed and the presence of calculi determined.

Small irregular kidneys are often seen in association with chronic damage secondary to *Encephalitozoon cuniculi* infection. There is typically a loss of boundary between the cortex and medulla or a thinning of the cortex in these cases (Figure 15.11). Bladder wall thickness may also be measured (Figure 15.12) and, if grossly thickened, measurements may be used for more long-term monitoring. The bladder needs to be full for this procedure.

Structures associated with the bladder neck may also be assessed, such as the uterus in entire females, the uterine stump in spayed animals and the prostate in males. Urethral calculi are more difficult to image using ultrasound, as the urethra passes into the pelvic area. Assessment of the urethra is best performed endoscopically in female rabbits (see Chapter 10) or using contrast radiography techniques (see above). Exploratory laparotomy may be required (see Chapter 13).

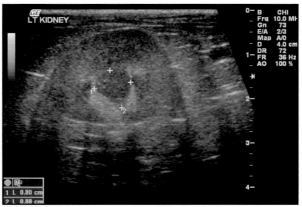

15.11 Transverse section ultrasound examination of the left kidney of a rabbit, showing slight dilation of the renal pelvis and mild mineralization of the renal crest.

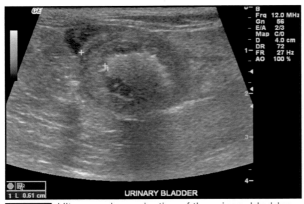

15.12 Ultrasound examination of the urinary bladder of a rabbit, showing a measurable wall thickness of 0.61 cm due to chronic inflammation.

Hypercalciuria and urolithiasis

These are the most common urinary tract disorders seen in pet rabbits in the authors' experience. Predisposing factors are outlined in Figure 15.13. Underlying causes should be investigated by careful history-taking, full clinical examination and further

Predisposing factor	Comments
Obesity	Animal often sedentary and retaining urine
Lack of exercise	Small cages may make urination difficult, so rabbit is less likely to urinate frequently or mark territory
Low fluid intake	Provide water in a bottle and a bowl; wet hay prior to feeding
Pododermatitis	Difficulty in adopting normal stance for urination; diagnose on clinical examination
Skeletal abnormalities, e.g. arthritis, hip dysplasia, vertebral spondylosis or scoliosis of the spine-	Difficulty in adopting normal stance for urination; urination may be painful due to posture adopted; less likely to urinate frequently. Diagnose on clinical and radiographic examination
Lack of behavioural stimuli	Neutered rabbits are less likely to mark territory with urine and so void urine less frequently; solitary animals are also less likely to mark their territory
Urinary incontinence due to e.g. neurogenic (upper or lower motor neuron) disorders, reflex dyssynergia, *E. cuniculi*, *Toxoplasma*, spinal luxation/fracture; paradoxical incontinence due to outflow obstruction (urethral calculi, neoplasia, polyps, inflammation, stricture formation, prostate disease)	Normal urine voiding does not occur and crystals accumulate in the bladder

15.13 Factors predisposing to the development of urinary tract calculi and hypercalciuria in the rabbit.

diagnostic investigations (such as radiography of the vertebral column and joints), in cases of urolithiasis and/or hypercalciuria.

Hypercalciuria
Normal rabbit urine is turbid and contains crystals, primarily calcium carbonate, but also ammonium magnesium phosphate and calcium oxalate (see Figure 15.7 for normal urinalysis in the rabbit). It is important to differentiate between normal urine-containing crystals and hypercalciuria or 'sludgy' urine. The latter is associated with clinical signs such as dysuria and straining: small amounts of urine may be passed with increased frequency. Rabbits may be depressed, adopt a hunched posture and be anorexic, with secondary intestinal ileus. A large intra-abdominal bladder is often found on examination, during which the rabbit resents palpation. Perineal scalding and urinary incontinence are commonly associated. Urine sediment analysis reveals large numbers of crystals, red cells and inflammatory cells, with or without bacterial infection, as a secondary cystitis develops. Radiography shows radiodense material in the bladder (Figure 15.14); ultrasonography may be used to assess bladder-wall thickness and rule out calculi (Figure 15.15).

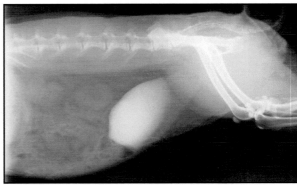

15.14 Lateral abdominal radiograph showing an abnormal accumulation of radiodense material within the rabbit's bladder, consistent with hypercalciuria.

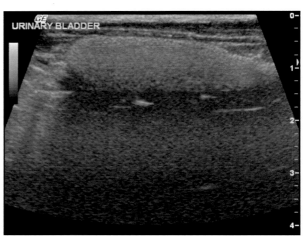

15.15 Ultrasound scan of the urinary bladder of a rabbit with hypercalciuria. Note the large amount of hyperechoic material (with associated acoustic shadow) filling the urinary bladder and proximal urethra. The bladder wall is not obviously thickened in this case.

Treatment should aim at first correcting any identified underlying causes. Secondary urine scalding of the perineum should be managed by clipping and bathing the affected area with dilute chlorhexidine and application of topical barrier or antibiotic creams. The rabbit should be sedated and a urinary catheter passed via the urethra and into the bladder for flushing with warm sterile saline. This process should be repeated until the aspirate is clear and radiodense material is no longer evident radiographically. In the authors' experience, cystotomy may be required in extreme cases if crystal deposits are too viscous and adherent to the bladder lining to achieve a resolution with flushing. Long-term analgesia is indicated in these cases and the authors typically prescribe oral meloxicam at 0.6 mg/kg q12h as long as renal function is normal.

Pre- and postoperative opiate analgesia should also be given (e.g. buprenorphine 0.05 mg/kg s.c. or i.v. q6–8h). Systemic antibiotics are usually indicated to treat secondary bladder and skin infections. These should be based on results of culture and sensitivity testing. Diuresis pre- and postoperatively is essential, with a combination of intravenous, subcutaneous and oral fluids.

The rabbit should be encouraged to increase its fluid intake, for example by wetting hay, increasing consumption of plant food with diuretic qualities (plantain, dandelion, goosegrass), offering fresh grass and providing water in a bowl as well as a bottle. The rabbit should be provided with the opportunity to exercise daily in order to encourage normal urination habits. A good quality high-fibre diet should be offered, consisting primarily of fresh grass and hay. A small amount of concentrates (the authors recommend 1 tablespoon maximum daily) and vegetables containing a moderate amount of calcium may also be offered. High-calcium items such as watercress, kale, Swiss chard, clover, alfalfa hay and broccoli should be avoided.

The rabbit should be monitored carefully for recurrence of the condition and regular repeat examinations and abdominal radiographs/ultrasonographic examinations of the bladder should be performed. The authors typically monitor cases every 3 months initially.

Urolithiasis

Calculi form commonly in rabbits since excess dietary calcium is absorbed from the intestine, resulting in variably high blood calcium levels. This process is not directly dependent on vitamin D. Calcium metabolism is regulated by the kidneys with excretion of excess calcium via the urine. Fractional excretion of calcium in rabbits is 45–60% compared with <2% in most mammals. Obese animals and those with low water consumption and/or limited exercise opportunities are predisposed to stone formation. Bacterial infection may also be present and sterile urine samples should be obtained for culture and sensitivity testing. Animals with restricted water intake, cystitis, urine retention problems or obstructions to urine flow (e.g. neoplasia, adhesions, abscesses, strictures, hypercalciuria) are also predisposed to stone formation.

Calculi may occur at any point along the urinary tract. If there is total blockage this constitutes an emergency since renal failure, hydronephrosis, hydroureter or bladder distension may result, with life-threatening consequences.

For small urethral calculi the rabbit can be sedated, catheterized and the stone flushed back into the bladder (retrograde urohydropulsion) prior to performing a cystotomy. Opiate and non-steroidal anti-inflammatory drugs (NSAIDs) should be provided for analgesia. Urination should be monitored following treatment. Calculi can recur and the rabbit should be regularly monitored using radiography and ultrasound examination. General dietary advice on provision of a good quality hay/grass-based diet and reduction in concentrates, regular exercise, weight reduction and increased fluid intake (wetting of hay and greens and provision of a water bowl) should be given to the owner.

Cystic calculi and hypercalciuria are often associated with urine retention disorders in the rabbit. This leads to inadequate voiding of urine, build-up of large amounts of crystals within the bladder and secondary lower urinary tract disease. Urine retention may be pathological or behavioural in origin.

Surgical removal of urinary tract calculi is discussed later in this chapter. The prognosis for bilateral renal calculi is poor long term, and surgery in this instance is not recommended since there is a high chance of post-nephrotomy complications and renal failure.

Lower urinary tract disease

Rabbits with lower urinary tract disease present with reduced appetite, lethargy, teeth grinding, dysuria, oliguria or anuria. Weight loss and intestinal ileus may also be present. Thorough patient evaluation is essential prior to surgery to determine the extent of the disease process and the suitability of the rabbit to undergo anaesthesia and surgery. It is also important to rule out other differential diagnoses which may present with similar clinical signs, such as dental disease (see Figure 15.6).

Urethral obstruction
It can be difficult to determine whether a rabbit has a complete urinary tract obstruction, since rabbits do not usually vocalize and the process of urination is less obvious than in cats and dogs. An observant owner may realize that the rabbit is straining but unable to pass urine, and if the rabbit is trained to use a litter tray this is much easier to determine. However, cystitis and hypercalciuria may also present with dysuria, and a partial urethral obstruction may still allow for small amounts of urine to be voided.

Urethral obstructions are more common in males and are usually associated with a urinary calculus, although other causes include strictures, inflammation or neoplasia. In the authors' experience calculi are most commonly found lodged at the distal urethral opening in male rabbits. A distended bladder may be palpable. If the rabbit is straining to urinate and no urine is voided this should alert the veterinary surgeon to the possibility of an obstruction and immediate diagnostic evaluations should be performed (radiography, ultrasonography, serum biochemistry, haematology). Aggressive fluid therapy is contraindicated until the blockage is removed. The bladder should be drained by cystocentesis if distended. Upper urinary tract obstructions (involving the renal pelvis or ureters), if unilateral, are usually less of an emergency as the contralateral kidney may compensate.

Medical management of urinary tract disease

There is a real lack of published, referenced and peer-reviewed data on the use of drugs in medical management of urinary tract disease in the rabbit. Much of the information in the literature is extrapolated from other species or is anecdotal. This makes it hard for the veterinary surgeon in practice to make an informed choice as to the most appropriate and effective therapeutic treatment in each case. The authors have attempted to summarize the information available and to indicate where this information is anecdotal or referenced.

- *N*-Acetylglucosamine is a nutraceutical that has anecdotally been reported as being beneficial in rabbits with cystitis or hypercalciuria/bladder calculi. It is proposed that it stimulates glycosaminoglycan formation, which aids in repair of the bladder uroepithelium (Gunn-Moore and Shenoy, 2004). Dose rates are extrapolated from feline medicine and are anecdotal ('Cystease' 125 mg capsules, ½ capsule per 2.5 kg rabbit daily for 14 days, then every other day, long-term if required).
- Injectable pentosan polysulphate has been reported to have no effect in treating feline idiopathic cystitis (Wallius and Tidholm, 2009) and, although the authors know of anecdotal reports of its use in rabbit hypercalciuria and cystitis cases, its use cannot be recommended due to a lack of data on its efficacy in this species.
- Omega-3 fatty acid supplements (flax seed and flax oil) have been shown experimentally in rats to reduce glomerular injury and slow down the progression of renal disease due to their anti-inflammatory and anti-atherogenic properties (Ingram *et al.*, 1995). There are no reports of their use in the rabbit or whether the addition of oil to the diet of a rabbit would have potential gastrointestinal and systemic side effects. This is an area in which further research is required.
- Potassium citrate is an alkalinizing salt that prevents calculi formation as it binds calcium and reduces ion activity, and so prevents calcium oxalate crystal formation. There is some debate as to its efficacy in rabbits where the urine pH is typically already alkaline. A dose rate of 33 mg/kg orally q12h has been anecdotally reported (Lightfoot, 2011). Care should be taken

when administering potassium to rabbits as side effects may occur with overdosage, and blood potassium levels should be closely monitored. It should not be used in rabbits with renal impairment or cardiac disease.
- Diuretics such as hydrochlorothiazide (a thiazide diuretic which inhibits resorption of sodium and causes secretion of potassium) may be of use in the prevention of urolithiasis and treatment of hypercalciuria. One of its uses in human medicine is in the treatment of hypercalciuria, as it is a calcium-sparing diuretic, reducing urinary calcium. Its use is anecdotally reported in the rabbit at a dose rate of 2 mg/kg orally q12h (extrapolated from feline medicine). Side effects include hyperglycaemia, hypercalcaemia, hypokalaemia, hyponatraemia and volume reduction. It is contraindicated in rabbits with renal disease as it reduces renal blood flow.
- Drugs to relieve urethral spasm such as dantrolene (0.5 mg/kg orally q12h) and prazosin (0.25 mg/rabbit orally q12h) may be beneficial in specific cases. Both these dose rates are extrapolated from feline medicine and the use of these drugs in rabbits is anecdotally reported. Potential side effects include hypotension, weakness and liver impairment.

Surgical considerations and specialist equipment

The basic principles of veterinary surgery described for other domestic species are applicable to rabbits. Surgical techniques and other considerations, however, may need to be modified to account for the unique anatomy, physiology and behaviour of the rabbit (see Chapter 11).

Rabbits can be challenging surgical patients but the chance of a successful outcome can be maximized by ensuring a good knowledge of regional anatomy, adequate patient preparation and suitable instrumentation. Pain, fear and stress should be kept to a minimum at all stages.

Equipment and tissue handling
A Lone Star veterinary retractor can be used to provide increased exposure to the abdomen in rabbits. Haemostatic clips are extremely useful where ligature placement is difficult due to poor surgical field exposure or small vessel size. Handling of tissues should be kept to a minimum to reduce the risk of adhesions; the use of sterile moistened cotton-tip applicators to handle and move organs out of the surgical field aids this process. Magnification and good illumination are essential for most of the procedures described in this chapter.

Suture materials
Suture material reactions are more common in rabbits than in some other species because of the response of the rabbit immune system to foreign material, with production of caseous pus, and a tendency to form adhesions. In rabbits, but not in cats

and dogs, formation of calculi commonly occurs along the suture line following cystotomy. These concretions were observed to resolve at 7 days after surgery if absorbable suture materials were used (Kaminski *et al.*, 1978). A further study concluded that the persistence of suture line calculi was dependent on the longevity of the suture material (Morris *et al.*, 1986).

Studies have been carried out to evaluate different suture materials for cystotomy closure in rabbits, their relative inflammatory response, formation of encrustations and healing time. Results indicated that reduced suture strength and use of suture material that is more rapidly absorbed are less likely to lead to post-cystotomy suture reactions and encrustations. Polyglactin 910 (e.g. Vicryl) provided sufficient firmness and was superior to other tested suture materials with regard to foreign-body reaction and inclination to encrustation. A thinner thread is recommended for sutures in the efferent urinary tract, such as poliglecaprone 25 (e.g. Monocryl) or polyglactin 910, as the bladder wall has usually healed by 3 days after surgery (Hanke *et al.*, 1994). The use of absorbable suture material in rabbit urinary tract surgery is therefore recommended; the present authors routinely use 1.5 metric (4/0 USP) suture material for cystotomy. It should be borne in mind, however, that while hydrolytically degraded suture materials may cause less reaction, the sutures may be weaker.

The authors prefer to use an intradermal suture pattern to close skin wounds, as rabbits are fastidious at grooming and commonly chew external sutures and remove dressings.

Surgical procedures

Kidney

Renal biopsy

Indications: Renal biopsy is generally performed in order to enable a diagnosis and determine the prognosis. Biopsy is indicated in cases of nephropathy,

kidney failure and renal tumours or masses. Although the technique described here is via laparotomy, in some instances it may be preferable to perform renal biopsy percutaneously with ultrasound guidance or via laparoscopy.

Approach: The rabbit is placed in dorsal recumbency and is surgically prepared from the sternum to the pelvis as for exploratory laparotomy. A midline incision is made from the sternum to the umbilicus and retractors are placed in order to improve visibility during the surgical procedure. The intestinal tract is gently removed and protected using abdominal swabs while the urinary tract is exposed. In obese rabbits, the perirenal fat can impede the visualization of the kidneys. Both kidneys should be sampled if systemic disease is suspected.

Technique:

1. The kidney is freed from the parietal peritoneum by blunt dissection and is then gently held between two fingers.
2. The greater curvature is exposed and a No. 15 scalpel blade is used to make two incisions at 60 degree angles in the cortical parenchyma to create a wedge (Figure 15.16a). The sample is then removed and the incision is closed with a simple interrupted suture pattern using 2 metric (3/0 USP) absorbable suture material.
3. If a smaller sample is needed, needle biopsy can be performed using a Tru-cut instrument (Figure 15.16b).
4. Haemorrhage is stopped by applying pressure using a finger, a swab or a sterile moistened cotton-tipped applicator.

Potential complications: Potential complications include postoperative bleeding, haematuria, leakage of urine (if a very large sample has been removed), peritonitis (where infection is present), excessive damage of the renal parenchyma and localized pain. Fluid therapy is advised during the surgical procedure in order to prevent obstruction of the urinary flow.

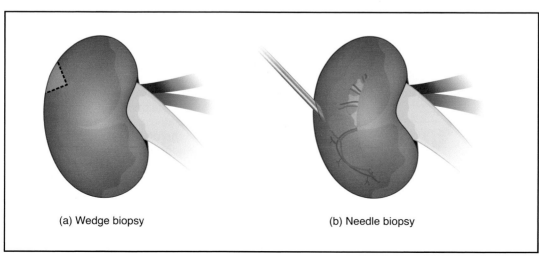

(a) Wedge biopsy   (b) Needle biopsy

15.16 Renal biopsy can be performed by removing a wedge of parenchyma or using a needle.

Nephrotomy

Indications: Nephrotomy is generally indicated for the extraction of calculi from the renal pelvis. It is also advised in cases of neoplasia, abscesses and bleeding within the renal pelvis. It is performed in uncontrolled and progressive conditions where the animal is deteriorating and medical management is not sufficient to control the clinical signs. It is not advised where there is advanced hydronephrosis, since the renal parenchyma is already damaged. In this case, the cause of the hydronephrosis should be addressed or, if the renal parenchyma is severely damaged, the kidney should be removed (see Nephrectomy, later).

Nephrotomy can reduce renal function by 30–50%. For this reason, it is important to evaluate kidney function fully prior to surgery, to confirm that no damage to the renal parenchyma has occurred. Kidney function can be evaluated by blood biochemistry, urinalysis, ultrasonography and IVU.

Approach: The anaesthetized rabbit is placed in dorsal recumbency and surgically prepared from the sternum to the pelvis as for exploratory laparotomy (see Operative Technique 13.1). A midline incision from the sternum to the umbilicus is made and retractors are placed in order to improve visibility during the surgical procedure. The intestinal tract is gently elevated out of the surgical view and protected using moistened abdominal swabs while the urinary tract is exposed. In obese rabbits, the perirenal fat can impede visualization of the kidneys; in this case, careful blunt dissection of the perirenal fat allows better visualization.

Recently, nephrotomy via a lateral approach has been reported (Martorell *et al.*, 2012). Those authors performed a laparotomy via a 4 cm incision over the kidney region, caudal to the last rib; this approach is illustrated in Figure 15.17.

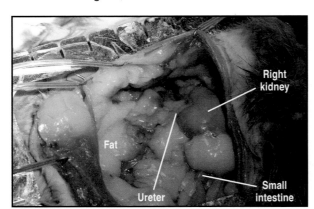

15.17 Post-mortem dissection showing the lateral (paracostal) approach to the kidney. (© John Chitty)

Technique:

1. The kidney is freed from the peritoneal attachment and carefully grasped between two fingers.

2. The greater curvature of the kidney, opposite the hilum, is visualized. The hilum, ureter and blood vessels are located to avoid damage during the procedure. Vessels are clamped using atraumatic clips (e.g. Hemoclips) or smooth microclips to reduce haemorrhage during the procedure.

3. A sagittal incision is made along the midline through the cortex to expose the pelvis (Figure 15.18).

4. The calculus is removed.

5. The pelvis and exposed parenchyma are swabbed to obtain culture samples and then flushed to remove any debris, sludge or clotted blood.

6. A 3 Fr catheter is inserted through the pelvis into the ureter to check patency.

7. The two halves of the renal parenchyma are then apposed and held together for a few seconds.

8. If necessary, a single horizontal mattress suture can be placed through the cortex before closing the capsule.

9. The capsule is closed with a simple interrupted suture pattern using 2 metric (3/0 USP) absorbable suture material. The vessel clips are removed and bleeding is evaluated.

10. Abdominal wound closure is routine (see Chapters 11 and 13).

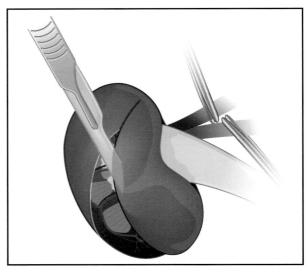

15.18 Nephrotomy is performed by making a sagittal incision along the greater curvature of the kidney, after atraumatic clamping of the vessels.

Potential complications: Potential complications include intra-renal bleeding, urine leakage, renal failure, adhesions and localized pain.

To minimize complications, it is important that renal function is evaluated prior to surgery. Factors likely to lead to postoperative complications can be identified by ultrasonography; if these are severe, a different technique such as nephrectomy should be considered.

The kidney should also be evaluated before abdominal closure, to ensure there is no leakage of urine or haemorrhage from the surgical site. Adhesions and localized pain can be reduced using anti-inflammatory and analgesic drugs.

Pyelolithotomy

Indications: Pyelolithotomy is advised when urinary calculi become lodged in the extra-renal region of the pelvis and the proximal ureter. It is not recommended for stones with minimal invasion into the ureter; in this case, a medical approach is preferable. Pyelolithotomy is possible when the area is distended due to obstruction; otherwise it is difficult to perform. However, when possible, pyelolithotomy is preferable to nephrotomy since it avoids damage to the renal parenchyma, making recovery smoother and minimizing postoperative complications; also, it is not necessary to occlude the renal vessels.

Approach: The anaesthetized rabbit is placed in dorsal recumbency and a routine midline laparotomy incision made.

Technique:

1. The kidney is freed from the peritoneal attachments by blunt dissection and rotated medially to allow visualization of the extra-renal region of the pelvis and the proximal ureter.
2. A longitudinal incision is made over the calculus (Figure 15.19).
3. The calculus is removed and the area is gently flushed with warm sterile saline solution.
4. The incision is then closed with either a longitudinal or a transverse interrupted single suture pattern, using 1 metric (5/0 USP) absorbable suture material.

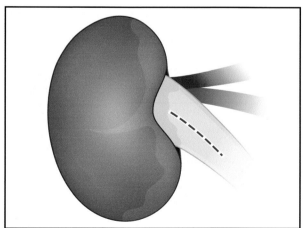

15.19 Pyelolithotomy is performed by making a longitudinal incision along the proximal ureter.

Potential complications: Possible complications include urine flow obstruction from blood clots, adhesions, or a reduced size of the lumen. Transverse closure is advised to avoid adhesions during healing and maintain a wider lumen. Renal pathology and any potential causes of calculus formation need to be addressed in order to avoid recurrence.

Nephrectomy

The procedure is illustrated in Operative Technique 15.1.

Indications: Complete nephrectomy is considered when there is extensive damage to the kidney. Possible causes are trauma, neoplasia, advanced hydronephrosis, pyelonephritis, calculi and obstruction. It is also considered in cases of polycystic kidneys, congenital abnormalities and severe nephropathies. This surgery is not advised if the function of the contralateral kidney is unknown, as kidney failure can occur if the contralateral kidney is not fully functional. Ideally, an excretory pyelogram should be performed prior to surgery to determine the full function of the contralateral kidney. A knowledge of kidney anatomy and topography is essential prior to undertaking this technique. Ureteronephrectomy (see below) should be considered if damage to the ureter is noticed.

Potential complications: Iatrogenic damage to the ureter is a potential complication during surgery, while internal bleeding and urine leakage from the surgical site is a potential postoperative complication.

Ureteronephrectomy

Indications: Ureteronephrectomy is considered when there is extensive damage to both the kidney and the ureter. Possible causes are trauma, neoplasia, hydroureteronephrosis, pyelonephritis, calculi and obstruction.

Approach: The rabbit is placed in dorsal recumbency and is surgically prepared from the sternum to the pelvis as for exploratory laparotomy. A midline incision is made and retractors are used to improve visibility during the surgical procedure. Moistened surgical swabs help to isolate the kidney and ureter from the abdominal contents and avoid damage to the gastrointestinal tract.

Technique:

1. The kidney is freed from its peritoneal attachment and the renal artery and vein are cauterized or ligated and removed.
2. The ureter is then gently removed and detached from the peritoneum along its length.
3. The distal ureter is cauterized or ligated approximately 1 cm from its insertion into the urinary bladder. It is then transected above the ligature. It is important to be careful not to damage the urinary bladder in order to prevent urine leakage.
4. Abdominal wound closure is routine (see Chapters 11 and 13).

Potential complications: Possible complications are internal bleeding, damage to the urinary bladder, urine leakage from the insertion of the resected ureter into the urinary bladder, renal dysfunction, adhesions and infections.

Ureters

To the authors' knowledge ectopic ureters have not been described in rabbits. It should, however, be considered as a differential diagnosis in rabbits born with urinary incontinence.

Ureterotomy

The term ureterotomy is used to describe an incision into the ureter. Ureterotomy is technically advanced surgery and is not to be undertaken lightly.

Indications: The most common indication in rabbits is for removal of calculi, and successful removal of ureteral calculi has been described (White, 2001). Obstruction of the ureter is usually associated with hydronephrosis, hydroureter and nephrolithiasis. Options for removal include retrograde flushing of calculi into the renal pelvis and subsequent removal via the pelvis (pyelolithotomy), ureterotomy and ureteronephrectomy. Flushing may be difficult since calculi are often adhered to the mucosa.

In non-obstructive cases where calculi are identified in the kidney or ureter, a medical approach should be considered first. Intravenous fluid therapy to increase the flow of urine through the urinary system may help dislodge calculi into the bladder. Muscle relaxants such as diazepam may also be useful. Ureterotomy should not be considered if an obstruction is present (see earlier) or likely (in cases of hydroureter or hydronephrosis).

Approach: The patient is surgically prepared for a routine midline abdominal incision. The length of the incision is dependent on the location of the calculus, but for proximal ureteral obstructions extends from the xiphoid process to just caudal to the umbilicus. A Lone Star or Balfour retractor should be used to retract the abdominal wall. Moistened surgical swabs help isolate the kidney and ureter from the abdominal contents.

Technique:

1. The affected ureter is visualized and the calculus located by palpation. Encircling stay sutures may be placed around the ureter, proximal and distal to the calculus, to isolate it and allow gentle elevation.
2. The peritoneum is incised over the ureter and a transverse or longitudinal incision made either directly over it or just proximal to it:
   - Transverse incisions have less tension across the suture line and therefore heal more quickly
   - In cases where the ureter is not dilated, there is a higher postoperative risk of stricture formation. These cases are best managed using a longitudinal incision (Figure 15.20).
3. The calculus is then removed. It is essential to ensure all calculi are removed and ureteral patency is checked prior to closure. To ensure this, a 3 Fr catheter can be placed via the incision and the proximal ureter and renal pelvis gently flushed with sterile saline. Small calculi from the renal pelvis or proximal ureter are flushed towards the incision and can be removed from there.
4. The incision is closed with a simple interrupted absorbable suture pattern (0.5 metric (7/0 USP) monofilament material). Where a longitudinal incision has been used, it is closed in a transverse manner to widen the lumen (Figure 15.20).
5. Abdominal wound closure is routine (see Chapters 11 and 13).

The calculus should be sent for analysis postoperatively.

Perioperative intravenous fluid therapy and analgesia (see Chapter 2) are essential in these patients. Systemic antibiotics, such as enrofloxacin prior to urine culture results, and benzodiazepine muscle relaxants may also be indicated.

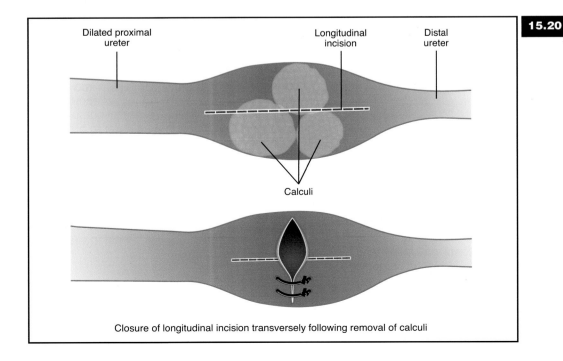

15.20 Ureterotomy to remove calculi.

Dilated proximal ureter — Longitudinal incision — Distal ureter — Calculi

Closure of longitudinal incision transversely following removal of calculi

Potential complications and postoperative care: These include postoperative leakage of urine and stricture formation due to intraluminal scar tissue formation. If a complete blockage has occurred there may be secondary renal damage. Assessment of normal renal function (by measurement of biochemical and haematological parameters) and normal urination is essential postoperatively. If hydronephrosis is diagnosed, nephrectomy may be indicated. Prior to this, assessment of normal renal function in the healthy kidney should be confirmed using IVU. Care should be taken since large volumes of contrast material can precipitate renal failure in otherwise mild to moderate renal disease. The rabbit should be hydrated prior to this procedure, and fluid therapy continued postoperatively.

Prognosis: Recurrence of calculi is common and appropriate husbandry changes should be instigated following surgery to reduce this risk (see earlier).

The bladder

Cystotomy

Indications: This is the treatment of choice for removal of large cystic calculi in the rabbit and is illustrated in Operative Technique 15.2. It is a relatively straightforward procedure with a good prognosis.

A knowledge of bladder anatomy is essential prior to undertaking this technique. The bladder is extremely thin-walled in rabbits and careful elevation using stay sutures to exteriorize it during cystotomy should prevent tearing of the wall. Often, however, in cases requiring cystotomy, the bladder wall is chronically thickened and inflamed and may haemorrhage easily. Suture placement is, however, less likely to result in tearing of the bladder wall in cases with chronic thickening.

Very small calculi and cases with hypercalciuria may be treated by catheterization of the bladder under sedation and careful flushing with saline, or by direct visualization and endoscopic removal. Premedication with opiates and benzodiazepines will provide analgesia and muscle relaxation to aid this procedure. For bucks, a 3.5–5 Fr catheter is used and catheterization is straightforward. In does a 5–8 Fr catheter is used. The doe is placed in sternal recumbency with a sandbag under the rear end to elevate the pelvis (Figure 15.21). A lubricated sterile catheter is carefully advanced along the vaginal floor, aiming ventrally into the urethra. Correct placement is confirmed by aspiration of urine. Flushing with warm sterile saline is carried out until the aspirate is clear of crystals. Gentle manipulation and agitation of the bladder will aid the process and encourage the expulsion of crystals.

Large calculi are easily identified by radiography, contrast cystography and ultrasonography, and are most commonly composed of calcium carbonate. Full urinalysis and urine culture should be performed to rule out concurrent bacterial infection in these cases prior to surgery, together with serum biochemistry and haematology to assess renal function.

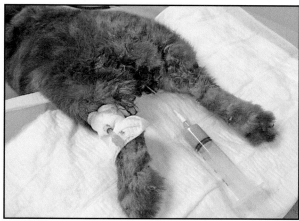

15.21 Urethral catheterization in the female rabbit is straightforward in a sedated animal, with slight elevation of the hindlimbs. Note the perineal scalding in this patient. The rabbit has been placed in sternal recumbency and the hindlimbs elevated by placement of a sandbag under the pelvic area. An absorbent pad has been placed over the sandbag to contain any urine passed around the catheter.

Other indications for cystotomy include biopsy for bladder masses, removal of excessive urinary sediment (hypercalciuria; Figure 15.22) and investigation of chronic refractory urinary tract infection.

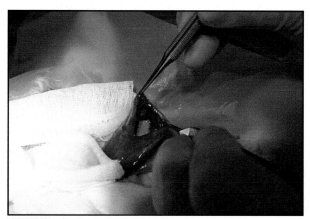

15.22 Cystotomy in a rabbit to remove excessive accumulation of calcium carbonate crystals. (Courtesy of Elisabetta Mancinelli)

Prognosis: The postoperative prognosis is generally good, although recurrence of the underlying condition may occur. Concretions of crystals along the suture line are also common after surgery and may cause complications at a later date.

Biopsy

Indications: Neoplasia of the bladder has been described in rabbits but is rare. Leiomyoma is most commonly seen and it is also possible for uterine adenocarcinoma to spread to the urinary system. Bacterial infections with *Pseudomonas* spp. and *Escherichia coli* can cause cystitis in pet rabbits, and bladder wall samples may be required for culture in chronic or resistant infections. Bladder mucosal biopsy samples are often positive on bacterial culture where urine culture has previously been negative. If full-thickness biopsy samples are not required, endoscopic biopsy is an alternative option in female rabbits (see Chapter 10).

Approach, technique and potential complications: These are as described for cystotomy in rabbits (see above). Multiple full-thickness bladder wall biopsy samples should be taken from grossly affected areas for bacterial/fungal culture and sensitivity and histopathological examination.

Cystectomy

Indications for cystectomy: Indications include bladder neoplasia, traumatic injuries and polyps.

Approach, technique and potential complications: These are as described for cystotomy in rabbits (see above). The bladder should be palpated prior to incision to identify any masses and the incision should be made 1–2 cm away from the mass margin. The use of stay sutures placed in normal bladder wall aids mass removal and enables the surgeon to gauge better how the bladder should be closed once the mass is resected. Bladder healing is rapid compared with other organs, and relatively large sections (65–70% of the urinary bladder) can be removed if the trigone remains intact and unaffected, since expansion of the remaining bladder occurs postoperatively. A composite membrane (e.g. collagen/Vicryl) may be used to repair full-thickness defects in the urinary bladder (Monsour *et al.*, 1987). This material is biodegradable and will prevent leakage of urine in large deficits. It is replaced by collagenous scar tissue lined with a urothelium. Regeneration of smooth muscle can also occur in the repaired area.

Cystopexy

Transurethral urinary bladder eversion may occur postpartum in does, and may be encouraged by multiple pregnancies in a young animal. It presents with straining to urinate, a hunched posture and a soft tissue mass protruding from the vulva. Animals are often in a state of hypovolaemic shock and are usually poor surgical candidates. Differential diagnoses include abortion, hernia, prolapse of other organs and trauma. Fluid therapy, analgesia and systemic antibiotics are all indicated.

Technique: A partial cystectomy and cystopexy is carried out via a routine midline incision, as for cystotomy. The prolapsed tissue is flushed with sterile saline. Gentle external pressure is applied to move the prolapsed bladder back into the vagina. Using atraumatic forceps (e.g. Babcock), the bladder should be gently grasped via the midline incision and pulled back into an abdominal position. Ovariohysterectomy may be performed if the prolapse includes reproductive structures (see Chapter 12). Partial cystectomy may be required if necrotic bladder tissue is present (see above). In one case

study the ventral serosal bladder surface was scarified and sutured in when closing the abdominal incision (Greenacre *et al.*, 1999).

Potential complications: Careful case selection is required since a poor prognosis is associated with this condition. Euthanasia should be considered in advanced/severe cases where there is significant contamination, trauma or necrosis of the prolapsed material. Full serum biochemistry and haematology should be performed prior to surgery to assess renal function. Presurgical problems include necrosis of the bladder mucosa and secondary renal failure due to ureteral constriction and hydronephrosis. Bladder dehiscence following surgery, bacterial contamination and urinary incontinence are potential complications.

Urethra

Urethrotomy

Indications: Urethral calculi and secondary blockage of the urethra is more common in male rabbits than in females. Most often, calculi become dislodged in the distal urethra (Figure 15.23). Manual expression of the bladder to force the calculi out via the urethra (urohydropulsion) is not recommended by the authors since there is a significant risk of bladder rupture and trauma, even in anaesthetized animals. Calculus removal may require surgical intervention via a urethrotomy incision. However, cystotomy should be performed in preference to urethrotomy if the stones can be flushed back into the bladder, since postoperative urethral stricture is a potentially serious complication following urethrotomy.

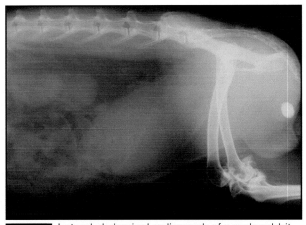

15.23 Lateral abdominal radiograph of a male rabbit, showing a large urolith lodged in the distal urethra. This was obstructing urine flow and a distended bladder is visible.

Technique: The area is surgically prepared including the scrotal area, which lies laterally on either side of the central urethra in intact male rabbits. The testicle within the scrotal sac may need to be reflected away from the surgical site to improve exposure. The deep inguinal skin folds, which lie on either side of the preputial orifice, should be draped such that they are outside the surgical site.

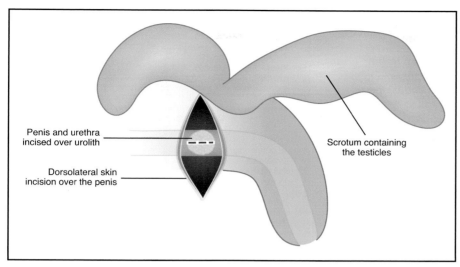

15.24 Diagrammatic representation of the urethrotomy technique. Gentle dissection exposes the body of the penis.

Penis and urethra incised over urolith

Dorsolateral skin incision over the penis

Scrotum containing the testicles

1. A sterile urinary catheter should be placed in the penile urethra at the level of the obstruction.
2. A dorsolateral incision is made in the skin over the urethra and the subcutaneous tissue is exposed.
3. The urolith should be located by palpation and an incision made in the penis directly over it (Figure 15.24).
4. Pressure should be applied to the site to control any haemorrhage. Haemorrhage is common in urethral surgery.
5. The urolith is removed with forceps and the urethra closed using 1–1.5 metric (5/0–4/0 USP) monofilament absorbable suture material in a continuous suture pattern.
6. Subcuticular continuous absorbable sutures are placed in the skin to close the incision and the catheter is removed at the end of the procedure.

Urethral mucosa can heal as rapidly as 7 days after surgery.

Potential complications and postoperative care:
Urination should be monitored carefully following surgery on the urethra, since obstruction to urine flow can occur secondary to tissue swelling, fibrosis or necrosis.

Stricture formation is more likely to occur if there is urine leakage from the wound, particularly if infection is also present. Fastidious suture technique, with particular care to close both ends of the wound completely, is essential to reduce the risk of peri-urethral urine leakage after surgery.

Fluid therapy should be instigated once any obstruction has been removed, and electrolytes should also be monitored as hypokalaemia commonly occurs following post-surgical diuresis. Appropriate antibiotic therapy should also be instigated to treat any existing infection that would delay wound healing and promote stricture formation.

Self-trauma is possible postoperatively and an Elizabethan collar may be necessary for the first 24 hours (but see Chapter 11). It is important to provide appropriate analgesia to encourage normal urination.

Manual bladder expression may be necessary if urine is not passed within 12 hours; however, extreme care should be taken in the rabbit as bladder rupture can occur with excessive digital pressure. Bladder atony may occur with urine retention following the procedure unless this is carefully monitored.

Preputial scarring
This condition occurs in male rabbits in association either with trauma to the prepuce from fight wounds or with urine scald. It may lead to abnormalities in urination due to alteration of the direction of urine flow. In some cases the urethra itself may be damaged and corrective surgery to reconstruct the urethral opening may be required (see Chapter 21). A technique has been described to lift the perineal area and the anal and urethral openings dorsally, such that the urine is directed away from the hindlegs and perineum. This should only be used as a last resort once other causes of urine scald have been eliminated, since it requires amputation of the tail (Jenkins, 1997).

Postoperative care

Antibiotics
Antibiotic therapy should be implemented when infection is present, e.g. bacterial cystitis. However, in order to prevent antimicrobial resistance, it is important to administer antibiotics only when there is evidence of bacterial infection. The choice of antibiotic should always be based on results of culture and sensitivity, although the authors commence broad-spectrum antibiotic treatment pending results. Two antibiotics are primarily advocated in cases with urinary tract infection: trimethoprim/sulfamethoxazole (30 mg/kg orally q12h) and enrofloxacin (20 mg/kg orally q24h). While enrofloxacin is excreted via both the liver and kidney, trimethoprim/sulfamethoxazole is excreted primarily by the kidneys at both glomerular and tubular levels. Long-term antibiotic use may be required for treatment of chronic bladder infections.

Chapter 15 Urinary tract surgery

Analgesia

Provision of analgesia is essential in rabbits with urinary tract disease, as clinical signs of discomfort are routinely observed. Response to treatment and recovery rate is improved with analgesia. Opioids such as buprenorphine or morphine should be used in the first instance. Once diagnostic testing for renal disease has been performed and the animal has been rehydrated, NSAIDs may be instigated. For example, the authors routinely use meloxicam at 0.6 mg/kg orally or s.c. q12h in cases of hypercalciuria, usually in combination with buprenorphine at 0.05 mg/kg s.c. q6–8h. The authors also advocate the use of constant rate infusion analgesia in bladder surgery cases.

Prokinetics

Prokinetics are required to stimulate gastrointestinal motility before and after surgery and to treat the side effects which are often associated with urinary tract disease in the rabbit.

Diet

Provision of a high-fibre diet is essential in the management of hypercalciuria and urinary calculi in the rabbit, and to stimulate normal gut motility after urinary tract surgery. A dietary source of both short and long fibres should be provided. While short fibres promote caecal fermentation and provide nutrients, long fibres promote gut motility. Appetite may be stimulated in the convalescing rabbit by provision of fresh greens, such as grass, dandelion leaves, parsley, coriander and kale. Grass and good quality hay should be available at all times as well as fresh water (see also dietary discussion under urolithiasis and hypercalciuria above).

Fluid therapy

Following urinary tract surgery it is essential to monitor urination closely and continue fluid therapy until the rabbit is voluntarily eating, urinating and passing droppings normally. The authors prefer intravenous fluid therapy, with catheter placement prior to surgery and the catheter maintained postoperatively.

Recent research has shown that rabbits greatly prefer drinking water from a bowl and are more likely to drink if offered water via this route than using a bottle (Tschudin et al., 2011). Both routes should be provided in the hospital environment to give the rabbit free choice. Litter trays should be provided if usually used by the rabbit, to encourage normal urination. Offering foods that have potential diuretic properties may also be beneficial, such as goosegrass, dandelion or plantain.

References and further reading

Capello V (2005) Diagnosis and treatment of urolithiasis in pet rabbits. Exotic DVM 6(2), 15–22
Douglas GC and Hossler FE (1995) Vascular anatomy of the rabbit ureter. Anatomical Record 242, 47–56
Dwyer TM and Schmidt-Nielsen B (2003) The renal pelvis: machinery that concentrates urine in the papilla. News in Physiological Sciences 18, 1–6
Eken E, Çorumluolu O, Paksoy Y, Befloluk K and Kalayc I (2009) A study on evaluation of 3D virtual rabbit kidney models by multidetector computed tomography images. Anatomy 3, 40–44
Fisher PG (2006) Exotic mammal renal disease: diagnosis and treatment. Veterinary Clinics of North America: Exotic Animal Practice 9(1), 69–96
Greenacre CB, Allen SW and Ritchie BW (1999) Urinary bladder eversion in rabbit does. Compendium on Continuing Education for the Practicing Veterinarian 21(6), 524–528
Gunn-Moore DA and Shenoy CM (2004) Oral glucosamine and the management of feline idiopathic cystitis. Journal of Feline Medicine and Surgery 6, 219–225
Hanke PR, Timm P, Falk G and Kramer W (1994) Behavior of different suture materials in the urinary bladder of the rabbit with special reference to wound healing, epithelization and crystallization. Urologica Internationalis 52, 26–33
Harcourt-Brown F (2002) Textbook of Rabbit Medicine. Butterworth-Heinemann, Oxford
Harcourt-Brown F (2007) Radiographic signs of renal disease in rabbits. Veterinary Record 160, 787–794
Harcourt-Brown F (2013) Diagnosis of renal disease in rabbits. Veterinary Clinics of North America: Exotic Animal Practice 16, 145–174
Holz P and Raidal SR (2006) Comparative renal anatomy of exotic species. Veterinary Clinics of North America: Exotic Animal Practice 9(1), 1–11
Hossler FE and Monson FC (1995) Microvasculature of the rabbit urinary bladder. Anatomical Record 243, 438–448
Hristov H, Kostov D and Vladova D (2006) Topographical anatomy of some abdominal organs in rabbits. Trakia Journal of Sciences 4(3), 7–10
Ingram AJ, Parbtani A, Clark WF et al. (1995) Effects of flaxseed and flax oil diets in a rat-96 renal ablation model. American Journal of Kidney Disease 25, 320–329
Jenkins J (1997) Soft tissue surgery. In: Ferrets, Rabbits and Rodents: Clinical Medicine and Surgery, 2nd edn, ed. K Quesenberry and JW Carpenter, pp. 228–229. Elsevier Saunders, St. Louis
Kaminski JM, Katz AR and Woodward SC (1978) Urinary bladder calculus formation on sutures in rabbits, cats and dogs. Surgery, Gynecology and Obstetrics 146, 353–355
Krautwald-Junghanns M-E, Pees M, Reese S and Tully T (2011) Diagnostic Imaging of Exotic Pets: Birds, Small Mammals, Reptiles. Schlütersche, Hannover
Lightfoot T (2011) Recognising and treating rabbit geriatric syndromes. Florida Veterinary Medical Association 82nd Conference Proceedings, Orlando, Florida, April 29–May 1, 2011, p.5
Martorell J, Bailon D, Majó N and Andaluz A (2012) Lateral approach to nephrotomy in the management of unilateral renal calculi in a rabbit (Oryctolagus cuniculus). Journal of the American Veterinary Medical Association 240, 863–868
Meredith A and Flecknell P (2006) BSAVA Manual of Rabbit Medicine and Surgery, 2nd edn. BSAVA Publications, Gloucester
Monsour MJ, Mohammed R, Gorham SD, French DA and Scott R (1987) An assessment of a collagen/vicryl composite membrane to repair defects of the urinary bladder in rabbits. Urological Research 15, 235–238
Morris MC, Baquero A, Redovan E, Mahoney E and Bannett AD (1986) Urolithiasis on absorbable and non-absorbable suture materials in the rabbit bladder. Journal of Urology 135, 602–603
Morton DB and Griffiths PHM (1985) Guidelines on the recognition of pain, distress and discomfort in experimental animals and a hypothesis for assessment. Veterinary Record 116, 431–436
Paul-Murphy J (2007) Critical care of the rabbit. Veterinary Clinics of North America: Exotic Animal Practice 10(2), 437–461
Porzio P, Pharr JW and Allen AL (2001) Excretory urography by intraosseous injection of contrast media in a rabbit model. Veterinary Radiology & Ultrasound 42, 238–243
Quesenberry KE and Carpenter JW (2012) Ferrets, Rabbits and Rodents: Clinical Medicine and Surgery, 3rd edn. Elsevier Saunders, St. Louis
Raidal SR and Raidal SL (2006) Comparative renal physiology of exotic species. Veterinary Clinics of North America: Exotic Animal Practice 9(1), 13–31
Reusch B, Murray JK, Papasouliotis K and Redrobe SP (2009) Urinary protein:creatinine ratio in rabbits in relation to their serological status to Encephalitozoon cuniculi. Veterinary Record 164, 293–295
Rodríguez-Antolín J, Xelhuantzi N, García-Lorenzana M et al. (2009) General tissue characteristics of the lower urethral and vaginal walls in the domestic rabbit. International Urogynecology Journal and Pelvic Floor Dysfunction 20(1), 53–60
Seifman BD, Rubin MA, Williams L and Wolf JS (2002) Use of absorbable cyanoacrylate glue to repair an open cystotomy. Journal of Urology 167(4), 1872–75
Sheehan HL and Davis JC (1959) Anatomy of the pelvis in the rabbit kidney. Journal of Anatomy 93, 499–502
Tschudin A, Clauss M, Codron D and Hatt JM (2011) Preference of rabbits for drinking from open dishes versus nipple drinkers.

Veterinary Record **168**(7), 190

Wallius BM and Tidholm AE (2009) Use of pentosan polysulphate in cats with idiopathic, non-obstructive lower urinary tract disease: a double-blind, randomised, placebo-controlled trial. *Journal of Feline Medicine and Surgery* **11**, 409–412

Warren HB, Lausen NC, Segre GV, el-Hajj G and Brown EM (1989) Regulation of calciotropic hormones in vivo in the New Zealand white rabbit. *Endocrinology* **125**(5), 2683–2690

White RN (2001) Management of calcium ureterolithiasis in a French lop rabbit. *Journal of Small Animal Practice* **42**, 595–598

OPERATIVE TECHNIQUES →

OPERATIVE TECHNIQUE 15.1:
Nephrectomy

Positioning and patient preparation

The rabbit is anaesthetized and placed in dorsal recumbency. The patient is clipped and surgically prepared for a routine midline abdominal incision.

Assistant

Optional.

Equipment extras

- Suction (may be required if bleeding or urine leakage occurs)
- Abdominal retractors such as Balfour or Gossett
- Ring retractors such as Lone Star
- Abdominal swabs
- Haemostatic clips

Procedure

1 Make a routine midline abdominal incision extending from the sternum to the pelvis.

2 Examine both kidneys and the rest of the upper urinary tract to check for gross lesions.

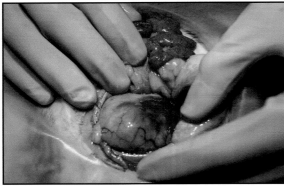

Midline abdominal incision with reflection of the viscera, showing a benign embryonal nephroma in a 3-year-old male neutered Dutch rabbit. The mass was detected on routine clinical examination with no other clinical signs reported by the owner. (© Mikel Sabater)

3 Pack around the kidney that needs to be removed with moistened abdominal swabs to prevent contamination of the abdomen.

4 Remove from the retroperitoneal space by blunt dissection using forceps or fingers for better manipulation and visibility.

> **WARNING**
> The adrenal gland should be gently freed away from the kidney and left in place.

5 Rotate the kidney medially to better identify the renal hilum, vessels and ureter.

6 The renal artery, renal vein and ureter are clamped distal to the kidney and each ligated using 1.5 or 2 metric (4/0 or 3/0 USP) absorbable suture material.

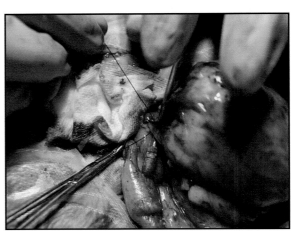

Kidney detached by blunt dissection, with vessels and ureter ligated. (© Mikel Sabater)

> **PRACTICAL TIP**
> The vessels and the ureter may be cauterized rather than ligated.

7 The blood vessels and the ureter are transected above the ligature and the kidney is then removed.

8 Check for any signs of bleeding or urine leakage from the ligature site.

> **PRACTICAL TIP**
> Store the kidney in both formalin and sterile saline solution for histopathology and culture if required.

9 Closure of the laparotomy wound is routine (see Chapter 13).

OPERATIVE TECHNIQUE 15.1 continued:
Nephrectomy

Postoperative management and potential complications

- There is a potential for electrolyte imbalance after surgery; fluid therapy should be carefully planned and instigated (see main text).
- Antibiotics and analgesics are required to prevent infection and localized pain (see main text).
- Internal bleeding and urine leakage from the

surgical site is a potential postoperative complication. Always check the seal formed by the sutures before closing the abdomen.
- Iatrogenic damage to the ureter is a potential complication of this surgery and care should be taken during surgery. Ureteronephrectomy should be considered if damage to the ureter occurs.
- Exercise is restricted for 2–3 days following surgery.

OPERATIVE TECHNIQUE 15.2:
Cystotomy

Positioning and patient preparation

The rabbit is anaesthetized and placed in dorsal recumbency. The patient is clipped and surgically prepared for a routine midline abdominal incision.

Assistant

Optional.

Equipment extras

- Suction
- Surgical spoon
- Urinary catheters

Procedure

1 Use a routine midline abdominal incision extending from the pubis to the umbilicus.

2 Exteriorize the bladder and pack around it with moistened laparotomy swabs to prevent contamination of the abdomen. Place stay sutures in the bladder wall, cranial and caudal to the incision site.

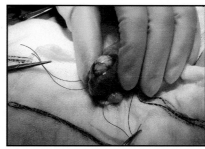

Exteriorized bladder with stay sutures. An incision has been made to reveal a urolith. (Courtesy of Joanna Hedley)

PRACTICAL TIP
A needle may be inserted into the bladder and any free urine aspirated prior to making an incision, as for dogs and cats.

3 Incise in an avascular location in the dorsal or ventral aspect away from the ureters (which enter the bladder dorsally) and the urethra. The bladder vascular supply comes from single left and right vesicular branches of the internal and external iliac arteries (see Chapter 12). These vesicular arteries lie laterally along the bladder borders running from the base to the apex and are just deep to the serosal surface. There are smaller dorsal and ventral branches supplying the dorsal and ventral bladder wall, respectively. In the rabbit bladder apex there is a dense complex of vessels which should be avoided. →

OPERATIVE TECHNIQUE 15.2 continued:
Cystotomy

4 Remove any calculi using a surgical spoon.

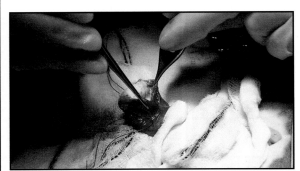

The urolith has been removed revealing the grossly thickened and oedematous mucosal layer of the bladder wall. (Courtesy of Joanna Hedley)

5 Pass a 3 Fr urinary catheter normograde down the urethra and gently flush with warm saline to remove any further calculi and check patency.

6 The bladder is flushed with isotonic sterile saline and gentle suction used to remove any fine granular material or blood clots.

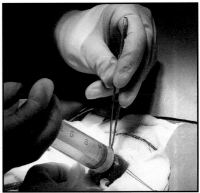

(Courtesy of Joanna Hedley)

PRACTICAL TIP
Biopsy samples of bladder wall can be taken for histopathology and culture if required.

7 The bladder is closed using a single continuous inverting suture pattern with absorbable monofilament suture material (1–1.5 metric, 5/0–4/0 USP).

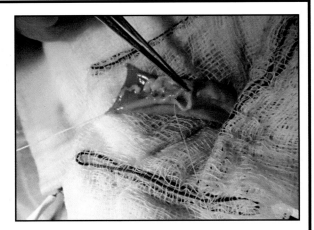

WARNING
Sutures should not penetrate full thickness to avoid suture material entering the bladder lumen as this predisposes to formation of concretions and may act as a nidus for infection.

A double suture layer may be required if the bladder wall is very thin to prevent urine leakage. Cystotomy wound closure has also been described in rabbits using absorbable cyanoacrylate glue (Seifman *et al.*, 2002), although the authors have no personal experience of this technique.

PRACTICAL TIP
Saline may be injected into the bladder after closure to check patency of the closure.

8 Closure of the laparotomy wound is routine (see Chapter 13).

Postoperative management and potential complications

- There is a potential for rupture of the thin-walled bladder if overdistended and handled roughly during surgery.
- In chronic cases it is more common to find thickening and inflammation of the bladder wall, which can be more friable than usual and haemorrhage easily on handling.
- Iatrogenic bladder perforation is possible on incision of the linea alba, especially if the bladder is full, as this tissue lies directly below the incision site.

OPERATIVE TECHNIQUE 15.2 continued:
Cystotomy

- Urine leakage from the surgical site is a potential postoperative complication. Always check the seal formed by the sutures (by expanding the bladder with saline) before closure of the abdomen.
- Calculi may form along the suture line within the bladder lumen (see earlier in chapter). There is less likelihood of this if a fine monofilament absorbable suture material is used, such as 1.5 metric (4/0 USP) poliglecaprone (e.g. Monocryl).
- Iatrogenic damage to the ureters is a potential complication of this surgery and care should be taken to identify these structures prior to bladder incision. Incisions into the dorsocaudal aspect of the bladder should be avoided, as this is associated with an increased risk of iatrogenic damage to the ureters.
- Recurrence of calculi is common and regular radiographic examinations should be carried out, as well as dietary modifications, weight reduction, increased exercise and increased fluid intake.

PRACTICAL TIP
Feed good quality grass/hay *ad libitum* and reduce the pelleted component of the diet. Increase fluid intake by wetting the hay and leafy greens and offering water from a bowl as well as a bottle.

16

Ear and sinus surgery

John Chitty and Aidan Raftery

Ear disease and surgery

Ear disease is a common presentation in rabbits; as in other species, it takes the form of otitis externa, media and/or interna. Medical management of these conditions has been discussed by Harcourt-Brown (2002) and Keeble (2006). In cases of otitis externa or otitis media, where medical management is either impossible or unsuccessful or the situation is recurrent, surgery may be indicated.

Anatomy of the ear

Knowledge of the relevant anatomy is essential to understand disease pathogenesis and to perform successful surgery.

The striking feature of the rabbit ear is the large pinna (Figure 16.1). In addition to ascertaining the direction of sound, this is used for thermoregulation and visual communication between rabbits. Occasionally young rabbits are presented with no pinnae. Generally, these have been chewed off by the mother rather than being a congenital defect.

The remainder of the external ear consists of the external auditory meatus and the external auditory canal. The vertical (distal) part of the external ear canal also has a deep pouch. The canal extends as far as the tympanic membrane. It is supported by three auricular cartilages that interlock and provide rigidity to the ear. The first (proximal) cartilage is a complete ring (the cartilaginous acoustic meatus) and interlocks with the vertical bony acoustic duct arising from the bulla. Distally there is a small dorsally placed scutiform cartilage and a much larger complex auricular cartilage. The portion adjacent to the cartilaginous acoustic meatus is the irregularly shaped tragus and this forms the distal portion of the ear canal.

In 'normal' prick-eared rabbits, these cartilages interdigitate, forming an almost vertical canal that is a rigid structure. In lop-eared rabbits there is a 3–5 mm gap between the cartilaginous acoustic meatus and the tragus (Figure 16.2). This portion, formed only of soft ear canal wall, therefore folds, forming the lop, and closing the external ear canal.

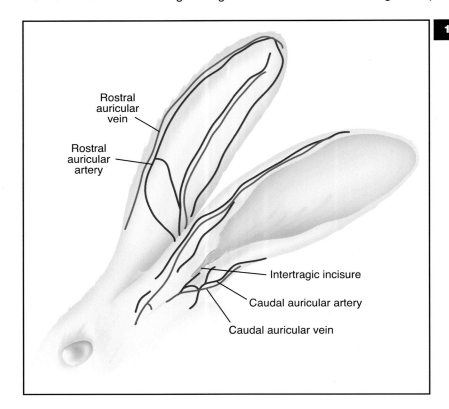

16.1 External ear canal anatomy and vasculature.

- Rostral auricular vein
- Rostral auricular artery
- Intertragic incisure
- Caudal auricular artery
- Caudal auricular vein

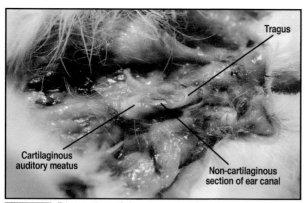

16.2 Dissection of the ear canal in a lop-eared rabbit, showing the gap between the cartilaginous acoustic meatus and the tragus. (© John Chitty)

In effect this creates a very short proximal horizontal canal (albeit oblique) and a distal vertical canal, similar to dogs. This closure of the canal makes it hard for normal discharges (cerumen) to be expelled from the canal. As a result there may be build-up of cerumen (Figure 16.3), increasing the risk of secondary bacterial/yeast infection. The concept of vertical and horizontal canals is controversial in rabbits, and most sources state that they do not have them. This may be because dissections have been performed on rabbits with 'normal' ear position. However, in the lop-eared rabbit the gap between auricular cartilages effectively divides the canal and functionally creates a situation similar to that in the dog.

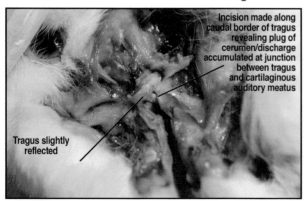

16.3 This dissection of the ear canal in a lop-eared rabbit shows where ear discharges tend to accumulate. (© John Chitty)

Normal cerumen in the distal ear canal appears golden yellow on otoscopy (Figure 16.4), while abnormal discharge/pus appears white (Figure 16.5), often with associated inflammation of the epithelium of the canal. It should be noted that in the deeper (proximal) parts of the ear, normal ceruminous discharges will also appear white, without any associated inflammation. All ear discharges should therefore be examined cytologically to distinguish pus from normal cerumen.

The tympanic membrane is elliptical, with the longest axis being nearly vertical. It is thin compared with that of dogs and cats and appears a translucent 'blue' on examination. It is located just

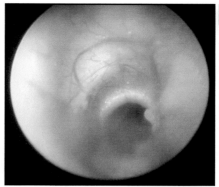

16.4 Otoendoscopic view of the normal ear canal, showing golden-coloured cerumen. (© John Chitty)

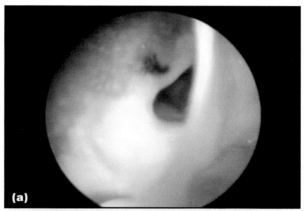

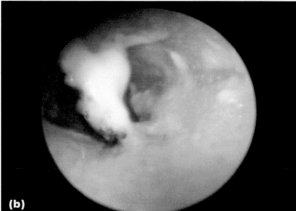

16.5 **(a)** Otoendoscopic view of the ear canal of a lop-eared rabbit, showing abnormal white purulent discharge. The fold in the ear can be seen on the right, running vertically. **(b)** In this case of otitis externa, the purulent discharge is associated with canal inflammation. When touched, haemorrhage occurred. (© John Chitty)

proximal to the interdigitation of the bony and cartilaginous acoustic meatus, making it hard to examine in the conscious prick-eared rabbit and impossible to examine in the conscious lop-eared rabbit.

The structure of the middle/inner ear behind the tympanic membrane is similar to that in dogs and cats, although the tympanic bulla is comparatively large in the rabbit. The bony walls are thicker on their lateral and rostral aspects. The facial nerve exits via the stylomastoid foramen and courses along the ventral surface of the horizontal ear canal (see Chapter 29).

Otitis

Underlying causes of otitis include:

- Mite infestation with *Psoroptes cuniculi*. This will cause a distinctive crusting otitis externa. Secondary bacterial infection may cause further external ear inflammation or a secondary otitis media
- Irritation (potentially caused by allergy, though as yet this is unproven) of the external ear canal. While analogous to the situation in other species, there is little evidence for this at present
- Amputation of or damage to the ipsilateral hindlimb. This makes it hard for the rabbit to scratch the ear as part of normal grooming
- Anatomy. Otitis externa and media are highly prevalent in lop-eared rabbits compared with rabbits with 'normal' ears (see above)
- Dental/upper respiratory infection. Tracking infection via the auditory tubes appears likely in some cases of otitis media/interna. In others, septicaemia or spread of bacteria seems likely. Rarely, infection tracking from a Eustachian foreign body may occur.

Clinical signs

Otitis externa may manifest as irritation of the ear or head shaking, or may be detected on auriscopic examination in asymptomatic rabbits. It should be stressed that subclinical otitis externa should not be treated but should be monitored on a regular basis. Therapy can be given either at the onset of clinical signs or if cytology of the exudates confirms inflammation rather than cerumen.

Subclinical otitis externa can be defined as:

- Presence of larger than normal amounts of white cerumen in the canal
- Variable degrees of canal wall erythema
- No clinical signs associated with the ears.

Otitis media may be seen as an underlying cause of chronic disease such as weight loss, persistent/recurrent gastrointestinal hypomotility, reduced appetite (possibly due to the proximity of the temporomandibular joint to the middle ear, or to facial neuritis) or parasitic dermatoses. It may also be seen as a cause of head tilt or torticollis. Atrophy of facial muscles caused by facial neuritis may be evident in some rabbits as a sequel to otitis media, though initially this may present as drooping of muscles on the affected side before atrophy results in 'twisting' of the face toward the affected side (see Chapter 29).

Signs of **otitis interna** are very similar to those of otitis media, with head tilt and torticollis and, potentially, evidence of a vestibular syndrome.

Diagnosis

Otoendoscopy: An otoendoscope, with channels for instruments and for flushing, is more effective than a handheld otoscope. The light source used needs to be very bright for good visualization.

Otoendoscopy also facilitates the accurate collection of samples for cytology and culture, and the biopsy of any abnormal mass.

Normal ears are a pink colour with a smooth lining and minimal exudate present (Figure 16.6). Lop-eared rabbits usually have much more ceruminous exudate than 'prick-eared' rabbits and the lining is often a red colour. Otoscopy may reveal abnormal discharge/exudate (see Figure 16.5), masses, ulceration, stenosis or foreign bodies.

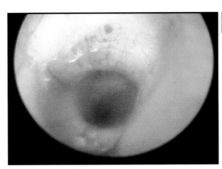

16.6
Otoendoscopic view of the normal ear canal. (© John Chitty)

In most cases of otitis the tympanic membrane is obscured by purulent accumulations and stenosis. General anaesthesia is required in most rabbits to evaluate the external ear canal and the tympanic membrane fully, especially if cleaning is required to allow visualization. Flushing may be necessary to view and evaluate the tympanum but the exudate is usually very thick and requires gentle removal with cotton tips. The lining of the external ear canal may be inflamed and a rough technique will cause further swelling and bleeding. If there is otitis media and the middle ear is filled with material, the tympanum will look darker than normal and sometimes bulge outwards.

Sample collection

- A swab inserted through a sterile otoscope cone can be used to obtain a sample suitable for culture.
- A sterile catheter (attached to a syringe) passed through the working channel of an otoendoscope can be used to aspirate a sample for cytology.
- If otitis media is present with no otitis externa, a deep nasal swab sample should be obtained in addition to a sample direct from the middle ear, via a myringotomy incision. The use of an otoendoscope facilitates safe myringotomy. A 3 Fr tomcat catheter is passed through the instrument channel and used to make an incision through the caudoventral quadrant of the tympanic membrane. Samples are collected by aspiration.

Imaging: Radiographs are essential in the investigation of otitis. With otitis media there may be increased fluid density in the bullae; lysis and remodelling of the bones may be visible in some cases.

The following views are usually required:

- Dorsoventral
- Lateral
- Oblique × 2.

Radiography often gives false negative results as the changes are not always sufficiently advanced or mineralized to be visible radiographically. Computed tomography (CT) and magnetic resonance imaging (MRI), if available, will provide further diagnostic information. In particular, CT can provide detailed information regarding the bullae and middle ear and is generally regarded as the most sensitive diagnostic tool in such cases (Love *et al.*, 1995; see also Chapter 9), especially as it shows the presence of soft exudates (pus/exudates) more clearly than radiography.

Contrast radiography: Canalography (see Chapter 3) may be used to provide information about the tympanic cavity and its margins when investigating otitis, e.g. whether the tympanic membrane is intact. This may produce deceptive images, however, due to the presence of thick exudate preventing the passage of contrast material.

Haematology, biochemistry and serology: These may be required to:

- Establish a possible underlying cause, e.g. serology for encephalitozoonosis; a negative result will effectively rule this out as a cause of neurological signs
- Identify other ongoing and/or underlying disease processes which may affect healing
- Assist with formulating a treatment plan in the best interests of the animal.

Neurological examination: It is important to identify any neurological deficits before surgery. They may alter the prognosis and may be misidentified after surgery as surgical complications. In particular, the following should be examined:

- Facial nerve
- Vestibular deficits
- Paralysis of the facial muscles and an exposure keratitis due to inability to blink (see complications after bulla osteotomy, later)
- Head tilt, nystagmus and torticollis
- Paralysis of the tongue
- Horner's syndrome.

Upper respiratory tract evaluation: Rabbits with otitis media should be investigated for signs of upper respiratory disease, as many cases are due to ascending infections of the auditory canal. Radiography, rhinoscopy and culture/cytology of deep nasal swabs may be helpful.

Treatment

All cases of otitis (other than those associated with *Psoroptes*) will require systemic antibiosis and non-steroidal anti-inflammatory drugs (NSAIDs). In some cases these will be sufficient to control clinical signs. These are difficult cases to manage; decision-making for antibiotic choice is similar to that for abscesses (see Chapter 29) but it is hard to determine how long these should be used for, as affected rabbits will always have subclinical aural disease.

Use of topical therapies is controversial, as the shape of the external ear canal (especially in lop-eared breeds) simply does not allow penetration of the therapy. Polypharmacy products marketed for dogs should be avoided as many contain corticosteroids; as mentioned earlier, the role of primary inflammatory disease (either allergic or irritant) is not clear, so the local immunosuppression induced by these products may not assist, or may even worsen, the situation.

Otherwise, the following treatments may be employed.

Syringing: General anaesthesia is normally required to allow full examination of the external ear canal and, especially, visualization of the tympanic membrane. Sampling of cerumen/aural discharges is essential at this stage. In severe cases it is also necessary in order to examine the ear canal properly.

Removal of pus and aural discharges will assist in management by reducing infective load, enabling better penetration of therapies (both topical and systemic) and reducing localized irritation caused by the build-up of discharge. In cases of otitis media with rupture of the tympanic membrane, syringing the ear will also remove debris from the bulla, thereby reducing pressure on the facial nerves. It is not, however, sufficient as primary therapy as it does not address the primary causes of otitis externa/media.

Syringing the ear is carried out in a similar fashion as for dogs and cats (see Technique 16.1). In mild cases, cleaning of the ears on a regular or irregular basis, along with systemic therapy, may provide reasonable control. In more severe cases, further invasive therapy is required.

Wick placement: Polyvinyl acetate sponges (e.g. Ear Wick, Dermapet) may be used in cases of both otitis externa and media. These are used following thorough cleaning of the ears under anaesthesia (described in Technique 16.1). In essence, they are dry sponges that are inserted in the ear canal (or deeper into the bulla if the tympanic membrane is ruptured) and then 'filled' using antibiotic solution (Figure 16.7). They are then held *in situ* over a period of time enabling continuous localized antibiotic therapy deep in the ear. For rabbits, the standard dog sponge is cut in half.

Choice of antibacterial is based, as always, on culture and sensitivity testing, combined with cytological findings. However, choices must be tempered with the need to avoid ototoxicity. Therefore trimethoprim/sulphonamide injectable solutions appear to be safe and suitable as a first choice in most cases. If required, Tris-EDTA solution may be added to the wick as well, in order to potentiate the antibiotic effect.

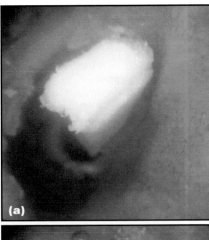

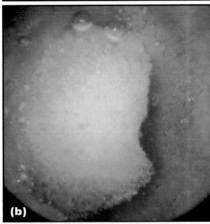

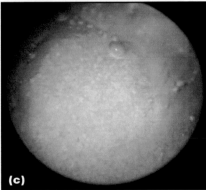

16.7 **(a)** Ear wick placed in the ear canal before addition of 'filling' antibiotic. **(b)** Once antibiotic has been added, the sponge swells to fill the ear canal. **(c)** Sponge fully swollen. (© John Chitty)

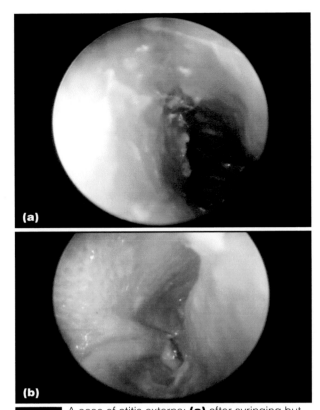

16.8 A case of otitis externa: **(a)** after syringing but before placement of an ear wick; **(b)** immediately after removal of the ear wick. Note the reduction in inflammation. (© John Chitty)

The wick should be removed after a week (Figure 16.8). Longer periods in place may result in excessive granulation around the wick, making it hard to locate and remove. In a case one author (JC) has seen, failure to remove the wick resulted in abscessation and 'expulsion' of the wick via the skin from the vertical canal. However, removal at 7 days is normally straightforward. Wick removal should be carried out under general anaesthesia, allowing for further cleaning of the ear at the same time. If necessary another wick may be placed at this stage.

In cases where the ear disease is suspected to be due to primary inflammatory disease or where cytology of pus/discharge reveals no microorganisms (and no suggestive cellular reaction to these), or where the ear canal is severely stenosed, then anti-inflammatory drugs may also be added to the wick. In general this author (JC) has used water-soluble carprofen. However, on at least one occasion, dexamethasone sodium phosphate solution has been used in severely inflamed ears with successful results. If corticosteroids are used, the ears should be monitored closely on a daily basis and the wicks removed after 3–5 days, i.e. once there has been sufficient reduction in inflammation to allow management using systemic drugs.

The main complications seen are:

* Irritation caused by presence of the wick. However, this is unusual and normally stops after the first 24–48 hours. If it continues the rabbit should be re-anaesthetized and the wick removed
* Premature loss of the wick. Some wicks may be removed by head shaking/grooming.

While this technique is relatively new and evaluation is largely subjective, it appears useful and certainly appears to prolong intervals between ear cleaning episodes in chronic otitis cases.

Aural diverticulosis

Lop-eared rabbits often present with fluid-filled swellings at the base of the ear. These are often described as 'abscesses' and treated by lancing or marsupialization (see Chapter 29) or lateral wall resection (see Operative Technique 16.2). In reality, they represent a build-up of cerumen at the junction of the cartilaginous auditory meatus and tragus (see Figure 16.3). As this region is soft-walled at this point in lop-eared rabbits it is liable to become distended, forming a diverticulum or even hernia of the ear canal wall. Some cases will become secondarily infected (and may then require interventional surgery). However, as the primary process is not infective, but an anatomical defect, these authors propose naming the syndrome 'aural diverticulosis'.

If there are no associated clinical signs, the lump may be left alone, other than teaching the owner to massage it gently to move the cerumen into the more distal parts of the ear canal. This may prevent 'stagnation' of the cerumen and also reduce the rate of further stretch of the ear canal.

If there are clinical signs, rather than lancing, which will further damage the ear canal wall, the material should initially be treated as in any case of otitis (see above). The presence of bacterial infection should be determined by culture and cytology. Otherwise material may be removed by syringing and wicks may be placed if necessary.

In cases that are refractory to this therapy or persistently recur, possibly due to chronic overdistension of the ear canal wall, lateral wall resection may be indicated (see Operative Technique 16.2).

Surgical considerations

Gentle tissue handling, avoiding important blood vessels, and good haemostasis are important during the surgery. The suture material selected should elicit minimal reaction and tissue drag. Suitable materials include: polydioxanone (e.g. PDS), polyglyconate (e.g. Maxon), glycomer 631 (e.g. Biosyn), poliglecaprone 25 (e.g. Monocryl) and polyglytone 6211 (e.g. Caprosyn).

In post-surgical care, NSAIDs should be used to control inflammation, and an effective analgesic protocol used to make the animal comfortable and reduce the risk of self-trauma (see Chapter 2).

Dehiscence is a commonly reported complication of surgery on the ear due to incisional infections. Avascular necrosis (see Figure 16.9), caused by either vascular damage during the surgery or secondary to post-surgical swelling, is more commonly reported as a surgical complication of ear surgery in rabbits than in other species.

Surgical procedures

Aural haematoma/oedema drainage

Aural haematomas are less common in rabbits than in cats and dogs. Oedema of the pinnae is a more common presentation. Trauma is the most common cause; for example, rabbits that have been picked up by the ears are sometimes presented with oedematous ears. Intravascular injections are a common cause of localized oedema of the pinnae, with severe oedema leading to avascular necrosis.

Aural haematomas are treated surgically by providing drainage:

1. The blood clot plus any fibrinous material are removed.
2. Suturing is performed to re-oppose the skin and cartilage, leaving a gap for drainage, using a similar technique to that for dogs and cats. Trans-illumination of the pinnae can be used to avoid incorporating blood vessels in the sutures.

Oedematous ears need to be treated with NSAIDs. Opioid analgesics are often also indicated, as this can be a very painful condition. Diuretics may help reduce the swelling.

If avascular necrosis develops, amputation of all or part of the pinna may be indicated (see below). The caudal and rostral auricular arteries, which branch off the maxillary artery, provide the blood supply to the pinnae, while the caudal and rostral veins provide drainage. Damage to any of these vessels can lead to oedema of a section or all of the pinna.

The ear may need to be bandaged after surgery in some cases to protect from self-trauma. Alternatively, the rabbit's hindfoot can be bandaged, although this is poorly tolerated by some rabbits.

Amputation of the pinna

Partial amputation: Partial amputation of a pinna is most commonly indicated for the management of neoplasia or to resect avascular traumatic flaps.

Attention must be paid to the vascular supply when planning surgery. Attempting to restore the normal contour of the ear will minimize the risk of avascular areas and of leaving edges prone to trauma.

The cartilage is shortened a millimetre more than the surrounding skin. Strict attention to haemostasis is essential. Suture material of 1.5 metric (USP 4/0) or smaller is used to close the skin with horizontal mattress sutures with either an interrupted or a continuous pattern. Skin must be sutured to skin as, if there is cartilage between the skin layers, healing will be compromised. Additionally the skin must not be under tension.

Pinnectomy: Full amputation of a pinna is sometimes necessary due to trauma, avascular necrosis (Figure 16.9) or neoplasia. Malignant melanomas are a relatively common neoplasm on the pinna in rabbits and require wide surgical excision. However, there is lymphatic invasion in a percentage of these, so a cautious prognosis should be given.

Sometimes the lesion extends into the auditory canal and pinnectomy must be combined with a lateral wall resection (see below) or a total ear canal ablation (TECA; see below). However, TECA carries a high risk of chronic complications in the rabbit, due to inadequate drainage if there is also otitis media. A bulla osteotomy should be combined with TECA if there is concurrent otitis media.

To remove the pinna, the intertragic incisure should be used as a guide and the incision made

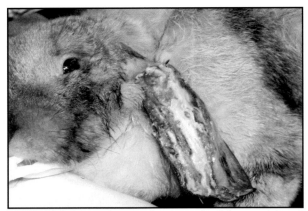

16.9 Advanced avascular necrosis of the cranial part of the pinna due to traumatic damage to the rostral auricular blood vessels. This is an indication for amputation of the pinna. (© Aidan Raftery)

horizontally through the skin and cartilage at this level (Figure 16.10).

It is vital that a patent auditory canal is maintained. As with partial resections, the cartilage and muscles should be removed approximately 1 mm below the skin level so that skin-to-skin closure can be achieved without tension. Extra sutures may be needed to eliminate any dead space.

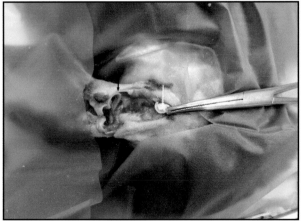

16.10 The proximal portion of the auricular cartilage has been removed in this rabbit because of neoplasia. The level of an incision for a full amputation of the pinna can be seen (black arrow). The cartilage of the remaining acoustic meatus is filled with ceruminous exudate (white arrow). (© Aidan Raftery)

Repairing lacerations of the pinnae

Lacerations and punctures of the pinnae are common and are mostly caused by bites from other rabbits. Many can be left to heal by second intention, but some will require antimicrobials in addition to cleaning.

Flaps of skin avulsed from the cartilage can be sutured back. Simple interrupted sutures are used to reattach the margins; sutures through to the cartilage will eliminate the potential for fluid to accumulate.

Full-thickness lacerations are repaired using simple interrupted sutures to re-oppose the skin on each side. Larger lacerations extending to the margin may benefit from the extra support of vertical mattress sutures on the medial side where there is less vasculature.

Lateral wall resection

In severe or chronic cases of otitis externa where regular cleaning and wick placement in combination with systemic therapy are not controlling the condition, or where cleaning is required at such frequency that it is felt the rabbit's welfare may be compromised, lateral wall resection may be considered. This procedure may also be indicated for tumours of the lateral wall of the ear canal, though these are extremely rare, and for aural diverticulosis see above). As in other species, this technique is not generally curative (other than for tumour removal and in aural diverticulosis); rather, it is designed to improve exposure of the vertical canal and improve access to the horizontal canal. This enables easier cleaning and application of topical therapies, greatly facilitating conservative management of these cases.

The technique (see Operative Technique 16.2) is similar to that used in dogs; this author (JC) uses a technique similar to that described by Capello (2004). In aural diverticulosis this is particularly effective, as it is easy to create a good-sized 'drainage board' from the lateral wall of the diverticulum.

A potential complication in lop-eared rabbits is caused by the unsupported region between the auricular cartilages. This can result in a tendency for the ear stoma to 'collapse', making it much more difficult to maintain an opening to the horizontal canal, especially where there is no diverticulum and hence only a small amount of tissue available for creating the drainage board. To assist in preventing this, this author (JC) also performs a slight modification where the medial wall of the region between cartilages is also incised. This enables the entire horizontal canal to be marsupialized to the skin (the dorsal attachment being the skin drawn across from either side of the incisions), i.e. a full stoma. The vertical canal is repaired as above but no longer communicates with the horizontal canal (Figure 16.11).

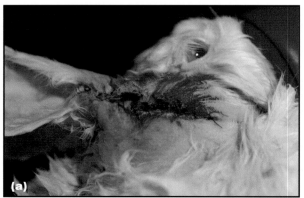

16.11 Postoperative images following lateral wall resection in a lop-eared rabbit. **(a)** The opening created in the lateral wall and the 'anastomosis' to the skin can be seen. (© John Chitty) (continues) ▶

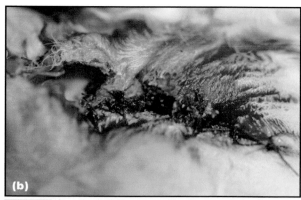

16.11 (continued) Postoperative images following lateral wall resection in a lop-eared rabbit. **(b)** Close-up of the area where the horizontal canal has been separated from the vertical canal and marsupialized to the skin. (© John Chitty)

Lateral wall resection may require a lot of postoperative care, especially in otitis cases where the lateral wall will have been chronically inflamed and there is less tissue available for the drainage board. In the authors' experience owners need to clean and maintain the wounds daily, as well as to flush the horizontal canal carefully with saline to avoid closure of the surgical stoma. Nonetheless, good results are readily achieved with careful technique. However, should stoma closure occur, repeat surgery is unlikely to be successful owing to scarring and loss of tissue in the initial operation. In these cases TECA is indicated (see below).

Total ear canal ablation

Indications:

- Otitis media non-responsive to non-surgical treatments
- Benign neoplasms, where there is a rational treatment plan.

Contraindications:

- Otitis interna
- Lytic bone changes of the medial aspect of the tympanic bulla or deeper
- Extensive proliferative bone changes
- Malignant neoplasia or benign neoplasia where tumour growth is too extensive
- Vestibular symptoms
- Other severe intractable disease processes.

Preparation: A comprehensive work-up is essential before embarking on surgery of the middle ear, including:

- Radiology of the skull – to review the extent of any bone changes. Lytic changes to the bone of the lateral wall of the bulla due to chronic osteomyelitis will require thorough debriding
- CT and MRI (if available) – can provide important information to aid decision-making. CT provides

details of osseous structures, while MRI allows visualization of the fluid-filled spaces and the vestibulocochlear nerve
- Neurological examination – important to identify any neuropathies already present before surgery
- Ideally, pathogenic bacteria present should be cultured and antimicrobial sensitivity identified before surgery.

See Chapter 11 for more detailed information on pre-surgical work-up for soft tissue surgery.

Surgical approach: If the tympanic membrane is ruptured, the surgeon should perform a TECA using the lateral approach (see Operative Technique 16.3). A ventral bulla osteotomy (see Operative Technique 16.4) is indicated when there is an intact tympanum and no involvement of the external ear canal. Compared to the lateral approach, the ventral approach provides better access to the bulla, facilitating a more reliable removal of tissue debris, necrotic material and the epithelial lining of the bulla. There is also better drainage after surgery and the risk of damage to the facial nerve is reduced. However, there is a risk of damage to the hypoglossal nerve. Occasionally, on curettage of the bulla, the tympanic membrane ruptures. This will increase the risk of ongoing chronic otitis media requiring a repeat procedure (Fossum, 2007).

Complications: Neurological deficits are common but will resolve within 14 days unless a nerve has been transected. Facial nerve deficits and peripheral vestibular signs are usually seen if that is the case.

The facial nerve can easily be damaged during the surgery as the external ear canal is being dissected. In some cases there is lysis of the lateral wall of the tympanic bulla which may just crumble during surgery. This poses a greater risk to the facial nerve as it exits through the stylomastoid foramen on the caudal border of the lateral wall of the bulla. The clinical signs seen include facial paralysis, an absent or reduced palpebral reflex, and exposure keratitis (Figure 16.12). If there is drooling due to facial nerve damage, regular cleaning of the chin will help prevent dermatitis in the area.

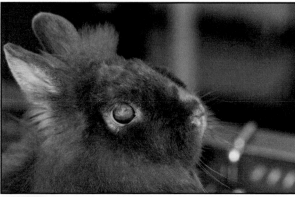

16.12 Exposure keratitis due to facial nerve damage. Ocular lubricants can be used to avoid the eye becoming dry during surgery. (© Aidan Raftery)

Peripheral vestibular deficits are caused by damage to the dorsomedial area of the bulla during curettage. Signs are horizontal nystagmus, ataxia and head tilt. Incisional infection, pinna necrosis, haematoma, hearing loss and salivary gland damage. Pinna necrosis is due to vascular damage and in the rabbit may require removal of the pinna.

Fistula formation is a chronic complication that can be seen months after an apparently successful surgery. A repeat bulla osteotomy is usually required to resolve it.

Postoperative care

Supportive care is especially important after major invasive surgery. A balanced analgesic plan should be in place and if necessary the rabbit should be provided with nutritional support; medical intervention may be needed to ensure normal gut motility (see Chapter 2).

Antimicrobial therapy based on culture and sensitivity testing will be needed for a minimum of 4 weeks. In most cases there is some osteomyelitis, in which case a 12-week course is advised.

Sinus disease and surgery

Chronic bacterial sinusitis is the most common indication for sinus surgery. It is a common sequel to upper respiratory tract infection. Sinusitis can also be secondary to dental disease, as an extension to pathology at the apex of the first maxillary cheek teeth into the ventral recess of the maxillary sinus. Neoplasia and foreign bodies are less common indications.

Anatomy and physiology

The paranasal sinuses are pneumatic areas lined with respiratory epithelium, which is continuous with that of the nasal cavity. The anatomy is detailed in Casteleyn *et al.* (2010). There are three paired structures: the maxillary sinuses; the dorsal conchal sinuses; and the sphenoid sinuses.

Maxillary sinus:
- The largest sinus, extending from the perforated area of the maxilla to the rostral orbital edge. Twice as long as the dorsal conchal sinus
- Ventral to the dorsal conchal sinus and lateral to the nasal cavity
- Divided into a dorsal and a ventral recess, the caudal halves of which are connected to each other by a large opening (Figures 16.13 and 16.14). The caudal half is ventral to the ethmoid meatuses and dorsal to the sphenoidal sinus
- Connected to the dorsal conchal sinus through a large opening in the rostral part of the dorsal recess (Figure 16.14)
- The ostium is a small slit-like opening which opens into the nasal cavity in common with the dorsal conchal sinus
- Maxillary premolars create impressions in the ventral floor of the ventral recess.

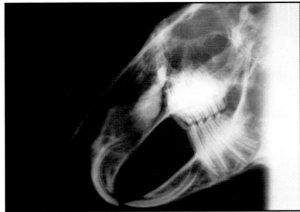

16.13 Contrast material leaking from the nasolacrimal duct and outlining the ventral recess of the maxillary sinus. (© John Chitty)

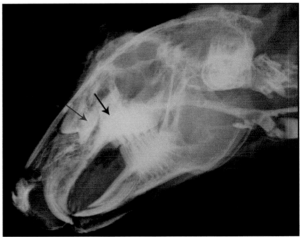

16.14 Contrast study of the sinuses in a cadaver to demonstrate their anatomy. The red arrow marks the position of the large opening from the dorsal conchal sinus into the dorsal recess of the maxillary sinus. The black arrow marks the position of the connection between the dorsal and ventral recesses of the maxillary sinus. (© Aidan Raftery)

Dorsal conchal sinus:
- A cavity in the dorsal nasal concha; in earlier literature it has sometimes been called the frontal sinus
- Situated dorsally in the middle third of the nasal cavity. Rostral border is level with the rostral border of the maxillary sinus. Caudal border is rostral to the ethmoturbinal bones, at approximately the middle of the dorsal recess of the maxillary sinus
- Connects with the dorsal recess of the maxillary sinus through a very large opening and has a single curved slit-like opening to the nasal cavity in common with the maxillary sinus.

Sphenoidal sinus:
- The most caudally and medially located of the sinuses
- Surrounded by the presphenoid bone
- Connects to the middle nasal meatus through a small slit-like rostral opening, often referred to as the ostium.

The paranasal sinuses are lined by ciliated respiratory mucosa; coordinated movements of these cilia aid removal of secretions, especially as positioning of the drainage opening requires the movement of secretions against gravity.

Nitrous oxide is produced within the sinuses to reach bacteriostatic levels and these high levels have been shown to enhance ciliary clearance (Chatkin *et al.*, 1999; Croen, 1993; Lindberg *et al.*, 1997; Lundberg *et al.*, 1995; Ozturk *et al.*, 2003). Excessive opening and surgical iatrogenic damage have been shown to affect ciliary flow and to reduce the ability to build up high concentrations of nitrous oxide (Lindberg *et al.*, 1997; Guevara *et al.*, 2006). Thus, surgery may inadvertently facilitate future problems by reducing local immunity. Surgical approaches to the sinuses should therefore be minimal, and designed to maintain integrity of as much of the sinus structure as possible (see below).

Sinus disease

Clinical signs
These include:

- Nasal discharge – often unilateral, although bilateral sinusitis also occurs
- Sneezing
- Staining and matting of the medial aspects of the front paws from rubbing the nares. If unilateral, this suggests a unilateral discharge
- Head tilt – usually as a result of pain, but extension via the auditory canal into the ears can result in head tilt due to vestibular signs
- Epiphora
- Skull deformity
- Epistaxis
- Dyspnoea
- Exophthalmos
- Erythema and exudates on the skin overlying the perforated part of the maxillary bone due to extension of the infection through the bone.

Diagnosis
Radiography (see Chapter 4) and rhinoscopy (see Chapter 10) are the primary diagnostic tools used to investigate clinical signs. CT and MRI will often give more information (see Chapter 9) as they show soft tissue pus/exudates more readily than radiography (Divers, 2011; Lennox, 2011).

Samples for cytology and culture and sensitivity testing should be collected by deep nasal swab from the nasal cavity and by needle aspiration from the sinuses, using the lateral approaches detailed later. The lateral approach to the ventral recess of the maxillary sinus will require a bone marrow biopsy needle.

The nasolacrimal duct should also be evaluated in the investigation of possible sinusitis. Dacryocystorhinography using contrast material may be needed to reveal areas of obstruction or perforation of the duct. For a very detailed description of the anatomy of the nasolacrimal duct see Burling *et al.* (1991).

Treatment
In milder cases (where the sinus is not completely filled with hard exudates) the sinus may be flushed by passing a hypodermic needle into the affected sinus (using the same entry site as for surgery – see later) and flushing with isotonic saline at body temperature. The rabbit should be anaesthetized and intubated (see Chapter 1). The rabbit's head is held such that flushed material passes down the nose and exits via the nares.

The aim of sinus surgery is generally to re-establish the patency of the normal physiological ostium, salvage the normal mucosa and provide an environment in which the mucosa may recover so that normal ciliary drainage can be re-established.

The normal principles of surgery should be followed. Appropriate antimicrobial medication, based on culture and sensitivity testing of the isolated microbes, should be prescribed. Analgesic and anti-inflammatory medications should also be used as required.

Surgical approaches: There are a number of approaches to the sinuses. The approach, or combination of approaches, chosen will depend on diagnostic findings.

Approaches may need to be modified to accommodate bone deformities, and the surgeon should review the relevant anatomy (see References and further reading).

Dorsal approach to the dorsal conchal sinus: The dorsal approach through the nasal bone into the dorsal conchal sinus (see Operative Technique 16.5) is the easiest to perform.

Lateral approach to the dorsal recess of the maxillary sinus: This approach is made through a perforated part of the maxillary bone (see Operative Technique 16.6). The opening will be through a part of the maxilla which is very thin in the rabbit and, depending on the size of the rabbit, may also include part of the nasal process of the incisive bone. The infraorbital neurovascular bundle is just ventral to the trephine site (see Chapters 2 and 24). This sinusotomy site is right over the curved slit-like common opening of the dorsal conchal sinus and the maxillary sinus into the nasal cavity.

Lateral approach to the ventral recess of the maxillary sinus: This approach involves entry just rostral to the facial tuberosity, just above the line of the diastema (see Operative Technique 16.7), through the body of the maxilla. This gives access to the most rostral point of the ventral recess of the maxillary sinus, which is the most ventral part of the maxillary sinus. This is the area in which discharges often accumulate when the ciliary clearance is not functioning. This lateral approach is the most difficult, due to the layers of levator muscles and the close proximity of the infraorbital nerve which passes close to the dorsal margin of the sinusotomy.

WARNING

It is important to avoid the nasolacrimal duct, which traverses a line between the two lateral approaches. After leaving the lacrimal sac, the nasolacrimal duct enters the maxillary bone just below the palpable lacrimal process at the rostral margin of the bony orbit. It traverses through the maxilla for 5–6 mm in a rostral and medial direction. Then it continues in a rostral direction approximately at the level of the boundary between the dorsal and ventral recesses of the maxillary sinus.

Trephination and flushing: The procedure is described in Operative Techniques 16.5 to 16.7. The following considerations should be noted.

- Samples for cytology and culture should be collected *before* the sinus is flushed. The mucosa of the sinuses and the incisional edges of the tissues are sprayed with local anaesthetic. Any haemorrhage can be controlled using gentle pressure with moist cotton tips. Use of a rigid endoscope through the sinusotomy openings will improve visualization of areas such as the ostium. Depending on the size of the opening, use of a sheath with a working channel can allow better targeted flushing and easier use of instruments to remove necrotic tissues, debride any lesions and collect biopsy samples as necessary. Fungal granulomas can sometimes be removed totally; appropriate medication can be injected directly into fungal granulomas that cannot be completely removed.
- Isotonic saline at body temperature should be used for flushing, so as not to compromise the mucosa. The rabbit should have an endotracheal tube placed and the oropharyngeal area packed with cotton wool or oral sponges to protect it from aspiration of the fluids used for flushing. Removal of the inflammatory exudate can be time-consuming. Moist cotton tips can be used to remove inflammatory exudate gently, where it can be reached.
- Special attention should be paid to the area of the normal ostium to try to re-establish a patent ostium. A normally functioning ostium is vital for long-term resolution. Clearance of discharges through the ostium into the nasal cavity relies on normal functioning of the cilliary circulation. The ostium is not in a position where gravity will result in drainage. An experimental procedure has been described to enlarge the physiological ostium, to try to improve drainage from the sinuses (Kennedy and Shaalan, 1989; Hassab and Kennedy, 1996). However, this procedure has been shown to interfere with normal ciliary drainage and result in recurring sinusitis. Removing the mucosal lining may result in short-term resolution but the sinusitis will have a high rate of recurrence (Perko and Karin, 1992). Procedures to create artificial drainage routes for the sinuses can be used. Creating an artificial ostium into the nasal cavity may help (Perko and Karin, 1992; Haight *et al.*, 1999).
- Any necrotic or loose bone should be debrided and removed; any severely diseased tissue and mucosal fragments should also be removed. Bony sequestra can be a cause of recurring sinusitis.
- Chronically diseased sinuses often have major alterations to their anatomy. Many of the thin bones separating the sinuses from the nasal cavity and each other may be eroded by the disease. The nasal and ethmoid turbinates may also be reduced with osteolytic areas which should be removed if they can be visualized during rhinoscopy or through the sinusotomy as a result of bone loss.
- On completion of the surgery, an ingress drain can be placed if necessary. It should be directed through a separate incision in the skin and overlying musculature but through the same trephine hole. It should be positioned well away from any nearby important neurovascular areas. It is usually sutured (or glued) to the skin at several positions as it travels to just behind the ears.

Postoperative flushing: The sinuses must be flushed at least twice daily with warm hypertonic saline for 5–14 days. Appropriate antimicrobials can also be applied directly into the sinus. If necessary an endoscope can be reintroduced through the trephine hole via a trocar in the skin to re-evaluate a lesion that has been debrided or to repeat intralesional medication.

References and further reading

Barone R, Pavaux C, Blin PC and Cuq P (1973) *Atlas d'Anatomie du Lapin*. Masson, Paris [in French; out of print but may be available in libraries]

Bensley BA (1910) *Practical Anatomy of the Rabbit*. University Press, Toronto

Burling K, Murphy CJ, da Silva Curiel J *et al.* (1991) Anatomy of the rabbit nasolacrimal duct and its clinical implications. *Progress in Veterinary and Comparative Ophthalmology* **1**, 33–40.

Capello V (2004) Surgical treatment of otitis media and externa in pet rabbits. *Exotic DVM* **6**(3), 15–21

Casteleyn C, Cornillie P, Hermens A *et al.* (2010) Topography of the rabbit paranasal sinuses as a prerequisite to model human sinusitis. *Rhinology* **48**, 300–304

Chatkin JM, Silkoff P, Qian W *et al.* (1999) The measurement of nitric oxide accumulation in the non-ventilated nasal cavity. *Archives of Otolaryngology – Head & Neck Surgery* **125**, 682–685

Chow EP (2011) Surgical management of rabbit ear disease. *Journal of Exotic Pet Medicine* **20**, 182–187

Croen K (1993) Evidence of an antiviral effect of nitric oxide. Inhibition of herpes simplex virus type 1 replication. *Journal of Clinical Investigation* **91**, 2446–2452

Divers SJ (2011) Rabbit rhinitis: the good, the bad, and the ugly. *Proceedings, AAV/AEMV Annual Conference 2011, Seattle* pp. 391–401

Fossum TW (2007) Surgery of the ear. In: *Small Animal Surgery, 3rd edn*, ed. TW Fossum *et al.*, pp. 289–316. Saunders Elsevier, St. Louis

Guevara N, Hofman V, Hofman P, Santini J and Castillo L (2006) A comparison between functional and radical sinus surgery in an experimental model of maxillary sinusitis. *Rhinology* **44**, 255–258

Haight J, Djupesland PG, Qian W *et al.* (1999) Does nasal nitric oxide come from the sinuses? *Journal of Otolaryngology* **28**, 197–204

Harcourt-Brown FM (2002) *Textbook of Rabbit Medicine*. Butterworth-Heinemann, Oxford

Hassab M and Kennedy DW (1996) Maxillary sinus osteoplasty versus nasal antral window in maxillary sinusitis: an experimental study. *American Journal of Rhinology* **10**, 357–63

Keeble E (2006) Nervous and musculoskeletal disorders. In: *BSAVA Manual of Rabbit Medicine and Surgery, 2nd edn*, ed. A Meredith and P Flecknell, pp. 103–116. BSAVA Publications, Gloucester

Kennedy DW and Shaalan H (1989) Re-evaluation of maxillary sinus surgery: experimental study in rabbits. *Annals of Otology Rhinology and Laryngology* **98**, 901–906

Lennox A (2011) Rhinostomy: adjunct treatment for treatment of chronic rhinitis in rabbits. *Proceedings, AAV/AEMV Annual Conference 2011, Seattle* pp. 141–143

Lindberg S, Cervin A and Runer T (1997) Low levels of nasal nitric oxide (NO) correlate with impaired mucociliary function in the upper airways. *Acta Otolaryngologica (Stockholm)* **117**, 728–734

Love NE, Kramer RW, Spodnick GJ and Thrall DE (1995) Radiographic and computed tomographic evaluation of otitis media in the dog. *Veterinary Radiology & Ultrasound* **36**, 375–379

Lundberg JON, Lundberg JM, Settergren G *et al.* (1995) Nitric oxide, produced in the upper airways, may act in an 'aerocrine' fashion to enhance pulmonary uptake in humans. *Acta Physiologica Scandinavica* **155**, 467–468

Melgarejo-Moreno P and Hellín-Meseguer D (2006) Submucosal glands and goblet cells in maxillary sinus surgery: an experimental study in rabbits. *Rhinology* **44**, 259–263

Oztürk M, Selimoğlu E, Polat MF and Erman Z (2003) Serum and mucosal nitric oxide levels and efficacy of sodium nitroprusside in experimentally induced acute sinusitis. *Yonsei Medical Journal* **44**(3), 424-428

Perko D and Karin RR (1992) Nasoantral windows: an experimental study in rabbits. *Laryngoscope* **102**, 320–326

Popesko P, Rajtova V and Horak J (1992) *A Colour Atlas of the Anatomy of Small Laboratory Animals. Vol. I: Rabbit, Guinea Pig.* Wolfe, London

OPERATIVE TECHNIQUES →

TECHNIQUE 16.1:
Ear syringing
John Chitty

Patient positioning and preparation

The procedure is carried out with the rabbit under general anaesthesia (see Chapter 1) and in lateral recumbency.

Assistant

An assistant is not required other than to monitor the anaesthesia.

Equipment

- Otoscope
- Alligator forceps
- Spreull needle
- 5 ml syringe
- Warmed saline. Saline is used because possible ototoxicity of the ear-cleansing solutions used in dogs and cats does not appear to have been evaluated in the rabbit. This is especially important where the tympanic membrane may be ruptured
- Instead of an otoscope, a 4 mm otoendoscope may be utilized with grasping forceps. However, this author (JC) finds this considerably more difficult than using an otoscope and Spreull needle. Rather, the endoscope should be reserved for examination of the ear, where it provides much better visualization of canal and tympanic membrane than an otoscope (see text)

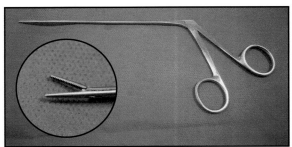

Alligator forceps suitable for use in rabbit ears via the otoscope. (© John Chitty)

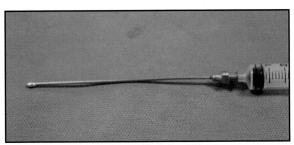

Spreull needle on syringe. (© John Chitty)

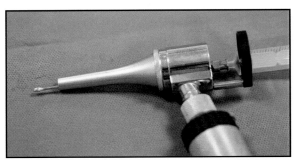

Spreull needle in position via otoscope cone. (© John Chitty)

Procedure

1 Large lumps of discharge and crust are removed using the forceps via the otoscope cone.

2 Warmed saline is inserted gently from the syringe and the remaining discharge removed using the Spreull needle via the otoscope cone.

3 The tympanic membrane should be assessed as soon as it becomes visible. If intact, it should be assessed for pus in the middle ear (see text). If this is present, the tympanum may be incised, allowing access to the middle ear.

4 If the tympanum is damaged, diseased portions may be removed using the alligator forceps. Normal-appearing remnants may be left *in situ*.

OPERATIVE TECHNIQUE 16.2:
Lateral wall resection
John Chitty

Patient positioning and preparation

The procedure is carried out with the rabbit under general anaesthesia (see Chapter 1) and in lateral recumbency. The skin over the ear canal is clipped and prepared aseptically.

Assistant

An assistant is not required other than to monitor anaesthesia.

Equipment

- Scalpel
- Basic surgery kit – straight scissors, fine mosquito forceps (curved and straight), longer straight artery forceps, rat-toothed forceps, Olsen–Hegar needle holders
- Suture material: polydioxanone 2 metric (3/0 USP)

Procedure

1 The ear canal is identified and parallel skin incisions made either side of the canal, from just ventral to the base of the vertical canal to the pinna.

2 The resultant skin flap is reflected and the incisions continued ventrally through the cartilage of the lateral wall of the vertical canal.

WARNING
- It is vital that the incisions are maintained parallel to each other and do not converge.
- It is also important that surrounding soft tissues are accurately identified and reflected in order to avoid damage to blood vessels and nerves.

3 The incisions are stopped when the horizontal canal is exposed.

4 The cartilage of the ventral horizontal canal is then sutured to the skin ventral to the canal (at the point of the original incision). This should be under sufficient tension that the resultant stoma is held open by the action of this 'drainage board'.

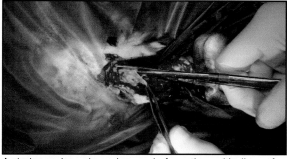

A drainage board can be made from the epithelium of the ear canal in lop-eared rabbits with a diverticulum that is causing a bulge at the base of the ear. Once the soft tissue over the swelling has been cleared away, two parallel incisions can be made to form a flap. (Courtesy of Frances Harcourt-Brown)

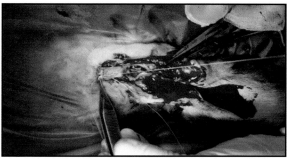

The flap of ear epithelium is reflected and sutured to the skin. It is important to ensure that the flap is stretched out but not under tension. In most cases an additional section of skin needs to be removed in order to place the flap correctly to form the drainage board. (Courtesy of Frances Harcourt-Brown)

5 Once this is achieved, the remaining skin and cartilage from the lateral wall of the vertical canal may be excised; this is not done earlier as determination of the size and tension of the drainage board is imperative in determining success of the surgery. This is more difficult in rabbits than in dogs as the horizontal canal of the rabbit is comparatively short.

6 The skin is then sutured to the exposed edges of cartilage and ear canal epithelium to create a continuous opening of vertical and horizontal canals.

OPERATIVE TECHNIQUE 16.2 continued:
Lateral wall resection
John Chitty

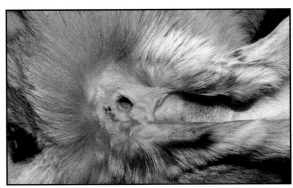

The end result of a lateral wall resection that was performed 3 years previously on this lop-eared rabbit. The surgery was carried out because the rabbit had a persistent ear infection and an aural diverticulosis at the ear base. Surgery was curative in this case. During the operation, care was taken to separate the epithelial lining of the ear from the cartilage along the cut edge of the ear canal. This meant that any excess cartilage could be trimmed away and the epithelium could be attached to the skin with no tension on the wound. A soft suture material (1.5 metric (4/0 USP) polyglactin 910 (Vicryl Rapide)) was used in this case. (Courtesy of Frances Harcourt-Brown)

OPERATIVE TECHNIQUE 16.3:
Total ear canal ablation via a lateral bulla osteotomy
Aidan Raftery

- Familiarity with the complex anatomy of this area is vital for a successful surgical outcome, especially if there are unexpected findings during the surgery such as osteomyelitis of the lateral wall of the bulla.
- See the main text for the comprehensive work-up necessary before embarking on this surgery and a discussion of the many possible complications.

Patient positioning and preparation

The procedure is carried out with the rabbit under general anaesthesia (see Chapter 1). The rabbit is positioned in lateral recumbency with the forelimbs extended caudally. A pad is positioned under the neck to create a convex profile of the proximal cervical area and improve exposure of the surgical site. The area prepared for surgery extends from the lateral canthus of the eye to the level of the intertragic incisures, and the same distance down the neck. The dorsal margin of the prepared area is the external sagittal crest and the ventral margin is the angle of the mandible.

Assistant

Not required other than for monitoring anaesthesia.

Additional instruments

- Small rongeurs to enlarge the external acoustic opening
- Curette for debridement of the bulla

Procedure

1 A horizontal skin incision is made from the dorsal surface of the tragus to encircle the ear canal.

WARNING
Great care needs to be taken at this point to preserve the blood vessels that supply the pinna. The caudal auricular vessels are found on the caudal aspect of the auricular cartilage (of the pinna); the rostral auricular vessels are on the rostral surface (see Figure 16.1). If any of these vessels is damaged, the entire auricular cartilage, i.e. the pinna, should also be removed. If it is left, there is a very high risk of avascular necrosis.

OPERATIVE TECHNIQUE 16.3 continued:
Total ear canal ablation via a lateral bulla osteotomy
Aidan Raftery

2 A vertical skin incision is made from the horizontal incision down to the level of the tympanic membrane.

3 The cartilages that comprise the external canal are bluntly dissected as one (i.e. the ventral part of the auricular cartilage, the scutiform cartilage and the cartilage of the acoustic meatus). Great care should be taken not to enter the canal.

4 The cartilaginous ear canal is transected at its junction with the bony acoustic canal.

5 Necrotic material is carefully removed from within the short bony acoustic canal and its lateral wall is then removed with rongeurs to provide better access to the tympanic bulla.

6 Samples are collected from within the bulla for cytology and culture.

7 Curettage of the bulla:

- Irrigate with warm saline
- Remove all the debris
- Occasionally the lateral wall of the bulla is necrotic, in which case all the infected bone has to be debrided
- Remove the epithelial lining gently with a curette.

WARNING
Avoid the area of the ossicles and the promontory (the dorsomedial area of the bulla). Damage to this area will result in vestibular signs.

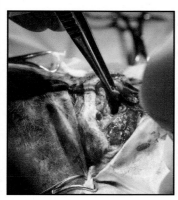

The lateral approach to the bulla. In this case there were severe changes of the lateral wall of the bulla caused by osteomyelitis. All the necrotic bone has to be carefully removed. The pinna has also been removed in this case. (© Aidan Raftery)

8 An active drain is positioned before closure. This should not have any fenestrations. The aim is to flush the bulla postoperatively to remove necrotic material and to maintain local high concentrations of the appropriate antimicrobial. Avoid aminoglycosides, alcohol or any other irritant drug in the flush. If the results of previous culture and sensitivity testing are not available, cytology can be used to inform the choice of antimicrobial until results are available. Lidocaine is sometimes added to this flush as part of the analgesic plan.

- A stab incision is made for the drain, separate from the skin incision.
- One end is placed within the bulla and the other attached to the skin using a Chinese finger-trap suture.
- The volume of fluid that will be required to fill the bulla cavity is measured using saline.
- The osseous cavity is flushed three times daily. Syringe in the calculated volume; wait 2–3 minutes; then aspirate. Repeat this three times at each flushing session.
- The drain is removed after 5 days.

9 The muscle and subcutaneous layers are closed over the bony deficit created by the surgery, at the level of the bony acoustic canal. The skin is closed over this layer in a standard fashion.

OPERATIVE TECHNIQUE 16.4:
Total ear canal ablation via a ventral bulla osteotomy
Aidan Raftery

See the main text for the comprehensive work-up necessary before embarking on this surgery and a discussion of the possible complications.

Patient positioning and preparation

The procedure is carried out with the rabbit under general anaesthesia (see Chapter 1). The rabbit is positioned in dorsal recumbency with the forelimbs extended caudally. The skin is prepared for surgery from the symphysis of the mandible extending back to the manubrium. The prepared area should extend just to the lateral aspect of the mandible on the normal side but on the diseased side continue the preparation up to and around the pinna.

Assistant

Not required other than for monitoring anaesthesia.

Additional instruments

- Intramedullary pin to penetrate into the bulla
- Small rongeurs to enlarge the opening
- Curette for debridement of the bulla

Procedure

1 Make a 3 cm incision between the wings of the atlas vertebra and the angular process of the mandible.

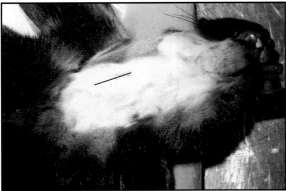

The position of the ventral approach incision is marked with a black line. Clipping of this patient is not complete. A sandbag has been placed under the neck to give better exposure. (© Aidan Raftery)

2 Incise through the subcutaneous tissues medial to the mandibular salivary gland.

3 Separate the digastricus muscle, which is reflected laterally, from the hypoglossal and styloglossal muscles, which are reflected medially. Avoid the hypoglossal nerve, which can be seen on the lateral aspect of the hypoglossal muscle and the medial aspect of the styloglossal muscle (between them).

4 Then dissect bluntly down to the bulla.

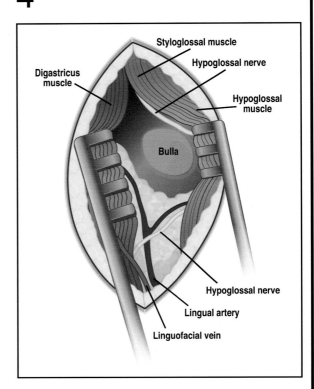

5 Incise the periosteum. The medial aspect of the ventral surface of the bulla is very thin and easily penetrated.

6 Use rongeurs to enlarge the opening.

7 Collect samples for culture and cytology.

8 Curettage of the bulla:

- Irrigate with warm saline
- Remove all the debris
- Remove the epithelial lining gently with a curette.

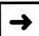

OPERATIVE TECHNIQUE 16.4 continued:
Total ear canal ablation via a ventral bulla osteotomy
Aidan Raftery

WARNING
Leave the area of the ossicles and the promontory (the dorsomedial area of the bulla). Damage to this area will result in vestibular signs.

9 An active drain is positioned before closure (see Operative Technique 16.3).

10 The muscle and subcutaneous layers are closed over the bony deficit created in the tympanic bulla. The skin is closed over this layer in a standard fashion.

OPERATIVE TECHNIQUE 16.5:
Flushing the dorsal conchal sinus via a dorsal approach
Aidan Raftery

Patient positioning and preparation

The procedure is carried out with the rabbit under general anaesthesia (see Chapter 1). The rabbit is placed in ventral recumbency on a tilted table, with the head lowest. The area from the rostral margin of the nasal bone to the level of the eye on the affected side down to a line from the medial canthus of the eye to the lateral commissure of the nose is shaved and surgically prepared.

Assistant

Required to provide a constant supply of irrigation fluid and suction.

Additional instruments

- A ball-tip seeker is used to explore the sinus and to loosen inflammatory material
- Bone trephine 6–8 mm

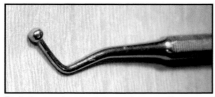

Ball-tip seeker instrument, sometimes called a frontal ostium seeker, used for atraumatic exploration of the sinus. The balls at either end of the handle are of different sizes and set at different angles.

Procedure

1 The surgical site is identified by imagining a line from the level of the medial canthi to the rostral margin of the nasal bone on the midline. The sinusotomy entry point is just caudal to the midpoint of this line, on the affected side.

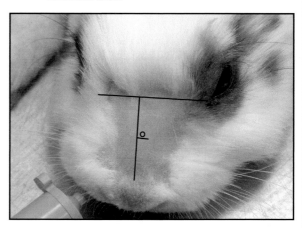

2 Incise the skin directly over the surgical site in the posterior rostral plane. Reflect the skin and the overlying soft tissues.

3 Using the trephine, make an opening into the sinus. The opening can be enlarged as necessary.

4 Samples are collected for cytology and culture.

OPERATIVE TECHNIQUE 16.5 continued:
Flushing the dorsal conchal sinus via a dorsal approach
Aidan Raftery

---

5 The ball-tip seeker is used to explore the sinus atraumatically. In advanced or chronic cases the thin medial wall may be missing in areas, leaving an abnormal ostium into the nasal cavity. The large opening into the dorsal recess of the maxillary sinus is in the floor of the dorsal conchal sinus. Following the floor of the dorsal recess of the maxillary sinus caudally will lead to the opening into the ventral recess of the maxillary sinus.

6 The sinuses are irrigated with isotonic saline at body temperature. *Note: From this dorsal approach it is not possible to access the rostral section of the ventral recess of the maxillary sinus, the most ventral part of the sinuses.*

7 Gentle suction, in combination with copious quantities of fluid, will help with the removal of inflammatory exudates.

8 Remove any areas of osteitic bone. These are usually on the medial wall. Preserve the mucosal lining of the sinus where possible.

9 A catheter can be positioned in the sinus for the direct administration of postoperative medication. It is placed through a separate skin incision and sutured (or glued) to the skin at several positions as it travels to just behind the ear. Choice of medication depends on the microbes identified. Irritant medication must not be used.

10 The skin is closed over the entry hole. No attempt is made to replace the bone.

Postoperative flushing

See Operative Technique 16.7.

OPERATIVE TECHNIQUE 16.6:
Flushing the dorsal recess of the maxillary sinus via a lateral approach
Aidan Raftery

Patient positioning and preparation

The procedure is carried out with the rabbit under general anaesthesia (see Chapter 1). The rabbit is placed in lateral recumbency on a tilted table with the head lowest. An area from the dorsal midline between the rostral margin of the nasal bone to the level of the eyes and down to the hair follicles of the whiskers on the upper lip and the ventral margin of the mandible is shaved and surgically prepared.

Assistant

Required to provide a constant supply of irrigation fluid and suction.

Additional instruments

- Ball-tip seeker (see Operative Technique 16.5)
- Bone trephine 4–6 mm

Surgical technique

1 The surgical site is identified by imagining a line from the middle of the eye to meet the commissure of the nose. The sinusotomy entry point is just dorsal to this line and rostral to the palpable rim of the bony orbit.

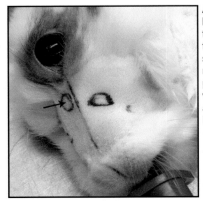

Anatomical landmarks for trephination of the maxillary sinus. The dorsal recess puncture point is marked with the black arrow. (© Aidan Raftery)

OPERATIVE TECHNIQUE 16.6 continued:
Flushing the dorsal recess of the maxillary sinus via a lateral approach
Aidan Raftery

2 Incise the skin directly over the surgical site in the posterior rostral plane. Reflect the skin and the overlying soft tissues.

3 Using the trephine make an opening into the sinus. The bone can be very thin here so care is needed not to damage the medial wall of the sinus, especially the ostium which is just under the sinusotomy entry point.

4 Samples are collected for cytology and culture.

5 The ball-tip seeker is used to explore the sinus atraumatically. In advanced or chronic cases the thin medial wall may be missing in areas. Ventral to the sinusotomy entry point is the large opening into the ventral recess of the maxillary sinus. It is difficult to get to the most ventral point of this recess, which is directly ventral and then rostral. The dorsal conchal sinus is rostral and then dorsal.

6 Gentle suction, in combination with copious quantities of isotonic saline at body temperature, will help with the removal of inflammatory exudates. Always attempt to preserve the mucosal lining of the sinus where possible.

7 Any areas of osteitic bone should be removed; this may create artificial openings into the nasal cavity.

8 A catheter can be positioned in the sinus for the direct administration of postoperative medication. It is placed through a separate skin incision and sutured (or glued) to the skin at several positions as it travels to just behind the ear. Choice of medication depends on the microbes identified. Irritant medication must not be used.

9 The skin is closed over the entry hole. No attempt is made to replace the bone.

Postoperative flushing

See Operative Technique 16.7.

OPERATIVE TECHNIQUE 16.7:
Flushing the ventral recess of the maxillary sinus via a lateral approach
Aidan Raftery

Patient positioning and preparation

The procedure is carried out with the rabbit under general anaesthesia (see Chapter 1). The rabbit is placed in lateral recumbency on a tilted table with the head lowest. An area from the dorsal midline between the rostral margin of the nasal bone to the level of the eyes and down to the hair follicles of the whiskers on the upper lip and the ventral margin of the mandible is shaved and surgically prepared.

Assistant

Required to provide constant supply of irrigation fluid and suction.

Additional instruments

• Ball-tip seeker (see Operative Technique 6.5)
• Bone trephine 4–6 mm

Surgical technique

1 The surgical site is identified just rostral to the facial tuberosity and just above the line of the diastema. The infraorbital neurovascular bundle is just dorsal to this in the triangular area formed by drawing a line from each canthus to the most caudal point of the commissure of the nose.

OPERATIVE TECHNIQUE 16.7 continued:
Flushing the ventral recess of the maxillary sinus via a lateral approach
Aidan Raftery

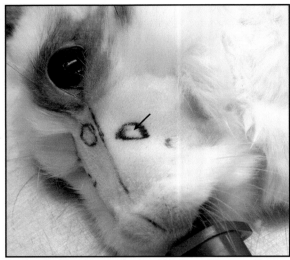

Anatomical landmarks for trephination of the maxillary sinus. The ventral recess puncture point is marked by the black arrow. (© Aidan Raftery)

2 Incise the skin directly over the surgical site in the posterior rostral plane. Reflect the skin.

3 Bluntly dissect between the levator muscles of the labiae to reach the maxillary bone.

4 Use the trephine to make an opening into the sinus. Very little force is needed as the bone is very thin here. Alternatively, in small rabbits, artery forceps can be pushed through the bone into the sinus.

5 Samples are collected for cytology and culture.

6 The ball-tip seeker is used to explore the sinus atraumatically and loosen the inflammatory exudate. From the entry point,

follow the floor of the recess rostrally to reach the rostral pole. The ventral floor of the caudal pole is elevated by the apical areas of the premolars, which also create impression marks in its floor. Travelling dorsally from the sinusotomy opening will lead into the dorsal recess of the maxillary sinus.

7 Use gentle suction, in combination with copious quantities of isotonic saline at body temperature, to remove the inflammatory exudates.

8 An ingress–egress drain is positioned to exit through a separate stab incision. It is attached to the skin in several places by either a suture or surgical glue as it travels to just behind the ear, enabling the sinus to be flushed. The volume of fluid needed to fill the conchomaxillary cavity is measured.

9 The skin is closed over the entry hole. No attempt is made to replace the bone.

Postoperative flushing

Hypertonic saline at body temperature, which may have antibacterials added, based on results of cytology and culture, is used by the author for flushing.

The conchomaxillary cavity is flushed two to three times daily:

- Syringe in the calculated volume; wait 2–3 minutes; then aspirate
- Repeat three times at each flushing session.

Flushing is continued for a minimum period of 3 days until no inflammatory material is aspirated.

17

Eye and eyelid surgery

Michael Fehr

Relevant anatomy

The rabbit eye shows several anatomical differences compared to other mammals, some of which are important for surgery.

Structures of the orbit

Optic foramen
The rabbit orbit communicates with the contralateral orbit through the optic foramen, an opening of about 5 mm. The communication can allow infection to pass from one side to the other, so the optic foramen is an important feature to recognize in cases of enucleation and during curettage of retrobulbar abscesses.

Retrobulbar venous plexus
Within the orbit, immediately adjacent to the periorbital membrane of the globe, lies the retrobulbar venous plexus (orbital sinus) which extends from the orbital apex to the equator of the globe. It is important to note the orbital sinus during enucleation because of its communications with major veins and the intracranial cavernous sinus.

Size of the globe
Ophthalmometric bulb measurements in rabbits with a bodyweight of 2 kg are: axial 16.95 ± 0.5 mm; equatorial 17.85 ± 1.0 mm (Uthoff, 1984).

Lacrimal glands and tear production

- The orbital lacrimal gland is situated dorsolaterally in the orbit and caudodorsal to the eyeball (Figure 17.1). Its multiple openings are situated in the lateral half of the superior conjunctival sac.
- The accessory lacrimal glands extend along the caudal and ventral orbital margins and protrude medially into the orbit. They have a single excretory duct opening into the lateral edge of the conjunctival sac.

All of the glands contribute to tear production. Reference values of 0–11.22 mm/min with a mean of 5.30 ± 2.96 mm/min for the Schirmer tear test have been reported in New Zealand White rabbits (Abrams *et al.*, 1990).

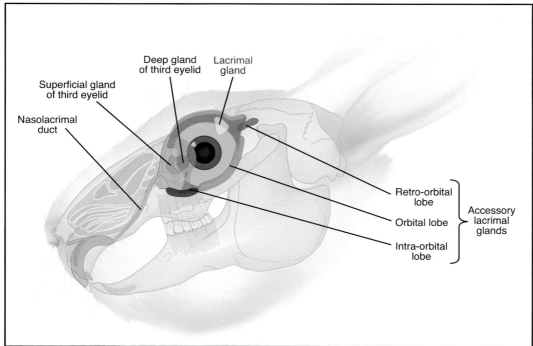

17.1 Anatomical structures surrounding the globe.

Glands of the third eyelid

The superficial gland of the third eyelid (also called the nictitans gland) lies against the convex surface of the cartilage within the lid (Figure 17.1). The deep gland of the third eyelid (also called the Harderian gland or the glandula palpebrae tertiae profunda) is located rostromedially in the orbit (Figure 17.1); it is composed of a dorsal white lobe and a ventral pink (red) lobe. Prolapse of the glands of the third eyelid (Figures 17.2 and 17.3) invariably involves the superficial gland, and often the ventral portion of the deep gland as well (Janssens *et al.*, 1999; Wagner and Fehr, 2007).

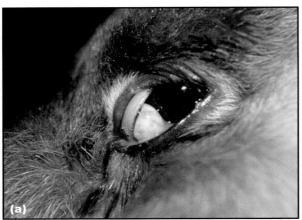
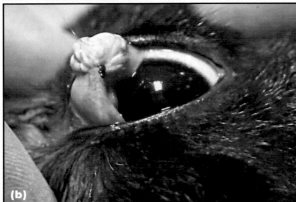

17.2 **(a)** Prolapse of the deep gland of the third eyelid, 'cherry eye'. **(b)** Prolapse of glandular tissue after incision through the capsule.

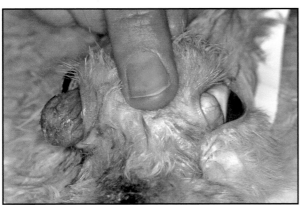

17.3 Prolapsed glands of the third eyelid (right eye) and protrusion (left eye).

Nasolacrimal duct

On each eye, a nasolacrimal duct drains the lacrimal fluid from the conjunctival sac to a nasal opening. The nasolacrimal duct starts with a single nasolacrimal punctum on the lower eyelid, approximately 3 mm from the medial canthus and about 3–4 mm ventral to the lid margin. The duct has a convoluted passage through the lacrimal and frontal bones, passing close to the molar and incisor tooth roots (see Figure 17.1). Dental diseases can affect the passage of lacrimal fluid and result in nasolacrimal occlusion with permanent epiphora (Burling *et al.*, 1998). Diseases of the nasolacrimal duct are described in Chapter 28.

Rectus dorsalis muscle

The rectus dorsalis muscle can be seen posterior to the dorsal limbus under the bulbar conjunctiva. It is a pale fleshy structure (Figure 17.4) that is sometimes misinterpreted as a pathological feature. The muscle can be used to stabilize the globe during ocular surgery, by placing an anchoring suture around the muscle, fixed with a clamp nearby.

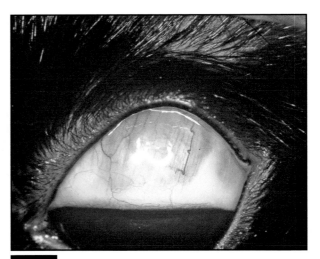

17.4 Rectus dorsalis muscle at the dorsal bulb.

Cornea, uvea and lens

Diseases of the cornea include trauma, ulceration, degeneration, dystrophy, abscess formation, dermoid cyst (see Figure 17.8) and inflammatory keratitis (Figure 17.5). The proximity of the intraocular tissues and their high vascularity means that uveal inflammation is a part of nearly all intraocular disease processes. Uveitis is most often caused by capsular rupture due to *Encephalitozoon cuniculi* infection (Wolfer *et al.*, 1993) or to *Pasteurella* or *Staphylococcus* infection.

Examination of the lens and vitreous can be performed after topical administration of tropicamide solution 0.5%. If dilation of the pupil is insufficient, a combination of atropine 1% and phenylephrine 10% solution can be added (Lee, 1983). Congenital and osmotic cataracts as well as lens luxations occur in rabbits.

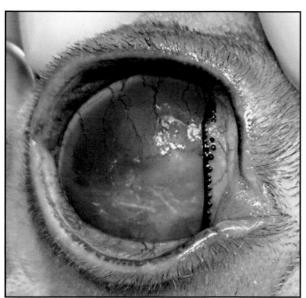

17.5 Phacoclastic uveitis with stromal diffuse keratitis.

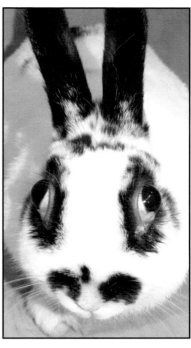

17.6 Bilateral exophthalmos due to thymoma.

Decision-making and treatment options

Exophthalmos (unilateral or bilateral)
Exophthalmos may be due to:

- Orbital cellulitis or retrobulbar abscessation, which is usually associated with dental disease and is common in pet rabbits (Bagley and Lavach, 1995) (see Chapter 29)
- Trauma with haematoma formation
- *Taenia serialis* (tapeworm) cysts, which can cause unilateral exophthalmos in pet rabbits (O'Reilly *et al.*, 2002)
- Malignant uni- or bilateral lymphoma-induced exophthalmos, due to infiltration of the lacrimal glands (Volopich *et al.*, 2005)
- Permanent (Kostolich and Panciera, 1992) and recurrent bilateral exophthalmos in rabbits with thymoma (Wagner *et al.*, 2005; Figure 17.6) or mediastinal lymphoma
- Fear (Harcourt-Brown, 2000)
- Glaucoma.

Comparison of the position, size, and shape of the left and right globes allows diagnosis (or ex-clusion) of a uni- or bilateral exophthalmos. Determination of the cause can be done by clinical investigation (protrusion of the third eyelid), tonometry, radiography of the skull (foreign body or tooth/bone involvement) or ultrasonography (abscess), with or without fine-needle biopsy (cytological evaluation, e.g. lymphoma), computed tomography (CT) or magnetic resonance imaging (MRI).

A position-induced exophthalmos through ventro-flexion of the head may be detected during clinical examination, which may be due to a mediastinal mass (Figure 17.6). Other ophthalmological tests are normal (Vernau *et al.*, 1995). Diagnosis depends on the radiographic and/or ultrasonographic confirmation of the mediastinal mass (see Chapters 5 and 19).

Diagnosis of a retrobulbar abscess depends on clinical examination (e.g. oral examination and tooth probing), ultrasonography of the orbit and radiography of the skull (see Chapter 29).

Cataracts
Although large numbers of laboratory rabbits have been used in ophthalmic studies, little information is available regarding the incidence and presentation of cataracts (Gelatt, 1975; Munger *et al.*, 2002). Congenital cataracts (Weisse *et al.*, 1974) and osmotic cataracts due to diabetes (Munger *et al.*, 2002; Williams, 2007) have been described, although diabetes in pet rabbits is rare (Harcourt-Brown and Harcourt-Brown, 2012).

Cataracts are often diagnosed in association with *E. cuniculi* infection of the lens (Wolfer *et al.*, 1993), which may rupture and cause uveitis. Testing for antibodies, especially of the IgM and IgG classes, should be considered for all cases of cataracts, to investigate the possibility of underlying *E. cuniculi* infection (Jeklova *et al.*, 2010). Although *E. cuniculi*-induced uveitis may not respond well to symptomatic medical therapy, cataract formation can be treated by intracapsular phacoemulsification (Felchle and Sigler, 2002). Because *E. cuniculi* infection can affect other organs in addition to the eye, evaluation of kidney, heart and liver function is recommended using ultrasonography, radiography and blood chemistry (e.g. glucose, fructosamine). Although cataract surgery in rabbits is possible, expensive ophthalmo-surgical equipment is necessary, and the anaesthetic risks have to be considered. There is also a propensity for regrowth of the lens cortex (Williams, 2007). Overall, blind rabbits living in well known surroundings with a convenient food supply manage well.

Corneal ulcers

Corneal ulceration (Figure 17.7) is frequently encountered in rabbits. There is a wide variety of underlying aetiologies: external trauma has been cited as the most important cause, but few owners report seeing a relevant incident (Andrew, 2002). The main causes of traumatic lesions are direct fight wounds, self-trauma due to irritation and/or pain with underlying eyelid deformities, chronic dacryocystitis or orbital diseases (Wagner and Fehr, 2007).

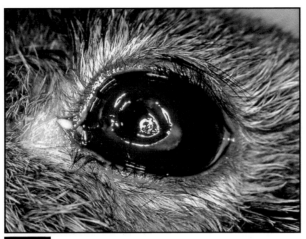

17.7 Deep corneal ulceration.

Diseased rabbits will be presented with external or internal ocular signs. External clinical signs include blepharospasm, epiphora, conjunctival hyperaemia and purulent secretions. A typical internal sign might be anterior uveitis. After application of fluorescein dye, biomicroscopic examination of the cornea can reveal the extent and depth of the ulcer. Complicated ulcers require culture of the ulcer bed for bacterial identification and antibiotic sensitivity testing of any isolate, although most cases require immediate medical therapy. Untreated, a corneal ulcer or infection can damage the cornea permanently or may progress to corneal perforation and spread of the infection within the eye, which increases the risk of permanent visual problems.

Treatment depends on the type of ulcer. Non-healing indolent ulcers are characterized by an undermined corneal epithelium (epithelial lips) and the absence of ingrowing vessels from the limbus. In these cases, the healing process can be induced by removal of all the loosely attached epithelium after applying topical anaesthesia (e.g. proxymetacaine (proparacaine) 0.5% eye solution) to the affected eye. After instillation of an eye drop, only 5% of the applied drug penetrates the cornea; the major fraction is resorbed and enters the systemic circulation, usually via the nasal mucosa. This can result in undesirable systemic side effects, e.g. cardiac effects, the incidence of which can be reduced using dropper bottles that deliver drops with an optimal drop volume of about 20 microlitres (Kumar *et al.*, 2011). Using a rolling movement, a dry cotton-tipped applicator can be used to remove any loose epithelial material from the centre of the ulcer to the periphery (see Operative Technique 17.1). To prevent secondary bacterial infection, topical broad-spectrum antibiotics are administered for 1 week, together with topical atropine for its cycloplegic and mydriatic properties (1% q12h for 2 days then q24h). If the mydriasis obtained is insufficient, topical phenylephrine 1% eye solution may be added.

Infective or progressive melting ulcers require aggressive and frequent administration of topical antibiotics based on cytological examination of a Gram-stained corneal scraping. Additional application of autologous serum q6h ensures the preservation of growth factors and anticollagenase activity (Akyol-Salman, 2006). Growth factors in autologous serum eye drops are stable at 4°C for up to 1 month (Phasukkijwatana *et al.*, 2011).

Cases that fail to respond to topical therapy, or severe ulcers that are more than half the corneal thickness deep, need a conjunctival pedicle graft into the ulcer region. If a corneal ulcer heals with re-epithelialization and the infection is sealed into the corneal stroma, a corneal abscess can develop. Stromal involvement may be demonstrated by slit lamp biomicroscopy; the lesion does not stain with fluorescein because epithelium has sealed it. Bacterial identification, sensitivity and cytological testing are only possible after removal of the epithelium. Complicated ulcers and stromal abscesses require aggressive treatment with topical chloramphenicol solution, which can penetrate intact epithelium. Improvement should be seen after a few days; if not, keratectomy and conjunctival grafting are indicated (Wagner and Fehr, 2007).

Dermoid cyst

Spontaneous congenital dysplasia of the cornea, including skin-like material, is occasionally seen in rabbits (Wagner *et al.*, 1998). As in dogs or cats the removal of the dermoid cyst is necessary (Figure 17.8). Superficial keratectomy is possible, using an operating microscope because of the thin corneal diameter.

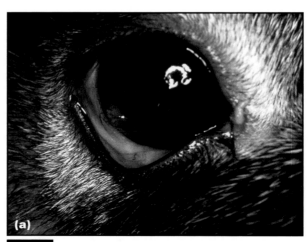

(a)

17.8 **(a)** Congenital dermoid cyst. (continues) ▶

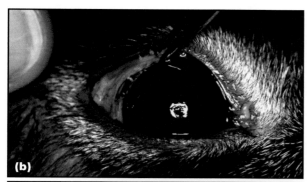

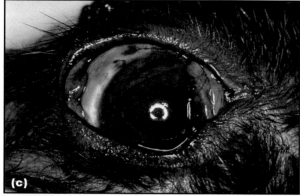

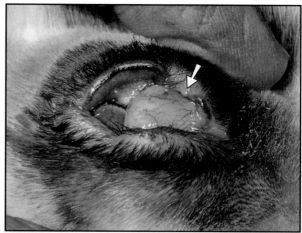

17.9 Eyelid dysplasia in a 2-year-old French Lop rabbit. There is an extra piece of eyelid (arrow) that lacks the normal rigidity and tends to roll in and cause discomfort and spastic entropion. A method of repair is described in Operative Technique 17.3. (Courtesy of Frances Harcourt-Brown)

17.8 (continued) **(b)** Corneal deficit after removal of dermoid cyst. **(c)** End result immediately after removal.

Entropion, ectropion and eyelid dysplasia

In rabbits ectropion, entropion, coloboma and eyelid dysplasia can be congenital (Fox *et al.*, 1979) or acquired. A primary keratitis may be induced by disorders of the eyelids (Wagner *et al.*, 1998).

Entropion is a relatively common disease in rabbits. Clinical signs are based upon the degree of in- or out-turning of the eyelid and vary from superficial irritation of the conjunctiva and/or cornea, producing epiphora and ocular discharge, to keratitis and corneal ulceration. Ectropion and entropion can occur separately or together. Distichiasis and trichiasis have also been described in rabbits with spastic entropion (Kern, 1997). Spastic entropion can often be seen in association with dacryocystitis and secondary keratitis. If in doubt, flushing of the nasolacrimal duct and local instillation of a topical anaesthetic eye solution (proxymetacaine 0.5%) can rule out the underlying disease. Other possible causes of ocular irritation should first be ruled out. Ocular lubrication can be helpful in protecting the ocular surface. In severe cases of ectropion and entropion, surgery is advised, according to the same principles used in dogs and cats (see Operative Technique 17.2). In cases of additional distichiasis, distichia can be removed by simple epilation, electro-epilation or cryoepilation (Kern, 1997).

A form of eyelid dysplasia is common in certain breeds, such as the French Lop, in which there seems to be an extra piece of lid due to loose skin formation (Figure 17.9). Surgical correction of eyelid defects depends on the size and localization of the defect. In most cases good apposition of the wound edges can be accomplished. In defects larger than one-third of the eyelid length, reconstruction is only possible with the aid of skin flaps (see Operative Technique 17.3).

Protrusion and prolapse of the gland of the third eyelid

Protrusion of the third eyelid caused by orbital gland tissue (see Figures 17.2 and 17.3) has been reported in rabbits as an occasional finding (Fehr, 1984). This condition, which may be uni- or bilateral, is clinically similar to 'cherry eye' in dogs. Recent studies in rabbits have demonstrated that, in most cases, protrusion of the deep gland of the third eyelid (Harderian gland) leads to prolapse, often accompanied by marked congestion of the venous plexus lying immediately beneath the prolapsed gland tissue (Figure 17.10). Direct prolapse of the deep gland lobe has also been reported, and it is speculated that this might be due to abnormal laxity of the connective tissue that attaches the gland to the surrounding orbital structures (Janssens *et al.*, 1999). Untreated, there is a risk of corneal irritation with the risk of permanent visual problems.

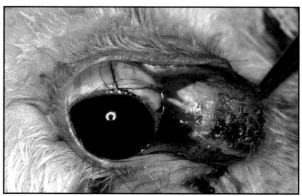

17.10 Prolapsed gland of the third eyelid, showing the close association with the retrobulbar venous plexus.

Prolapse of the gland of the third eyelid can be surgically corrected using a procedure to resect the prolapsed glandular tissue and/or reattach the gland (see Operative Technique 17.4). Theoretically, resecting the gland could carry a risk of kerato-conjunctivitis sicca, although the author's experience does not bear this out, and nor is it documented in the literature; the large lacrimal and Harderian glands remain, meaning that significant tear deficiency is unlikely.

An alternative approach is to retain the prolapsed gland and reattach it to the third eyelid using the Morgan pocket technique (see Operative Technique 17.5). If recurrence occurs, the suturing technique can be repeated.

Aberrant conjunctival growth

An aberrant conjunctival overgrowth or stricture (Williams, 2007; Allgoewer *et al.*, 2008) is a lesion unique to the rabbit. It has also been called a precorneal membranous occlusion (Wagner and Fehr, 2007), pseudopterygium conjunctivae (Arnbjer, 1979) or pseudosymblepharon (Yata *et al.*, 1995). These terms describe the location and tissue involvement.

Little is known about the pathogenesis of this particular condition. Most cases present bilaterally, as a membrane emanating from the bulbar conjunctiva (Allgoewer *et al.*, 2008). The membrane formation of the conjunctiva starts from the limbal circumference and progresses centripetally to cover the cornea, without scar tissue forming a connection to the corneal surface (Figure 17.11). Because of the remaining central aperture, vision is only partially impaired, and the animal seldom becomes blind due to complete coverage. Corresponding conjunctivitis is minimal or absent, although there may be corneal oedema in the central opening. A high incidence has been reported in young dwarf rabbits and there is also one case report of a congenital defect (Wagner and Fehr, 2007; Williams, 2007; Allgoewer *et al.*, 2008). Surgery is indicated to solve the problem (see Operative Technique 17.6). The prognosis depends upon the extent of the resected membrane margins (4–5 mm posterior to the limbus) or upon the performance of the

'Allgoewer technique' (Wagner and Fehr, 2007). The latter technique is more demanding but has been performed without relapse in six rabbits (Allgoewer *et al.*, 2008).

Enucleation or exenteration

- Ocular enucleation is the removal of the eyelids, globe, conjunctiva and third eyelid from the orbit.
- Exenteration is the removal of the eyelids, globe, adnexa and as much as possible of the associated structures.

Enucleation is indicated in diseases confined to the globe, e.g. endophthalmitis, intraocular neoplasia/melanoma, perforating trauma. It gives a better postoperative cosmetic appearance because only the globe and conjunctiva are removed, leaving the extraorbital tissues and other orbital tissues *in situ*. Exenteration is indicated in diseases involving tissues outside the globe and should be performed in cases of panophthalmitis with orbital involvement, abscessation and orbital neoplasia.

The transpalpebral enucleation–exenteration technique is preferred. This starts with suturing the eyelids together with a simple continuous suture or clamping them together with two 'mini' Allis forceps (see Operative Technique 17.7).

References and further reading

Abrams KL, Brooks DE and Funk RS (1990) Evaluation of Schirmer tear test in clinically normal rabbits. *American Journal of Veterinary Research* **51**, 1912–1913

Akyol-Salman I (2006) Effects of autologous serum eye drops on corneal wound healing after superficial keratectomy in rabbits. *Cornea* **26**, 1178–1181

Allgoewer I, Malho P, Schulze H *et al.* (2008) Aberrant conjunctival stricture and overgrowth in the rabbit. *Veterinary Ophthalmology* **11**, 18–22

Arnbjer J (1979) Pseudopterygium in a pygmy rabbit. *Veterinary Medicine, Small Animal Clinician* **79**, 737–738

Andrew SE (2002) Corneal diseases in rabbits. *Veterinary Clinics of North America: Exotic Animal Practice* **5**, 341–356

Bagley LH and Lavach D (1995) Ophthalmic diseases of rabbits. *Californian Veterinarian* **49**, 7–9

Boydell P (1991) Fine needle aspiration biopsy in the diagnosis of exophthalmos. *Journal of Small Animal Practice* **32**, 542–546

Burling K, Murphy CJ, daSilva Curiel J *et al.* (1998) Anatomy of the rabbit nasolacrimal duct and its clinical implications. *Veterinary Ophthalmology* **1**, 33–40

Dupont C, Carrier M and Gauvin J (1995) Bilateral precorneal membranous occlusion in a dwarf rabbit. *Journal of Small Exotic Animal Medicine* **3**, 41–44

Fehr M (1984) Augenanomalien beim Zwergkaninchen. *Kleintierpraxis* **29**, 129–132

Felchle LM and Sigler RL (2002) Phacoemulsification for the management of *Encephalitozoon cuniculi*-induced phacoclastic uveitis in a rabbit. *Veterinary Ophthalmology* **5**, 211–215

Fox JG, Shaley M, Beaucage CM *et al.* (1979) Congenital entropion in a litter of rabbits. *Laboratory Animal Science* **29**, 509–511

Gelatt KN (1975) Congenital cataracts on a litter of rabbits. *Journal of the American Veterinary Medicine Association* **167**, 598–599

Harcourt-Brown F (2000) *Textbook of Rabbit Medicine.* (p. 294) Butterworth-Heinemann, Oxford

Harcourt-Brown FM and Harcourt-Brown SF (2012) Clinical value of blood glucose measurement in pet rabbits. *Veterinary Record* **170**, 674

Janssens G, Simoens P, Muylle S and Lauwers H (1999) Bilateral prolapse of the deep gland of the third eyelid in a rabbit: diagnosis and treatment. *Laboratory Animal Science* **49**(19), 105–109

Jeklova E, Jekl V, Kovarcik K *et al.* (2010) Usefulness of detection of specific IgM and IgG antibodies for diagnosis of clinical encephalitozoonosis in pet rabbits. *Veterinary Parasitology* **170**(1/2), 143–148

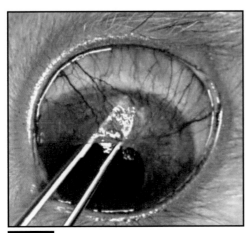
17.11 Aberrant conjunctival overgrowth.

Kern TJ (1997) Rabbit and rodent ophthalmology. *Seminars in Avian and Exotic Pet Medicine* **6**, 138–145

Kostolich M and Panciera RJ (1992) Thymoma in a domestic rabbit. *Cornell Veterinarian* **82**, 125–129

Kumar S, Karki R, Meena M and Acharya BM (2011) Reduction in drop size of ophthalmic topical drop preparations and the impact of treatment. *Journal of Advanced Pharmaceutical Technology and Research* **2**, 192–194

Lee VHI (1983) Esterase activities in adult rabbits' eyes. *Journal of Pharmaceutical Science* **72**, 239–248

Munger RJ, Langevin N and Podval J (2002) Spontaneous cataracts in laboratory rabbits. *Veterinary Ophthalmology* **5**, 177–181

O′Reilly AO, McCowan C, Hardman C and Stanley R (2002) Taenia serialis causing exophthalmos in a pet rabbit. *Veterinary Ophthalmology* **5**, 227–230

Phasukkijwatana N, Lertit P, Liammongkolkul S and Prabhasawat P (2011) Stability of epitheliotrophic factors in autologous serum eye drops from chronic Stevens-Johnson syndrome dry eye compared to non-autoimmune dry eye. *Current Eye Research* **36**, 775–781

Reiser BJ, Ignacio TS, Wand Y *et al.* (2005) In vitro measurement of rabbit corneal epithelial thickness using ultrahigh resolution optical coherence tomography. *Veterinary Ophthalmology* **8**, 85–88

Roze M, Ridings B and Lagadic M (2001) Comparative morphology of epicorneal conjunctival membranes in rabbits and human pterygium. *Veterinary Ophthalmology* **4**, 171–174

Sakai T (1989) Major ocular glands of the musk shrew with a review on the comparative anatomy and histology of the mammalian lacrimal glands. *Journal of Morphology* **201**, 39–57

Toni MA, Meirelles AE, Gava FN *et al.* (2010) Rabbits' eye globe sonographic biometry. *Veterinary Ophthalmology* **13**, 384–386

Uthoff D (1984) Biometric studies on the rabbit's eye. *Klinische Monatsblatter fűr Augenheilkunde* **185**, 189–192

Vernau KM, Grahn BH, Clarke-Scott HA and Sullivan N (1995) Thymoma in a geriatric rabbit with hypercalcaemia and periodic exophthalmos. *Journal of the American Veterinary Association* **206**, 820–822

Volopich S, Gruber A, Hassan J *et al.* (2005) Malignant B-cell lymphoma of the Harder′s gland in a rabbit. *Veterinary Ophthalmology* **8**, 259–263

Wagner F, Beinecke A, Fehr M *et al.* (2005) Recurrent bilateral exophthalmos associated with metastatic thymic carcinoma in a pet rabbit. *Journal of Small Animal Practice* **46**, 393–397

Wagner F and Fehr M (2007) Common ophthalmic problems in pet rabbits. *Journal of Exotic Pet Medicine* **16**, 158–167

Wagner F, Heider HJ, Görig C and Fehr M (1998) Ophthalmic diseases in dwarf rabbits. Part I: Anatomy, examination procedure, diseases of the eye lids, conjunctiva, and of the nasolacrimal duct. *Tierärztliche Praxis* **26**, 205–210

Weisse I, Niggeschulze A and Stözer H (1974) Spontane, congenitale Katarakte bei Ratte, Maus und Kaninchen. *Archives of Toxicology* **32**, 199–207

Williams D (2007) Rabbit and rodent ophthalmology. *European Journal of Companion Animal Practice* **17**, 242–252

Wolfer J, Grahn B, Wilcock B and Pery D (1993) Phacoclastic uveitis in the rabbit. *Progress in Veterinary and Comparative Ophthalmology* **3**, 92–97

Yata S, Hara H, Kitano H *et al.* (1995) Treatment of a rabbit with pseudosymblepharon. *Journal of the Japanese Veterinary Medicine Association* **48**, 335–337

OPERATIVE TECHNIQUES →

OPERATIVE TECHNIQUE 17.1:
Corneal ulcer treatment
Michael Fehr

Patient preparation and positioning

For debridement, sternal recumbency and topical anaesthesia (in rare cases midazolam) are advised. For temporary tarsorrhaphy (conjunctival grafting), general anaesthesia is necessary (see Chapter 1).

Equipment

For debridement:
- Topical anaesthetic, e.g. proxymetacaine 0.5% eye solution
- Cotton-tipped applicator
- Sterile water

For temporary tarsorrhaphy:
- Suture material: silk 2–3 metric (3/0–2/0 USP)
- Buttons

For conjunctival grafting:
- Small Stevens tenotomy or Mayo scissors
- Small plain and rat-toothed forceps
- Small straight and curved haemostats
- Small needle-holder
- Swabs (sterile cotton and gauze)
- Suture material: polyglactin (e.g. Vicryl) or polyglecaprone (e.g. Monocryl) 0.4–1 metric (8/0–5/0 USP)

Procedures

Gentle debridement

Any non-adherent corneal epithelium can be debrided with a cotton bud or a suitable cotton brush. The dry tip of the cotton bud is lightly rubbed back and forth along the margin of the ulcer before rinsing the cornea with sterile water.

The application of carbomer gel (e.g. Viscotears) for a few days helps to stabilize the tear film and improve the epithelialization process.

Surgery

Keratectomy is indicated if the ulcer is more than half the thickness of the cornea.

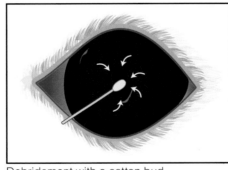

Debridement with a cotton bud.

Temporary tarsorrhaphy

During the healing process, the cornea can be protected by: application of a contact lens; covering the cornea by a third eyelid flap; a temporary tarsorrhaphy; or rotating a conjunctival advancement graft sutured into the defect. The graft should be harvested from the conjunctiva adjacent to the corneal defect.

Lateral cross-sectional view of suture placement through the upper and lower eyelids. The compression forces of the knot can be reduced by an underlying button.

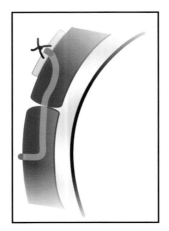

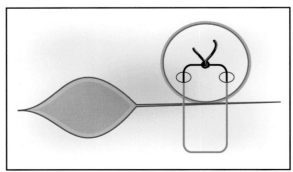

Eyelid view after placement of first suture. Knot compression is reduced by a button. Depending on the size of the eyelid and button, one or two suture/button combinations may be necessary.

OPERATIVE TECHNIQUE 17.1 continued:
Corneal ulcer treatment
Michael Fehr

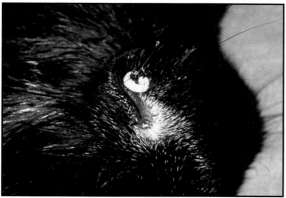

Postoperative appearance following temporary tarsorrhaphy.

Conjunctival grafting
This technique is the same as that performed on a dog or cat (see *BSAVA Manual of Canine and Feline Ophthalmology*).

Complications

The following complications may be seen after debridement of ulcers:

- Self-trauma
- Scar formation on cornea
- Loss of vision/loss of eye.

OPERATIVE TECHNIQUE 17.2:
Correction of entropion or ectropion
Michael Fehr

Patient preparation and positioning

In cases of entropion, prior to induction of general anaesthesia (see Chapter 1), the affected eyelid is everted manually with small Halsted or rat-toothed forceps at the point of maximum lid inversion, in order to estimate the amount of skin that will need to be removed.

Equipment

- Small straight Mayo scissors
- Small Halsted forceps or rat-toothed forceps
- Small straight and curved haemostats
- Small needle-holder
- Swabs (sterile cotton and gauze)
- Suture material: nylon or silk 0.7–1.0 metric (6/0–5/0 USP)

Procedures

Correction of entropion
The correction of entropion can be managed by the Hotz–Celsus procedure.

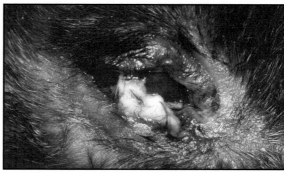

Entropion.

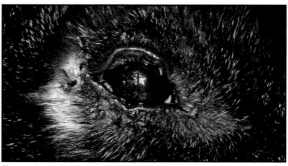

Entropion after cleaning the eye.

OPERATIVE TECHNIQUE 17.2 continued:
Correction of entropion or ectropion
Michael Fehr

1 Place a pair of Halsted forceps on the skin area to be resected, 3–4 mm from the lid margin.

2 Remove the forceps, grasp the strip of the lid with forceps and hold it in the jaws of straight Mayo scissors before excising it.

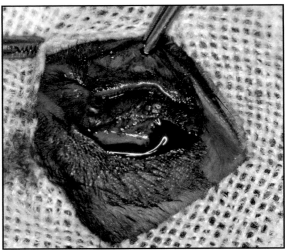

A strip of the upper lid has been excised.

3 Close the wound with simple interrupted sutures placed 1.5–2 mm apart.

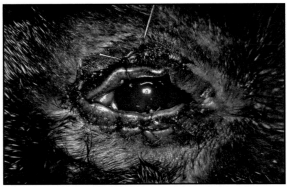

After wound closure following excision of strips from upper and lower lids.

4 Remove the sutures after 10 days.

Correction of combined ectropion/entropion

In cases of combined entropion/ectropion, a combination of the Hotz–Celsus procedure and the arrowhead procedure can fix the problem.

1 Create folds of upper and lower lid of necessary sizes, which meet at the lateral canthus so that a large arrowhead-shaped wedge is created.

2 Resect strips of skin terminating in a single base and dissect strings of orbicularis muscle, terminating in a single base near the lateral canthus.

3 Retract the muscle strings laterally and suture them to the periosteum of zygomatic and temporal bone.

4 Accurately appose the skin margins and suture with appositional sutures.

Complications

Over-correction of entropion can result in ectropion.

Postoperative care

The postoperative care is the same as for any rabbit undergoing surgery (see Chapter 2). Systemic antibiotics are indicated depending on practice policy and presence of infection. Topical ofloxacin is indicated for 7–10 days following surgery. Analgesia with non-steroidal anti-inflammatory drugs (NSAIDs) with or without opioids is indicated.

OPERATIVE TECHNIQUE 17.3:
Correction of eyelid dysplasia
John Chitty

Patient preparation and positioning

The rabbit is anaesthetized and intubated (see Chapter 1). Lubricating jelly (e.g. K–Y) is applied to the eye. The skin over the periorbital area and dorsal head is shaved and aseptically prepared. Diluted povidone–iodine is used to clean the cornea.

Equipment

Standard rabbit surgical kit; no special equipment required.

Procedure

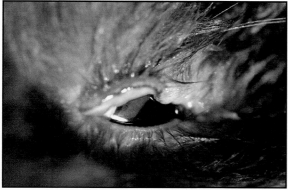

Dysplasia of the upper lid of the right eye (the ear is to the left, the nose to the right). The region of dysplastic lid can sometimes be described as entropion. However, this effect is due to lack of support where there is no cartilage in this region. The condition is typified by the abrupt demarcation between normal and abnormal eyelid.
© John Chitty

1 The defect from the medial canthus to the edge of the lesion is removed as a full-thickness wedge resection.

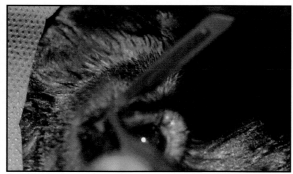

© John Chitty

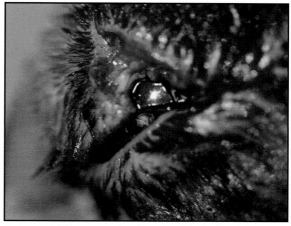

© John Chitty

2 The caudal part of the upper lid from the edge of the lesion to the lateral canthus is split along the margin.

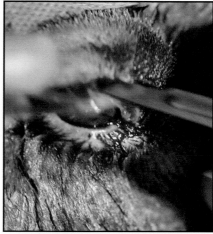

© John Chitty

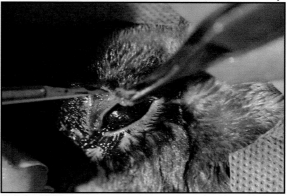

© John Chitty

OPERATIVE TECHNIQUE 17.3 continued:
Correction of eyelid dysplasia
John Chitty

3 The wound is extended caudally then dorsally from the lateral canthus, and dorsally from the cranial edge of the wound to prepare a skin flap.

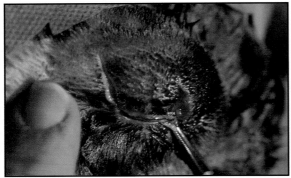

© John Chitty

4 The skin is dissected clear of conjunctiva and subcutaneous fibrous tissue.

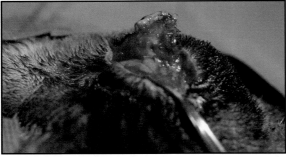

© John Chitty

5 The conjunctival defect is repaired using 1 metric (5/0 USP) polyglactone. Sutures are placed carefully so that they do not pass through the full thickness, and avoid contact with the cornea.

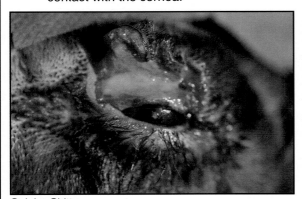

© John Chitty

6 The flap is advanced and the ventral cranial corner is sutured to the medial canthus using 1 metric (5/0 USP) polyglactone.

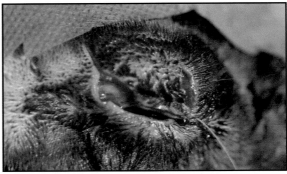

© John Chitty

7 A new eyelid margin is made by suturing the flap to the conjunctiva. Care is taken to avoid the suture ends contacting the cornea.

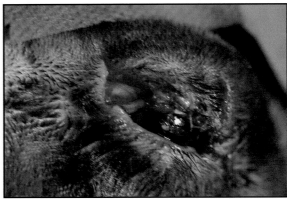

© John Chitty

8 The skin flap is advanced to remake the lateral canthus.

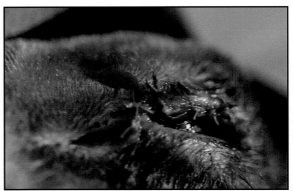

© John Chitty

OPERATIVE TECHNIQUE 17.3 continued:
Correction of eyelid dysplasia
John Chitty

---

9 Skin wounds are closed routinely.

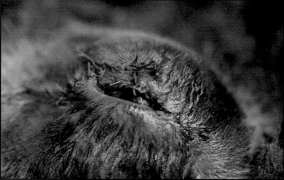

Appearance immediately following routine closure of the skin wounds. © John Chitty

10 Artificial tears are applied to the cornea.

Postoperative care

Systemic NSAIDs are given for 5 days post-operatively. Topical emollient and antibiotic creams are used twice daily until healing. Sutures are removed after 10 days.

OPERATIVE TECHNIQUE 17.4:
Removal of prolapsed superficial gland of third eyelid
Frances Harcourt-Brown

All photographs courtesy of Frances Harcourt-Brown

Patient preparation and positioning

After induction of general anaesthesia (see Chapter 1), the rabbit is placed in lateral recumbency. The fur is clipped from around the eye. The third eyelid and prolapsed gland are cleansed with warm water. The area is draped. No assistant is necessary.

Equipment

- Fine surgical instruments
- Optical loupes (optional)

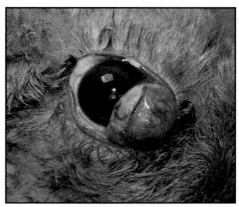

Prior to surgery the prolapsed gland can be seen as a pale fleshy structure displacing the third eyelid.

Procedure

1 The prolapsed gland is grasped and pulled away from the globe.

OPERATIVE TECHNIQUE 17.4 continued:
Removal of prolapsed superficial gland of third eyelid
Frances Harcourt-Brown

2 The conjunctiva over the gland is incised and split to expose the glandular tissue. A large branch of the venous plexus may be seen (arrow).

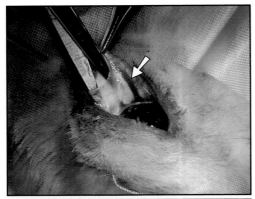

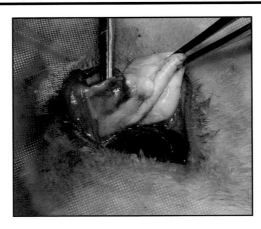

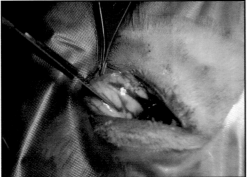

3 While traction is applied, the gland is carefully dissected away from the conjunctiva and cartilage of the third eyelid.

4 As the gland is freed from the surrounding tissues, artery forceps may need to be applied to any bleeding vessels but ligatures are not necessary. The blood clots quickly.

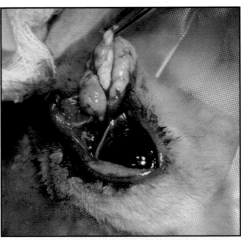

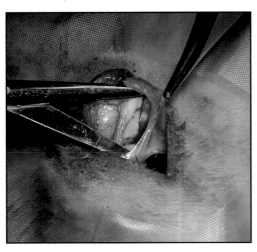

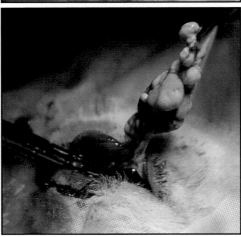

OPERATIVE TECHNIQUE 17.4 continued:
Removal of prolapsed superficial gland of third eyelid
Frances Harcourt-Brown

5 The gland is eventually freed and removed. Any blood is wiped away before replacing the third eyelid and applying pressure for a moment or two.

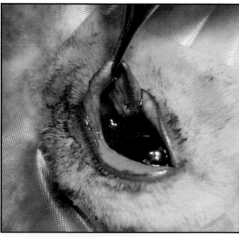

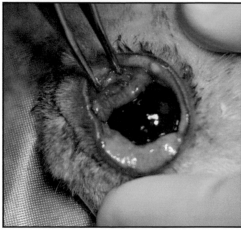

Postoperative care

Topical antibiotic eye ointment (e.g. Fucithalmic Vet) is applied twice a day for 5 days postoperatively. Analgesia (NSAIDs such as meloxicam) and systemic antibiotics (e.g. enrofloxacin or trimethoprim/sulphonamide) are also administered.

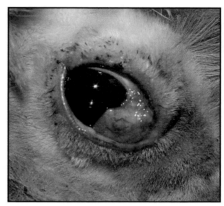

Appearance of the eye on the day after surgery.

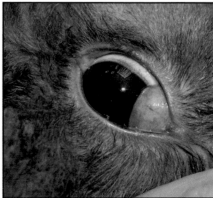

Appearance of the eye 10 days after surgery.

Wound closure

No sutures are necessary.

Potential complications

Keratoconjunctivitis sicca is a theoretical complication but has not been encountered.

OPERATIVE TECHNIQUE 17.5:
Pocket technique for re-placement of prolapsed gland of third eyelid
Michael Fehr

All photographs courtesy of Frances Harcourt-Brown

Patient preparation and positioning

After induction of general anaesthesia (see Chapter 1), the rabbit is placed in lateral recumbency. The fur is clipped from around the eye. The third eyelid and prolapsed gland are cleansed with warm water. The area is draped. No assistant is necessary.

Equipment

- Topical anaesthesia, e.g. proxymetacaine 0.5% eye solution (additional topical anaesthesia is advised to prevent unexpected reactions)
- Small Stevens tenotomy or Mayo scissors
- Small plain and rat-toothed forceps
- Small straight and curved haemostats
- Small needle-holder
- Swabs (sterile cotton and gauze)
- Sterile transparent drapes
- Suture materials: polyglactin (e.g. Vicryl) or polyglecaprone (e.g. Monocryl) 1–1.5 metric (5/0–4/0 USP)

Surgical procedure

1 Place a suture from outside the nasal third of the third eyelid into the nasal fornix and hold the suture end by fixation with a clamp.

2 Evert the third eyelid. Make a first incision into the epithelial layer of the third eyelid, parallel to its edge, at the base of the enlarged protruded tissue mass.

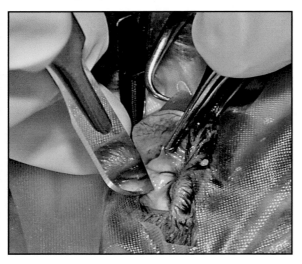

3 Make a second skin incision parallel to the first, above the enlarged tissue mass.

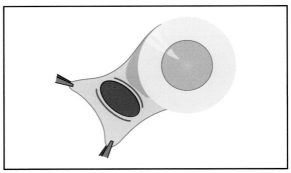

4 Create a pocket using small Metzenbaum scissors to undermine the first incision in the direction of the medial lower conjunctival fornix.

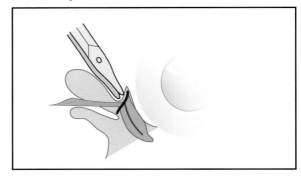

5 Place the gland into the pocket and suture the two incisions together using a continuous (Cushing) suture pattern. To allow drainage of tears from the pocket, thus preventing the formation of a pseudocyst, the suture should not be tightened too much.

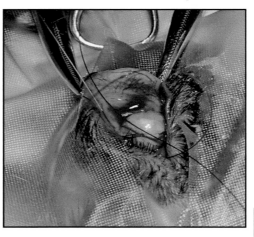

OPERATIVE TECHNIQUE 17.5 continued:
Pocket technique for re-placement of prolapsed gland of third eyelid
Michael Fehr

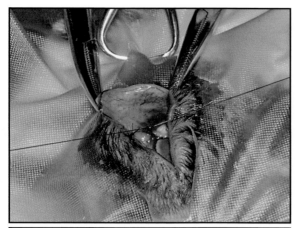

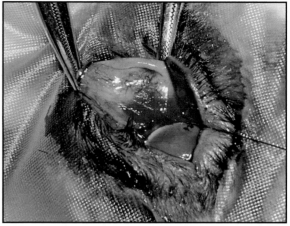

End result after re-placement of the gland.

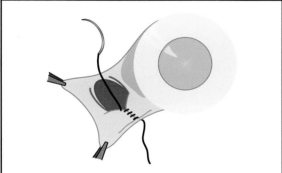

6 Starting and final knots should not irritate the cornea; knots should therefore be placed into the fornix. In some cases it is advised to fix the third eyelid with an anchor suture to the periosteum of the anterior ventral fornix.

Complications after Morgan pocket technique

- Rubbing by the suture knot.
- Recurrence of prolapse.
- Keratoconjunctivitis sicca.

Postoperative care

The postoperative care is the same as for any rabbit undergoing surgery (see Chapter 2). Systemic antibiotics are indicated depending on practice policy and presence of infection. Topical preparations containing fusidic acid (e.g. Fucithalmic Vet) or gentamicin (e.g. Tiacil) are indicated for 7–10 days following surgery. Analgesia with NSAIDs with or without opioids is indicated.

OPERATIVE TECHNIQUE 17.6:
Surgical treatment of aberrant conjunctival overgrowth
Michael Fehr

Patient preparation and positioning

After induction of general anaesthesia (see Chapter 1), the rabbit is placed in lateral recumbency, and the eyeball, conjunctiva and fornix are irrigated with sterile physiological saline or eyewash solution.

Equipment

- Topical anaesthesia, e.g. proxymetacaine 0.5% eye solution (additional topical anaesthesia is advised to prevent unexpected reactions)
- Small Stevens tenotomy or Mayo scissors
- Small plain and rat-toothed forceps
- Small straight and curved haemostats
- Small needle-holder
- Swabs (sterile cotton and gauze)
- Suture materials: polyglactin (e.g. Vicryl) or polyglecaprone (e.g. Monocryl) 0.7–1 metric (6/0–5/0 USP); polypropylene (e.g. Prolene) 0.5 metric (7/0 USP)

Procedure

Two methods have been described for the treatment of this condition. The first is removal of the conjunctival overgrowth. The second is radial resection of 4–6 sections of the membrane and suturing them to the conjunctival fornix.

Simple excision of the membrane

Technique
1. Lavage the conjunctival fornix with Ringer's solution.
2. Elevate the membrane with fine forceps.
3. Excise the membrane along the limbus corneae using small scissors.
4. Take care at the nasal canthus to preserve the third eyelid.
5. Small bleeds can be controlled by compression with an adrenaline-soaked swab.

Prognosis
There is a high rate of regrowth with this technique.

Radial resection (the Allgoewer technique)

The high rate of regrowth with simple resection of the membrane may be avoided by radial incisions of at least 4 mm of bulbar conjunctiva adjacent to the limbus, pulling them back under the eyelids and suturing the remnants into the fornix (Dupont et al., 1995; Roze et al., 2001; Wagner and Fehr, 2007; Allgoewer et al., 2008).

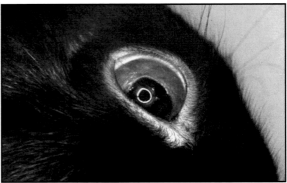

Aberrant conjunctival overgrowth before surgery.

Technique

1 Divide the occluding membrane from the central aperture into different parts with 4 or 6 straight incisions using small scissors (Stevens tenotomy).

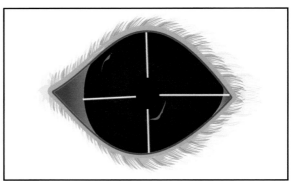

2 Suture each part back into the fornix conjunctivae by re-placing the central rim of the segment into its normal position in the fornix. This is achieved using mattress sutures (polypropylene), penetrating the upper (then the lower) lid at a distance of 6–8 mm from the eyelid margin from

OPERATIVE TECHNIQUE 17.6 continued:
Surgical treatment of aberrant conjunctival overgrowth
Michael Fehr

outside to inside through the fornix, then through the conjunctival fold of the segment and back through the fornix, exiting approximately 5 mm from the entrance of the suture. The procedure is finished by grasping the conjunctiva with fine forceps, folding it back into the fornix and tying off the suture. All remaining parts must be sutured similarly.

Prognosis
Prognosis depends largely on the care with which the procedure is carried out. If the resection of the membrane is meticulous, this technique may give good results, though it remains to be tested in a larger study.

Postoperative care

The postoperative care is the same as for any rabbit undergoing surgery (see Chapter 2). Antibiotics are indicated depending on practice policy and presence of infection. Analgesia with NSAIDs with or without opioids is indicated. Eye drops containing dexamethasone, neomycin and polymyxin should be administered twice daily (Allgoewer *et al.*, 2008). Sutures are either removed after 3 weeks or left in place until they drop out.

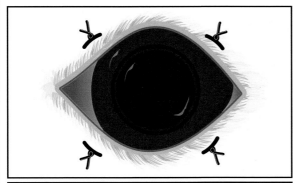

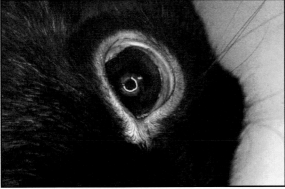

OPERATIVE TECHNIQUE 17.7:
Enucleation and exenteration
Michael Fehr

Patient preparation and positioning

These procedures are carried out with the rabbit under general anaesthesia (see Chapter 1). For the transpalpebral approach the rabbit is placed in lateral recumbency. The head can be fixed to the underlying table by a piece of tape, which is placed caudal to the nostrils around the upper and lower jaws. The eyeball, conjunctiva and fornix are irrigated with sterile physiological saline or eyewash solution.

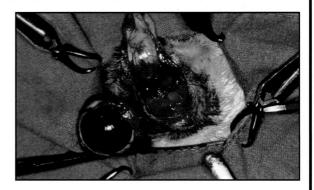

Equipment

Essential equipment:
* Standard enucleation set
* Small Stevens tenotomy or Mayo scissors
* Small plain and rat-toothed forceps
* Small straight and curved haemostats
* Small needle-holder
* Swabs (sterile cotton and gauze)
* Iodoform solution, honey, etc.
* Suture materials: polyglactin (e.g. Vicryl) or polyglecaprone (e.g. Monocryl) 0.7–1 metric (6/0–5/0 USP); nylon (e.g. Supramid), 1–1.5 metric (5/0–4/0 USP)

Additional equipment:
* Magnification instruments may be helpful when dealing with small animals
* Thermal cautery, bipolar radiosurgery to facilitate haemostasis
* Eyelid speculum

Surgical procedure

Enucleation

1 Close the eyelids with a small Allis clamp or haemostat.

2 Create a transpalpebral approach by placing one incision into the upper eyelid and another into the lower lid 1–2 mm outside the lid margin.

3 Grasp the conjunctiva near the limbus with toothed forceps, create a 360 degree perilimbal incision and separate the sclera, extraocular muscles and Tenon's capsule using curved Metzenbaum scissors around to the optic nerve. Remove the globe.

4 After removal of the globe, remove the third eyelid and the lid margins completely and close the wound with absorbable suture material in a continuous pattern.

5 Close the skin incision with nylon.

Exenteration

1 For removal of all tissues within the orbit, dissect along the border of the sclera through the extraocular muscles to the orbital apex. Remove the Harderian gland if necessary.

2 Sever the optic nerve with scissors, avoiding traction on the nerve. A ligature may be placed if possible, but is not mandatory. Remove the globe.

3 If bleeding occurs due to laceration of the venous sinus, attempt to control it by placing cotton swabs temporarily in the orbit; rabbit blood clots rapidly.

4 Look for abscess formation, bone perforation or protruding teeth. Remove any abscess capsule, clear the pus and extract the teeth that are within it.

5 If infection is present, the socket may be packed with iodoform- or honey-impregnated collagen sponges or antibiotic-impregnated polymethylmethacrylate beads. (Treatment of retrobulbar abscesses is covered in more detail in Chapter 29.)

OPERATIVE TECHNIQUE 17.7 continued:
Enucleation and exenteration
Michael Fehr

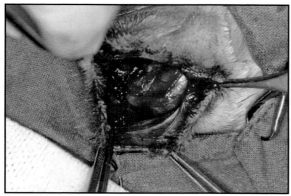

Orbit packed with honey-impregnated sponges.

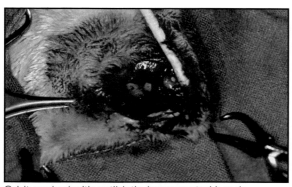

Orbit packed with antibiotic-impregnated beads.

6 Close the subcutis with absorbable suture material in a continuous pattern and then close the skin incision with nylon.

Postoperative care

The postoperative care is the same as for any rabbit undergoing surgery (see Chapter 2). Antibiotics are indicated depending on practice policy and presence of infection. Analgesia with NSAIDs with or without opioids is indicated.

The wound should be inspected daily for at least 3–7 days after surgery. Healing will depend on the reason for enucleation or exenteration. Healing by first intention will occur if no infection is present. If infection is present, the wound may need periodic debridement or further exploratory surgery to look for infected tooth roots. Removal of sponges, curettage and lavage depend on the situation.

Complications

The following complications may occur infrequently during or after enucleation:

*   Haemorrhage, rupture of venous sinus
*   Infection, abscess, orbital cyst formation
*   Wound dehiscence
*   Postoperative gut stasis, ileus.

Prognosis

Prognosis depends on the underlying disease and the extent of orbital involvement. In cases of neoplasia, the tendency of local recurrence may require adjuvant chemotherapy. In cases of severe abscess formation, healing can be prolonged or impossible due to food and saliva contamination through bone perforations of the orbit as a consequence of infected molar tooth roots, which may need to be extracted (see Chapter 29).

18

Anorectal papilloma

Anna Meredith

Anorectal papillomas in rabbits are benign, well differentiated epithelial tumours of the anorectal junction. Their aetiology is unknown but they have not been associated with any papilloma viruses, and transmission experiments have been unsuccessful (Weisbroth, 1994).

Relevant anatomy

Anorectal papillomas arise from the squamous columnar epithelium at the mucocutaneous junction of the rectum and anus. They can extend within the rectum but, once large enough, often protrude out through the anus, interfering with the function of the anal sphincter. The attachment at the mucocutaneous junction may be stalk-like or broad-based and the papillomas are friable and easily traumatized.

Clinical signs

Anorectal papillomas present as proliferative cauliflower-like growths protruding from the anus (Figure 18.1). Many are small and do not cause any clinical signs but they can be a source of discomfort and, due to their friable nature, can bleed easily and profusely. The presence of a papilloma at the anorectal junction, especially if large, can cause persistent contractions or spasms of the rectum, leading to

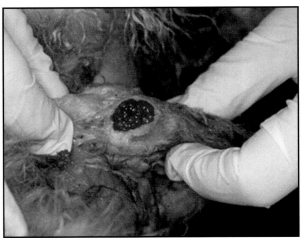

18.1 An anorectal papilloma *in situ* prior to surgery. (Courtesy of Kevin Eatwell)

inability to defecate normally. Presenting signs in affected rabbits include:

- Presence of a red friable mass at the anus
- Bleeding from the anus
- Faecal tenesmus and inability to defecate
- Caking of faecal and caecotroph material around the anus
- Excessive grooming of the perineum.

Differential diagnosis and diagnostic procedures

Differential diagnoses to be considered include other causes of lack of defecation or faecal tenesmus, such as gastrointestinal stasis and colitis, anal bite wounds, and other tumours (Figure 18.2).

- Gastrointestinal stasis
- Gastrointestinal impaction
- Colitis
- Other colonic/rectal or anal mass (abscess, polyp, neoplasia)
- Anal bite wounds
- *Treponema cuniculi* (rabbit syphilis)
- Myxomatosis
- *Passalurus ambiguus* (pinworm)

18.2 Main differential diagnoses for anorectal papilloma.

Diagnosis is frequently presumptive, based on location and appearance of the mass. Examination of the rectum under sedation or general anaesthesia, using eversion or a speculum, may occasionally be necessary if the papilloma is located only within the rectum and not externally. Definitive diagnosis is made by biopsy (generally excisional biopsy) and histopathological examination.

Treatment options

Spontaneous regression of anorectal papillomas can occur in some cases, but if associated clinical signs are present surgical removal is generally required and is the treatment of choice (see Operative Technique 18.1). Removal techniques include classical surgical excision, excision using radiosurgery, or destruction of the tumour using laser or liquid nitrogen.

Prognosis

Removal is usually successful and uncomplicated. However, with all techniques it is important to ensure the base of the tumour is completely removed or destroyed, otherwise the papilloma may recur. Even after complete removal, recurrence is still possible at other sites around the anorectal junction.

References and further reading

Jenkins JR (2004) Soft tissue surgery and dental procedures. In: *Ferrets, Rabbits and Rodents: Clinical Medicine and Surgery,* ed. EV Hillyer and KE Quesenberry, pp. 227–239. WB Saunders, Philadelphia

Weisbroth SH (1994) Neoplastic diseases. In: *The Biology of the Laboratory Rabbit, 2nd edn,* ed. PJ Manning *et al.*, pp. 227–239 Academic Press, New York

OPERATIVE TECHNIQUE 18.1 ➜

OPERATIVE TECHNIQUE 18.1:
Surgical removal of anorectal papillomas

Patient preparation and positioning

Anaesthetize the rabbit according to standard protocols (see Chapter 1) and position in dorsal recumbency with the pelvis slightly elevated. Clipping of fur may not be necessary but, if required, carefully clip any perianal fur, avoiding the papilloma as it is easily traumatized. Remove any faecal material and clean and prepare the surgical site using standard surgical skin antiseptic preparations. Avoid alcohol-containing solutions.

Assistant

An assistant is required either to hold an appropriately sized speculum (e.g. canine vaginal speculum) within the anus, or to hold two or three stay sutures placed around the anus, in order to dilate the anus. For some papillomas, manual pressure by an assistant either side of the anus is all that is required to evert the anus and papilloma and expose the base. For very small papillomas, especially if well pedunculated, an assistant may not be required.

Equipment extras

- Canine vaginal speculum (optional)
- Radiosurgery (preferable)

Procedure

1 Dilate the anus using the speculum or sutures, to expose the base of the papilloma at the mucocutaneous junction.

2 Remove the papilloma in its entirety from the base. If the tumour is very large, removal in sections may be appropriate.

PRACTICAL TIPS
- Gentle handling of the papilloma is essential to minimize trauma and bleeding.
- Radiosurgery is preferable to sharp dissection in order to control bleeding. Laser therapy or cryosurgery may also be employed if available.
- Care must be taken not to damage the anal sphincter muscle.

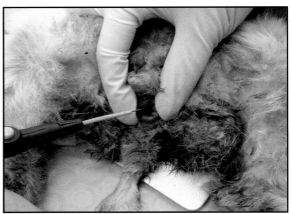

Anorectal papilloma being removed by radiosurgery. (Courtesy of Kevin Eatwell)

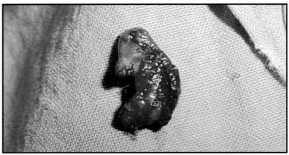

A typical red and friable papilloma that was removed by radiosurgery. (Courtesy of Kevin Eatwell)

3 After sharp dissection, suture the anorectal mucosa using a simple continuous pattern, with absorbable material (e.g. polydioxanone or poliglecaprone 1 or 0.7 metric (5/0 or 6/0 USP)). If radiosurgery, laser or liquid nitrogen is used, mucosal closure is not generally necessary.

Postoperative care

Standard postoperative care includes use of NSAIDs and provision of a high-fibre diet. An Elizabethan collar may be necessary in some rabbits to prevent trauma of the surgical site or suture removal. Motility modifiers such as cisapride may be necessary to support hindgut function in the postoperative period.

19

Mediastinal masses and other thoracic surgery

William Lewis

Considerations for thoracic surgery in rabbits *versus* cats and dogs

Rabbits have small thoracic cavities compared to dogs and cats; the thoracic cavity of a rabbit is also much smaller than its abdominal cavity. There are either 12 or 13 pairs of ribs: the first (cranial) six pairs are attached by costal cartilage to the sternum while the last (caudal) two pairs have no attachment to the sternum. The right lung comprises four lobes: cranial, middle, caudal and accessory (see Chapter 5). The left side comprises the cranial and caudal lobes. The left cranial lobe is divided into cranial and caudal sections by a fold. The lungs are not divided into lobules, which results in most cases of pneumonia being lobar or generalized rather than localized. Rabbits primarily use the diaphragm for breathing, whereas dogs and cats rely largely on the intercostal muscles.

The thymus of dogs and cats typically involutes with age, whereas that of rabbits persists into adulthood. It is found cranial and ventral to the heart on both the left and right sides of the thoracic cavity. The large stomach and caecum of rabbits places pressure on the diaphragm. This creates important considerations for anaesthesia, e.g. positioning of the patient in order to decrease pressure on the diaphragm.

Many rabbits are carriers of infections such as *Pasteurella multocida*, *Bordetella bronchiseptica* and *Moraxella catarrhalis*. Some of these organisms may be commensals but may still become a problem due to immune suppression as a result of other disease processes or husbandry. Many of the infections are subclinical or inapparent but can result in significant pulmonary pathology, which leads to an increased risk for general anaesthesia in these patients.

Diagnosis of surgical thoracic disease

Several clinical signs may alert the clinician to the presence of thoracic disease. The main signs are dyspnoea and tachypnoea and there are several differential diagnoses for these signs.

Respiratory noise, poor exercise tolerance, cyanosis, muffled and other heart sounds (e.g. murmurs or dysrhythmias), syncope, lethargy and bilateral exophthalmos are other signs of possible thoracic cavity disease.

Differential diagnoses for dyspnoea and tachypnoea:
- Upper respiratory infection
- Lower respiratory infection
- Mediastinal neoplasia, e.g. lymphoma, thymic lymphoma, thymic carcinoma
- Mediastinal lipomas, cysts and abscesses
- Pulmonary neoplasia or abscessation
- Collapsing trachea (lateral collapse)
- Lung lobe torsion
- Spontaneous or traumatic pneumothorax
- Bronchiopulmonary foreign body
- Ruptured diaphragm
- Congestive heart failure
- Pleural effusion
- Chylothorax.

Exophthalmos (Figure 19.1) occurs due to the presence of the large orbital venous sinus in rabbits and compression of the cranial vena cava (precaval syndrome), which can also lead to oedema of the head, neck and front limbs as well as jugular distension. There are other conditions that can cause exophthalmos in rabbits (see below and Chapter 17).

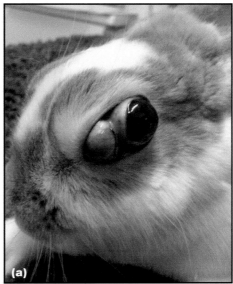

19.1 **(a)** A 5-year-old neutered doe with thymoma, prior to surgery, showing exophthalmos and protrusion of the superficial gland of the third eyelid. (continues) ▶

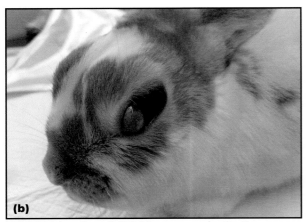

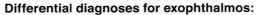
19.1 (continued) **(b)** After surgery for the thymoma the exophthalmos has been resolved but the gland is still prolapsed.

Differential diagnoses for exophthalmos:
- Congestive heart failure
- Occlusion of jugular veins, e.g. as a result of perivascular necrosis
- Thymomas – usually bilateral exophthalmos
- Salivary mucocele
- Orbital abscess
- Orbital cellulitis
- Orbital cysts
- Retrobulbar fat prolapse
- Other orbital neoplasia
- Glaucoma.

Several diagnostic procedures can assist in the diagnosis of surgical thoracic cavity disease.

Radiography

Interpretation of thoracic radiographs is discussed in Chapter 5. In the case of thymomas, lateral and dorsoventral radiographs readily show the presence of a large cranial thoracic mass (Figure 19.2). This may be differentiated from cardiomegaly or pericardial effusion using ultrasonography. The presence of fat in the thoracic cavity of obese rabbits and the persistence of the thymus can make interpretation of thoracic radiographs challenging. Pulmonary abscesses are visible as consolidated lung lobes.

Ultrasonography

Thymomas show a mixed echogenicity and cavitations (Figure 19.3), whereas thymic lymphomas tend to be more homogeneous and hypoechoic without the cavitations. In the case of lung abscesses, ultrasonography will reveal a cavitated lesion in the affected lung (see Chapter 8).

Fine-needle aspiration and core biopsy

Cytology based on samples obtained by fine-needle aspiration (FNA; see Chapter 5) cannot easily differentiate between thymomas and thymic lymphomas but may be used to rule out other conditions. Ultrasound-guided core biopsy samples submitted

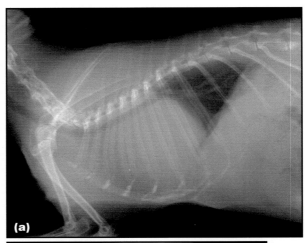

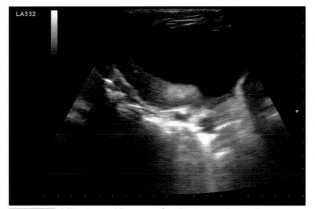

19.2 Radiographic appearance of a thymoma in a 6-year-old rabbit. Lateral and dorsoventral views show a large space-occupying mass in the cranial thoracic cavity. Note the elevation and constriction of the trachea in (a) and the restricted lung volume on both views.

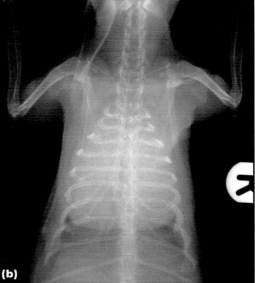

19.3 Ultrasound image of a thymoma in an 8-year-old male neutered rabbit. There was a large hypoechoic cystic structure within it, which was drained with a needle as soon as the mass was surgically exposed. It was not drained prior to surgery because of the risk of leakage of tumour cells through the puncture hole into the mediastinal cavity. (Courtesy of Frances Harcourt-Brown)

for histopathology are more likely to yield a diagnosis. Biopsy should be performed under general anaesthesia by a competent operator. Ultrasound-guided aspirates of consolidated lung lobes may be obtained for cytology as well as for culture and sensitivity testing. This will also help to differentiate abscesses from pulmonary neoplasia. Aerobic and anaerobic as well as fungal cultures should always be performed. Acid-fast stains may prove useful if mycobacteria are suspected.

Bronchoalveolar lavage

Bronchoalveolar lavage may be performed under general anaesthesia in order to obtain samples for microbiology, cytology or histopathology. A sterile endotracheal tube should be used and the rabbit placed in lateral recumbency with the affected lung lobes on the dependent side. A sterile urinary catheter is advanced into the distal airway and 1–2 ml/kg bodyweight of sterile saline is instilled. As much of the fluid as possible should be retrieved. Elevating the caudal part of the rabbit may aid this process.

Thoracoscopy and endoscopy

Endoscopy of the trachea may be useful to diagnose foreign bodies and tumours, collapsing trachea and the presence of pus or discharges. Thoracoscopy allows visualization of lung lobes and masses and may afford the opportunity to obtain diagnostic samples (see Chapter 10).

Magnetic resonance imaging and computed tomography

These modalities have become more readily available both in referral centres and general practice. They may prove useful aids to surgeons in planning their surgical approach and in differentiating operable from inoperable masses (see Chapter 9).

Indications for thoracic surgery

Thoracic surgery is not commonly performed in rabbits. The removal of mediastinal masses, usually thymomas or thymic lymphomas, and pulmonary abscesses are the most common reasons for such surgery. Other possible indications include: correction of congenital cardiac defects such as patent ductus arteriosus; removal of neoplastic lung lobes; intrathoracic tracheal surgery for a laterally collapsing trachea; lung lobe torsion; spontaneous or traumatic pneumothorax; and bronchopulmonary foreign bodies that cannot be retrieved endoscopically.

Thymomas

Thymomas are the most common mediastinal tumours in rabbits. Thymomas are considered to be histologically benign but have a tendency to recur. This is usually due to incomplete removal at the time of initial surgery; it is very rare that they will metastasize.

The clinical signs that may alert the clinician to the presence of a thymoma are listed in Figure 19.4. Thymomas frequently present with signs of

- Exophthalmos
- Protrusion of nictitating membranes
- Increased respiratory effort
- Dyspnoea on exertion
- Oedema of head, neck and forelimbs
- Jugular vein distension
- Muffled heart and lung sounds
- Caudal displacement of the apex beat
- Reduced compliance of cranioventral thorax
- Sebaceous adenitis
- ? Myasthenia gravis (suspected; Harcourt-Brown, personal communication)

19.4 Clinical signs that may be associated with thymomas in rabbits.

increased respiratory effort and bilateral exophthalmos (see Figure 19.1) and protrusion of the nictitating membrane with exertion or stress. In rabbits with thymomas, the heart and lung sounds may be diminished in the cranial and ventral lung fields and there may also be reduced compressibility of the cranioventral thorax due to the presence of the mass. There are no particular biochemical or haematological changes associated with thymomas in rabbits.

Sebaceous adenitis is a paraneoplastic syndrome that may be associated with thymomas in rabbits (Figure 19.5). Signs may include non-pruritic scaling and alopecia. Treatment with essential fatty acids and retinoids has not proved universally successful. Sebaceous adenitis has been known to resolve after thymoma removal and to recur upon reappearance of the tumour. Myasthenia gravis has not been documented in rabbits with thymomas but is suspected to occur (Harcourt-Brown, personal communication).

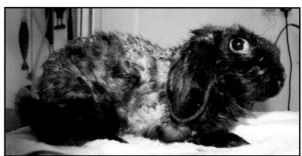

19.5 Sebaceous adenitis in a 5-year-old male neutered rabbit with a thymoma. Following surgical removal of the tumour the sebaceous adenitis improved, but it relapsed when thymoma recurred 2 years later. (Courtesy of Frances Harcourt-Brown)

Treatment options

Surgery: Surgery is considered to be the treatment of choice in rabbits and is a feasible option because the majority of thymomas are not invasive, making it possible to 'shell' them out. The surgery should be approached via a midline thoracotomy, which allows access to both sides of the thoracic cavity and exposure of the jugular veins, cranial vena cava, brachiocephalic vessels, aorta, vagus nerves, trachea and oesophagus (see Operative Technique 19.1). Wherever possible, the tissue that has been removed (Figure 19.6) should be placed in formalin

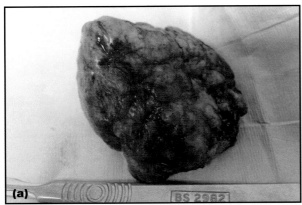

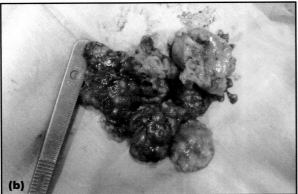

19.6 **(a)** A thymoma that has been surgically removed. Such masses should be submitted for histopathology. **(b)** A second, recurrent mass removed from the same rabbit 1 year after the initial surgery was more infiltrative and less well defined.

and submitted for histopathology. The prognosis after thymoma removal is variable. Clinicians have reported a good long-term survival rate in approximately 50% of cases following surgery. Complications are most likely to occur during surgery and in the 10-day postoperative period. Rabbits that survive this period can live for several years (Harcourt-Brown, 2013). The author's cases have survived for 12–22 months.

Chemotherapy: Chemotherapy has not proved effective in cases of thymoma in rabbits, although anecdotally it appears that prednisolone given postoperatively slows the rate of recurrence.

Radiation therapy: Radiation therapy has been described by several authors. There is an 80% chance of the rabbit surviving the procedure, but the chance of recurrence and post-treatment complications is greater than with surgical removal of the tumour.

Antinoff (2009) presented a case study of five rabbits treated with radiation therapy. The patients received 600 cGy weekly for 6 weeks, giving a total dose of 3600 cGy. They were all treated with prednisolone for 7–30 days, commencing at induction of the radiation therapy. Two patients had recurrence of their masses at 12 and 25 months and survived another 17 and 25 months, respectively, after a second course of radiation therapy. This small study

indicates that radiation therapy could be considered for the non-surgical management of these masses.

There is an anecdotal report on the House Rabbit Society website of a case in which 2 weeks of treatment with two cycles per week resulted in a 77% reduction in tumour size on follow-up CT scan.

Thymomas are radiosensitive tumours but the proximity to critical normal tissues (e.g. heart, lung) may limit the radiation dose that can be delivered. Radiation pneumonitis (inflammation of the lung tissue) and fibrosis (scarring of the tissue) may develop with radiation treatment. If facilities are available, radiation therapy is recommended after incomplete surgical resection of thymomas or if the patient is not considered a good surgical candidate.

Lung lobe abscesses

Abscesses of lung lobes occur fairly frequently in rabbits and may be underdiagnosed. Many cases are not visibly symptomatic. It is generally accepted that *Pasteurella multocida* is the most common cause of pneumonia and lung abscessation in rabbits. The capsule of *P. multocida* consists largely of hyaluronic acid which inhibits phagocytosis and opsonization. This results in the formation of thick pus and consequently it is rare for medical therapy to be successful. Other organisms shown to cause pneumonia include *Bordetella bronchiseptica, Staphylococcus aureus, Chlamydophila* spp., *Mycobacterium tuberculosis, M. bovis, M. avium* and *Pseudomonas aeruginosa*.

Clinical signs of pulmonary abscesses may include lethargy, depression, decreased appetite, weight loss, sneezing and increased respiratory effort with diminished lung sounds in the affected lung field. Rabbits may also show a fever and heterophilia on haematology. Radiographs may show evidence of consolidated lung lobes. This may also be visualized with ultrasonography. Magnetic resonance imaging (MRI) or computed tomography (CT) may be able to provide additional information or detail as to which lung lobes are affected. This may be of use in deciding whether surgery is feasible and may aid in planning the surgical approach.

If surgery is performed, the lung lobe that has been removed should be examined for the presence of a foreign body. The pus (Figure 19.7) and lung parenchyma should be cultured for the presence of

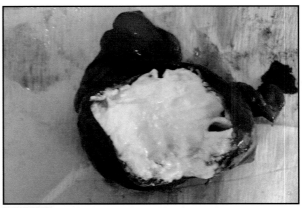

19.7 Excised lung lobes containing caseous pus.

aerobic and anaerobic bacteria as well as the presence of fungi. Lung tissue should also be submitted in formalin for histopathological analysis, particularly if neoplasia is suspected.

Principles of thoracic surgery

Thoracotomy can be performed through a sternal or lateral approach. The sternal approach is used for thymoma removal. The main indication for a lateral thoracotomy in general practice would be lung lobectomy (see Operative Technique 19.2).

Pre-anaesthetic assessment and preparation for surgery

A thorough clinical examination, paying particular attention to the thoracic cavity, should be performed on any rabbit likely to undergo thoracic surgery (Figures 19.8 and 19.9). Consolidation or abscessation of lung lobes may result in the absence of lung sounds. The rectal temperature should also be noted (normal is 38.5–40.0°C).

Intravenous access is useful for the administration of emergency drugs or for blood transfusions if these prove necessary. The marginal ear vein is the most easily accessed blood vessel for the placement of a catheter. Fluids should be administered at 10 ml/kg/h.

Anaesthesia

Surgeons contemplating thoracic surgery in a rabbit need to be confident of their ability to intubate their patient as endotracheal intubation is essential for thoracic surgery. For rabbits <5 kg it is preferable to use an uncuffed endotracheal tube, due to its slightly larger internal diameter. For further information on premedication and induction and maintenance of general anaesthesia see Chapter 1.

Upon entering the chest cavity, mechanical or manual ventilation will need to be initiated. This can be performed manually or with the use of a ventilator that will cope with small patients. There is a general tendency to overinflate the lungs. They should not be inflated to a pressure higher than 20 cmH$_2$O. It may not be possible to measure the pressure, in which case care should be taken to inflate the lungs only to overcome atelectasis. At no time should the lungs appear pale or white in colour or billow out of the chest. Careful manual ventilation may be a safer option.

If staff and facilities allow, it is ideal to monitor body temperature, end expiratory CO$_2$, blood pressure, and haemoglobin saturation with O$_2$ and blood gas levels. It would also be useful to monitor the heart with an electrocardiogram. It is, however, possible to perform thoracic surgery safely in rabbits without measuring these parameters (see Chapter 1 for further information on anaesthesia).

Postoperative considerations

Postoperative analgesia is paramount. Chapter 2 presents further details of opioid and non-steroidal anti-inflammatory analgesia. The author's choice of opioid is buprenorphine administered every 6–8 hours as deemed appropriate. Bupivacaine at 2 mg/kg can be instilled into the chest cavity every 8 hours. It should be diluted with saline to

Examination	Comments
Observation of breathing	Open-mouth breathing or breathing with extended neck is a poor prognostic sign. In dyspnoea, breathing is primarily diaphragmatic with minimal movement of chest wall
Respiratory rate and rhythm	Normal respiratory rate 30–60 breaths/min
Nares	Twitch at rate of 20–120 times per minute. May stop when relaxed or under anaesthetic
Sneezing	Note frequency, and presence or absence of discharge
Larynx and trachea	Palpate for symmetry and presence of swelling or masses
Auscultation of chest	Identify crackles, wheezes or absence of lung sounds
Palpation of chest	Note changes in compliance of thoracic cavity which could indicate presence of thoracic masses

19.8 Clinical examination of the respiratory system prior to thoracic surgery.

Examination	Comments
Resting heart rate and rhythm	Normal heart rate 150–300 beats/min
Resting pulse rate	Use femoral or central auricular artery and note any deficit
Auscultation	Heart murmurs should be further investigated using ultrasound techniques
Capillary refill time	Use gingivae
Mucous membrane colour	Use oral or conjunctival mucosa. Normally slightly paler than in dog or cat

19.9 Clinical examination of the cardiovascular system prior to thoracic surgery.

ensure that good contact is made inside the thoracic cavity. If this is instilled through a chest drain then a note should be made of the volume in order that the same volume can be removed via the chest drain.

Postoperative radiographs will show the presence and extent of air in the pleural cavity. The air can be removed by thoracocentesis if a chest drain has not been placed. Indwelling chest drains are not always necessary, and have advantages and disadvantages (Figure 19.10). If used, they should be placed prior to closure of the sternotomy and will enable air to be evacuated from the chest cavity. Alternatively, the air may be carefully extracted after closure using a hypodermic needle, syringe and three-way tap. The presence of a chest drain will create an inflammatory response which may produce up to 2 ml/kg per day of fluid. This should be borne in mind when evaluating the volume of fluid removed from the chest. Chest drain placement is described in Operative Technique 19.3.

Advantages
• Management of postsurgical pneumothorax
• Removal of accumulated fluid
• Flushing of pyothorax

Disadvantages
• Prolonged surgical time
• Risk of iatrogenic pneumothorax if poorly placed and/or managed
• Prolonged hospitalization and expense
• Intense, regular management required
• Risk of infection, which increases with time that drain is in place
• Excessive suction pressure may lead to lung injury
• Risk of re-expansion pulmonary oedema if air evacuated too quickly from chest
• Phrenic nerve irritation, Horner's syndrome or cardiac arrhythmias may be caused by presence of drain

19.10 Advantages and disadvantages of chest drains in rabbits following thoracotomy.

It is sensible to use a broad-spectrum antibiotic given intravenously 60–90 minutes prior to the surgery and at intervals during prolonged surgery. Antibiotics should be continued for at least 5–7 days postoperatively. The course may be prolonged if deemed necessary, especially in cases of pulmonary abscessation.

Acknowledgement

The author would like to thank Liz Sinclair MRCVS for her help with the surgical cases.

References and further reading

Antinoff N (2009) Mediastinal masses in rabbits: another therapeutic option. In : *Pre Conference Program AEMV (Association of Exotic Mammal Veterinarians)* pp. 69
Bellah JR (1993) The thymus. In: *Textbook of Small Animal Surgery, 2nd edn,* ed. D Slatter, pp. 977–983. WB Saunders Company, Philadelphia
Clippinger TL, Bennett RA, Alleman AR, Ginn PE and Bellah JR (1998) Removal of a thymoma via median sternotomy in a rabbit with recurrent appendicular neurofibrosarcoma. *Journal of the American Veterinary Medical Association* **218**, 1140–1143
Deeb BJ (2003) Respiratory disease and pasteurellosis. In: *Ferrets, Rabbits and Rodents: Clinical Medicine and Surgery, 2nd edn,* ed. KE Quesenberry and JW Carpenter, pp. 172–182. WB Saunders, Philadelphia
Deeb BJ and DiGiacomo RF (2000) Respiratory diseases of rabbits. *Veterinary Clinics of North America: Exotic Animal Practice* **3**, 465–480
Deeb BJ, DiGiacomo RF, Bernard BL and Silbernagel SM (1990) *Pasteurella multocida* and *Bordetella bronchiseptica* infections in rabbits. *Journal of Clinical Microbiology* **28**, 70–75
Florizoone K (2005) Thymoma associated exfoliative dermatitis in a rabbit. *Veterinary Dermatology* **16**, 281–284
Fossum TW (2007) Thymomas, thymic branchial cysts, and mediastinal cysts. In: *Small Animal Surgery, 3rd edn,* ed. TW Fossum. Mosby Elsevier, St. Louis
Fox RR, Meier H, Crary DD, Norberg RF and Myers DD (1971) Hemolytic anemia associated with thymoma in the rabbit. *Oncology* **25**, 372–382
Greene H and Strauss J (1949) Multiple primary tumors in the rabbit. *Cancer* **2**, 673–691
Harcourt-Brown FM (2002) Surgical removal of a mediastinal mass. *Exotic DVM* **4**, 59–60
Harcourt-Brown FM (2013) Complications and outcome of thymic mass removal in rabbits. *Proceedings of 1st International Conference on Avian, Herpetological and Exotic Mammal Medicine, Wiesbaden, Germany* pp. 185–185
Harcourt-Brown FM and Harcourt-Brown NH (2009) Thymoma in rabbits. In: *Proceedings of Soft Tissue Surgery in Exotic Pet Animals, Brno, Czech Republic* 121–124
Heatley JJ and Smith AN (2004) Neoplastic diseases of rabbits. *Veterinary Clinics of North America: Exotic Animal Practice* **7**, 561–577
Hernandez-Divers SJ and Murray M (2004) Small mammal endoscopy. In: *Ferrets, Rabbits and Rodents: Clinical Medicine and Surgery,* ed. KE Quesenberry and JW Carpenter, pp. 392–394. WB Saunders, Philadelphia
Kostolich M and Panciera RJ (1991) Thymoma in a domestic rabbit. *Cornell Veterinarian* **82**, 125–129
Meredith A (2006) Respiratory disorders. In: *BSAVA Manual of Rabbit Medicine and Surgery, 2nd edn,* ed. A Meredith and P Flecknell, pp. 67–73. BSAVA Publications, Gloucester
Morrisey JK and McEntee M (2005) Therapeutic options for thymoma in the rabbit. *Journal of Exotic Pet Medicine* **14**(3), 175–181
Popesko P, Rajtova V and Horak J (1992) *A Colour Atlas of Anatomy of Small Laboratory Animals.* Wolfe, London
Thurston JR, Cysewski SJ and Richard JL (1979) Exposure of rabbits to spores of *Aspergillus fumigatus* or *Penicillium* sp: survival of fungi and microscopic changes in the respiratory and gastrointestinal tracts. *American Journal of Veterinary Research* **40**, 1443–1449
Vernau KM, Grahn BH, Clarke-Scott HA and Sullivan N (1995) Thymoma in a geriatric rabbit with hypercalcaemia and periodic exopthalmos. *Journal of the American Veterinary Medical Association* **206**(6), 820–822
Wagner F, Beinecke A, Fehr M *et al.* (2005) Recurrent bilateral exophthalmos associated with metastatic thymic carcinoma in a pet rabbit. *Journal of Small Animal Practice* **46**, 393–397
Weisbroth SH (1994) Neoplastic diseases. In: *The Biology of the Laboratory Rabbit, 2nd edn,* ed. PJ Manning, DH Ringler and CE Newcomer, pp. 259–292. Academic Press, San Diego
White SD, Linder KE, Schultheiss P *et al.* (2000) Sebaceous adenitis in four domestic rabbits. *Veterinary Dermatology* **11**, 53–60
Withrow SJ (2001) Thymoma. In: *Small Animal Clinical Oncology,* ed. SJ Withrow and EG MacEwan, pp. 646–651. WB Saunders, Philadelphia

OPERATIVE TECHNIQUE 19.1:
Median sternotomy for thymoma removal

Patient positioning and preparation

General anaesthesia is induced with the surgeon's drug of choice and the rabbit is intubated with a non-cuffed tube (anaesthesia for thoracotomy is described in detail in Chapter 1). The rabbit is placed in dorsal recumbency.

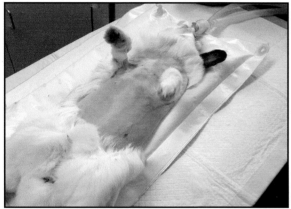

Patient clipped and prepared for surgery. The forelimbs will be extended and tied securely.

Assistant

Required.

Additional equipment

- Gelpi or Lone Star retractors
- Oscillating saw or Dremel drill with sterile diamond disc
- Radiosurgical equipment
- Suction
- Chest drain
- Three-way tap

Procedure

1 Inject bupivacaine (2 mg/kg) into all intercostal spaces due to the length of the incision.

2 Make a ventral midline skin incision starting 2–3 cm cranial to the manubrium and extending back to the xiphoid.

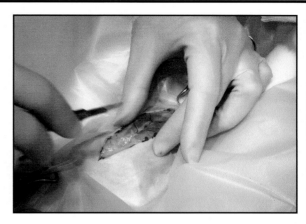

3 Continue the incision through the thin muscle layers.

4 Separate the sternohyoideus and sternocephalicus muscles from the sternum using blunt dissection and controlling bleeding with radiosurgery.

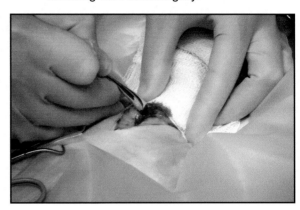

5 Score the midline of the sternum with the scalpel blade and continue the incision with an oscillating saw or a Dremel drill with a sterile diamond disc.

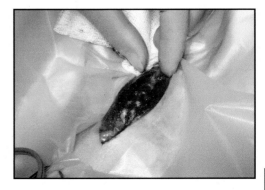

OPERATIVE TECHNIQUE 19.1 continued:
Median sternotomy for thymoma removal

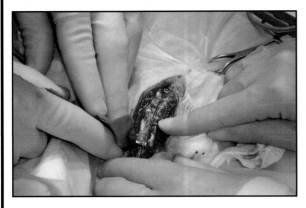

6 Narrow sternebrae may necessitate transection of costal cartilages.

7 Insert retractors after the incision of the first few sternebrae. This stabilizes the sternum and allows easier transection of the midline.

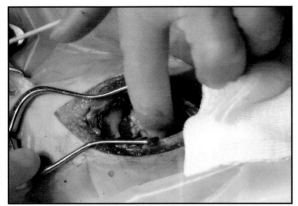

Gelpi retractors used to aid visualization of the thymoma.

8 Leave the last one or two costal cartilages intact.

9 Initiate intermittent positive pressure ventilation as soon as the thoracic cavity is entered.

10 Place moist laparotomy sponges along the edges of the wound and open it as wide as possible with retractors.

11 Dissect the mass away from the surrounding tissue slowly and meticulously using fingers, sterile cotton buds or haemostats. Use radiosurgery or sutures to control bleeding.

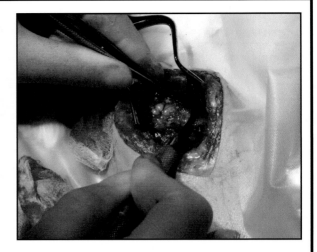

12 Carefully dissect the mass free from the subclavian arteries and veins, jugular veins and carotid arteries in the cranial thoracic inlet. Gently elevate the mass out of the thoracic cavity.

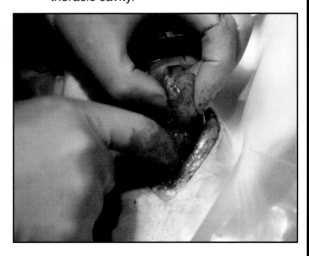

13 Meticulously control bleeding and flush the thoracic cavity with warm saline to remove blood clots, debris and assess lungs for leakage of air. Remove the saline with suction.

14 Place a chest drain if considered necessary.

15 The sternebrae should be apposed using preplaced sutures of polydioxanone (e.g. PDS) or polypropylene (e.g. Prolene).

OPERATIVE TECHNIQUE 19.1 continued:
Median sternotomy for thymoma removal

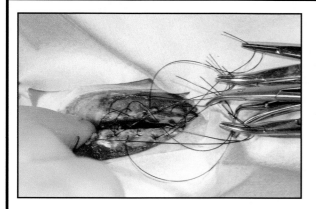

16 Tie knots in the preplaced sutures.

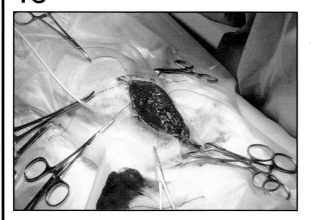

17 Appose overlying muscles, using 2 metric (3/0 USP) polyglactin 910 (e.g. Vicryl) or poliglecaprone (e.g. Monocryl).

18 Close dead space with subcuticular sutures and close the skin with intradermal sutures, using 2 metric (3/0 USP) polyglactin 910 (e.g. Vicryl) or poliglecaprone (e.g. Monocryl).

19 Remove excess air via a chest drain if placed (see Operative Technique 19.3) or via a needle with a three-way tap attached.

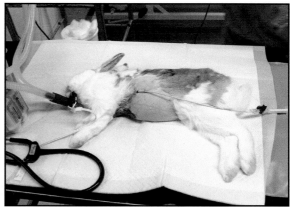

Chest drain in place and air being gently removed via syringe and three-way tap.

Postoperative care

The rabbit should be kept warm, intravenous fluids continued, oxygen supplementation given if necessary and careful attention given to providing analgesia. Radiographs may be taken to check that the lungs are fully inflated postoperatively.

OPERATIVE TECHNIQUE 19.2:
Lung lobectomy via a lateral thoracotomy

Patient positioning and preparation

General anaesthesia is induced with the surgeon's drug of choice and the rabbit is intubated with a non-cuffed tube (anaesthesia for thoracotomy is described in detail in Chapter 1). It is placed in lateral recumbency with forelimbs restrained cranially. Clip the hair over the left (for right-handed operators) lateral chest wall, including the entire rib area, prior to thoracotomy.

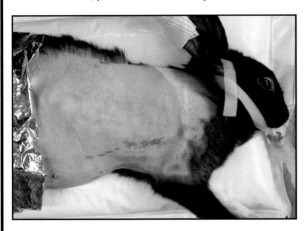

Assistant

Required.

Additional equipment

- Gelpi or Lone Star retractors
- Radiosurgical equipment
- Suction
- Chest drain
- Three-way tap

Procedure

Lung lobectomies are best performed via the 4th or 5th intercostal space.

1 Incise through the skin and subcutaneous tissue at the caudodorsal border of the scapula, which lies at the 4th intercostal space. The latissimus dorsi muscle is incised from ventral to dorsal.

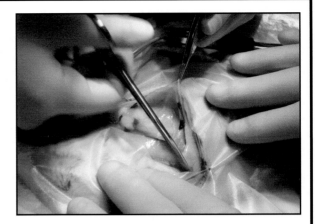

2 Palpate underneath the lattisimus dorsi to identify the thoracic inlet and 1st rib.

3 Separate the serratus ventralis muscle and transect the scalenus muscle along the 5th rib.

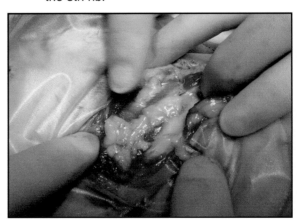

4 Transect the external and internal intercostal muscles and spread the ribs with a retractor.

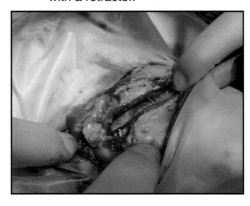

OPERATIVE TECHNIQUE 19.2 continued:
Lung lobectomy via a lateral thoracotomy

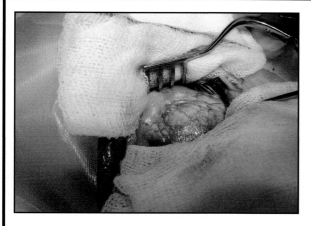

5 Initiate mechanical or manual ventilation upon entering the chest.

6 Elevate the abscessed or neoplastic lung lobe gently out of the chest cavity.

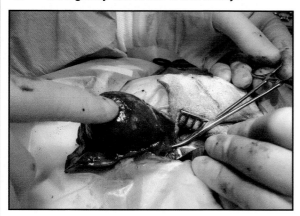

7 The artery, vein and bronchus are all very small and may be sealed, ligated or clipped as a single unit using polydioxanone, polypropylene, haemoclips or a Ligasure device. The bronchus is sectioned. A harmonic scalpel may be used. The lobe is removed and the ligated bronchus is checked for air leakage.

8 A chest drain can be placed if desired at this point (see Operative Technique 19.3).

9 Sutures should be preplaced before the knots are tied and should encircle the ribs cranially and caudally.

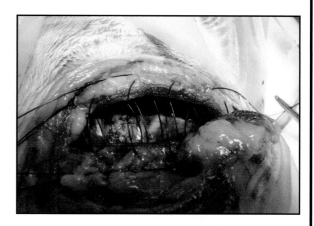

10 The scalenus, serratus ventralis and lattisimus dorsi muscles can be closed with absorbable sutures such as 2 metric (3/0 USP) poliglecaprone (e.g. Monocryl) or polyglactin 910 (e.g. Vicryl). A simple continuous suture pattern may be used. Intradermal sutures should be used for closure of the skin.

Postoperative care

The rabbit should be kept warm, intravenous fluids continued, oxygen given if necessary and analgesia provided. Radiographs may be taken to assess the presence of air in the thoracic cavity, or the chest should be drained with the preplaced chest drain or a needle and three-way tap.

OPERATIVE TECHNIQUE 19.3:
Placing a chest drain

A drain should be placed after closure of a ventral sternotomy or prior to closure of a lateral thoracotomy.

Assistant

A surgical assistant may help with placement. A second assistant is required to manage the anaesthetic.

Additional instruments

- Trocar chest drain (14–16 Fr)
- Chest drain connectors
- Three-way tap
- Bungs
- Gate clamp
- 2, 5 and 10 ml syringes

The tip of the drain should be long enough to reach the 2nd rib.

Surgical approach

1 A small stab incision is made through the skin two-thirds of the way up the chest at the level of the 10th intercostal space.

2 The tip of the drain is advanced under the skin in a cranioventral direction to approximately the 8th intercostal space.

3 The drain with trocar is held perpendicularly at the 8th intercostal space and introduced with a short sharp stabbing motion using the heel of the hand. Take care to ensure that only a short section of trocar is introduced into the thoracic cavity to avoid damage to thoracic organs.

4 The drain is advanced a short distance over the end of the trocar to protect the sharp tip.

5 The drain and trocar are advanced parallel to the ribs up to the level of the 2nd rib.

6 The trocar is removed while the drain is held firmly in position and the tube is then occluded temporarily with forceps.

7 Place a gate clamp on the drain and attach a connector and three-way tap.

8 Remove the forceps and gently drain the chest with a 2 or 5 ml syringe, taking care to avoid too much suction.

9 Close the three-way tap and place bungs on the two ports.

10 Secure the drain to the chest wall using a Chinese fingertrap suture.

11 Place a dressing over the site of insertion of the chest drain and cover with a chest bandage.

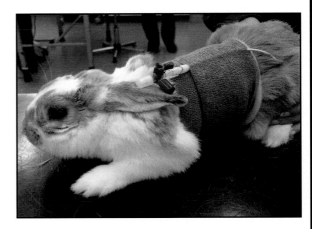

Postoperative care

- Check all connections and change the dressing and bandage at least once a day.
- Consider use of a soft Elizabethan collar but take care to manage caecotrophy.
- Monitor the patient throughout the day and night for any complications.

20

Surgical treatment of adrenocortical disease

Angela M. Lennox

Post-gonadectomy adrenal hyperplasia and/or neoplasia with overproduction of sex hormones have been recognized in a number of laboratory species (Reincke *et al.*, 1997; Bernichtein *et al.*, 2008). In pets, the disease is well documented in the ferret but still poorly described in the rabbit, although Lennox and Chitty have reported two cases in castrated male rabbits (Lennox and Chitty, 2006).

Presenting signs

Adrenocortical disease (ACD) is suspected in any neutered rabbit exhibiting the onset of unusual aggressive or sexual behaviour, especially in older animals. Owners may describe the following behaviours: aggression in the form of chasing other pets and/or humans; biting, scratching and mounting other pets and/or humans, especially the feet; and urinating over other pets, the owners or objects. The average age at diagnosis in the six cases summarized in this chapter was 7.6 years.

Diagnostic procedures

Diagnosis of ACD is suspected based on history and demonstration of elevated testosterone or other sex hormones, and confirmed via histopathology. All cases presented in Figure 20.1 featured elevated testosterone; however, there is early evidence that elevations in other hormones, including progesterone, may also occur. Sex hormone reference ranges for neutered rabbits of both sexes were reported by Fectau *et al.* in 2007 (Figure 20.2). Results were pooled, as there was no significant difference between genders.

Age (years)	Sex	Condition	Testosterone (ng/ml)	Treatment/outcome	Source
9	M	Right adrenocortical hyperplasia	2.67	Attempted subtotal right adrenalectomy, no response; did not respond to deslorelin	Paolo Selleri
7	M	Right adrenocortical hyperplasia	3.96	No response to leuprorelin; responded for 3 months to right adrenalectomy, then clinical signs recurred; no response to finasteride	Angela Lennox
8	M	Left adrenocortical neoplasia; possible carcinoma	0.80	Attempted removal of left adrenal gland; elected euthanasia	John Chitty
6	F	Left adrenal adenocarcinoma	0.68 initially; 0.57 after medical therapy; 0.02 after adrenalectomy	No response to deslorelin or trilostane; good response to adrenalectomy	Robert Wagner
8	M	Left adrenal hyperplasia	0.52 initially; 0.57 after flutamide and trilostane; 0.04 after leuprorelin (leuprolide acetate; 100 μg/kg of a human 1-month depot preparation); 0.03 after adrenalectomy	Responded to leuprorelin and adrenalectomy	Robert Wagner

20.1 Features of adrenal hyperplasia/neoplasia in selected cases.

Hormone	Concentration (reference values in parentheses)	
	ng/ml	*nmol/l*
Progesterone	0.25 ± 0.02 (0.11–0.46)	0.79 ± 0.06 (0.35–1.46)
Testosterone	0.02 ± 0.00 (0.02–0.04)	0.07 ± 0.00 (0.07–0.14)
Cortisol	7.28 ± 0.40 (4.64–11.2)	20.10 ± 0.10 (12.80–30.91)
17-Hydroxyprogesterone	6.46 ± 1.35 (0.75–22.2)	19.75 ± 4.09 (2.27–67.27)
Androstenedione	2.47 ± 0.22 (0.80–4.0)	8.62 ± 0.77 (2.79–13.96)

20.2 Serum hormone levels reported in male and female neutered rabbits (Fectau *et al.*, 2007).

It is uncertain whether ultrasonography may be a useful diagnostic tool; features of histopathologically confirmed abnormal adrenal glands are uncertain, due to the limited number of cases.

Relevant anatomy and surgical landmarks

The adrenal glands of the normal rabbit are relatively large (Figure 20.3), and proportionately larger than those of the ferret. Actual measurements vary significantly with the size of the animal. The appearance is pink, smooth and slightly rounded.

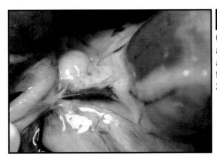

20.3 Grossly normal-appearing left adrenal gland in the cadaver of a 3-year-old rabbit.

Exact anatomical descriptions of the normal adrenal gland and vasculature vary slightly between sources (Harrison, 1951; Barone *et al.*, 1973; Popesko *et al.*, 1992). The left adrenal gland lies in an angle between the aorta and the left renal vessels, and is easily separated from the vasculature, while the right gland is closely associated with the caudal vena cava (Figure 20.4). The right adrenal gland is supplied by the right cranial and right caudal adrenal arteries from the abdominal aorta and the right renal artery, respectively. The blood supply to the left adrenal gland consists of the left cranial and left medial adrenal arteries from the aorta. The left adrenal gland is connected to the caudal vena cava via the left adrenal vein (Popesko *et al.*, 1992).

Adrenalectomy

Adrenalectomy for treatment of ACD is well described in the ferret. While reported and anecdotal cases of surgical adrenalectomy in the rabbit are few, these cases utilized similar techniques, including total or subtotal excision with the use of sutures and/or haemostatic clips (e.g. Hemoclips) (Lennox and Chitty, 2006; Wagner, personal communication).

- As in the ferret, removal of the left adrenal gland is by complete excision. The left adrenal gland is identified within the perirenal fat, and bluntly dissected. The vessels are isolated and ligated with 1.5–2 metric (4/0 to 3/0 USP) sutures or haemostatic clips. In the author's experience, the use of haemostatic clips is preferable.
- Right adrenalectomy is challenging, due to the association of the gland with the vena cava. However, in the author's experience, a single attempt to remove an abnormal right adrenal

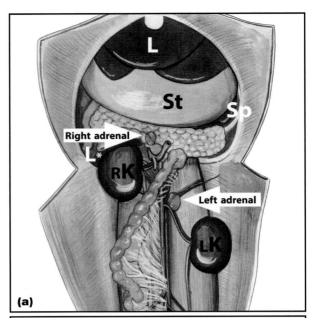

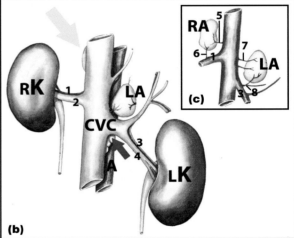

20.4 Anatomy of the normal rabbit adrenal glands. **(a)** Position of the adrenal glands in the abdominal cavity, and anatomical relationship with other organs. The silhouette of the right adrenal gland is a projection, since it is dorsal to the cranial vena cava. L = liver; LK = left kidney; RK = right kidney; Sp = spleen; St = stomach. **(b)** Kidneys and adrenal glands, ventral view. The right adrenal gland is located dorsal to the caudal vena cava (arrow). A = aorta; CVC = caudal vena cava; LA = left adrenal gland; LK = left kidney; RK = right kidney; 1 = right renal artery; 2 = right renal vein; 3 = left renal artery; 4 = left renal vein. **(c)** Blood supply of the adrenal glands after removal of the caudal vena cava, ventral view. LA = left adrenal gland; RA = right adrenal gland; 1 = right renal artery; 3 = left renal artery; 5 = right cranial adrenal artery; 6 = right caudal adrenal artery; 7 = left cranial adrenal artery; 8 = left caudal adrenal artery. (Reproduced with permission from Popesko (1992) *A Colour Atlas of Anatomy of Small Laboratory Animals*, plate 7; arrows and labels modified by by Vittorio Capello)

gland was easier than in the ferret due to larger gland size, and less close association with the vena cava. In this case, and one other case, Hemoclips were placed between the right gland and the vena cava. It is uncertain in either case whether the gland was removed in its entirety.

Total excision utilizing vascular clamps and re-suturing of the wall of the vena cava, using lasers, cryosurgery, or ameroid constrictor rings, as reported in the ferret, have not been reported in the rabbit.

In ferrets, there is evidence that partial occlusion of the vena cava by an adrenal tumour promotes the formation of collateral circulation via the vertebral venous sinus and the azygous vein; therefore, resection of the adrenal gland and associated vena cava may not result in severe circulatory disturbances or death. There is no information on similar development of collateral circulation in the rabbit; therefore, ligation of the vena cava cannot be recommended.

Figure 20.1 describes selected cases and their outcomes. There are very few descriptions and illustrations of histologically confirmed abnormal rabbit adrenal glands, and their appearance in these few cases was variable; the surgical appearance of some representative cases is shown in Figure 20.5. Three rabbits underwent successful full or partial adrenalectomy (Figure 20.6) resulting in at least temporary resolution of clinical signs. Two other cases featured local invasion that was determined to be non-resectable. In all cases, a standard midline approach to the abdomen was utilized, and closure was accomplished in two to three layers using 1.5–2 metric (4/0 to 3/0 USP) absorbable sutures. Abnormal adrenal glands were, in most cases, two to four times larger than the contralateral gland. One contained a small, firm nodule.

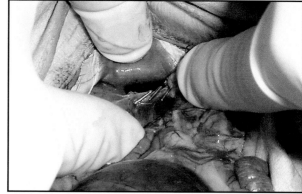

20.6 Appearance of the right vena cava and placement of haemostatic clips after debulking of the abnormal adrenal gland pictured in Figure 20.5a. (Reprinted with permission from Lennox and Chitty (2006) © Elsevier)

Other treatment options

Non-surgical therapies, including leuprolide acetate and deslorelin, have been utilized alone and in conjunction with surgery. Response to medical therapy is variable (see Figure 20.1).

Prognosis

Due to low case numbers, prognosis is uncertain, and there is not enough information to determine the advantages or disadvantages of any particular

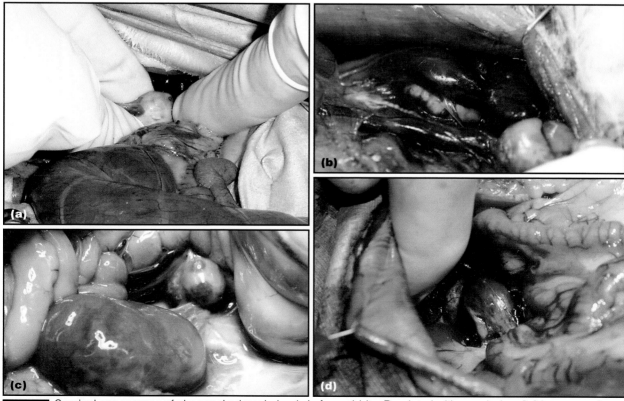

20.5 Surgical appearance of abnormal adrenal glands in four rabbits. Reprinted with permission: **(a)** Lennox and Chitty (2006) © Elsevier; **(b,c)** © Vittorio Capello; **(d)** © Paolo Selleri.

approach. However, it is clear even from these limited reported cases that response to medical and/or surgical therapy is variable.

References and further reading

Barone R, Pavaux C, Blin PC and Cuq P (1973) *Atlas D'anatomie du Lapin*, p.189. Masson, Paris

Bernichtein S, Petretto E, Jamieson S *et al.* (2008) Adrenal gland tumorigenesis after gonadectomy in mice is a complex genetic trait driven by epistatic loci. *Endocrinology* **149**, 651–661

Fectau JA, Deeb BJ and Rickel JM (2007) Diagnostic endocrinology: blood steroid concentrations in neutered male and female rabbits. *Journal of Exotic Pet Medicine* **16**, 256–259

Harrison RG (1951) A comparative study of the vascularization of the adrenal gland in the rabbit, rat and cat. *Journal of Anatomy* **85**, 12–23

Lennox AM and Chitty J (2006) Adrenal neoplasia and hyperplasia as a cause of hypertestosteronism in two rabbits. *Journal of Exotic Pet Medicine* **15**(1), 56–58

Popesko P, Rajtova V and Horak J (1992) *A Colour Atlas of Anatomy of Small Laboratory Animals, Vol.1. Rabbit, Guinea pig*, p. 92. Wolfe, London

Reincke M, Mora P, Beuschlein F *et al.* (1997) Deletion of the adrenocorticotropin receptor gene in human adrenocortical tumors: implications for tumorigenesis. *Journal of Clinical Endocrinology and Metabolism* **82**, 3054–3058

OPERATIVE TECHNIQUE 20.1:
Adrenalectomy

Patient positioning and preparation

Place the patient in dorsal recumbency. Clip and prepare the entire ventral abdomen in the event that additional exposure is required. The procedure is carried out under general anaesthesia (see Chapter 1).

Assistant

May help to improve visualization by reflecting viscera.

Equipment extras

- Retractor
- Haemostatic clips and applicator

Procedure

1 Make an incision on the ventral midline from the xiphoid to the umbilicus. The use of a retractor improves visibility.

2 Identify the abnormal-appearing gland.

Left adrenal gland

3 Using blunt dissection, identify the vasculature to the gland.

4 Ligate with haemostatic clips and excise the gland.

5 Check carefully for bleeding.

Right adrenal gland

3 Using blunt dissection, carefully isolate the gland and its attachment to the vena cava.

4 Carefully place haemostatic clips between the gland and the vena cava.

5 Carefully excise the gland distal to the haemostatic clips and monitor for bleeding.

Closure

6 Close as for any abdominal suture. The author prefers a simple continuous pattern, followed by a continuous subcuticular closure of the skin in order to prevent patient disruption of the sutures.

Postoperative care

Monitor the patient carefully for any complications after abdominal surgery. General complications include hypovolaemia and haemorrhage.

21

Removal of perineal and other skin folds

Alessandro Melillo

Chronic perineal dermatitis

Chronic perineal dermatitis is a common problem in pet rabbits and may be a consequence of prolonged contact with urine, caecotrophs or both. It can be the result of urinary or reproductive tract disease that causes incontinence, or conditions that result in soft caecotrophs or impair the rabbit's ability to ingest them. Rabbits with dental disease or spinal problems (such as spondylosis) are often unable to reach the perineum to groom themselves and any condition that prevents a rabbit from rotating its pelvis during urination can result in urine scald. Urine scald is a 'vicious circle' problem because the more the skin gets inflamed and painful, the less the rabbit is able to move its pelvis freely, so that even more urine and faeces contaminate the area.

Many cases of chronic perineal dermatitis are simply due to obesity. Fat rabbits can develop a large fold of skin which covers the genital area (Figure 21.1). Myiasis can be a further complication.

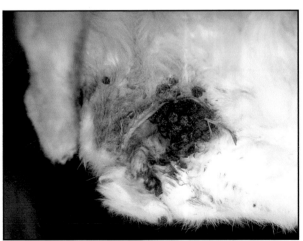

21.1 Some rabbits, especially loose-skinned breeds that were obese and then lost weight, can develop a large fold of skin covering the genital area. Faeces and skin debris can collect under the fold. Secondary infection and moist dermatitis develop readily.

Initial treatment

Initially, rabbits with urine scald and/or caecotrophs under the tail should be treated conservatively by clipping the hair over the affected skin and allowing it to dry. Rabbits with urine scald may benefit from topical ointments or powders and general antibiotic therapy, cytology, culture and sensitivity tests may help in choosing the most appropriate antibiotic. Non-steroidal anti-inflammatory drugs (NSAIDs) are useful and can be combined with the topical preparation or administered systemically. Increased exercise should be encouraged and the diet modified to promote weight loss. Fibre intake should be increased to make the caecotrophs firmer, and any dental and mobility issues managed as far as possible. Addressing the underlying problem is the first and most important part of treatment, but in some cases the problem is not curable and surgery is indicated.

Skin fold resection

Resection of the skin around the genitalia is a straightforward procedure that varies with the severity of the problem. In simple cases, only the surplus fold of skin needs to be removed.

1. Following induction of general anaesthesia, the rabbit is positioned in dorsal recumbency and the area between the navel and the tail, including the medial thigh region to the stifle, is shaved and prepared for surgery.
2. A crescent-shaped area cranial to the genitourinary area, large enough to remove all the excess skin, is marked with a pen, then cut with a blade and removed. The surgeon must be careful not to damage the lateral abdominal vein, which lies lateral to the nipple but quite deep to the mammary tissue.
3. Under the excess skin a large adipose body is found, whose partial or total removal is advised. The remaining skin should be taut but without tension on the incision.
4. Closure in two layers is advised:
   - The deep layer is closed with horizontal 'U' or 'X' stitches, which are good for relieving tension. Poliglecaprone (Monocryl), polydioxanone (PDS) or polyglactin (Vicryl) are suitable materials, although Vicryl may be associated with a greater inflammatory response
   - The skin is closed with staples or the same tension-relieving suture pattern. Monocryl is the author's choice of suture material.

Postoperatively, the most important point is to keep the skin clean and soft, paying attention to the hygiene of the area and of the cage. The use of softening creams, with or without antibiotics, is advised.

Skin fold resection with inguinal pouch removal

Rabbits have two deep hairless pouches on either side of the genital orifice (Figure 21.2) that contain the inguinal scent glands. Each gland consists of a superficial pale spherical lobe and an adjacent deeper-lying dark brown lobe (Martinez-Gomez *et al.*, 1997). Ducts from the gland open into the deep part of the hairless pouch, which fills with plugs of waxy exudate. In rabbits with perineal infections these pouches easily become infected (Figure 21.3). Removal of the pouches and associated scent glands can be performed in addition to removal of extra skin folds (see Operative Technique 21.1).

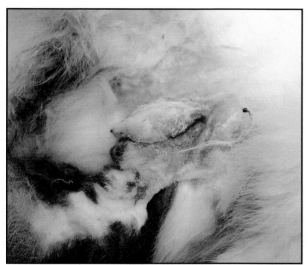

21.2   Rabbits have two deep hairless pouches on either side of the genital orifice that contain the inguinal scent glands.

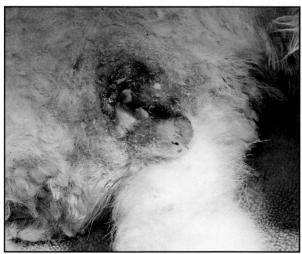

21.3   The inguinal pouches easily become infected, especially in rabbits with moist dermatitis in the perineal area.

Skin fold problems in male rabbits

Most skin fold problems are seen in female rabbits, although they occasionally occur in neutered males.

In older entire male rabbits, dermatitis can develop under the scrotum if the rabbit has difficulty grooming the area. This problem is more likely to develop if neoplasia is present; removal of the scrotal skin is necessary in addition to castration (Figure 21.4).

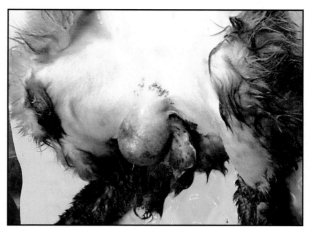

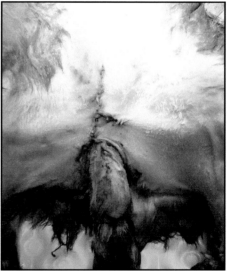

21.4   In rabbits with testicular neoplasia, removal of some scrotal skin may be necessary, in addition to castration.

Dermoplasty and tail amputation

A more radical and difficult procedure is indicated in rabbits that cannot direct the urine stream away from their body during urination. This may be the consequence of spinal cord disease and other neurological problems, severe arthritis or misaligned spinal/pelvis fractures.

Preoperatively, these patients may benefit from a course of antibiotics and anti-inflammatories if they are showing signs of infection or inflammation.

1. Following induction of general anaesthesia the rabbit is positioned in ventral recumbency with its legs extended backwards (Jenkins, 2012).

2. An area 6–8 cm in diameter around the tail and anus is clipped and surgically prepared.

3. A crescent-shaped area, including the tail, is marked, with its ventral curvature just tangent to the dorsal limits of the external anal sphincter muscle, the tips lateral and ventral to the urethral opening and its dorsal curvature cranial to the tail. The crescent should be broad enough that, when removed, the anus and urethral opening will be lifted dorsally at the most caudal end of the rabbit's body.

4. The skin is incised and the coccygeal and sacrocaudal muscles removed from their insertion on the caudal vertebrae.

5. The tail is amputated at the third or fourth vertebra, having ligated the medial sacral artery and the other tail vessels. In some male rabbits the retractor penis muscle must be dissected as well.

6. All the dissected muscles are reattached at the dorsal caudal origin of the semitendinosus muscle using a strong monofilament suture.

7. The wound edges are pulled near by vertical mattress suture, against tension, and the incision is closed in two layers, as described above.

Postoperative care is as described above.

Reconstructive surgery in the perineal area

Correct positioning of the urethral opening is important to ensure that the rabbit directs the stream of urine away from the body during urination. Many conditions can damage or inflame the external genitalia and alter the direction of urine flow, or result in abnormal folds of skin. Extensive wounds, chronic urine scalding, burns, fight wounds, myiasis, surgical complications or any other accident can cause the formation of scar tissue, which distorts the genitalia so the rabbit urinates down its leg or dribbles urine.

Many affected rabbits will heal well, even if the injuries are extensive, if all the wet and soiled fur is clipped off and antibiotic and analgesic therapy is provided. Some cases, however, require more treatment, sometimes involving surgery.

Severe flystrike can result in large areas of full-thickness skin loss (Figure 21.5), which need to be covered as they heal. Initially, hydrogels (e.g. Intrasite) can be covered with a moisture vapour-permeable dressing (e.g. Opsite) to absorb bacteria and hydrate the area (Cousquer, 2006) before a more permanent dressing, such as Granuflex, is sutured over the skin deficit to protect exposed nerve endings and provide a healthy bed of granulation tissue. Alternatively, if sufficient loose skin is available, it can be moved over the skin deficit. After healing has taken place, scar tissue may need to be removed to restore normal anatomy as far as possible.

Each case is individual, so providing exact guidelines can be difficult. Close examination of the area and consideration of the anatomy and underlying problem is required for successful surgery

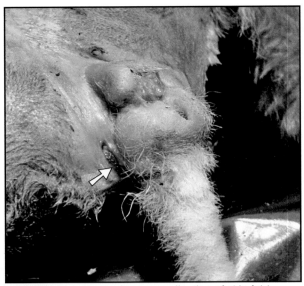

21.5 Myiasis can be a complication of skin fold infections and result in full-thickness skin loss, especially in the area between the tail and the back (arrow). In severe cases, reconstructive surgery may be required.

(Figure 21.6). The surgeon should always consider the lines of tension and the forces applied on the part during normal rabbit movements. As mentioned earlier, it is important to keep the area clean and soft, using creams with or without antibiotics.

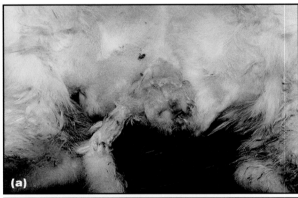

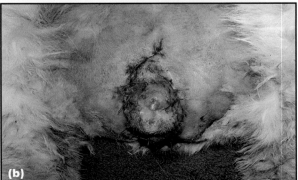

21.6 **(a)** In some older rabbits, the tail becomes deformed and twists to one side so the genital mound is rotated and the direction of urine flow is altered. Urine scald is the result. **(b)** The same rabbit after reconstructive surgery, which can be used to correct the problem and may require tail amputation. (Courtesy of Frances Harcourt-Brown)

Dewlap surgery

Many female rabbits have a large fold of skin over the throat, which is called a dewlap (Figure 21.7), even though most of the breed standards regard it as undesirable. It is more developed in heavily built rabbits and in older does. Some owners worry about its presence and request surgical removal but the dewlap is a natural structure and in most cases, even if looks quite cumbersome, it does not need treatment.

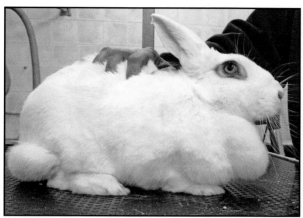

21.7 The large fold of skin over the throat in some female rabbits is called a dewlap.

Sometimes a lot of fat accumulates in the dewlap, which may be confused with an abscess or a tumour by the owner. Areas of fat necrosis can feel hard and solid. Moist dermatitis can occur on the dewlap, either as a consequence of drooling secondary to dental disease or of being constantly wet by drinking from dirty water bottles or bowls. In the latter case *Pseudomonas aeruginosa* is often involved in skin infection and the condition is referred to as 'blue fur disease' because the pigment produced by the bacteria stains the skin and the hair blue–green. In some cases the deep skin folds under the dewlap get infected because the rabbit does not groom properly and flystrike is a risk.

Dewlap surgery is sometimes tempting in rabbits that have moist dermatitis and lick or chew their dewlap. This self-mutilation can be a displacement activity because the rabbit cannot reach another area of its body, such as the perineum. Resolving the underlying problem, which may be pain (arthritis, spondylosis), obesity, pruritus (dermatitis, cheyletiellosis) or dental disease, is far more important than surgery in resolving the condition.

A fat rabbit that loses a lot of weight in a short time can maintain a huge dewlap and other skin folds that may benefit from corrective surgery, although these cases are uncommon. If surgery is required, it is performed using a technique similar to resection of a perineal skin fold, though the large amount of fat within the dewlap can cause problems. This fat is present in large pads or cushions that are attached to the nerves and blood vessels in the neck. Exteriorizing the fat pad to remove it in its entirety can stretch the nerves. Therefore, care is needed to avoid cutting any nerves or major blood vessels, especially the jugular vein. Transecting the fat pads may be preferable but fat and oil tends to seep into the operation site, making visualization difficult. After removal of the fat, there may be a large amount of dead space that needs to be reduced to prevent seroma, or even abscess formation postoperatively.

Dewlap removal is not a procedure that should be undertaken lightly. Weight loss prior to surgery, to reduce the amount of fat in the fat pads, is recommended so that the skin and a minimal amount of fat can be removed (see Operative Technique 21.2).

References and further reading

Cousquer G (2006) Veterinary care of rabbits with myiasis. *In Practice* **28**, 342–349

Jenkins J (2012) Soft tissue surgery. In: *Ferrets, Rabbits and Rodents: Clinical Medicine and Surgery, 3rd edn*, ed. KE Quesenbery and JW Carpenter, pp. 275–277. Elsevier, St. Louis

Martínez-Gomez M, Lucio RL, Carro M, Pacheco P and Hudson R (1997) Striated muscles and scent glands associated with the vaginal tract of the rabbit. *Anatomical Record* **247**, 486–495

OPERATIVE TECHNIQUES ➜

OPERATIVE TECHNIQUE 21.1:
Removal of perineal skin fold and inguinal pouches
Frances Harcourt-Brown

Preoperative assessment and preparation

After it has been anaesthetized (see Chapter 1), the rabbit is placed in dorsal recumbency. The fur is clipped away from the perineal area, so that it can be examined carefully to decide how much skin should be removed and from where.

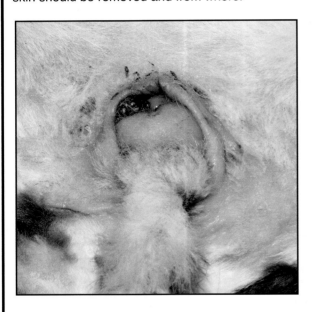

The area is cleaned, clipped, surgically prepared and draped. Skin preparation may cause a mild degree of soft tissue swelling, which is why close examination prior to preparation is necessary.

Equipment extras

- Cradle to maintain the rabbit in ventral recumbency
- Fine surgical kit
- Polyglactin (e.g. Vicryl Rapide) 1.5 metric (4/0 USP)

Procedure

1 A crescent-shaped incision is made at the periphery of the skin fold that is to be removed.

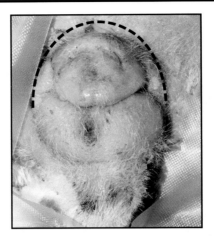

2 Further incisions are made along the boundaries of the inguinal pouches. These incisions extend to the original crescent-shaped incision.

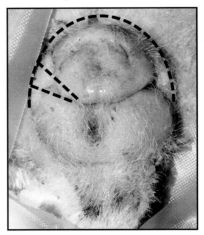

3 The interior of each pouch is exposed to reveal the pale superficial lobe of the scent gland (arrowed).

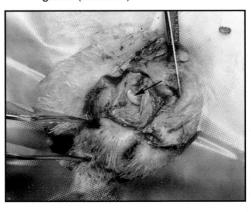

OPERATIVE TECHNIQUE 21.1 continued:
Removal of perineal skin fold and inguinal pouches
Frances Harcourt-Brown

4 The epithelium of the pouch is carefully dissected away from the underlying tissue by careful blunt dissection, keeping close to the epithelium. The dark deep lobe of the scent gland (arrowed) is identified and removed.

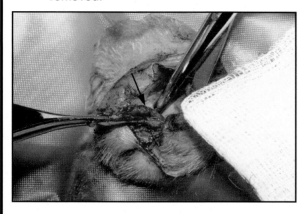

5 After the epithelium has been completely removed, the edges of the pouch are apposed with loose skin sutures.

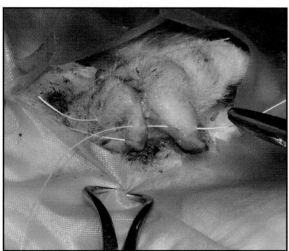

6 The fold of skin around the genitalia is stretched out so the surgeon can decide how much to remove. It is important that no tension is placed on the incision. If too much skin is removed the urethral opening may be everted to expose the mucosa which can cause urethritis, but if too little skin is removed, a fold may still be present postoperatively. The surplus skin can be removed in sections, while deciding how much to take.

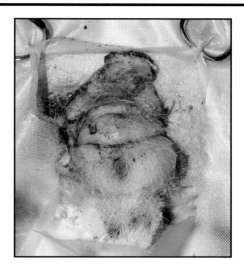

7 Sufficient skin should be removed to leave the edges of the incision in perfect apposition before the sutures are placed.

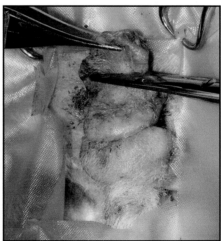

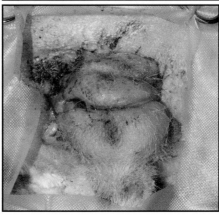

OPERATIVE TECHNIQUE 21.1 continued:
Removal of perineal skin fold and inguinal pouches
Frances Harcourt-Brown

8 The wound is closed with a single layer of skin sutures to maintain apposition of the skin. There must be no tension on the stitches, so that the rabbit will be comfortable. Subcuticular sutures are not placed because of the risk of stitch abscesses developing in the postoperative weeks or months. Vicryl Rapide is the author's preferred suture material because it is soft and comfortable for the rabbit and the sutures wipe off after 10–14 days without leaving any residual foreign material to act as a nidus of infection.

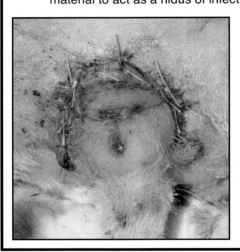

Postoperative care

Postoperative antibiotics are used. The author generally selects daily injections of penicillin/ streptomycin (e.g. 0.2 ml/kg Streptocare) for 7–10 days if purulent infection was present in the inguinal pouches or skin folds prior to surgery. If no pus was present, enrofloxacin or trimethoprim/sulphonamide is used. Concurrent analgesia using an NSAID (e.g. meloxicam) is given.

The rabbit is bedded on soft absorbent bedding (e.g. towel) that does not stick to the wound and can be kept clean postoperatively. Sawdust or wood shavings should not be used and hay should be provided in a rack or bowl rather than as bedding. If necessary, any blood or exudate from the wound can be gently cleaned away each day with warm water and antiseptic. Otherwise the wound is left alone. Patient interference does not occur if the wound is comfortable. Many of the rabbits that are affected by this condition cannot reach their perineum, so any form of Elizabethan collar is unnecessary and may stress the rabbit.

Postoperative healing is generally good.

OPERATIVE TECHNIQUE 21.2:
Dewlap removal
Frances Harcourt-Brown

In most cases removal of the dewlap is unnecessary and should be avoided, but occasionally the skin fold is so large that the rabbit cannot groom, especially if it is affected by other mobility problems. Removal of the skin is technically easy but is time-consuming, both in preparation time and suturing. Removal of the fat pads increases the risk of the procedure. It is preferable to reduce the amount of fat in the dewlap by dietary modification prior to surgery.

Positioning and patient preparation

The anaesthetized patient is positioned in a trough in dorsal recumbency and the area from the chin to midway down the chest is clipped. The area should extend from one shoulder to the other.

The dewlap is examined and the amount of skin that needs to be removed is determined and marked.

The skin is aseptically prepared.

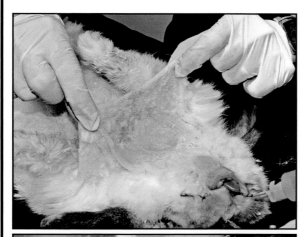

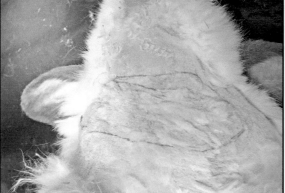

Equipment extras

- Fine surgical kit
- Pen

Procedure

1 The marked area of skin is removed to expose the cushions of fat beneath.

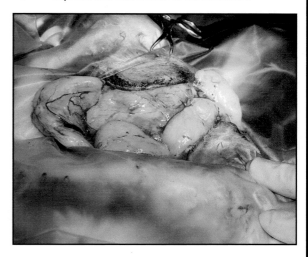

2 Ideally the fat pads are left *in situ* to avoid damage to the deeper structures of the neck, i.e. the nerves, such as the vagus, and major blood vessels, such as the jugular vein (arrowed).

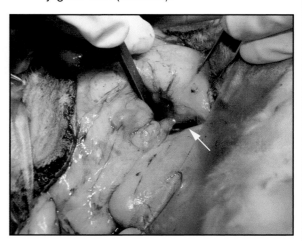

OPERATIVE TECHNIQUE 21.2 continued:
Dewlap removal
Frances Harcourt-Brown

3 The skin is closed routinely. The wound is often large. If there is no tension on the wound, skin sutures can be placed to keep the edges in apposition. If there is tension, or the rabbit has been licking or chewing the area preoperatively, subcuticular sutures are required.

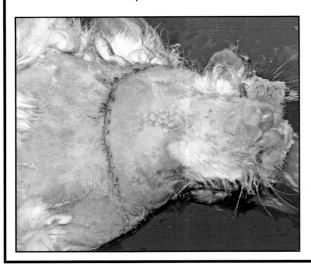

Postoperative care

Analgesia and antibiotic cover is essential (see Chapter 2). Some rabbits do not eat postoperatively and require treatment to prevent gut stasis (see Chapter 14).

22

Fracture management

Sorrel Langley-Hobbs and Nigel Harcourt-Brown

Rabbits are popular pets and many are presented to veterinary surgeons with a history of sudden lameness caused by a fracture. For many clinicians this is a daunting prospect. Some dedicated surgeons will have the expertise necessary to negotiate the 'minefield' of managing a rabbit through anaesthesia, surgery and postoperative care. Their expertise can, however, be an expensive option due to the techniques used, the need for qualified staff, expensive equipment and implants, postoperative radiographic monitoring and implant removal, etc.

At the time of writing, information on orthopaedic surgery in rabbits is sparse; there is little guidance on repair techniques and no peer-reviewed literature on outcomes of fracture repair. Hence, this chapter is based on the experience of the authors. Hopefully, more evidence-based information on rabbit orthopaedics, describing treatments and their outcome, will be published in the future, allowing us to treat these animals more confidently. At the present time, however, much of the information available is anecdotal.

Types of fracture in rabbits

Many rabbits are presented with no obvious reason for their broken bones and the owner was not present when the fracture occurred. Fractures in rabbits can be categorized into one of three categories:

- **Low-energy fractures**, e.g. caused by the rabbit being stood upon, or dropped or falling or jumping from a low height. In these cases the fracture is usually closed, has little soft tissue trauma and the vascular supply is relatively undamaged. These fractures carry a good prognosis. They often involve the long or distal bones (radius and ulna, tibia and tarsal bones) where there is usually no ancillary support and very little soft tissue between the bone and skin. These fractures may be simple or comminuted with fissures. Smaller bones (e.g. scapula, pelvis, metacarpals, metatarsals, digits) often have support from adjacent unfractured bones and/or surrounding swollen soft tissue
- **High-energy fractures**, e.g. caused by explosive movements when the leg is trapped. These injuries often involve the femur or humerus and the fractures are usually severely comminuted, with fissures in the large fragments. They are

often open with significant soft tissue damage caused by the splintered bone. These cases have a graver prognosis, with a higher risk of infection, neurological deficits and tissue necrosis.
- **Pathological fractures** – these occur in bone weakened by, for example, infection, bone neoplasia or osteoporosis.

Once the fracture type has been identified, the appropriate treatment should be selected. It is common for there to be several approaches that could be applied to the same fracture.

Formulating a treatment plan

Most practitioners are familiar with fracture repair in dogs and cats and can easily formulate a treatment plan for those species. As with dogs and cats, the cost of treatment is often an issue, especially if the outcome of a procedure is in doubt. Many fractures in rabbits require complex orthopaedic surgery to obtain a perfect repair and the costs may be prohibitive for some owners. The ease of treatment and outcome depend on:

- Whether the fracture is low-energy, high-energy or pathological
- Whether the fracture is open or closed
- Which bone is involved
- The age, demeanour, activity and general health of the rabbit
- How long the fracture has been present
- The degree of soft tissue damage
- The commitment of the owners
- The orthopaedic skills of the surgeon
- The availability of specialized equipment and implants.

There are also some rabbit-specific considerations to take into account. Rabbits' bones are brittle and prone to fissure formation, and also seem more subject to fracture at the implant site than those of dogs or cats (stress riser). Rabbits also appear to be more affected by osteomyelitis, and any infection is more challenging to treat because of the effects of oral antibiotics on the gut flora.

However, pet rabbits do have some advantages with regard to fracture repair, compared to dogs and cats. The small size and high metabolic rate of rabbits allows rapid healing, given the right environment of stability and preservation of blood supply. In adult rabbits, fractures will heal in 6–8 weeks. Rabbits can also manage with more skeletal deformity than a dog or cat. They do not have to go for walks, dodge cars or climb trees; most are house rabbits or spend much of their time in a confined space, so return to full function may be less important than for a wild animal or some other domestic species. It is important that the rabbit is free from pain, and lameness with pain is unacceptable; however, pain-free lameness caused by functional or mechanical problems may be an acceptable condition.

Treatment options

Cage rest and no stabilization
This option is simple and is inexpensive for owners. However, for cage rest to be the first line of treatment, there should be minimal displacement of bone fragments. The treatment requires:

- A suitable cage
- Comfortable soft bedding that can be easily changed (e.g. short pieces of hay)
- Analgesia
- Owners motivated to take good care of the rabbit.

This is an option for fractures of the scapula, humerus, distal humeral condyles, radius and/or ulna, comminuted femoral fractures, metacarpal, metatarsal, or digital fractures involving one to three bones out of four or five. It is not indicated for tibial fractures. The advantage of this approach is that it is inexpensive, easy, and leaves the rabbit with four legs. The end result can be surprisingly good, with minimal impairment of limb function and mobility. The disadvantages include:

- Initial pain from a mobile fracture
- Skin penetration from a bone fragment
- Malunion and permanent limb deformity
- Non-union and loss of limb function
- Arthritis if a joint was involved in the fracture.

Incomplete (simple) splint
Rabbit bone heals quickly and supporting a fracture often allows the bone to heal. An incomplete splint does not need to be above and below the joints of the affected bone. A simple small splint made from a syringe case or barrel, cut to fit and strengthened with adhesive bandage (Figure 22.1), has many advantages:

- It is comfortable for the rabbit
- It is cheap and easy to apply
- Anaesthesia is not usually required to change it.

Such a splint is suitable for closed fractures that are not displaced (mostly involving the radius and ulna). If the fur is not clipped, it acts as padding under the splint. The adhesive bandage can be applied directly to the fur to keep the splint in place.

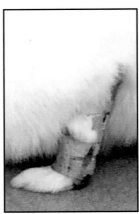

22.1 An incomplete splint made from half a 5 ml syringe case has been used to stabilize a minimally displaced fracture of the radius and ulna; the splint was applied to counteract bending forces across the fracture. The splint allows movement at the carpus and elbow and therefore minimizes fracture disease such as joint stiffness; in addition the foot is left uncovered. However, the splint does not provide stability against rotational or shear forces at the fracture site.

The disadvantages of an incomplete splint are: it does not provide adequate support for more serious fractures; and it can be removed by the rabbit. The inside of the bandage must be kept clean and dry or infection will occur. The rabbit should be checked, and the splint and dressing changed, at least every week.

Complete splint
Complete splints are made from formed casting material. Waterproof casting material should be used – fibreglass-impregnated polyurethane or thermoplastics are used in preference to plaster of Paris. The splints are padded and placed to immobilize the bone by including the proximal and distal joints (Figure 22.2) and can be full cylinder, caudal, lateral or medial gutter. The advantage of these splints is that they result in good alignment and immobilization of the fracture, so if they are applied well there is less likely to be permanent deformity of the leg. However, there are a number of disadvantages:

- They are more expensive to apply, as the rabbit requires anaesthesia

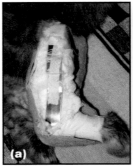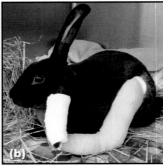

22.2 A complete splint immobilizes the joint above and below the fracture site but the anatomy of both the fore- and hindlimbs makes placement of these splints difficult in rabbits. **(a)** A piece of finger splint has been used to encircle a fractured tibia by being bent under the hock and over the stifle. This was used to immobilize a serious distal tibial fracture temporarily prior to repair with external fixation the following day. **(b)** This rabbit has a distal tibial fracture that was treated by intramedullary pinning and external skeletal fixation (see Figure 22.18). The bandage was placed around the limb to reduce swelling for 48 hours postoperatively. The ear is also bandaged to keep an intravenous cannula in the ear vein.

• They are more difficult to manage, as problems can occur related to joint movement, e.g. at the olecranon
• They are uncomfortable and may be stressful for the rabbit, with the potential to cause gut stasis and patient interference
• They may need to be adjusted or changed if they are rubbing against the skin or causing pressure sores, and this will require general anaesthesia.

External fixation

External fixation is often seen as the method of choice for fracture repair in rabbits (see Figures 22.11, 22.14 and 22.18 and Operative Technique 22.1). Its main advantage is in the outcome: if the procedure goes well, the rabbit can be left with a fully functional, anatomically realigned leg. The disadvantages are: the potential for infection; the cost of the procedure and implants; and the skill required to place the pins perfectly. Rabbits seem to be prone to haematogenous spread of bacteria, which can often settle around implants to produce osteomyelitis at a later date. The hard, brittle and fragile nature of rabbit bone also tests the ability of the implants to maintain their position in the bone. External fixation in combination with a tied-in intramedullary pin makes implant removal a relatively easy procedure; cerclage wire is more complicated to remove.

Internal fixation

Intramedullary pins (see Figures 22.11 and 22.18) are useful if there is no tendency for rotation around the fracture site. Plates are useful and are available in several sizes and lengths, used with 1.5, 2.0, 2.4 and 2.7 mm diameter screws. It can be helpful to combine the plate with an intramedullary pin; this increases the strength of the fracture repair and helps to prevent fracture through the proximal or distal screw.

Amputation

This is a controversial topic and there are two views within the profession. One view is that amputation is a safe, humane way of saving the rabbit's life without difficult (and expensive) surgery with an uncertain outcome. The other view is that amputation, especially of a hindleg, can be a disaster. If the rabbit is overweight, or has spondylosis or arthritis in other joints, it will already struggle to keep the area around its genitalia clean. Amputation will only add to its problems as it will need to place the remaining hindleg in the midline in order to move and the leg will then become contaminated with urine and caecotrophs, which will make the skin sore. A rabbit with pododermatitis is also going to be made worse by amputation, as all the weight of the hindquarters will be on one leg. Rabbits benefit from the presence of the fourth leg, even if it is slightly deformed, as it can be used to take some of the animal's weight. There is merit in the arguments both for and against amputation. As most of the bodyweight is taken by the hindlegs, the results of forelimb amputation are much better than for a hindlimb. Careful assessment of the patient is required before making the decision, which can be made at any time and should not be rushed into. Amputation usually goes well if it involves the front leg of a young, fit rabbit of normal bodyweight. If the hindleg of an old, fat, inactive rabbit is amputated, however, it will probably go badly. The veterinary surgeon must assess each patient fully rather than just respond to the fracture. If the decision is made to amputate, it is essential that the owner keeps the rabbit slim and ensures good husbandry postoperatively. Amputation procedure is discussed later in the chapter.

Assessment of the patient and fracture

Clinical examination

Severe single-leg lameness in rabbits is usually indicative of either a fracture or an infection. In most cases, diagnosis of a broken leg is not difficult, as the rabbit will not bear weight on the leg and the break is often obvious, with instability and crepitus at the site. In addition to examining the lame leg, it is important to carry out a full clinical examination and to assess the general health of the rabbit. For example: a thin rabbit with tooth problems may be on an inadequate plane of nutrition and have osteoporosis; an entire female rabbit with a uterine mass may have an adenocarcinoma with metastases in the bones.

A full assessment of the patient includes age, gender, weight, diet, housing and husbandry. Old fat rabbits are less likely to heal than young fit rabbits; however, older rabbits are often more amenable to handling, confinement, nursing, etc. Ancillary diseases are a real problem in any rabbit, but older animals usually have more problems than young ones. Other than a toe pinch, neurological examination of a rabbit can be difficult, especially if the rabbit is lame and stressed.

Lame limbs must be investigated properly but it is preferable to sedate or anaesthetize the rabbit first. Rabbits are strong and often anxious; they have large powerful muscles in the pelvic limb and if not handled carefully they can panic during the examination and cause further injury to themselves or to the owner or clinician.

> **PRACTICAL TIP**
> Examination of the site of injury is aided by wetting or clipping the hair. Use scissors rather than clippers in a conscious rabbit, as the sound of the clippers can cause the rabbit to panic.

Survey radiography

Once the initial examination is complete it is useful to obtain a whole body radiograph as well as at least two views of the fracture. This may be conducted with the rabbit conscious or sedated (see Chapter 3). If the rabbit needs to be anaesthetized immediately (e.g. to immobilize the leg) it is easier to take correctly positioned radiographs once it is unconscious (see Chapter 3).

- **Whole body radiography** allows evaluation of all the injuries but also shows concurrent problems, such as cardiothoracic or renal disease.
- **The overall bone quality should be assessed** by viewing the first three lumbar vertebrae (see Chapter 6). This will give an idea of the generalized bone density, although studies in humans have shown that a substantial amount of bone loss (35–40%) has to occur to be noticeable on a radiograph. Bone disease is common in rabbits and can be seen in otherwise apparently healthy individuals. If undiagnosed, it can cause major complications in fracture management. Increased bone density and brittle bones are features of chronic renal failure in some rabbits (Harcourt-Brown, 2007) that may show few other clinical signs. Conversely, decreased bone density (Figure 22.3) is common in rabbits that are fed on muesli mixes and kept confined to a house or hutch with no exposure to sunlight. Age is also a consideration: very young or very old rabbits may have decreased bone strength. Isaksson et al. (2010) showed that the strength of normal bone was fully developed by 6–7 months; although collagen was mature by 3 months, further mineral deposition was needed for full bone strength.

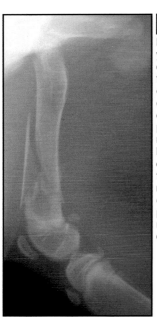

22.3 Lateral radiograph of a young rabbit with a comminuted femoral fracture. There is poor bone density associated with a diet containing insufficient calcium with high phosphorus. This caused nutritional secondary hyperparathyroidism and osteopenia, and resulted in fractures occurring after minimal trauma. There is a double cortical line in the proximal femur, which is a radiological sign of osteopenia (Lamb, 1990).

- **The fractured limb** should be examined closely and carefully on radiographs. In addition to assessing the fracture, the bones should be examined for:
  - **Fissures:** If present, these can make surgery difficult (Figure 22.4)
  - **Epiphyseal plates:** As with all mammals, immature growing rabbits have growth plates that are obvious radiographically as radiolucent lines (the physis) at the ends of the long bones; there is also a radiopaque ossification centre (the epiphysis).

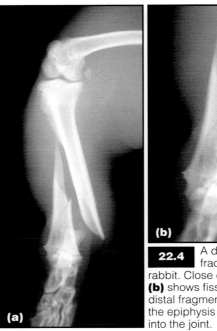

22.4 A distal tibial fracture in a rabbit. Close examination **(b)** shows fissures in the distal fragment, extending to the epiphysis and possibly into the joint.

A longitudinal study on rabbits (Masoud et al., 1986) showed that 95% of tibial and femoral bone growth had occurred by 16 weeks, although the growth plates are open radiologically and histologically until 28–30 weeks (except those of the distal tibia, which are truly closed by 16 weeks). Other bones are expected to be similar

- **Focal lesions of osteolysis or osteosclerosis:** Evidence of infection (Figure 22.5) or bone tumours (Figure 22.6) that will complicate fracture repair may be seen on radiographs. Bone tumours are seen regularly in rabbits, and any rabbit presented with a spontaneous fracture of a long bone

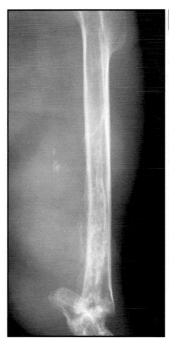

22.5 This 3-year-old male neutered Dwarf Lop had osteomyelitis and a septic arthritis originating from the os calcis. The affected area was opened on the lateral aspect, and radical debridement of necrotic tissue performed. Over the next 6 weeks the owners diligently removed all the necrotic tissue, pus and fibrin twice daily and covered the wound with Manuka honey; daily injections of penicillin/ streptomycin were given subcutaneously for a month. The rabbit recovered from the infection.

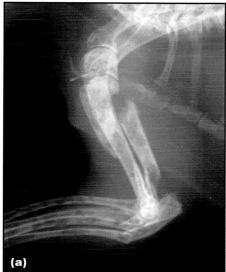

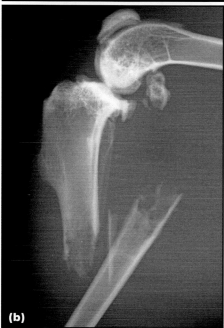

22.6 **(a)** Forelimb radiograph from a 6-year-old male Dwarf Lop that was presented moribund. There were multiple fractures throughout the skeleton. The 'punched hole' appearance' of the bones is highly suggestive of plasmacytic lymphoma. **(b)** Radiograph of the tibia of a 7-year-old neutered female Dutch rabbit that presented with sudden-onset lameness. Soft tissue swelling and the 'moth-eaten' radiographic appearance of the bone around the fracture made a tumour the most likely differential diagnosis. Cytological analysis of a fine-needle aspirate showed cells with typical signs of malignancy. The histopathological diagnosis was squamous cell carcinoma. The rabbit was euthanased.

that looks on first examination to be a simple fracture may have a bone tumour. Fractures may occur through the weakened area of the neoplasm. Because rabbit bone can be thin and often osteoporotic normally, bone tumours can be a challenge to diagnose. Radiographic diagnosis is facilitated if there is periosteal reaction but with some tumours lysis is the only feature. Most bone tumours

are considered to be primary although secondary tumours are seen. There is a tendency for uterine adenocarcinoma to spread to the bones: this is a common malignant tumour in older entire female rabbits (see Chapter 12).

Clinical assessment of the fracture site

General anaesthesia is needed for full assessment of difficult fractures, especially those involving the long bones. Once the rabbit is anaesthetized, any infected wounds can be examined, with removal of pus and other necrotic debris. Culture and sensitivity testing should be carried out if the fracture site is infected. Immobilization of the radius and ulna or the tibia is necessary as soon as possible to prevent the sharp edges of the bone penetrating the skin and making a point of entry for infection.

If neoplasia is suspected, palpation of the bone under anaesthesia allows the soft tissue swelling to be assessed; this is usually firmer than that around a traumatic fracture if a tumour is present. Cytology of a carefully targeted fine-needle aspirate usually confirms the presence of malignant cells.

Orthopaedic surgery

Equipment

The surgeon's preference predicts much of the choice and use of surgical instruments. Most orthopaedic surgery in rabbits requires appropriately sized instruments for gaining access through the soft tissue, as well as for manipulating the hard tissue. The authors' choice of instruments is listed below.

Useful instruments for rabbit orthopaedic surgery

For soft tissue manipulation and surgical access:
- Backhaus paediatric towel clamps 7.5 cm
- Bard–Parker scalpel handle No.9 and blades
- Stevens tenotomy scissors, straight pointed 10 cm
- Metzenbaum scissors, straight 15 cm
- Iris scissors, fine-pointed straight 11.5 cm
- DeBakey tissue forceps, straight 15 cm, atraumatic 1.6 mm jaws
- Gillies dissecting forceps, 15 cm, 1 into 2 teeth
- McIndoe tissue forceps, 15 cm non-toothed serrated jaws
- Halsted mosquito artery forceps, straight 11.5 cm jaws
- Halsted mosquito artery forceps, curved on flat jaws 11.5 cm
- Halsted mosquito artery forceps, curved on flat jaws, 11.5 cm, 1 into 2 teeth
- Fosters needle-holders 12.5 cm
- Ryder (micro) needle-holders 15 cm
- Allis tissue forceps, American pattern 15 cm
- Alm retractor 10 cm
- Mini Weitlaner retractor
- Mini West retractor.

For bone manipulation and removal:
- Rongeurs, e.g. mini Friedmann and bone cutters in small sizes
- Dandy arthroscopy hook
- Dental excavators, Ash Patt 125/126 and Ash Patt G2
- Dental periosteal elevators, No.9 and Clappison CA/OA
- Small pointed reduction forceps for bone – spinlock
- Crab claw forceps, small
- Small Hohmann's retractors of various widths
- Small vice (chuck) for pins up to 2.5 mm diameter
- Pin driver with an attachment for wire sizes 0.6–1.6 mm
- Junior hacksaw (with blade for cutting metal, not wood).

Implants that are useful in the repair of rabbit fractures are listed below; implants need to be small in rabbits, and care is needed when using screws and positive profile external fixation pins.

Implant sizes and types useful in rabbit orthopaedic surgery

Pins:
- Positive-profile threaded half-pins (e.g. IMEX, inter-face): 0.9, 1.2, 1.6, 2.0 mm
- Positive-profile threaded full-pins (e.g. IMEX centre-face): 2.0 mm
- Negative-profile end-threaded pins (e.g. ELLIS): 1.2, 1.6, 2.0 mm
- Kirschner or arthrodesis wires: 0.6–2.0 mm.

External skeletal fixation bar:
- Chemical metal (Henkel Home Improvements) or methylmethacrylate
- Kirschner Ehmer or IMEX mini clamps and rods.

Orthopaedic wire (cerclage malleable wire):
Sizes 0.4 mm (24 gauge), 0.6 mm (22 gauge), 0.8 mm (20 gauge).

For some surgical techniques it is helpful to use magnification. An economic way of achieving this is to use a magnifying lens surrounded by a circular fluorescent light, which can be used like an operating light. Care must be taken to avoid the exposed tissues drying out under the light, rehydrating regularly with warm sterile normal saline dripped onto the desiccating tissues. Some practices have an operating microscope, which may be useful, but they are large and expensive and in most cases give too small a field of view for rabbit orthopaedics. Optical loupes are the best compromise: they are small (presenting no storage problems), convenient to use and reasonably priced. Panoramic loupes (e.g. Keeler, Windsor UK) with 3X magnification work well but there are many other brands. Some loupes have lighting integrated into the equipment.

Surgical considerations

Anatomy
Knowledge of normal anatomy is important.

Forelimb: The anatomy of the rabbit forelimb (Figure 22.7) differs from that of the cat in that the rabbit does not have a supracondylar foramen in the distal humerus. Most of the vital structures are on the medial aspect of the limb. The brachial artery and radial nerve cross from caudal to cranial on the

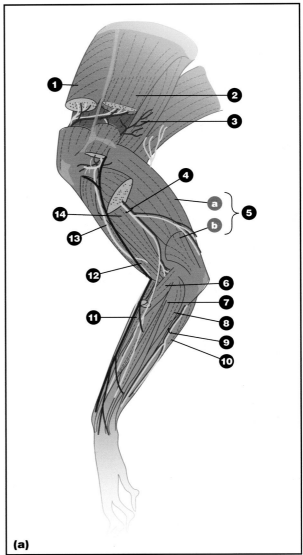

(a)

22.7 Surgical anatomy of the forelimb. The nerves, arteries and veins have more branches than shown in these diagrams; only the major branches are illustrated. Anatomy is variable between individuals; these illustrations are only a guide. **(a)** Lateral view. 1 = Supraspinatus muscle; 2 = Deltoid muscle overlying infraspinatus muscle; 3 = Teres major muscle; 4 = Radial nerve and artery; 5 = Heads of the triceps muscle (a = long; b = lateral); 6 = Adductor pollicis longus muscle; 7 = Lateral digital extensor muscle; 8 = Lateral ulnar muscle; 9 = Ulnar artery and nerve; 10 = Flexor carpi ulnaris muscle; 11 = Extensor carpi radialis muscle; 12 = Biceps muscle; 13 = Cutaneous branch of axillary nerve; 14 = Brachialis muscle. (continues) ▶

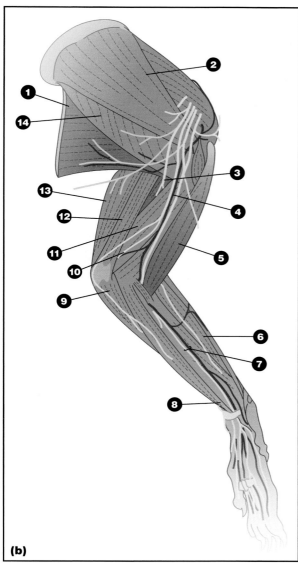

Hindlimb: The major arteries and veins are medial to the femur (Figure 22.8). In the distal third of the femur the saphenous branch goes caudomedially and runs caudal to the tibia; the femoral branch goes caudal to the stifle, crosses the tibia in its proximal third, between the tibia and fibula, and then runs cranial to the tibia. The nerves are mostly lateral. The sciatic nerve runs close to the hip, passing caudal to the joint and running about 1 cm caudal to the femur; it branches in the distal third of the femur, the fibular nerve running superficially over the gastrocnemius and then deeper but cranial to the tibia. The tibial nerve is caudal to the stifle and runs deeper and caudal to the tibia. Some nerves are contained within the retinaculum on the cranial distal tibia.

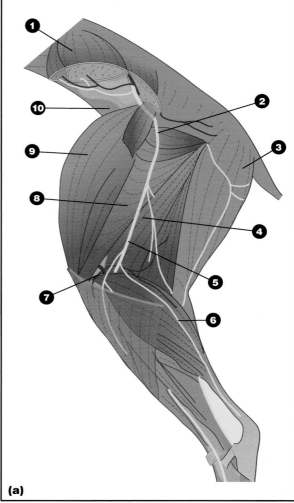

22.7 (continued) Surgical anatomy of the forelimb. The nerves, arteries and veins have more branches than shown in these diagrams; only the major branches are illustrated. Anatomy is variable between individuals; these illustrations are only a guide. **(b)** Medial view. 1 = Latissimus dorsi muscle; 2 = Subscapularis muscle; 3 = Radial nerve; 4 = Brachial artery; 5 = Biceps brachii muscle; 6 = Radial carpal extensor muscle; 7 = Median artery and nerve; 8 = Superficial digital flexor tendon; 9 = Deep digital flexor muscle; 10 = Ulnar nerve; 11 = Medial head of triceps muscle; 12 = Tensor of the antebrachial fascia; 13 = Long head of triceps muscle; 14 = Teres major muscle.

medial aspect of the distal third of the humerus. The brachial vein crosses from caudal to cranial medial to the humerus in the proximal third; the cephalic vein runs lateral but quite cranial. The humerus has two areas that are close to the skin with a minimum of tissue overlying the bone: the major tubercle and some shaft proximally, the lateral epicondyle and whole condylar region distally. The radius is palpable in the craniomedial distal third; the ulna is palpable in the lateral third. The accessory carpal bone is prominent. Branches of the median and ulnar nerves run through the carpal tunnel.

22.8 Surgical anatomy of the hindlimb. The nerves, arteries and veins have more branches than shown in these diagrams; only the major branches are illustrated. Anatomy is variable between individuals; these illustrations are only a guide. **(a)** Lateral view. 1 = Middle gluteal muscle; 2 = Sciatic nerve; 3 = Semitendinosus muscle; 4 = Semimembranosus muscle; 5 = Tibial nerve; 6 = Fibular nerve; 7 = Popliteal artery; 8 = Adductor brevis et magnus muscles; 9 = Vastus lateralis of quadriceps muscle; 10 = Rectus femoris muscle. (continues) ▶

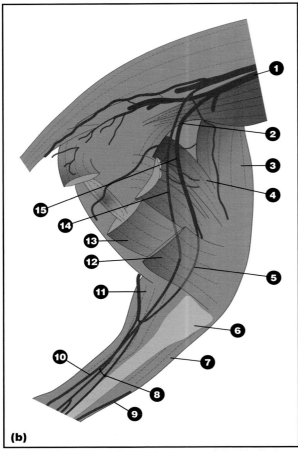

22.8 (continued) Surgical anatomy of the hindlimb. The nerves, arteries and veins have more branches than shown in these diagrams; only the major branches are illustrated. Anatomy is variable between individuals; these illustrations are only a guide. **(b)** Medial view. 1 = Caudal vena cava; 2 = External iliac vein; 3 = Tensor fascia lata muscle; 4 = Vastus medialis of quadriceps muscle; 5 = Medial saphenous vein; 6 = Tibia; 7 = Cranial tibial muscle; 8 = Caudal and cranial medial saphenous vein; 9 = Cranial tibial artery; 10 = Saphenous artery; 11 = Gastrocnemius medial head; 12 = Gracilis muscle; 13 = Semitendinosus muscle; 14 = Femoral artery; 15 = Femoral vein.

The nature of the bone

Rabbit bone is very brittle and shatters easily. Rongeurs and bone cutters should be used carefully, with small deliberate bites; large bites of tissue are much more likely to cause shattering.

The brittle nature of rabbit bone means that fissures are often present (see Figure 22.4), even in fractures that appear to be simple on radiographs. Fissures and brittleness can make internal fixation challenging, as the fissures may open up during implant application or be a cause of re-fracture if their presence is not noticed or treated. Whatever your plan, be prepared for unexpected fissures!

When drilling holes in small bones it must be borne in mind that, without care, these holes will be disproportionately large and, if drilled in normal bone such as the olecranon, calcaneus and even long bones, they can themselves cause fractures. Threads in the bone can strip easily, especially with 2.0 or 1.5 mm screws. Rabbits have a tremendous

power-to-weight ratio, which exacerbates this risk. Barron *et al.* (2010) showed that in electively fractured femurs, a bone plate and screw repair withstood 35.1 lb (47.6 N) of compressive and bending force while intramedullary pin and external skeletal fixation withstood 67.7 lb (91.8 N). A normal rabbit femur can withstand 148.4 lb (120.1 N).

Bone plates are seldom recommended as, on their own, they are a weak form of fixation even when it is possible to place them. Fissures that are undetected may lead to re-fracture during or after the surgery, or the femur may fracture due to weakening of the bone by the drilling of screw holes in brittle bone, or by the stress riser effect at the end of the bone plate (Figure 22.9).

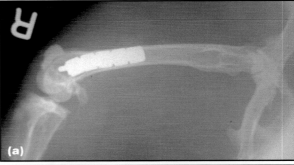

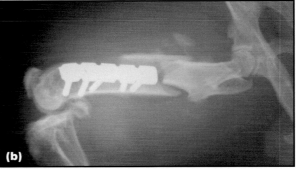

22.9 **(a)** The femur of a giant continental rabbit with a distal femoral intracondylar fracture that was plated with a 2.7 mm reconstruction plate and screws. **(b)** Postoperatively, an additional fracture occurred proximal to the plate. This fracture was possibly a result of the screw hole causing a stress riser in the brittle rabbit bone, or of an unrecognized fissure.

When placing external skeletal fixation (ESF) pin) it is often necessary to use power tools to drill into the bone but these must be used with care to prevent thermal necrosis. When using positive-profile pins, the hardness of the bones of adult rabbits makes it necessary to drill a hole with a sharp drill bit in the bone before inserting the pin. Without pre-drilling it is easy either to strip the near cortex thread or to split the bone as the pin enters the far cortex. For small diameter pins the bone hole can be made using the unthreaded end of the positive-profile external fixator pin, which has a trocar point, even though these are not designed to cut bone. It is possible to use a proper drill bit but these are brittle and the small diameter drill bits are prone to breakage. Saline can be dripped on to the pin or drill bit to prevent overheating during drilling.

The small size of some bones precludes the use of positive-profile threaded centre-face pins, so Kirschner wires must be used. If only unthreaded pins are used they must be placed at an angle to each other or the bone will slide along the pins.

It is not always essential to use power tools to drive pins into rabbit bones. However, drilling small holes by hand can be difficult and will invariably result in an eccentric hole. The use of trocar-pointed pins and a sensitive hand with a bone chuck can work well but a power tool with a suitable pin driver is best (e.g. DeSoutter MPZ motor with appropriate pin drivers).

Suture materials
Suitable suture materials include polydioxanone (e.g. PDS), poliglecaprone (e.g. Monocryl) and polyglyconate (e.g. Vicryl Rapide). Generally, small sizes such as 2 metric (3/0 USP) or 1.5 metric (4/0 USP) will be most suitable. Although rabbits tend to form adhesions in their body cavities, these do not tend to be a problem with careful orthopaedic surgery.

Infection
The development of infection during the healing period is common in rabbits with open fractures or external fixation. The skin and fascia around an external fixation pin can be very mobile, especially in the proximal femur or humerus, and in the femoral condylar region, which may prevent the skin/pin interface closing. The constant movement and resulting tissue fluid encourages infection that tracks down the pin into the bone, causing the pin to loosen.

Management of specific fractures

Jaw
Both upper and lower jaws can be fractured and may be a challenge to fix. Crushing injuries (e.g. between a predator's jaws) are the most serious and can include both fractures and soft tissue trauma. Nerve damage may also occur but may not be obvious for several days.

In general, the bone is too thin for fixation by implants, so assisted feeding, analgesia and time form the best option. An oesophagostomy tube may be necessary (see Chapter 2). An additional complication is the rapid growth of the teeth; their length and shape is normally kept in check by the grinding of the upper arcade against the lower (see Chapter 24). While in the short term there is a problem dealing with this level of force, in the long term any misalignment may result in lifelong dental problems that can be at least as bad for the rabbit as was the original fracture. The prognosis for jaw fractures is therefore guarded.

- **Maxilla:** Fractures of the incisive bone can affect the growing incisor teeth as well as the nasolacrimal duct and zygoma.
- **Mandible:** The most common fracture is in an area just caudal to the body of the mandible, across the mandibular angle (see Chapter 4).

In rabbits, the body of the mandible contains the incisor and, more caudally, the molariform teeth. There is a massive difference in thickness of bone: in 2–3 kg rabbits, the body of the mandible is 5–6 mm thick and the ramus 0.3–0.8 mm thick. This can be difficult to see radiographically as the bone is so thin. The caudal mandible is impossible to stabilize using an implant, as the ramus is so insubstantial. It is, however, covered laterally by the masseter and medially by the pterygoid muscles; because of their support, unilateral fractures often recover with careful nursing (see Chapter 2).

- **Separation of the mandibular symphysis** can be overcome by gluing the incisors together. These teeth grow at a rate of 2 mm per week, so a substantial portion of the incisors should be glued.

Vertebral fractures or dislocations
Fractured or dislocated vertebrae (Figure 22.10) are usually the result of incorrect handling or predator attack. If a rabbit is pinned down across its shoulders or by the scruff, it will often kick and suddenly extend its long hindlegs. This sudden explosive force has to be dissipated. The vertebral column is relatively inflexible, so a vertebral fracture or dislocation somewhere between the 5th lumbar vertebra and the sacrum is often the result.

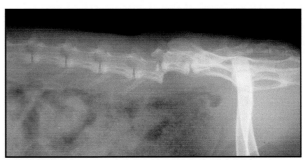

22.10 This young Minilop female rabbit had been restrained during its stay in boarding kennels. After a brief struggle it was unable to use its hindlegs. There is a fracture/luxation between the 6th and 7th lumbar vertebrae.

If the spinal cord is not transected, some of these cases have feeling and movement in their legs and may improve with cage restraint. Most, however, have major spinal cord injury. There are no accounts of a successful technique for repairing these fractures, although spinal fusion has been described in laboratory rabbits (Higashino *et al.*, 2010). The brittle nature of the bone, loss of bone density, and strength of the rabbit makes the prognosis for successful surgery poor.

Scapula
Most fractures are insignificant but occasionally the scapular body is so displaced that it has to be straightened. In rabbits, the scapula is a small fine bone, which is too small to plate. Repair of the broken scapular body can be achieved, however, with

polydioxanone sutures and reliance on the surrounding muscle mass. A hole is made at the junction of the spine and the body of the scapula, in both the proximal and distal fragments. A figure-of-eight suture is placed, with the cross-over part in the remaining fibrous tissue on the spine. Realigning the scapula and tightening the suture pulls the blade back into approximate apposition. The supraspinatus muscle (cranial) and the infraspinatus muscle (caudal) are then sutured to each other, including the fibrous tissue on the spine that is the origin of the deltoideus pars scapularis muscle. This strengthens the repair.

Surgical repair of the scapular neck would be a challenge. However, rather than performing amputation or euthanasia it would be worth resting the animal for 6 weeks. The subscapularis muscle has a tendon that occupies a groove in the neck which will give some stability to the area. Do not try to immobilize this area by bandaging.

Humerus

External fixation of the humerus is most easily performed through a lateral surgical approach, allowing open reduction of the fracture. It is unusual to encounter any vital structures.

- **Proximal fractures:** The head and greater tubercle can be fractured from the shaft. This fracture can be stabilized using one or two pins from the greater tubercle into the shaft, combined with a figure-of-eight tension band wire.
- **Shaft of the humerus:** Most fractures of the shaft of the humerus can be repaired using an intramedullary pin with proximal and distal positive-profile external fixation pins. Although tying the whole construct into a single lateral bar (Figure 22.11) gives a very firm fixation, the mobile skin around the shoulder can cause the pins to become infected. If the fracture looks stable at the time of surgery, the intramedullary pin should be buried rather than tied in. Placing the intramedullary pin retrograde is easier than doing it normograde. Avoid the temptation to place cerclage wire or other implants and do the minimum of manipulation necessary to avoid removing the last vestiges of blood supply from the fragments. A positive-profile interface pin across the condyles or distal shaft and one into the proximal diaphysis of the humerus prevent rotation and collapse of the bone.
- **Condylar fractures** can be repaired with a cortical bone screw but this is so difficult in small rabbits that serious consideration should be given to the advisability of using internal fixation. Rabbits with condylar fractures (Figure 22.12) can do well with conservative treatment through cage rest. This leaves the rabbit with a restricted elbow joint but for most pet rabbits it is adequate and better than no leg at all. In the cases that the authors have seen there seems to be no discernible sign of pain after the first few days.

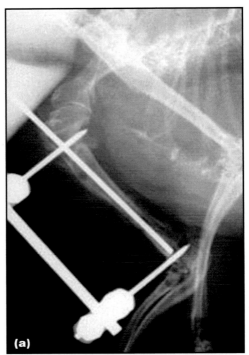

(a)

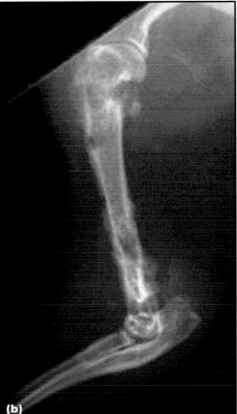

(b)

22.11 **(a)** A fracture of the distal third of the humerus was stabilized by an intramedullary pin tied into an external fixator frame, with two negative-profile threaded pins above and below the fracture. Insufficient care and cleaning allowed infection to track in along the pins, which all loosened. Because of the mobility of the tissues surrounding the shoulder, a protruding intramedullary pin must be kept clean and removed as soon as possible. **(b)** Removing all the pins plus a long course of penicillin/streptomycin gave the rabbit a functional leg.

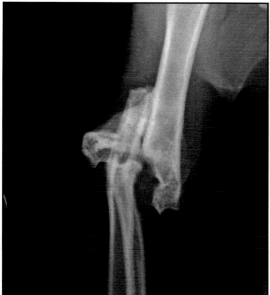

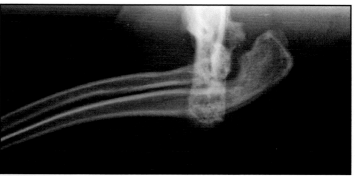

22.12 This rabbit sustained a condylar fracture at one year of age. Surgical fixation was considered too expensive by the owner so the rabbit was cage rested. After 6 weeks it had regained good mobility considered equivalent to that of a companion rabbit. Radiographs taken 6 weeks after the fracture radiographs are shown here. The rabbit's progress was monitored over the following 8 years. Although the elbow joint was palpably deformed and the leg slightly shorter than the contralateral limb, the rabbit never showed any obvious signs of pain after the first 6 weeks.

Radius and ulna

- **Olecranon:** The olecranon is a common fracture site, usually an avulsion fracture distracted by the triceps tendon. Ideally it is stabilized with an intramedullary pin (0.9–1.2 mm) and a figure-of-eight tension band wire (0.6 mm orthopaedic wire). Care must be taken to place the tension band wire through the smallest possible hole, as it is possible for the olecranon to break through a large hole after fracture repair. A pin without the tension band wire will bend. Cage rest without fixation gives an aesthetically poorer result but the leg is still functional and this is preferable to amputation.

- **Antebrachial fractures:** Antebrachial fractures are usually mid to distal diaphyseal fractures. Conservative management is generally unsatisfactory as it results in further displacement due to weight-bearing and the fracture will heal with a malunion. These fractures are amenable to splinting (Figure 22.13) if displacement is minimal. A 5 or 10 ml syringe can be cut in half longitudinally, padded and placed on the caudal surface of the antebrachium from the elbow to below the carpus. Owners need to be diligent with splint/cast care. Alternatively, it is possible to use external fixation. The radius is small but 0.9–1.2 mm smooth pins can be placed through

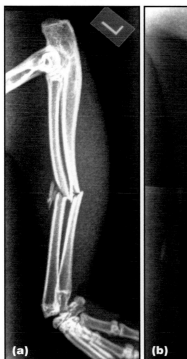
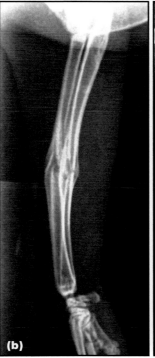
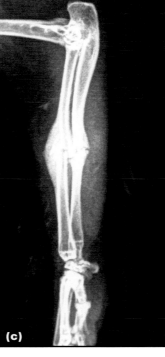

22.13 Fractured radius and ulna managed by external coaptation. The splint was created from a padded 5 ml syringe (see Figure 22.1). **(a)** The original fracture with a minimally displaced radius and ulna. **(b)** The fracture 4 weeks after splinting. **(c)** The healed fracture 8 weeks after treatment.

the bones and stabilized on both sides (Figure 22.14). It is best to provide as low profile a bar as possible on the medial aspect, as this bone sits close to the rabbit's body when at rest.

The brittle nature of the bone must be considered. High-quality radiographs should be examined carefully for the presence of fissures and these avoided when placing transosseous fixation pins. Small pins (e.g. 1.2 or 1.6 mm negative- or positive-profile threaded pins) or smooth Kirschner wires are used in dwarf and normal-sized rabbits. In giant breeds, 2.0 mm pins may be used – the pin size should not exceed 25% of the diameter of the bone in which it is placed. Pins should be placed at an angle to each other to prevent loosening (Figure 22.14). Usually a full pin above and below the fracture should be used in combination with half pins. Once the fracture is reduced, temporary external skeletal fixation clamps can be used to hold the bone in place. Alignment is checked radiographically. When this is satisfactory the clamps and bar can be replaced with an acrylic bar (e.g. made of epoxy resin from Veterinary Instrumentation or Chemical Metal from Henkel Home Improvements). This provides a light frame, is relatively radiolucent and covers the sharp ends of the protruding pins to prevent self-trauma. It also allows pins to be placed closer together than would be possible with clamps.

In small rabbits, a fracture of the distal third of the radius and ulna can be stabilized with an intramedullary pin in the radius. A 0.9 mm pin is introduced in a retrograde manner, carefully running down the cranial surface of the intramedullary cavity and exiting the radius with the carpus flexed. With care, this only involves a tiny part of the joint. The pin should be bent away from the joint before it is cut. The radius is so curved craniocaudally that the pin will only occupy the distal half of the cavity. An incomplete ('easy') splint is applied and, as soon as there is reasonable radiographic union, the pin should be removed. Larger rabbits can have this fracture stabilized using external fixation.

Metacarpi and metatarsi

Fractures involving some but not all of the metacarpals or metatarsals will heal with an incomplete splint. The remaining metacarpals/metatarsals augment the splint.

External coaptation is unlikely to result in healing if the fractures involve all the metacarpals or metatarsals. Although these bones can be extremely small in cross-section, in many cases it is possible to use intramedullary pins placed in a dowel fashion (Figure 22.15). A small pin is inserted into the intramedullary cavity of the proximal or larger fragment and cut so that a few millimetres protrude from the fracture. The distal or other part of the bone is then levered onto the protruding pin. The drawback is that the pins are extremely difficult to remove if there are postoperative complications, but this is a quick and easy technique that is frequently used in cats, where the results are very encouraging (Degasperi *et al.*, 2007; Zahn *et al.*, 2007). Burring a window into the bone so that the pins can be inserted and removed later is difficult due to the small size of these bones.

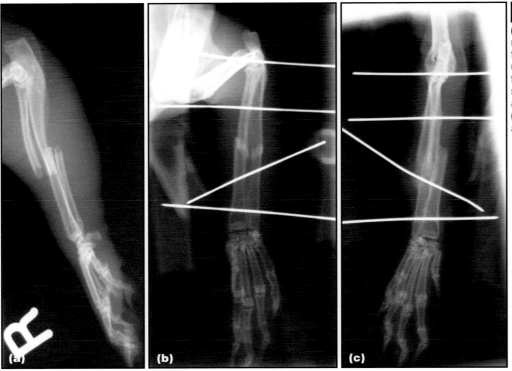

22.14

(a) Mid-diaphyseal radial and ulnar fracture. **(b)** Repair using external skeletal fixation with four smooth full pins and acrylic bars. **(c)** Fracture healing after 8 weeks.

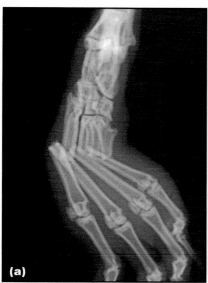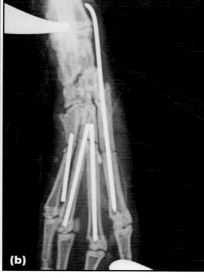

22.15 The fractured metatarsus in this rabbit was stabilized by first placing a pin in the 5th metatarsal in a retrograde manner. Metatarsals 3 and 4 were then toggle-pinned. This was attempted in metatarsal 2 but an intraoperative radiograph showed the pin to be outside the distal medullary cavity, so it was replaced. The foot was splinted in a padded gutter splint for 4 weeks. The long pin in the 5th metatarsal was removed when the bones had healed; the rest were left *in situ*.

Digits

Fractures of digits are not common. Single digits may fracture as a result of trauma, such as catching the toe in the cage mesh. A concurrent luxation may be present. Most injuries involving the digit are either trivial and will resolve with rest or are so severe that the toe requires amputation.

Pelvis

It is unusual to see this bone with a fracture without other bony injuries. It is less commonly injured than in cats, and repair is rarely performed.

Femur

Midshaft femur

Fractures of the midshaft femur seem to carry the worst prognosis of all the long bone fractures. Many occur with no history of trauma. While some of these are induced by tumours, many are probably due to osteopenia, coupled with restricted movement of the leg or vertebral column caused by age-related changes. Conservative treatment may not be the obvious choice for a femoral fracture but it can be considered. Femoral fractures often occur in older rabbits that seem content in a small cage for 4–6 weeks. Analgesia should be prescribed during the initial phases of healing. The large amount of surrounding musculature will splint the bone, limiting movement and pain from the fracture, as well as providing a good blood supply for the healing callus. Given the high metabolic rate and good healing potential in rabbits, healing may occur (Figure 22.16); a malunion may result but the limb can still be functional.

It can be useful to place a single 1.2 or 1.6 mm intramedullary pin to maintain alignment. Normograde placement is desirable but there is often sufficient displacement to make this extremely difficult. Retrograde placement of an intramedullary pin

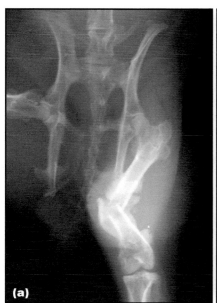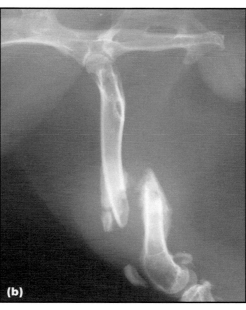

22.16 (a) Craniocaudal view and (b) mediolateral view of a femoral fracture, which was treated conservatively. There is evidence of callus formation and healing.

through a minimal incision is feasible. In severe fractures full stabilization can be attempted using an intramedullary pin tied in to external fixation positive-profile interface pins. The blunt distal end of the intramedullary pin (fashioned by removing the sharp tip of the pin) is used to make the length of the femur match that of the contralateral bone. Care must be taken not to push the blunt pin end into the stifle joint, which is possible if the rabbit is osteoporotic. Once the bone is the correct length, close the small wound, resisting the temptation to manipulate any small fracture fragments. This intramedullary pin must not fill the cavity, as an external fixation pin will need to bypass it within the cavity. The bone is stabilized by positive-profile threaded pins, one placed across the femoral condyle, and at least one in the proximal fragment, across the femur at the level of the greater trochanter where it unites with the femur.

The condylar pin is introduced through a stab incision using a No.15 scalpel blade. The proximal pin is also placed through a stab incision over the gluteal tuberosity (which is distal to the trochanter) and is directed ventromedial to miss the trochanteric fossa and exit on the medial aspect of the bone just distal to the neck of the femur (the calcar) where there is an area of relatively dense bone that is good for pin holding. For comminuted fractures in large rabbits, or where the fracture is more distal or proximal, it may be beneficial to add external skeletal fixation pins. The ideal of transfixing six cortices above and below the fracture is very difficult in the femur. The lateral profile of the femur is normally a curve; however it does not appear to affect function if this curvature is not retained after fixation. Follow-up radiographs are necessary to assess healing and staged destabilization. The intramedullary pin can also be left long and tied into the external skeletal fixator, which makes removal easy and adds to the fixation stability.

In many cases further fractures occur after fixation, especially in the proximal part of the bone. The same will happen with a bone plate, even if augmented with an intramedullary pin. The moving skin in the areas over the trochanter and the condyles can lead to infection that loosens the pins before bony union has taken place. However, enough cases heal with external fixation to make it worthwhile. Amputation can be carried out at any time if deemed necessary.

Physeal fracture

Recent capital physeal fractures can be missed on both lateral and ventrodorsal views of the pelvis. If they are suspected it is usually diagnostic to take a mediolateral view of the whole femur, including the hip joint. Fractures of the femoral diaphysis usually result in widely displaced fracture fragments due to the large muscles that both cross the bone and insert and originate on it. The high displacement forces on the bone and the inability to stabilize it sufficiently by external coaptation means that internal fixation should be considered.

One case of capital physeal fractures has been reported in the literature, affecting a giant white

rabbit (Knudsen and Langley-Hobbs, 2010). The rabbit had marked bilateral pelvic limb lameness and radiographs showed radiolucency at the capital physis bilaterally. The condition has some similarities to slipped capital femoral physis seen in both cats and humans, and in this giant rabbit it may have been related to its rapid growth rate and large size. Bilateral femoral head excision was performed but unfortunately this was not successful in that the rabbit was very reluctant to ambulate postoperatively. The present authors recommend attempting surgical repair by placing several small pins across the fracture, in a similar manner as for treating these injuries in cats (Voss *et al.*, 2009), rather than femoral head and neck excision. A case of a physeal fracture that must have healed with conservative treatment has also been encountered (Figure 22.17).

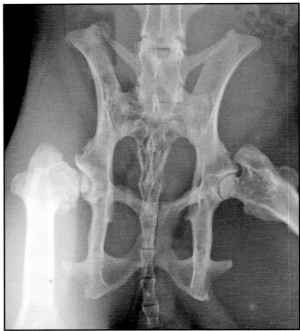

22.17 Healed fracture of the femoral neck. This radiograph of the pelvis of a young male was taken while he was anaesthetized for castration. The owner had noticed a strange gait.

Tibia

Compared with femoral fractures, most tibial fractures managed surgically have a good outcome although they can be challenging to repair. The fracture is nearly always comminuted and even cases that are not obviously comminuted on first inspection should be considered comminuted (fissured) until proven otherwise.

Proximal tibia

Simple proximal tibial fractures can be repaired with an intramedullary pin and tension band wire. The pin can be placed normograde or retrograde but in either case should be as close to the tibial crest as possible – i.e. running on the cranial surface of the medullary cavity. The distal part of the figure-of-eight wire can be placed through the medullary cavity as a hemicerclage wire so that it engages the pin and pulls it towards the cranial bone surface, which helps to prevent rotation of the distal part of fractured limb and avulsion of the proximal fragment. All this metalwork can be removed once healing is complete.

Midshaft tibia

Midshaft fractures are invariably comminuted and should be repaired by external fixation and an intramedullary pin. Rabbits sit with their legs flexed and their knees (stifles) held close to the body. It is therefore better for the rabbit if the external fixation is placed laterally, although it is easier for the surgeon to place the pins medially as the tibia is closer to the skin with no significant muscle mass. The major muscle mass is lateral and if the lateral surgical approach is taken it is important that careful blunt dissection is used to find the bony surface and avoid injuring arteries, veins and nerves.

The intramedullary pin is introduced in retrograde or normograde fashion; it is very easy to miss the distal fragment's cavity, as this may not be obvious. The triangular shape of the tibial crest has not got enough bone to hold the external fixation pin in the cranial aspect, so the pin must be placed more caudally in the proximal fragment. A surgical tip – if the proximal pin wobbles when placed, it is too far cranial. The fibular (peroneal) artery, vein and nerve run in this area and must be avoided; if the external fixator is placed laterally, blunt dissection is important. A drill guard should be used to protect the tissues as the pin is drilled in. Although the intramedullary pin can fill the distal medullary cavity, this is not possible in the proximal part of the fracture. A single threaded pin can be drilled through the distal part of the tibia, close to the condylar area. Again, blunt dissection is used to clear a path to the bone; medially there is a single tendon and laterally two tendons in close contact with the bone. In most pet rabbits, the intramedullary pin needs to be retracted proximally to allow the external fixator pin to pass through the medullary cavity. The intramedullary pin can be tied into the frame or left protruding through the tibia proximally – this is possible in rabbits, as opposed to cats and dogs, as rabbits sit with the stifle flexed and do not extend it sufficiently for the pin to cause problems. Alternatively the intramedullary pin can be cut short and left in the bone, also a successful technique.

Distal tibia

Distal tibial fractures can have many complications and may be difficult to repair. The fracture is often open and the injury may have compromised the blood supply to the skin and surrounding tissues. Serious injury can occur to the skin, nerves, tendons and blood vessels in this region, and it is important to immobilize the fracture carefully and quickly. A temporary splint may be necessary if surgery is not scheduled immediately. The fracture is generally displaced, unstable and open; cage rest is not an option because of the mobility of the fracture and the importance of the surrounding structures. External coaptation is unlikely to be successful, although it could be considered in a young rabbit with a minimally displaced, uninfected fracture (see Figure 22.2a). Given

the flexed nature of the stifle and hock of the rabbit and its hopping gait, placing a splint that will effectively immobilize the stifle and hock and not adversely affect the ability to hop around is difficult. In cases with an open comminuted fracture, amputation or surgical repair are the only options. Surgical repair is possible by placing an intramedullary pin from the proximal medullary cavity into the small distal fragment combined with a linear external fixator (Figure 22.18). In very distal fractures where it is not possible to stabilize the distal fragment, a transarticular ESF frame is placed in combination with the tibial intramedullary (IM) pin. Full ESF pins are placed through the calcaneus and the tarsal bones in a stable manner. The frame is made in either an L or triangular shape on both lateral and medial sides, so that the tarsus stabilizes the distal fragment. It is important to try to preserve the fur on the plantar aspect of the hock; it is possible to clip the fur from lateral to medial dorsally, leaving the pad on the plantar aspect. The rabbit should be kept quiet and confined postoperatively. This method of repair has been successful in three extreme distal tibial fractures and one case has been reported in the literature (Pead and Carmichael, 1989); failures have been due to infection or avascular necrosis of bone and/or soft tissues in two rabbits.

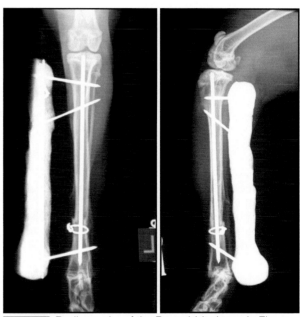

22.18 Radiographs of the Rex rabbit shown in Figure 22.2, taken 8 weeks postoperatively. The distal tibial fracture was treated by intramedullary pinning and external skeletal fixation. A small fissure fracture was present in the distal fragment and one cerclage wire was placed around this to prevent its dissipation. The fracture had healed uneventfully and the external fixator was removed at this stage.

Hock

Infected fractures

Fractures of the hock can be the endpoint of ulcerative pododermatitis (see Chapter 23) where infection has gained entry to the joint and eroded the bone

(Figure 22.19). Treatment is unlikely to be successful in these cases and euthanasia should be considered. Amputation may be tempting but the contralateral hock is very likely to be affected too and needs to be examined closely if amputation is the option the owners (and/or veterinary surgeon) wish to take.

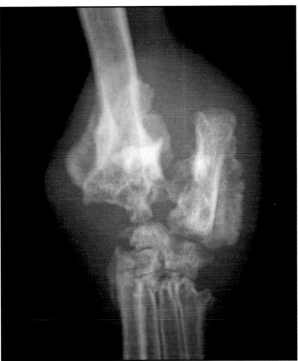

22.19 Radiograph of the fractured hock of an adult spayed female Dwarf Lop rabbit that was 10/10 lame with a hot, swollen, painful hock that was discharging pus. There was evidence of severe ulcerative pododermatitis on the contralateral hock. The rabbit was euthanased.

Calcaneus

The most usual uninfected acute fracture of the hock involves the calcaneus (Figure 22.20). This is a brittle bone and an apparently simple fracture can turn out to be severely comminuted. There is often a puncture wound from bone penetration to complicate matters. In dogs and cats the hock is upright and has to be correctly aligned or the animal is chronically lame. In rabbits, however, these fractures are extremely challenging to repair and, although most small animal surgeons would like to stabilize the fracture, this may not always be the best option or even necessary. A pet rabbit does not need to have a perfectly aligned hock and some cases have managed well with conservative treatment – bandage and cage restraint. At the end of the healing process the hock is deformed but the rabbit is pain-free and functional, although it needs to be kept permanently on soft bedding.

If surgery is performed, pin and tension band wire fixation is the best option. It is important to try to leave the plantar pad of fur. A lateral approach is used. Temporarily displacing the superficial flexor tendon from the tuber calcaneus allows an intramedullary pin to be introduced down the medullary

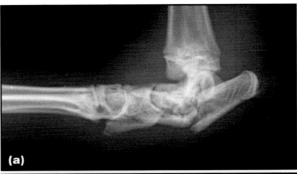

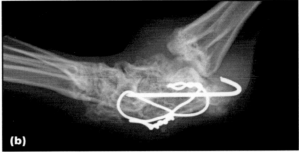

22.20 Calcaneal fracture repair in a young Flemish Giant. Whilst not obvious on the initial radiograph **(a)**, the fractured calcaneus was severely fissured and therefore difficult to stabilize. Small-gauge cerclage wire pulled through the bone and did not stabilize the fracture **(b)**. Postoperative infection led to a septic arthritis that resolved on long-term penicillin/streptomycin injections. The rabbit had a functional end result, with 1/5 lameness; this was considered satisfactory and preferable to amputation.

cavity to reduce the fracture. Orthopaedic wire must be used to counteract the huge forces on this bone. Displacing the tendon further from the plantar aspect of the bone allows the figure-of-eight wire to be placed. The most difficult part of the procedure is finding a secure anchor for the distal part of the wire, either through the calcaneus or the proximal or even distal rows of tarsal bones. Careful comparison with a lateral radiograph of the normal contralateral limb and a 25 G hypodermic needle to find the joints is useful. Once the distal part of the wire is secured, the proximal part is either looped around the pin or, in larger rabbits, placed through a drill hole in the calcaneus. Because of the risk of the calcaneus fracturing through this hole, the wire is placed around or craniodorsal to the pin. The wire is tightened and the tip of the pin bent over so that it can be removed later, even if the wire is placed through the bone. The superficial digital flexor tendon should be returned to its normal position and a small slit may need to be made for the pin to protrude through to allow for easy removal at a later date. If a compression bandage is used, great care must be taken that it does not cause skin necrosis on the cranial surface of the tibio-tarsal joint. The bandage should be inspected and probably changed daily. Even if this exacting surgery is carried out perfectly, many cases collapse around the pin and wire, leaving the rabbit with a deformed hock. When the bone has healed the pin and wire should be removed. Many rabbits manage well with this deformity provided it is not infected.

Metatarsi and digits
Fractures of these bones can be managed in a similar fashion to metacarpal and forelimb digital fractures (see earlier).

Ribs
Fractured ribs are usually an incidental finding on radiographs. They can be the result of a rabbit being crushed in a predator's mouth. Treatment is seldom necessary. The underlying injuries to the lungs and intrathoracic structures are usually more serious.

Limb amputation
Some fracture cases require amputation (see discussion earlier in the chapter). The surgery is straightforward and similar to that done in cats.

1. Dissect down to and ligate the large arteries and veins and sever the nerves with a sharp scalpel blade early on during the procedure.
2. Cut the bone (femur or humerus) with a 'Junior' hacksaw metalwork blade; these are close-toothed. Amputation saws have teeth that are too coarse for small rabbit bones. Power saws with a fine-toothed blade are a luxury but not necessary. Leave the proximal third of the bone intact. For those inexperienced with amputation in other small animals it is advisable to leave all the soft tissue, including the skin, with as great a length as possible while you dissect down to the bone. After cutting the bone it is far easier to shorten muscles etc. that are too long than to try to make do with too little muscle or skin!
3. Cover the bone stump with muscles, trying to oppose groups of muscle with antagonistic actions.
4. Reduce all the dead space with subcutaneous sutures.
5. Finally reconstruct the skin.

Postoperative complications

Osteomyelitis
Rabbits with bone infections tend to produce purulent material that is relatively caseous and does not flow easily. Infection, either postoperatively or as the initial presentation, causes a swollen painful limb. Radiography usually reveals a periosteal reaction as well as areas of bone lysis. Heat and pain are usually present; if there is doubt about the diagnosis a fine-needle aspirate can be examined. Surgical exploration is required for extensive cases. The purulent and necrotic tissue must be removed and the wound left open for treatment. It is more important to remove all the infected tissue than be concerned about the size of the wound. Manuka honey can be applied to the open wound daily.

Soft tissue injury
Immobilization of joints can allow adhesions to form; it is better to prevent them than to try to resolve the problem once it has occurred. Over-tight bandaging leading to skin and deeper tissue necrosis will cause these adhesions. Free movement of the joints

with appropriate fixation is the best method of prevention. Splints and bandages should be checked regularly. Cage hygiene should be good: wet dirty bandages lead to deep pressure sores and infection. Waterproof bandages prevent water from penetrating but will also prevent evaporation and alter the skin microflora, encouraging pathogens.

Postoperative care

Analgesia and prevention of gut stasis or wound interference are especially important for rabbits with fractures, so good postoperative care is essential (see Chapter 2). As well as opioids and NSAIDs, local anaesthesia is useful for pain relief postoperatively. Bupivacaine can be used during surgery, either infused locally at the operation site or injected around the nerves supplying the surgical wound (see Anatomy, earlier).

Antibiotic choice
Postoperative antibiotics are usually indicated following orthopaedic surgery.

- Oral enrofloxacin is authorized for use in rabbits and is good for superficial skin infection. However, when bone is infected, it seldom seems to stop the infection.
- Daily injections of penicillin/streptomycin have proved to be a useful regime. Cephalosporins or penicillin and its derivatives are most effective in the face of purulent infection, which is often a concern with rabbit fractures, especially if they are open or have implants.
- Amoxicillin/clavulanate seems to penetrate bone effectively. It can be given parenterally to rabbits without causing enterotoxaemia, although there is always a small risk of disruption of the gut flora associated with any antibiotic use in rabbits, especially penicillin (see Appendix 1).

Cages and bedding
Whichever method is chosen to manage a fracture, rabbits with broken legs will need to be restrained for some time, which means cage confinement.

- A quiet secluded environment is essential; worried rabbits tend to stamp their feet as a warning sign, which can have a serious effect on some fracture repairs, so circumstances that cause stamping should be minimized.
- A small cage is also useful to restrict movement.
- It is not a good idea to place rabbits on mesh floors while they are recovering from orthopaedic surgery (or probably at any other time) and wood-shavings and sawdust coat wounds and get inside bandages. Clean towels and soft bedding are best. A thick layer of newspaper underneath helps absorb urine, etc.
- Hay and leafy green vegetables should be provided postoperatively. The hay should be cut into approximately 10 cm lengths to prevent strands wrapping around injured legs or ESF frames.

- Cage hygiene is important and the cage should be completely cleaned out at least once daily. Unsoiled hay can be returned but everything else needs renewing.

Wound care and pin cleaning

The rabbit needs to be examined daily by nurses or owners. If there is external fixation, the pin/skin interface needs cleaning daily and the clamps and frames need cleaning too.

Cleaning small pins in a small leg can be challenging:

1. Use a 25 cm strip of white, open-weave 2.5 cm wide bandage.
2. Soak this in dilute povidone–iodine (chlorhexidine solution tends to sting) and put one end round the pin and under the bar/clamp.
3. Hold both ends and pull to and fro around the pin. It is possible to clean the pin/skin interface thoroughly using an action similar to towelling your back. Rabbits tolerate this very well.

The fixator bar and clamps should be wrapped in bandage to prevent them getting caught in cage doors.

Splint management

When external coaptation is used, the bandage or splint can get soiled by urine or faeces, even in a well cleaned cage. A waterproof or water-repellent covering can be applied to prevent bandage maceration (e.g. Vetwrap or duct tape). Casts, splints and bandages must be changed regularly to check for infection. Waterproof bandages are more susceptible to infection occurring underneath them, as the skin on the leg is not allowed to 'breathe'.

Postoperative radiography

Radiographs should be taken every 2–3 weeks postoperatively to monitor healing and to enable informed decisions to be made regarding removal of implants or external coaptation. Where external fixation has been used, the bone should be examined radiographically regularly and when healing is progressing well, the bone must be loaded by staged destabilization of implants (see Operative Technique 22.1).

References and further reading

Aron DN, Foutz TL, Keller WG *et al.* (1991) Experimental and clinical experience with an IM pin external skeletal fixator tie-in configuration. *Veterinary Comparative Orthopaedics and Traumatology* **4**, 86–94

Barone R (1986) *Anatomie Comparée des Mammifères Domestiques. Vol. I. Osteology.* Vigot Frères, Paris [in French; comprehensively illustrated]

Barone R (2000) *Anatomie Comparée des Mammifères Domestiques. Vol. 2. Arthrologie et Myologie.* Vigot Frères, Paris [in French; comprehensively illustrated]

Barone R (1996) *Anatomie Comparée des Mammifères Domestiques. Vol. 5. Angiologie.* Vigot Frères, Paris [in French; comprehensively illustrated]

Barone R (2010) *Anatomie Comparée des Mammifères Domestiques. Vol 7. Neurologie II.* Vigot Frères, Paris [in French; comprehensively illustrated]

Barone R, Pavaux C, Blin PC and Cuq P (1973) *Atlas d'Anatomie du Lapin.* Masson, Paris [in French; out of print but may be available in libraries]

Barron HW, McBride M, Martinez-Jimenez D *et al.* (2010) Comparison of two methods of long bone fracture repair in rabbits. *Journal of Exotic Pet Medicine* **19**, 183–188

Davies RR (2003) Surgical approaches to the bones of the rabbit forelimb. *Exotic DVM* **5**(3), 38–42

Degasperi B, Gradner G and Dupré G (2007) Intramedullary pinning of metacarpal and metatarsal fractures in cats using a simple distraction technique. *Veterinary Surgery* **36**, 382–388

Harcourt-Brown F (2007) Radiographic signs of renal disease in rabbits. *Veterinary Record* **160**, 787–794

Higashino K, Hamasaki T, Kim JH *et al.* (2010) Do the adjacent level intervertebral discs degenerate after a lumbar spinal fusion? An experimental study using a rabbit model. *Spine* **15**(35), 22

Isaksson H, Harjula T, Koistinen A *et al.* (2010) Collagen and mineral deposition in rabbit cortical bone during maturation and growth: effects on tissue properties. *Journal of Orthopaedic Research* **28**, 1626–1633

Knudsen CS and Langley-Hobbs SJ (2010) Spontaneous femoral capital physeal fractures in a Continental giant rabbit. *Veterinary Record* **166**, 462–464

Lamb CR (1990) The double cortical line: a sign of osteopenia. *Journal of Small Animal Practice* **31**, 189–192

Lawrie RD (2006) *Surgical Approaches to the Hindlimb of the Rabbit (Oryctolagus cuniculus).* Final Year Project, Edinburgh University

Masoud I, Shapiro F, Kent R *et al.* (1986) A longitudinal study of the growth of the New Zealand White rabbit: cumulative and biweekly incremental growth rates for body length, body weight, femoral length and tibial length. *Journal of Orthopaedic Research* **4**, 221–231

Pead MJ and Carmichael S (1989), Treatment of a severely comminuted fracture in a rabbit using a Kirschner–Ehmer apparatus. *Journal of Small Animal Practice*, **30**, 579–582

Tiraloche G, Griard C, Chouinard L *et al.* (2005) Effect of oral glucosamine on cartilage degradation in a rabbit model of osteoarthritis. *Arthritis and Rheumatism* **52**, 1118–1128

Voss K, Montavon P and Langley-Hobbs SJ (2009) *Feline Orthopedic Surgery and Musculoskeletal Disease.* Saunders Elsevier, London

Wang SX, Laverty S, Dumitru L *et al.* (2007) The effects of glucosamine hydrochloride on subchondral bone changes in an animal model of osteoarthritis. *Arthritis and Rheumatism* **56**, 1537–1548

Zahn K, Kornmeyer M and Matis U (2007) Dowel pinning for feline metacarpal and metatarsal fractures. *Veterinary Comparative Orthopaedics and Traumatology* **20**, 256–263

OPERATIVE TECHNIQUE 22.1:
External fixation of a tibial fracture

External fixation is a useful technique for some fractures, especially the commonest rabbit fracture – a fractured tibia. It is usually used in combination with an intramedullary pin. Success with this technique depends on several factors that are common to all fractures repaired with external fixation.

Considerations for external skeletal fixation

- If only external fixation is used to stabilize the fracture, the bone should have support distributed over four to six cortices (two or three pins per fragment) above and below the fracture.
- An intramedullary pin will give line and length as well as additional stability if is tied in to the frame. It also reduces the number of external skeletal fixator pins required above and below the fracture.
- Pin loosening is caused by thermal injury, poor shape of pre-drilled holes, infection and opening of fissures around the pin holes. Pin holes should be pre-drilled with a sharp drill bit to avoid thermal injury.
- Stability of the fracture site is the aim.
- The further away the clamp is from the bone, the lower the stability of the frame.
- The closer the clamp is to the bone, the more stable the fracture will be but the more difficult it is to keep the skin/pin interface clean.
- Bone heals in proportion to load. Sudden removal of all support may allow the bone to break at its weakest point. This can be avoided by a gradual increase in loading through staged disassembly of the external fixator.
- Positive-profile pins are superior to negative-profile pins – they hold better and are less inclined to break at the junction between the threaded and unthreaded pin.
- Clamps and bars have some advantages over tubing and methylmethacrylate, etc. Clamps can be removed and replaced easily. Pins can also be removed and even re-inserted. However, tubing plus acrylic has the advantage of being cheaper and lighter.

Positioning and patient preparation

The procedure is carried out with the rabbit under general anaesthesia (see Chapter 1). Position the rabbit in dorsal recumbency – on its back – with the contralateral leg held slightly caudal. Suspend the fractured leg for surgical preparation and aseptic preparation only. Clip the hair from the hip to just above the hock. Take care not to clip away hair that protects the calcaneus and tarsus, etc. Use sterile plastic drapes and a spirit-based chlorhexidine skin scrub (e.g. Vetasept, AnimalCare).

Assistance

It can be useful to have an assistant for this surgery. They can support the leg whilst holes are being drilled and prevent longitudinal rotation of the distal limb, as well as overseeing general alignment.

Equipment extras

- A suitable surgical kit, bone manipulating and holding instruments, especially small reduction forceps with a ratchet lock
- A power drill and pin driver are very useful
- Positive-profile threaded pins 0.9–2.0 mm, depending on the size of the patient
- Intramedullary pins, 1.6 or 2.0 mm
- Small pin vice
- Clamps and bars or tubing and methylmethacrylate or Chemical Metal, etc.

Surgical procedure

1 A lateral or medial approach to the tibia is made. A medial surgical approach is preferable as there is less soft tissue to dissect through.

2 The fracture is reduced and stabilized with a 1.2–2.0 mm intramedullary pin. Either place in a retrograde manner, running up the cranial aspect of the medullary cavity exiting from the cranial aspect of the tibial plateau (do not enter the joint), or make a stab incision medial to the straight patellar ligament and introduce the pin

→

OPERATIVE TECHNIQUE 22.1 continued:
External fixation of a tibial fracture

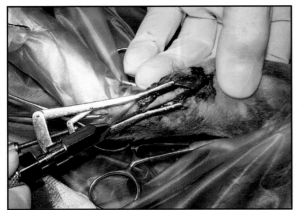

Retrograde pin insertion using a small vice and Alm retractors.

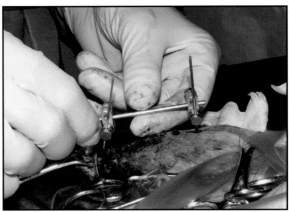

The clamps are placed and tightened, and the pins can then be cut.

normograde; this makes sure that the pin misses the joint.

3 Make stab incisions through the skin over the proximal and distal tibia.

4 Clear the tissue by blunt dissection to expose the bone. Drill a pilot hole of the same size as the shank of the pin, i.e. slightly smaller than the positive-profile threads so that they have bone to grip but will not force the bone apart.

7 Suture the surgical site but leave the holes around the pins to close by secondary intention unless they are very large, in which case they can be reduced by skin sutures. Skin sutures of polyglactin are the most suitable, but most suture materials can be used.

8 A bandage can be placed on the external fixator to prevent the frame catching in the kennel/cage bars.

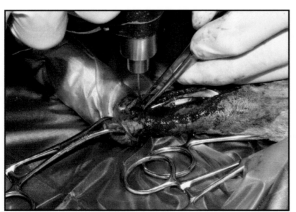

Pre-drilling with the smooth trocar-tipped end of the threaded pin; small artery forceps are used to retract the tendons and skin.

5 Place the pins one proximal and one distal.

6 Connect the clamps and bars. If further pins are to be inserted, these should be placed through clamps on the partially assembled frame to ensure correct alignment.

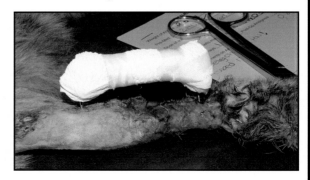

Postoperative care

Prophylactic antibiotic therapy is given until the wounds have healed and the risk of infection has gone. If infection is present, penicillin/streptomycin or amoxicillin/clavulanate by intramuscular injection is recommended, perhaps for several weeks. Enrofloxacin is not usually effective.

Daily cleaning of the pin/skin interface with dilute povidone–iodine solution is essential. All the crust around the pin must be removed.

OPERATIVE TECHNIQUE 22.1 continued:
External fixation of a tibial fracture

Fixator removal

Bone strength is dependent upon the load the bone receives. The external fixation pins share the load and remove it from the fracture site, which reduces the strength of the repair. Healing requires the pins to be removed in stages, each stage making the fracture site take more load and therefore become stronger. Premature, complete implant removal could allow the bone to re-fracture.

The bone must be regularly examined radiographically, taking orthogonal views (see below). When healing is progressing well, usually 4–5 weeks postoperatively, the first implants can be removed.

1 Carefully remove the clamps and test each pin to see if it is loose. If external fixation pins are surrounded by bone lysis on the radiograph, they are loose. It can be difficult to be certain, however, without palpation. Remove any loose pins first.

2 Ideally, remove the intramedullary pin in the first stage. This pin usually causes most problems at the skin/pin interface, as the skin is often mobile around the pin, which can lead to discharge and potential infection that can track down around the pin and cause loosening. As this pin only occupies part of the medullary cavity, it relies on engaging against the transosseous external fixation pins for the stiffness of the repair; it often contributes little without them. If the intramedullary pin is not tied into the frame but has been cut short and is buried beneath the skin, it can be left until last for removal.

3 Sometimes many of the external fixation pins are loose and most have to be removed. In these cases, leave any that are firm and tie them back in with the intramedullary pin if it has not already been removed. Once sufficient pins have been removed, the clamps and bar are reapplied to the remaining transosseous pins.

4 Three to four weeks later, repeat examination will show whether the external fixation pins can then be removed completely. Radiographic union dictates the speed and number of pin removals. Two or three sessions are usually needed. As a general rule it is good practice to remove all the implants once the bone has healed. Rabbits seem to be prone to haematogenous spread of bacteria and these can often settle round implants, producing osteomyelitis at a later date.

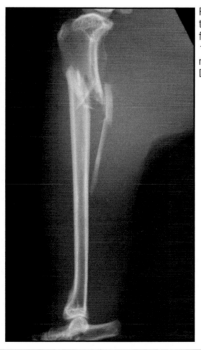

Radiograph of a traumatic fractured tibia in a 10-month-old male Netherland Dwarf rabbit.

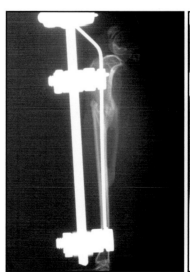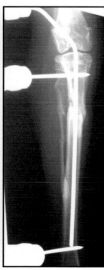

The tibial fracture was stabilized by placing two 1.2 mm IMEX interface pins tied into a 1.2 mm Kirschner wire. Mediolateral and craniocaudal radiographs taken at 5 weeks postoperatively showed healing to have progressed sufficiently to allow the intramedullary pin to be removed.

→

OPERATIVE TECHNIQUE 22.1 continued:
External fixation of a tibial fracture

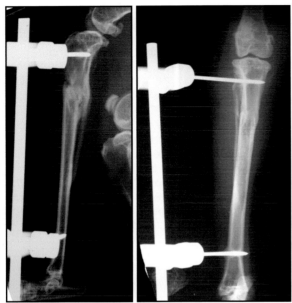

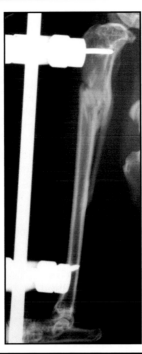

Final tibial radiograph taken at 14 weeks. The external skeletal fixator pins were removed at this time.

Mediolateral and craniocaudal views showing good evidence of tibial healing at 9 weeks; there was insufficient union to remove all external fixator pins.

23

Joint disease and surgery

Nigel Harcourt-Brown and Sorrel Langley-Hobbs

Rabbits suffer from a variety of different joint diseases. The recent increase in popularity of rabbits as pets means that the incidence and diagnosis of joint disease is also likely to increase. While some conditions can be treated successfully and appropriately with medical management, other joint problems will benefit from surgical correction. Some other periarticular conditions in rabbits, such as tendinopathies and intervertebral disc disease, are also briefly covered in this chapter.

Localization of lameness

A diagnosis of lameness is often based on the history given by an owner. Observation of the rabbit's movement is helpful, although it is difficult to 'run' a rabbit up and down on command. Placing the rabbit on the floor of the consulting room and watching it hop around while taking the history often works well. It is unusual to see single-leg lameness unless there is a fracture, septic arthritis or osteomyelitis. Palpation of the joints and legs may or may not show abnormalities. It can be difficult to assess a rabbit's joints, especially using flexion and extension tests. Examination of the fur on the hocks or front feet (Figure 23.1) can give some clues about weight-bearing and the source of lameness.

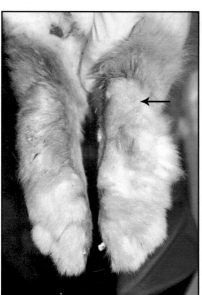

23.1

This rabbit was lame on its left leg and was not placing full weight on the foot. The contralateral leg showed hair loss over the calcaneus (arrow) and greater wear of the pad of hair covering the whole foot. This foot has the potential to develop pododermatitis.

Osteoarthritis

Osteoarthritis is rarely reported in rabbits. This may be due to lack of observed clinical signs rather than lack of occurrence, because rabbits have only recently been subjected to the level of care that is extended to dogs and cats. Large breeds of rabbit, such as English Giants and Belgian Hares, seem to be prone to osteoarthritis, especially in the stifle (Figure 23.2) and elbow joints, although it is possible for the condition to occur in any size of rabbit as a sequel to joint injury – either treated or untreated.

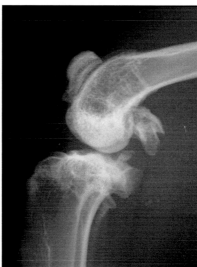

23.2

Radiograph of the stifle joint of a 3-year-old Belgian Hare with apparently stable stifle joints that had reduced flexion and extension. Osteoarthritic changes can be seen.

At the time of writing, the cause of osteoarthritis in rabbits is not known. It is more likely to occur with increasing age and is exacerbated by being overweight. All-in-one diets for rabbits tend to be very palatable and high in calories. Many owners offer them *ad libitum* and many rabbits eat them happily. There is a low-calorie all-in-one diet for rabbits, but grass and hay will be better.

Diagnosis

Diagnosis of osteoarthritis can be challenging. The condition may be found on survey radiographs or in a joint adjacent to a fracture. Affected rabbits often do not appear lame because of the bilateral nature of the disease. The owners may report that the rabbit is less agile, unwilling to play, sleeps for longer or has difficulty grooming its entire body, which leaves patches of ungroomed and occasionally parasitized fur. Abnormal urination and defecation, sludgy urine and/or a soiled perineum can indicate underlying disease. Signs of arthritis include a stiff gait or reluctance to get up and walk. Palpation alone may not be sufficient to determine whether an apparently normal joint is arthritic, although it may be possible to palpate swelling in a joint that shows radiographic changes of osteoarthritis. It may also be the case that, as in cats, not all joint changes are visible radiographically. Rabbits can show radiographic signs of osteoarthritis of the articular facets of the vertebrae, but there are also several degenerative conditions of the vertebrae that can cause the same signs as generalized osteoarthritis (see below). Radiography is the best method of diagnosis; a whole-body survey radiograph should first be obtained, followed by targeted radiography of suspicious joints.

Management
Multimodal medical management is the first-choice treatment for osteoarthritis. Gene therapy and joint replacement are unlikely. Arthrotomy or arthrodesis is theoretically possible.

Environmental adjustment
The rabbit's environment can be altered to avoid exacerbating lameness or exertion of an arthritic joint, for example by installing a ramp to aid access to the cage or sleeping quarters rather than expecting the rabbit to jump.

Exercise
Exercise can be encouraged by providing a larger area to move around in and encouraging distant foraging. Providing a shed and/or enclosed runs outside, or allowing the rabbit the freedom of some rooms in a house, will enable it to take more exercise. Providing a bonded companion can be helpful to encourage the rabbit to move around.

Diet
Ideally, overweight rabbits should be placed on a weight management regime but this requires dedicated owners who understand the importance and significance of an overweight animal. Weight reduction is not too difficult if the rabbit has good dentition and can eat hay; a diet of exclusively hay and leafy green vegetables provides sufficient nutrients and is low in calories (see Chapter 24). Rabbits with dental disease are more problematical as they cannot eat hay, and soft foods tend to be more fattening; chopped or shredded green vegetables, herbs, dried or fresh grass and low-calorie complete diets can be helpful.

Pharmacological treatment
Oral preparations are required for long-term medical management of osteoarthritis. Analgesia is discussed in more detail in Chapter 2.

- **Non-steroidal anti-inflammatory drugs**: NSAIDs are very useful. In particular, meloxicam seems to be effective and can be given orally. Although its effects are difficult to assess, owners seem to think it makes a difference to the activity of their pet; further investigations such as a movement sensor study would be needed to confirm efficacy.
- **Tramadol**: In severe cases, tramadol can be used for long-term pain management.
- **Corticosteroids**: These should be avoided as they have deleterious effects on cartilage, as well as other side effects.
- **Nutraceuticals**: Glucosamine and chondroitin have been suggested for other species but there is little evidence they have much effect (Wandel et al., 2010; Vanderweered et al., 2012), although they have not been shown to be toxic. Similar results could be expected in the rabbit. In extensive research on the use of nutraceuticals in laboratory rabbits that had been made acutely lame, there was some useful improvement in the early stages of joint inflammation (Tiraloche et al., 2005; Wang et al., 2007).

Physiotherapy
Physiotherapy is of questionable value in comparison with weight reduction and increased exercise. There are reports of hydrotherapy but rabbits are not natural swimmers and this is likely to be a stress-producing exercise rather than a help. It is not recommended.

Acupuncture
Acupuncture has been carried out on rabbits as an experimental model and, more recently, as a treatment for osteoarthritis and related conditions. Owners and the veterinary surgeons that have carried out the procedure have been happy with the results. The methods are similar to those used on other animals.

Septic arthritis
Septic, or infective, arthritis can be a sequel to a penetrating injury or haematogenous spread. *Pasteurella multocida* and *Staphylococcus* spp. are common isolates, but culture and sensitivity testing should be carried out if treatment is contemplated. Therapy involves performing an arthrotomy followed by irrigation and debridement to remove all the purulent material, which can be difficult as rabbit pus is often very thick and caseous; in some cases dilution by joint fluid makes the pus more liquid and easier to remove. Many cases have bone loss and periosteal reaction affecting adjacent bones of the affected joint; the chance of a successful outcome in these cases is poor, though treatment with long-term injections of penicillin and streptomycin or amoxicillin/clavulanate can be attempted. Limb amputation is a last resort. If only a digit is affected then it can be amputated (Figure 23.3).

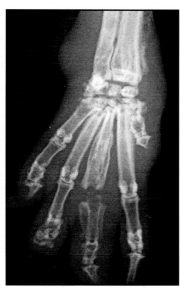

23.3
Radiograph of a rabbit with a swollen distal limb. There is periosteal new bone formation on the 3rd digit and distal radius, as well as some radiolucency in the carpus. These radiographic changes were suggestive of septic arthritis and osteomyelitis. Amputation of the 3rd digit through the proximal part of the 1st phalangeal bone, and a long course of penicillin/streptomycin resolved the problem.

Sore hocks (ulcerative pododermatitis)

Ulcerative pododermatitis is a term that describes inflammatory or degenerative lesions on the plantar aspect of the tarsal region. Rabbits have no digital pads and take a lot of their weight on their claws, especially when moving. At rest, some weight is distributed through the thick pad of hair on the plantar aspect of the foot. This is easily worn away, which happens as soon as this area takes extra pressure, e.g. due to obesity, lameness on the other leg, Achilles tendon injury, and sometimes poor cage flooring or lack of grooming of this area.

The first signs are hair loss over the region of the calcaneus. Subsequently, a pressure sore forms due to compromised blood supply to the area (Figure 23.4). The skin becomes thinner and erodes at the point of maximum pressure, exposing the soft tissue beneath, which can easily become infected. Infection

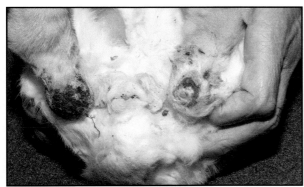

23.4 Ulcerative pododermatitis. This rabbit was presented with sore hocks; both hocks were affected, and the avascular necrosis had caused a deep ulcer in spite of treatment. The rabbit was also overweight. Radiography showed deformity of the calcaneus and the superficial flexor tendon had displaced. Although the hocks were bandaged (see right hock) with a flexible bandage, non-adherent dressing and antiseptic, there was very little padding and the condition was progressive.

causes septic arthritis, tendinitis and sometimes dislocation of the superficial digital flexor tendon from its normal path over the calcaneus, which causes the digitigrade stance to be lost (Harcourt-Brown, 2002). At this stage, excessive pressure is placed on the tarsal region (Figure 23.5), resulting in an intractable pressure sore. Careful examination under anaesthesia will allow the clinician to appreciate the lack of flexion of the digits in the affected limb.

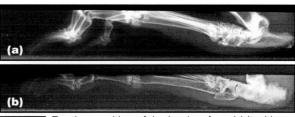

23.5 Resting position of the hocks of a rabbit with unilateral ulcerative pododermatitis.
(a) Unaffected leg. A lateromedial radiograph of the 'good' hock of the rabbit shows that the leg is positioned normally and there are only mild changes in the tibiotarsal joint. The plantar aspect of the hock adjacent to the calcaneus is very close to the ground. The digits are flexed normally, so the superficial flexor tendon is unaffected. This leg might still benefit from a padded 'shoe' (see Figure 23.6) as it is the major weight-bearing hindlimb and therefore at risk of developing pododermatitis. **(b)** A standing lateromedial radiograph of the affected hock shows that the digits are over-extended in a normal standing position. This is a sign of rupture or displacement of the superficial digital flexor tendon, the result of osteomyelitis of the calcaneus. The hock was hot, swollen and painful. Pressure caused pus to discharge from the tendon sheaths around the hock. Although antibiotics, analgesics, topical medication, weight loss, soft bedding and wound protection with a shoe may alleviate some of the clinical signs associated with these changes, the rabbit is permanently disabled by the displacement or rupture of the superficial flexor tendon. It will distribute its weight incorrectly, so that pressure is applied to the point of the hock.

Treatment of sore hocks and its outcome are dependent on the stage of the condition at presentation. Initially, a decrease in weight and better flooring may suffice. Lameness in both legs must be attended to. If a pressure sore is developing or has occurred, the treatment should be extended to removal of the crust, dressing the exposed soft tissues with a suitable antiseptic such as Manuka honey or Dermisol, parenteral antibiotic therapy to prevent tendon sheath or joint infection, and a bandage that removes the pressure from the hock.

Medical management

Ulcerative pododermatitis is essentially a pressure sore over the plantar bony prominence of the hock. It is a progressive condition that can lead to permanent disability. Medical management is an important part of treatment. The key points of medical management include the following.

- **Preserving the fur** on the plantar aspect of the tarsus: this is especially important in the early stages of the condition. The fur in this region is naturally thick and lies across the pressure point over the tarsometatarsal joint, acting as a cushion; clipping the fur away increases the pressure on the skin.

- **Increasing the activity** of the rabbit by providing it with a larger area to move around in.
- **Analgesia** (e.g. meloxicam) to reduce the pain of the condition, so the rabbit is more likely to move around.
- **Weight reduction:** this is important if the rabbit is overweight.
- **Providing soft, compliant, clean bedding:** this is very important, as sitting on carpet, vinyl, tiles or wooden floors seems to exacerbate the condition. A bed of hay in a large litter tray or stuffed into a pillowcase can be a satisfactory solution. Towels, bathmats, cushions or pieces of soft commercial bedding are less satisfactory alternatives.
- **Topical wound treatment:** if the pressure sore is not infected, the application of a non-stinging 'liquid bandage' (e.g. Cavilon spray) can protect the area of thin skin. If the pressure sore has penetrated through the skin, topical honey and/or antibiotic or antiseptic creams can help to eliminate infection and encourage a healthy bed of granulation tissue.
- **Systemic antibiotics** are indicated if the skin is broken and there is evidence of infection.
- **Fitting a protective shoe:** bandaging the foot can be counterproductive because it can increase pressure on the ulcerated area and the bandage can easily slip and/or become soiled with urine or faeces. A good alternative is to bandage a protective shoe to the foot (Vladimir Jekl, personal communication) so that the pressure point is alleviated and the weight spread again over the entire foot. Pipe insulation material is very suitable here as it is cheap and easily applied (Figure 23.6). The bandage is easy to change and leaves the wound visible for topical treatment. It is important to cut the hole in the correct place and to position the shoe correctly; it is held in place by tape. The fur is not clipped away, so the tape adheres to fur, not skin, which is likely to be more comfortable and less likely to cause patient interference. An Elizabethan collar is not necessary.

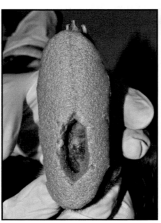

23.6 A protective shoe made from pipe insulation material can be helpful for the management of sore hocks, as it will alleviate pressure and spread the rabbit's weight over the entire foot. (Courtesy of Vladimir Jekl)

Surgery

If the tendon has displaced, treatment is unlikely to be successful unless it is re-placed and maintained in position. The superficial digital flexor tendon spreads out as it runs over the calcaneus and covers it like a cap. Repair of the lateral and medial aspect of this region will anchor the tendon in place. Do not attempt to screw the calcaneus to the tibia to take the strain off the tendon; this would be very disabling for the rabbit and the calcaneus would almost certainly fracture through the screw hole. Surgery is not usually easy to accomplish due to the chronicity of the lesion and the tendency for associated infection.

Conditions affecting the hip joint

Hip dysplasia

Hip dysplasia may occur in pet rabbits. Morphological changes include coxofemoral subluxation, shallow acetabulum, thickening of the hip joint and stifle joint capsules, lateral patellar luxation, valgus deformity, and slight bowing of the tibia (Innes *et al.,* 1957; Arendar *et al.,* 1966).

There is evidence that hip dysplasia may be linked with the surface on which young rabbits are raised. Hip dysplasia has been studied in laboratory rabbits raised on different flooring surfaces to see whether the surface influenced the development of hip dysplasia. The surfaces included waxed cardboard, Plexiglas (perspex), and Plexiglas covered by textured adhesive strips. Of 296 rabbits, 7% on cardboard and 22% on Plexiglas developed hip dysplasia but no animals on the non-slip surface developed the condition (Owiny *et al.,* 2001).

It can be difficult to decide whether a pet rabbit has hip dysplasia. Radiographic signs should be interpreted with caution, as hips that appear dysplastic on a ventrodorsal view with extended femurs can be seen in rabbits without any clinical signs of hip problems; re-evaluation using other views often shows that the hips look more normal. It is unusual to see arthritic changes.

Dislocation of the hip

Dislocation of the hip is a relatively common injury in rabbits and can be unilateral or bilateral (Figure 23.7). Unilateral dislocation usually occurs after a struggle with an owner or veterinary surgeon and causes sudden lameness. In general, rabbits resent extension of their hindlegs to compare leg length, so this test is not useful. Careful examination of the rabbit in its normal standing position will reveal displacement of the greater trochanter relative to the wing of the ilium and tuber ischium. Dislocation is easily confirmed by dorsoventral and lateral radiographs of the pelvis (see Operative Technique 23.1). The dislocated hip can displace in a craniodorsal or cranioventral direction and it may be necessary to take an oblique lateral view of the pelvis to confirm the condition. If there is no obvious fracture or other pathology the hip can be reduced in a closed fashion, although this seems to be more difficult than in dogs or cats. In some cases

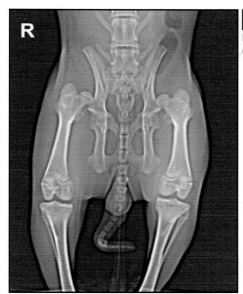

23.7
Bilateral hip dislocation.

radiography may indicate the presence of under-lying hip dysplasia but it is still worth reducing the dislocated hip, as the femoral head will often remain in the joint despite its radiographic appear-ance, and further radiography may show the hip to be relatively normal.

Manual reduction is described in Operative Technique 23.1. In the author's (NHB) experience of 10 rabbits with hip dislocation, reluxation after man-ual reduction does not occur. Two of these rabbits dislocated their other hip. Cases in which the hip will not stay in the joint after manual reduction will need surgical reduction and stabilization. Although this has yet to be described in the literature, it should be pos-sible to make a craniolateral approach to the joint that allows it to be checked for any chip fractures, etc., that have prevented it from staying in the joint. The middle gluteal muscle is very large and the hip is covered by it. A good proportion of this muscle needs to be incised to gain access to the joint and the body of the ilium; it has a substantial tendon insertion that may be cut and reattached, or the muscle belly can be incised. After re-placement of the femoral head, the joint capsule and the iliofemoral ligament should be repaired as fully as possible. A permanent suture (either monofilament polypropylene or braided such as braided terylene) should be placed through two holes drilled into the greater trochanter, and anchored to the origin of the head of the quadriceps just proximal to the joint; this mimics the iliofemoral ligament. Tying the suture reasonably tight pulls the trochanter cranially, rotating the head of the femur and holding it into the joint. Cage rest should allow the hip to stay in place. Any non-absorbable suture may cause problems, such as chronic calcifying inflammation or be a nidus for infection; a suitable warning should be given preoperatively.

'Splay leg'
Splay leg is a catch-all name for any condition that causes the rabbit to be unable to adduct the leg (Innes *et al.,* 1957; Arrendar *et al.,* 1966; Joosten *et*

al., 1981; Figure 23.8). The diagnosis has usually been made by a lay person and it is therefore important to keep an open mind about it. Lindsey and Fox (1994) surmised that splay leg remains a descriptive clinical term without clearly established pathological meanings and suggested that it is a manifestation of several disease entities. It is often bilateral, although it can be unilateral.

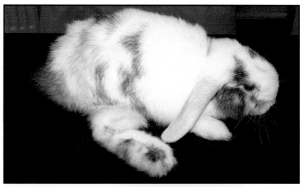

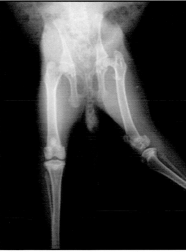

23.8
This 10-week-old female rabbit was presented by the breeder for treatment for 'splay leg'. The rabbit was lost to follow up. It is difficult to know whether the femoral deformity was a cause or effect of the condition.

The majority of these cases are brought for examination with little useful history. The rabbit is usually young and still growing. It is often unable to stand on its hindlegs, which just trail to the side or behind. There is usually a response to the patellar reflex as well as to a toe-pinch. At this stage a poor prognosis can be given.

For treatment to have any chance of success a diagnosis should be made. A lateral radiograph of the whole rabbit should first be taken. If still appro-priate, two views of the pelvis, vertebral column and each hindleg should then be obtained. The uncon-scious rabbit should be examined to ascertain joint movement and rotational limb deformity. Some rab-bits will show vertebral injury or deformity; others show hip dysplasia or other problems such as septic arthritis. A few rabbits appear to have muscle con-tracture and concomitant hip deformity. Many cases have longitudinal rotation of the femur and/or tibia. Others seem to have extreme joint laxity, often allowing severe and apparently uncontrollable rota-tion at the stifle joint. It is very difficult in many cases to know what is cause and what is effect.

Hobbling the legs together, or physiotherapy such as massage and passive flexion and extension, may be useful in some cases. Dietary correction is also indicated. If a rabbit does not have any apparent radiographic abnormalities, it is worth considering encephalitozoonosis.

It is unusual to find an easily correctable problem. In some cases these paraplegic rabbits are managed by their owners who are adamant that their pet appears to be pain-free and is 'happy' and functioning normally, i.e. it is able to eat, urinate, and defecate and has a reasonable quality of life.

Elbow luxation

Unilateral or bilateral elbow luxation is occasionally seen in practice (Figure 23.9). Caudal elbow luxation was most commonly seen in one review; the elbow functions as a 'snap joint' because of the eccentric origin of the collateral ligaments (Ertelt *et al.*, 2010). Although manual reduction is often easy, reluxation is common.

Lateral elbow luxation has been seen in two unrelated dwarf rabbits (SLH) and successfully treated by closed reduction in both rabbits. The

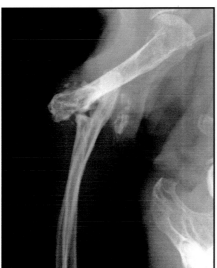
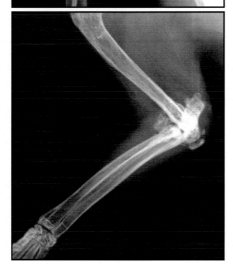

23.9 This 1.6 kg Netherland Dwarf was suddenly lame after a fall that resulted in a luxated elbow. The chronic arthritic changes made manual reduction impossible.

reduction was maintained temporarily by bandaging for several days until sufficient healing and fibrosis had occurred to prevent recurrence. For anatomical reasons, in the rabbit the elbow has to be bandaged in flexion to maintain elbow reduction, which is the opposite of the recommendation in the dog where the elbow is bandaged in extension. For many rabbits, it is difficult to maintain the leg in this position until sufficient healing has taken place to hold the joint together. Rabbits do not tolerate bandaging well and it is difficult or impossible to place a comfortable, stable bandage that does not move or slip from the elbow. When closed reduction and a Velpeau sling do not provide adequate stabilization for the treatment of elbow luxation, transosseous replacement of the humero-ulnar collateral ligaments may be indicated (Ertelt *et al.*, 2010).

Internal fixation to keep the elbow luxation reduced has been described by several authors (Mehler, 2006; Ertelt *et al.*, 2010; Zehnder and Kapatkin, 2012). Techniques described include placing a transarticular pin from the caudal olecranon through the bone into the humeral condyle to stabilize the dislocation. The elbow is also splinted and the pin is removed after 3 weeks, leaving the splint in place for a further 3 weeks to allow fibrosis to maintain the joint. The authors also describe placing a transarticular fixator for 2–4 weeks and splinting the elbow after the fixator was removed. Potential complications of these procedures are fracture of the olecranon or fracture of the pin at the interface between the ulna and humerus. Both of these complications are a challenge to correct.

An alternative method of repair is to close the torn ligaments and muscle mass around the dislocated joint. No splints or implants are required, although strict postoperative cage rest is essential. The procedure is described in Operative Technique 23.2.

Intervertebral disc disease

It is common for an apparently normal rabbit to have severe vertebral deformity and narrowed disc spaces (see Chapter 6), although neurological signs due to spinal cord compression from disc extrusion or protrusion appear to be uncommon. Narrowed intervertebral spaces, and other changes that would be highly suspicious of significant intervertebral disc protrusion, are often seen on plain lateral radiographs, but myelography often shows little compression. Magnetic resonance imaging (MRI) scans may be carried out but these rabbits are often small and many scanners are unable to give diagnostic resolution, even if the owners can afford the procedure. In contrast to the apparently normal rabbit with radiographic evidence of intervertebral disease, there are many severely paretic or ataxic rabbits with no radiographic signs of spinal cord injury or compression. *Encephalitozoon cuniculi* can complicate any diagnosis of spinal cord disease. Serological testing and/or MRI or computed tomography (CT) scanning may help in the differential diagnosis but many cases remain undiagnosed and unresolved.

Diseases of the stifle

Patellar luxation

A case of medial patellar luxation was diagnosed in a giant rabbit that was presented with a history of unilateral hindlimb lameness (Riggs and Langley-Hobbs, in press; Figure 23.10). The patella was classified as a grade II/III luxation. It was treated successfully by recession sulcoplasty and capsular overlap in a very similar fashion to treating patellar luxation in cats (Voss *et al.*, 2009). It was not necessary to perform a tibial tuberosity transposition, and it was thought prudent to avoid doing this as it was anticipated that complications might occur as a result of trying to cut this brittle dense bone and then stabilizing it, particularly given the large and powerful quadriceps muscle that would be acting to avulse it postoperatively.

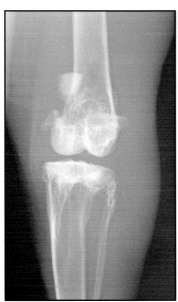

23.10
Craniocaudal view of the right stifle of a giant rabbit, showing medial dislocation of the patella and mild periarticular osteophytosis.

Cruciate ligament rupture

Rupture of the anterior cruciate ligament is regularly diagnosed in rabbits (Pizzi and Lawrie, 2006). It can occur as a unilateral problem but some rabbits have successive ruptures (van Zuijlen *et al.*, 2010). The rabbit is presented with acute-onset hindlimb lameness. Clinical examination followed by anaesthesia, palpation and radiography confirms the suspected diagnosis. The affected rabbit has a positive cranial draw sign. In cases of acute rupture there are usually no radiographic signs of injury or arthritis; it therefore appears to be a spontaneous or traumatic rupture. Partial tears are not recognized in the rabbit but it is very likely that they occur, and chronically lame rabbits, especially those with arthritic changes, should be examined with this in mind. Treatment is by extracapsular stabilization, in a very similar fashion to that in dogs and cats (see Operative Technique 23.3).

Rupture of the posterior cruciate ligament has been reported in the rabbit as an experimental procedure (Kim *et al.*, 2011). In this experiment, transection of the ligament was treated with an intra-articular injection of autogenous bone marrow.

It was interesting to note that the ligament in the knee with the injection healed more quickly but also that in both knees the ligament healed.

Dislocation of the hock

Jenkins (2006) reported dislocation of the hock as a commonly seen injury in rabbits. He suggested that closed reduction was easy to perform but difficult to keep stable, and open reduction should be accompanied by a cranial half-cast. He notes that the majority do not stabilize.

It would be worth considering immobilizing the area by applying full external skeletal fixation pins in the proximal tibia and the distal row of tarsal bones and bolting them into a triangular transarticular external skeletal frame. This has worked well for fractures (see Chapter 22). The frame can be left in place for 2–6 weeks as the limb should be immobilized in a normal standing position so the rabbit should cope well. Once the frame is removed, the animal will regain some of the normal range of movement in the joint. The proximal tibial pin should be placed in the upper 20% of the tibia at the wider part of the bone, or metaphysis, or there is a risk that the bone will fracture across the pin hole.

Carpal and digital luxation

Dislocation of the carpus (Figure 23.11) is an uncommon injury.

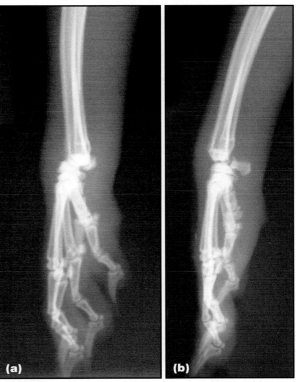

(a) (b)

23.11 This dwarf rabbit was presented lame with a sore, swollen carpus. **(a)** The radiograph shows cranial dislocation of the carpus. This was corrected and the leg splinted. **(b)** The rabbit made a good recovery within a few weeks.

Digital luxation can occur subsequent to catching toes in hay or cage netting, or wire floors (Figure 23.12). It is more likely to occur if the claws are not kept short. Closed reduction can be attempted. If luxation is recurrent or the toe is painful then amputation of the digit can be performed if necessary.

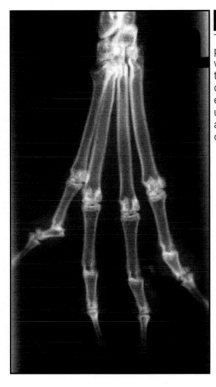

23.12

This rabbit was presented lame, with a dislocated toe. The dislocation was easily reduced under general anaesthesia and did not recur.

References and further reading

Arendar GM and RA Milch (1966) Splay-leg. A recessively inherited form of femoral neck anteversion, femoral shaft torsion and subluxation of the hip in the laboratory lop rabbit: its possible relationship to factors involved in so-called 'Congenital dislocation' of the hip. *Clinical Orthopaedics and Related Research* **44**, 221–229

Ertelt J, Maierl J, Kaiser A and Matis U (2010) Anatomical and pathophysiological features and treatment of elbow luxation in rabbits. *Tierärztliche Praxis Kleintiere* **38**, 201–210

Harcourt-Brown FM (2002) Skin diseases. In: *Textbook of Rabbit Medicine*, pp. 224–248. Butterworth-Heinemann, Oxford

Innes JRM and O'Steen WK (1957) Splayleg in rabbits. An inherited disease analogous to joint dysplasia in children and dogs. *Laboratory Investigations* **6**, 171–186

Jenkins J (2006) Conditions of the feet of rabbits and rodents. *BSAVA Congress 2006, Scientific Proceedings: Veterinary Programme* pp. 253–257

Joosten HE, Wirtz P, Verbeek HO *et al.* (1981) Splayleg: a spontaneous limb defect in rabbits. Genetics, gross anatomy and microscopy. *Teratology* **24**, 87–104

Kim E, Jeong HJ, Park SJ *et al.* (2011) The effect of intra-articular autogenous bone marrow injection on healing of an acute posterior cruciate ligament injury in rabbits. *Arthroscopy* **27**, 965–977

Lindsey JR and Fox RR (1994) Inherited diseases and variation. In: *The Biology of the Laboratory Rabbit*, ed. PJ Manning *et al.*, pp. 293–319. Academic Press, San Diego

Mehler S (2006) Common surgical procedures. In: *BSAVA Manual of Rabbit Medicine and Surgery, 2nd edn*, ed. A Meredith and P Flecknell, pp. 166–183. BSAVA Publications, Gloucester

Owiny JR, Vandewoude S, Painter JT *et al.* (2001) Hip dysplasia in rabbits: association with nest box flooring. *Comparative Medicine* **51**, 85–88

Pizzi R and Lawrie R (2006) Stifle instability and caudal cruciate ligament disease in pet rabbits. *British Veterinary Zoological Society and Rabbit Welfare Trust Conference, 11–12 November, Bristol University*, p. 41

Riggs J and Langley-Hobbs SJ (in press) Surgical correction of a patella luxation in a rabbit. *Case Reports in Veterinary Medicine*

Tiraloche G, Griard C, Chouinard L *et al.* (2005) Effect of oral glucosamine on cartilage degradation in a rabbit model of osteoarthritis. *Arthritis and Rheumatism* **52**, 1118–1128

Van Zuijlen MA, Vrolijk PWF and van der Heyden (2010) Bilateral successive cranial cruciate ligament rupture treated by extracapsular stabilization in a pet rabbit (*Oryctolagus cuniculus*). *Journal of Exotic Pet Medicine* **19**, 245–248

Vandeweerd JM, Coisnon C, Clegg P *et al.* (2012) Systematic review of efficacy of nutraceuticals to alleviate clinical signs of osteoarthritis. *Journal of Veterinary Internal Medicine* **26**, 448–456

Voss K, Montavon P and Langley-Hobbs SJ (2009) *Feline Orthopedic Surgery and Musculoskeletal Disease*. Saunders Elsevier, London

Wandel S, Jüni P, Tendal B *et al.* (2010) Effects of glucosamine, chondroitin, or placebo in patients with osteoarthritis of hip or knee: network meta-analysis. *British Medical Journal* **341**, 4675

Wang SX, Laverty S, Dumitru L *et al.* (2007) The effects of glucosamine hydrochloride on subchondral bone changes in an animal model of osteoarthritis. *Arthritis and Rheumatism* **56**, 1537–1548

Zehnder A and Kapatkin A (2012) Orthopaedics in small mammals. In: *Ferrets, Rabbits and Rodents: Clinical Medicine and Surgery, 3rd edn*, ed. KE Quesenbery and JW Carpenter, pp. 472–484. Saunders Elsevier, London

OPERATIVE TECHNIQUE 23.1:
Reduction of a dislocated hip

It is far more difficult to relocate the head of the femur of a rabbit than that of a dog or cat. However, it is worth persevering as once the hip is reduced it is unusual for it to reluxate, provided the animal is confined with careful nursing after reduction.

Dislocation of the hip is easily confirmed by dorsoventral and lateral radiographs of the pelvis. The dislocated hip may displace craniodorsally or cranioventrally. An oblique lateral view of the pelvis may be necessary to confirm the direction of dislocation, which aids reduction.

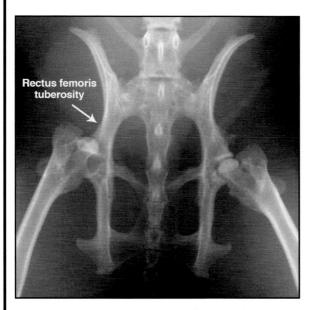

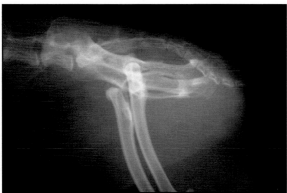

Positioning and patient preparation

Reduction of the dislocated joint is carried out with the rabbit under general anaesthesia (see Chapter 1). The rabbit is placed in lateral recumbency with the dislocated hip uppermost.

Assistance

An assistant is required.

Technique

The obstacles to reduction are the very steep cranial aspect of the acetabulum, the bony rectus femoris tuberosity and the massive gluteal muscles, all of which hamper both palpation and reduction.

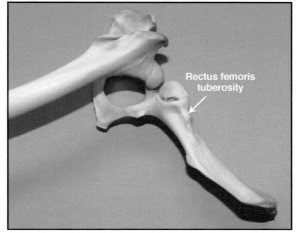
Hip bones of a rabbit, showing the natural articulation.

Because of the anatomical features of the rabbit's hip, in order to relocate it, the leg must be held with the fingers of the hand on the medial aspect of the femur so that the femur, and therefore the femoral head, can be lifted as well as rotated. This allows the head of the femur to be lifted over the cranial edge of the acetabulum; because of the large middle gluteal muscle it is difficult to feel that this is happening. A piece of 5 cm white open-wove bandage is looped around the leg and held dorsocranial to the hip joint by an assistant, to oppose the force used to relocate the hip.

Craniodorsal dislocation
Use one hand to hold the leg at the level of the mid to distal femur, to allow lifting and rotation of the femoral head. Use the other hand to guide the head by placing the thumb on and just cranial to the greater trochanter. The head of the femur must be pulled ventrocaudally as well as lifted, and then rotated so that the head is moved caudally towards the acetabulum. It is possible to position the femoral head over the acetabulum and rotate the femur so that the head is moved into the joint.

→

OPERATIVE TECHNIQUE 23.1 continued:
Reduction of a dislocated hip

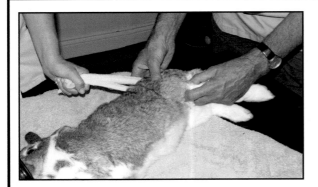

Cranioventral dislocation

Support the pelvic/hip region with one hand, and hold the stifle joint and distal limb in the other. Pull the femur distally and lift it laterally to bring the head from beneath the ilium. If this is successful, the hip usually displaces cranially. The hip is then reduced in a similar manner to that described above.

Postoperative care

After the dislocation has been reduced, an oblique view radiograph of the pelvis is taken to confirm that reduction has been successful. The oblique view is preferred because a true lateral view can sometimes be difficult to interpret due to the overlying limb.

The rabbit should be given analgesia, and care should be taken to stop it making violent or sudden movements. Hay should be cut into short

lengths so that it will not become entangled around the rabbit's legs, and the rabbit should be isolated from anything that might make it 'thump' its back legs. Food intake and faecal production must be monitored. The rabbit will require strict cage rest for at least a week.

Another pelvic radiograph should be taken after 7 days. The rabbit should be allowed to stand on the cassette and a dorsoventral view will show the hips well enough to confirm that the femoral head is still in place. The rabbit can then be sent home and kept quiet for a further week.

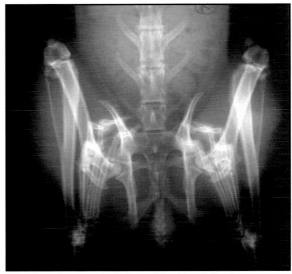

Standing dorsoventral view of the hips following reduction after a dislocation.

OPERATIVE TECHNIQUE 23.2:
Surgical repair of a dislocated elbow

Dislocation of the elbow may be the result of degenerative joint disease or, more usually, trauma. In the case illustrated here, preoperative radiographs show a dislocated elbow with no obvious fractures. The joint was easy to reduce but reduction could not be maintained. This was due to torn collateral ligaments and joint capsule. The ligaments were torn away from their origin on the epicondyle, leaving a fibrous remnant.

Anatomy

The lateral collateral ligament arises from the epicondyle and inserts on both the radius and the ulna. The joint capsule is also thick enough to be obvious.

OPERATIVE TECHNIQUE 23.2 continued:
Surgical repair of a dislocated elbow

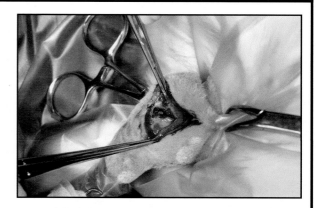

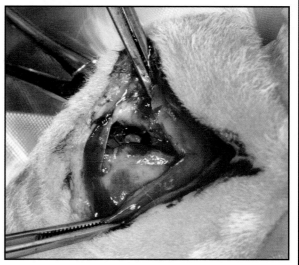

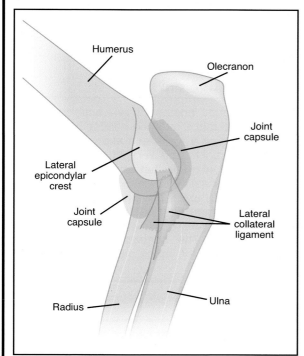

The rabbit elbow.

Positioning and patient preparation

The procedure is carried out with the rabbit under general anaesthesia (see Chapter 1). The rabbit is placed in lateral recumbency and the limb is prepared for surgery from the proximal humerus to the distal radius/ulna.

Assistance

No assistance is needed.

Equipment extras

A set of instruments suitable for small animal surgery plus some probes, etc., as listed in Chapter 22 is used.

Surgical procedure

1 A lateral incision is made over the lateral aspect of the elbow. The fascia overlying the elbow joint is incised to reveal the dislocated elbow and traumatized tissue. Once opened, the joint needs to be checked for small chip fractures that can be removed. In the illustrated case, none were present so the joint was reduced.

2 Two sutures (polydioxanone 2 metric (3/0 USP)) can be used to stabilize the joint:
   a. The first is applied as a near–interlocking loop–near–far suture; the first part goes through the tissue, remaining at the origin of the collateral ligament and then as an interlocking loop suture through the long distal part of the collateral ligament; the second part is put through the fibrous parts of the origin of the deep digital flexor muscle. This stabilizes the joint quite well.
   b. A second double suture can be placed through the origin of the muscles and then into the body of the muscles, as shown.

OPERATIVE TECHNIQUE 23.2 continued:
Surgical repair of a dislocated elbow

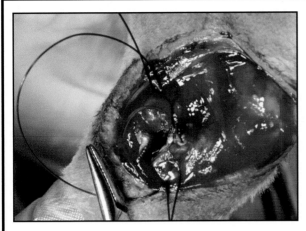

3 Polydioxanone 2 metric (3/0 USP) is used in a continuous pattern to close the subcutaneous tissue.

4 The skin is sutured in a simple interrupted pattern using polyglactin 2 metric (3/0 USP).

Postoperative care

Analgesia and postoperative antibiosis are required. The rabbit must be confined to a small cage for at least a week and exercise restricted for at least 1 month. It is very difficult to bandage the legs in a manner that provides support to the joint. In the illustrated case, both elbows were dislocated and repaired. It proved impossible to place the bandage high enough up the humeral region to give adequate support and allow the rabbit to walk. The bandages were removed the next day and the rabbit made a full recovery without them.

OPERATIVE TECHNIQUE 23.3:
Cruciate ligament repair

The aim of the procedure is to stabilize the joint with laterally placed stabilizing suture(s).

Anatomy

Two sutures were used in the repair illustrated. This picture of a stifle of a rabbit cadaver shows the relevant anatomy. The first part of the suture is placed in the origin of the lateral head of the gastrocnemius muscle (red arrow), incorporating

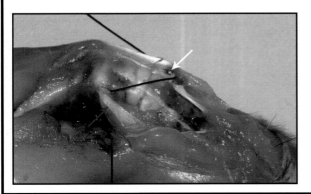

as much of the tendinous origin as possible. The next part of the suture is placed through two holes in the tibial crest (white arrow). It is tied firmly but not tightly.

Positioning and patient preparation

The procedure is carried out with the rabbit under general anaesthesia (see Chapter 1). The rabbit must be placed in lateral recumbency and the leg prepared for surgery from the hock to the hip. The leg should be suspended for aseptic skin preparation.

Assistant

Although some surgeons may feel that they require an assistant, the leg is small and the surgical site can easily become crowded. An assistant may be helpful to aid the suturing process.

→

OPERATIVE TECHNIQUE 23.3 continued:
Cruciate ligament repair

Equipment extras

- A standard surgical kit suitable for rabbits is required (see Appendix 2).
- Mayo needle-holders, or similar, to hold the first tie of the stabilizing suture, or a set of crimps and pliers are needed.
- Whilst surgical drills can be used, the technique described here uses a large triangular straight-cutting needle (No. 6, 55 mm long) in a small hand chuck/vice to drill the holes in the proximal tibia.

Suture materials

The choice of suture material for stabilizing the joint is dictated by the surgeon's preference. NHB uses braided terylene (W 969 Ethibond); SLH prefers 50 lb leader line and a crimp or large gauge monofilament nylon. The strength of the suture is less important in the rabbit than in the dog, as the origin of the gastrocnemius muscle is relatively weak. The hope is that fibrosis provides support for the suture over time.

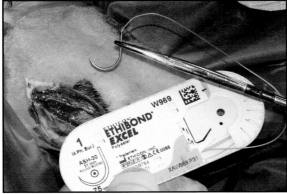

This Ethibond comes with a swaged-on J-shaped needle that is ideal for passing through the gastrocnemius insertion.

Surgical procedure

1 A lateral parapatellar skin incision is made.

2 The underlying fascia is incised in a similar direction to the skin incision and bluntly dissected back to the region of the fabella in the lateral head of the gastrocnemius muscle.

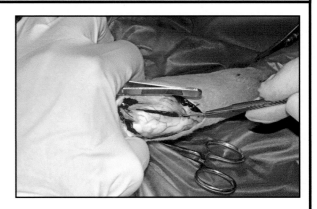

3 A suture is placed medial to the lateral fabella using curved mosquito forceps, a small wire passer, or swaged-on needle.

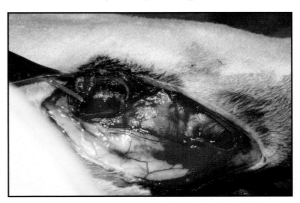

4 Two holes are drilled, one proximal and one cranial through the tibial crest.

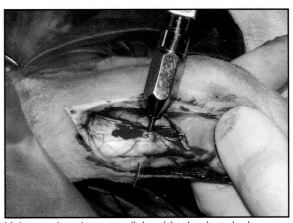

Holes made using a small Jacob's chuck and a large straight-cutting needle.

OPERATIVE TECHNIQUE 23.3 continued:
Cruciate ligament repair

5 Suture material is passed through the holes in the tibia.

PRACTICAL TIP
A hypodermic needle passed through the bone tunnels can be helpful for passing the suture material back through.

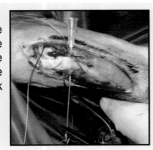

6 The suture can be knotted with two throws on the first loop followed by 1,1,2, and finally 1 loop with polydioxanone around the cut ends to prevent the knot untying. Do not tie the suture too tightly. It just needs to prevent the draw sign (negate the tibial thrust) which it can do without being so tight that it compromises extension and flexion of the stifle.

PRACTICAL TIP
When the first throw is tied it is useful if a gloved assistant can hold the first tie with some needle-holders (not artery forceps, which would damage the suture). This allows the joint to be fully flexed and extended to check that the suture is isometric before placing the next throw; it also keeps the correct tension on the suture when the next part of the tie is made.

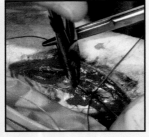

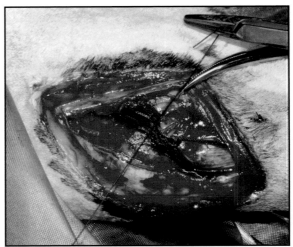

Braided terylene forms a knot that tends to come undone. Using a polydioxanone (e.g. PDS) suture to hold the ends of the tie prevents this from happening. Some surgeons choose to melt the knot partially with diathermy.

7 The fascia is closed using polydioxanone 2 metric (3/0 USP); the subcutaneous tissue is closed with polydioxanone 2 metric; and the skin is closed with simple interrupted sutures of polyglactin 2 metric. The leg is not bandaged.

Postoperative care

Tramadol and NSAIDs should be given immediately postoperatively, for 5–7 days. After 7 days no further analgesia should be required. The rabbit usually makes an uneventful recovery and should use the leg well within a few weeks. It must be kept in a small cage to limit movement for at least 4 weeks.

24

Normal rabbit dentition and pathogenesis of dental disease

Frances Harcourt-Brown

The structure of teeth

Teeth are composed of several types of tissue.

- Enamel covers part or most of the tooth, depending on the species. It is a hard crystalline, dense structure, which is almost entirely acellular, inorganic and mainly composed of calcium and phosphorus. Approximately 96% of enamel is hydroxyapatite, <1% is organic matter and the rest is water (Hillson, 2005). Enamel is formed by ameloblasts, which line the internal enamel epithelium. Amelogenesis is rhythmical, which results in microscopic cross-striations in the enamel.
- Cement or cementum may cover the enamel above and/or below the gingiva.
- Beneath the cementum and enamel, dentine forms the main structure of the tooth and encloses the pulp chamber that contains the blood and nerve supply to the tooth plus odontoblasts that form the dentine. Unlike enamel, dentine is living tissue, composed of

approximately 72% inorganic calcium phosphate molecules plus 18% organic matter, especially collagen. Tubules extend from the pulp chamber into the dentine.

Terminology

The standard description of a tooth that is used by anatomists and dentists is based on human teeth and divides the tooth into three parts: the crown, the neck and the root (Figure 24.1a). Some teeth have more than one root. The term 'crown' refers to the part of the tooth that protrudes into the mouth and, in humans, this part of the tooth is covered in enamel. The neck is the intermediate part between the crown and the root or roots. The root of the tooth is embedded in the jaw; in humans, the root is not covered in enamel so the root and crown can be distinguished by the presence or absence of enamel. The roots of human teeth and those of many other mammals are cone-shaped, so the term 'apex' aptly describes the pointed end of the root.

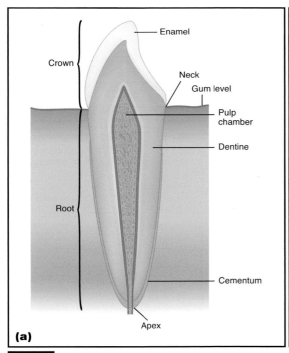

(a)

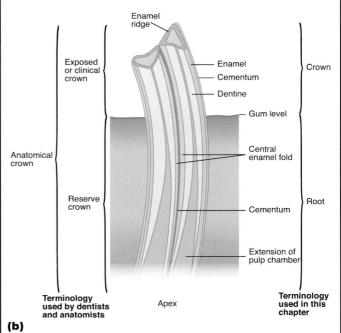

(b)

24.1 Dental terminology. **(a)** Human tooth. **(b)** Rabbit tooth

This standard description does not fit easily with some species, especially rabbits, whose teeth are very different from those of humans. Enamel is continually formed at the end of the tooth that is buried in the jaw. This buried section of tooth erupts continually from the socket and is eventually exposed in the oral cavity, to be worn away by attrition against the opposing teeth. Enamel covers both the exposed and the buried parts of the tooth, so there is no distinguishable root and crown and there is no neck (Figure 24.1b). The teeth of rabbits are also cylindrical in shape and do not have an apex. These features have led to the use of alternative terminology to describe the parts of lagomorph teeth. The terms 'exposed' or 'clinical' crown are often used for the supragingival section of the tooth, and 'reserve crown', 'submerged crown' or 'clinical root' for the subgingival section of the tooth. The term 'anatomical crown' is sometimes used to describe the whole tooth, including the part that is buried in the jaw. This terminology can be confusing. It is simpler to use 'root' to refer to *that part of the tooth that is buried in the tissues* and 'crown' to describe *the exposed part of the tooth within the mouth*. These definitions are acceptable and are given in *Saunders Comprehensive Veterinary Dictionary* (Blood *et al.*, 2007). 'Apex' can be used to refer to the extremity of the tooth that is embedded in the jaw, even though, strictly speaking, this is incorrect because this end of a rabbit's tooth is not conical.

Identification of teeth

Rabbits have two sets of teeth. A deciduous set is present in fetal rabbits and is shed just before or just after birth (Horowitz *et al.*, 1973). The permanent set of teeth erupts during the first 5 weeks of life and comprises:

$$I: \frac{2}{1} \quad C: \frac{0}{0} \quad P: \frac{3}{2} \quad M: \frac{3}{3} = 28$$

where I = incisors, C = canines, P = premolars and M = molars.

Several systems can be used to identify individual teeth in rabbits. Some authors use a Triadan system of identification in which the teeth are numbered with three digits representing the quadrant, position and whether it is a primary or secondary tooth. The use of the tTriadan system is illustrated in Chapter 25.

An alternative system is to divide the mouth into the four quadrants, i.e. right and left maxillary (upper) and right and left mandibular (lower) arcades. Individual teeth are numbered according to their type:

- As there are two maxillary (upper) incisors in the upper quadrants, these are numbered I1 and I2 for the large (1st) incisor and the small (2nd) one. In the mandible there is only a single mandibular incisor (I1).
- The cheek teeth are numbered from the rostral end and there are two methods of identification:
  - Because the cheek teeth are composed of four rows of premolars and molars that are indistinguishable from each other, some texts refer to them as 'molariform' teeth and make no distinction between the molars and premolars. In this case the cheek teeth are referred to as upper (or maxillary) cheek teeth 1–6 and lower (mandibular) cheek teeth 1–5
  - Alternatively, the numbering can differentiate between premolars and molars. The most caudal premolar is always designated P4. Thus, the maxillary teeth are numbered P2, P3, P4, M1, M2, M3 and the mandibular teeth are numbered P3, P4, M1, M2, M3.

Features of normal lagomorph dentition

Visual and radiological features of normal lagomorph dentition are summarized in Figure 24.2.

Domestic rabbits are descended from the European rabbit *Oryctolagus cuniculus*; the species

Site	Radiological and anatomical features		Significance
Incisor crowns	Curved, but upper and lower primary incisors have similar degree of curvature. Crowns have a smooth surface, with hard enamel and sharp chisel-shaped tips. Pulp cavities are large, open and tapering. Normal occlusion is with the tips of the lower incisors resting against the peg teeth		Sharp tips of the incisors allow effective biting, grooming and fighting. Open pulp cavities show tooth is growing (white arrow)
Apex of 1st upper incisor	Visible gap between apex of upper incisor and line of palatine bone. Bony nasolacrimal canal can be seen		Nasolacrimal duct is not obstructed by apex of incisor. Bone density is good enough to show bony canal (yellow arrow)
Line of palatine bone	Thick and straight (red arrow)		Strong cortical bone

24.2 Features of normal rabbit dentition. (continues) ▶

Site	Radiological and anatomical features		Significance
Apices of maxillary cheek teeth in alveolar bullae	Layer of undulating bone over apices		Maxillary cheek teeth do not extend into orbit
Occlusal line	Edges of upper cheek teeth occlude with enamel ridges of lower to form a regular zigzag line on same horizontal plane		Upper and lower teeth of equal hardness and wearing against each other. Teeth in occlusion and forming an effective system for cutting through fibre and reducing it to small particles before it is swallowed
Roots of the cheek teeth	Narrow interdental spaces with smooth edges to the teeth. Radiodense white lines of enamel at edge of teeth and in the longitudinal central enamel fold. This fold divides the pulp cavity into two tapering chambers. Apices do not penetrate ventral alveolar bone (red arrow). Clear radiodense line of alveolar bone (lamina dura) can be seen around each apex (white arrows)		Strong alveolar bone supporting teeth in mandible. The mandibular alveolar nerve and apices of cheek teeth are separated by bone so nerve is protected. This enables the rabbit to chew hard food (e.g. hay) without pain
Ventral mandibular border	Thick smooth layer of cortical bone (red arrow)		Good bone density

24.2 (continued) Features of normal rabbit dentition.

belongs to the order Lagomorpha, which also includes hares and pikas. All members of the lagomorph order are terrestrial and eat only vegetation, and their teeth are adapted for the ingestion of a fibrous diet. In lagomorphs, all the teeth erupt and grow continuously and the rate of growth is fast; incisor growth has been measured at 2–2.4 mm per week and is influenced by pregnancy, age and diet (Shadle, 1936; Ness, 1956; Lowe, 1998). The constant process of growth and dental wear demands a continual supply of calcium and other minerals and nutrients for the formation of dentine and enamel.

Each tooth socket is surrounded by the lamina dura, which is a layer of highly calcified alveolar bone that can be seen as lines of increased radiodensity on radiographs. Wild rabbits and those pet rabbits that eat grass and natural vegetation sometimes have brown staining on the supragingival crowns of the cheek teeth (Figure 24.3), which is caused by chlorophyll and porphyrin pigments from the herbage (Jubb *et al.*, 1985).

A characteristic of lagomorphs is the presence of a second set of small incisors, or 'peg teeth', situated just behind the large upper 1st incisors (Figure 24.3). The upper 1st incisors have a single deep groove on the labial aspect that runs longitudinally along the length of the tooth and locks the tooth into the socket by fitting into a corresponding ridge in the alveolar bone. These teeth also have a thick layer of enamel on the labial aspect but little on the lingual side. The lower incisors have enamel on both the labial and lingual aspects, and this distribution of

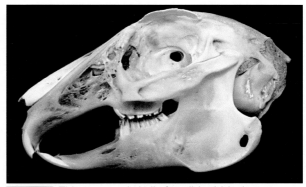

24.3 This prepared skull of a wild rabbit shows normal dentition and occlusal relationship between the upper and lower arcades.

enamel permits the formation of sharp cutting edges at the tips of the teeth (Hirschfield *et al.*, 1973). The incisors are primarily used for biting through vegetation, although they are also used for gnawing, fighting, grooming and gripping objects to move them.

The cheek teeth are used to cut food into small pieces before it is swallowed. The maxillary arcade is wider than the mandibular arcade (Figure 24.4) and the mandibular cheek teeth are arranged in a straight line. The maxillary cheek teeth are similarly arranged, except that the intermediate premolars and molars are wider than the 1st premolar and the last molar, giving the buccal side of the alignment a slightly convex shape (Figure 24.5). The circumference of each cheek tooth exhibits a deep longitudinal groove, which fits into a corresponding groove in

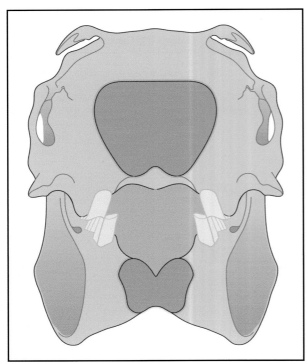

24.4 Resting occlusal position of cheek teeth. The maxilla is wider than the mandible, so the lower arcade of cheek teeth rest with their buccal edges just occluding with the lingual edges of the upper arcade.

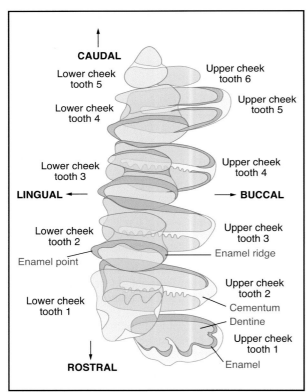

24.5 Relationship of upper and lower occlusal surfaces of the cheek teeth. This drawing shows the occlusal surfaces of the upper cheek teeth superimposed on those of the lower cheek teeth (shaded). The dark grey lines show the lines of enamel that are present on the occlusal surfaces. The enamel edges of the teeth occlude against the central enamel ridges on the opposing teeth.

the alveolar wall to lock the teeth firmly in place. There is a longitudinal fold of enamel that runs down the centre of each tooth and survives as a sharp enamel ridge at the occlusal end of the tooth (see Figure 24.1b and 24.2), which is important for slicing through fibrous food.

Occlusal relationship

At rest, the cutting edges of the lower incisor teeth are situated just caudal to the upper first incisors. They are in contact with, or just separated from, the small pair of 2nd incisors (see Figure 24.3).

The resting occlusal relationship of the cheek teeth is with the enamel ridge across the centre of the occlusal surface of each tooth, interlocking with the opposing interdental space (Figure 24.5). This results in a rostrocaudal succession of transverse ridges and valleys with the upper ridges reciprocal with lower valleys and *vice versa*, which gives a characteristic zigzag pattern on lateral skull radiographs (see Figure 24.2).

Dental wear

Rabbits' teeth are kept in shape by the continual processes of growth, attrition and abrasion.

Dental attrition is the physiological wearing away of the teeth as a result of tooth-to-tooth contact during mastication. This contact is evident from the smooth facets on the occlusal surfaces of the teeth. Contact with food also contributes to the process of attrition in rabbits because their natural diet is abrasive owing to the presence of lignin, cellulose and silicate phytoliths in grass and other plants. Rabbits can strip the bark from trees and chew through tree roots, in addition to grazing and browsing, and this fibrous diet blunts the teeth, so deliberate planing movements are necessary to bring the upper and lower teeth in contact and move them against each other to maintain the shape and sharpen the edges of the teeth.

The shape of the tips of the incisors is maintained by protruding the mandible so the lingual edge of the lower incisor is sharpened by contact with the tip of the upper first incisor (Figure 24.6). The shape of the cheek teeth is maintained by a short series of silent chewing movements when there is no food in the mouth. Rabbits exhibit these movements when they are at rest and this type of tooth grinding (bruxism) is

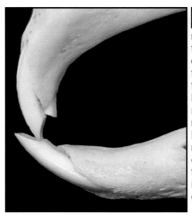

24.6 Periodic planing movements maintain the shape of the occlusal surfaces of the teeth. To maintain the sharp tip of the lower incisor, the rabbit protrudes the mandible to bring the labial surface of the mandibular incisor in contact with the tip of the first maxillary incisor as the mouth closes.

very different from the audible tooth grinding that occurs when rabbits are suffering from a painful abdominal condition such as mucoid enteropathy. There is even evidence of dental wear from bruxism on the non-functional deciduous teeth of neonatal rabbits (Wiggs and Lobprise, 1995).

The rate of growth of the teeth is not only determined by the rate of eruption and the rate at which dental tissue is worn away during attrition; it is also influenced by occlusal force. Taking teeth out of occlusion hastens the rate of eruption (Ness, 1956), which is evident in cases of congenital incisor malocclusion when the upper and lower teeth do not meet at all and grow very quickly.

Innervation of the teeth

The nerve supply to the teeth is from the mandibular and maxillary branches of the trigeminal nerve (Figure 24.7). The innervation of the cheek teeth of rabbits is from a mixed population of myelinated and unmyelinated nerve fibres that enter the tooth through the apical foramen and extend into the odontoblastic layer before terminating in tubules in the dentine. The nerve fibres at the occlusal surface of the tooth are protected by atubular dentine. There is an increasing proportion of unmyelinated fibres towards the occlusal end of the tooth, which are believed to be nociceptive (Bishop, 1995).

Mastication

There have been several studies of mastication in rabbits. Some authors have used cinematoradiography (Ardran and Kemp, 1958; Weijs and Dantuma, 1981) to monitor jaw movement. Others have used electromagnetic sensors placed at various sites on the head (Schwartz *et al.*, 1989; Yamada and Yamamura, 1996). During mastication of grass, it has been shown there may be 300–380 chewing cycles per minute (Ardran and Kemp, 1958). During each type of masticatory cycle, there are three types of jaw movement, as described below.

Type I: Biting

This is a preparatory phase when food is cut into pieces of manageable size between the incisors before transporting them, using the tongue, to the cheek teeth for reduction to smaller particles. The action of the incisors of rabbits during biting was analysed by Ardran and Kemp (1958), who trained rabbits to feed in the presence of photographic or radiographic apparatus. Their studies showed that, during grazing, if the grass was less than 2 inches (<5 cm) long, the stems were taken into the mouth and cut between the incisors. During this biting action, the lower jaw moves forward so that the incisors meet edge to edge. If tough stems are eaten, they may be detached by gripping the stem between the incisors and pulling. If long stems are eaten, the rabbit will cut off a length approximately 5 cm long by cutting it between the incisors. The stem is then turned so that one end projects from the mouth while the other end is ground between the cheek teeth. After stems have been sectioned between the tips of the incisors, the lower incisors slide along the caudal surface of the upper first incisor as the mouth closes. This sliding movement can also be used to take bites out of solid food such as a carrot or to gnaw hard material such as bark.

Type II: Chewing

Because the mandibular arcade is narrower than the maxillary arcade, chewing food between the cheek teeth can only take place on one side of the mouth. Lateral excursion is wide, and the jaw follows a unidirectional crescent-shaped movement throughout the chewing cycle. During the chewing cycle, the sharp enamel ridges and edges of the teeth effectively act as a series of sharp blades to cut the food into small pieces before it is swallowed (Figure 24.8). The tips of the lower incisors are swept transversely across the upper 2nd incisors (peg teeth) during the lateral jaw movements that take place, which helps to maintain their shape (Ardran and Kemp, 1958).

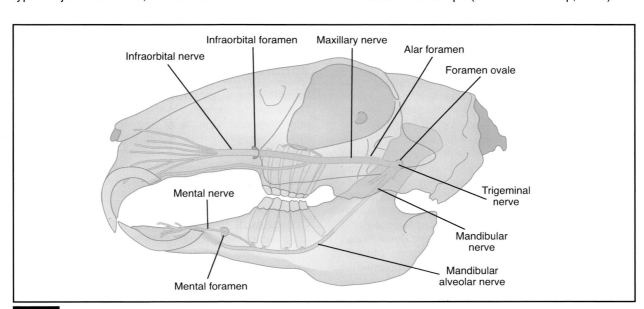

24.7 Innervation of the teeth by branches of the trigeminal nerve.

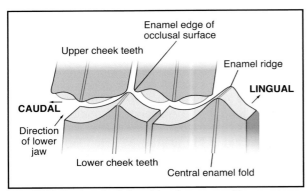

24.8 Occlusal relationship of upper and lower cheek teeth during chewing. The sharp enamel ridges that run across the centre of each cheek tooth occlude with the sharp enamel edges of the opposing teeth and effectively act as a series of sharp blades to cut the food into small pieces before it is swallowed. Reducing fibrous food to small particles aids digestion because more food enters the caecum to be degraded by the caecal microflora.

Type III

This is the pre-swallowing sequence of jaw movements.

Effect of food texture on chewing

Rabbits have evolved to eat a variety of vegetation. They are able to survive in a number of habitats on a range of foods that change with the season. Wild rabbits will select from a variety of plants in the environment. They will eat fallen fruit and cultivated vegetables. Monocotyledonous species, mainly grasses, form the major part of the diet of wild rabbits during the summer but they will eat mosses and dicotyledonous species in the spring and summer (Bhadresa, 1977).

The anatomy of the mandible and the site of the temporomandibular joint make the lower jaw an effective lever, so considerable force is applied between the upper and lower cheek teeth during chewing, which enables the teeth to cut through tough vegetation as well as to slice softer food. Laboratory studies have shown that the jaw movement and force that is applied by the teeth vary with the type of food that is eaten. Sensory input to the feedback mechanism comes from receptors in the periodontal ligament and muscle spindles in the muscles of mastication. Although the basic chewing rhythm is not affected by food texture (Yamada and Yamamura, 1996), the force that is applied by the teeth increases in proportion to the hardness of the food. Weijs and Dantuma (1981) compared the jaw movements of rabbits eating hay, pellets and carrots and identified two types of power stroke that varied with diet. The first type is a shearing stroke in which the mandibular cheek teeth are moved lingually and rostrally with minimal vertical and maximal transverse jaw excursion. This shearing action prevails during mastication of hay. It occurs sometimes in pellet mastication but never when rabbits are eating carrots. The second type is a crushing stroke that involves a lingually directed movement of the cheek teeth without the rostromedial shearing action. This

is always seen in carrot mastication, sometimes in pellet mastication but never when eating hay. Both these actions are normal and give rabbits the ability to eat and utilize a wide range of foods.

Relationship of the nasolacrimal duct to the 1st upper incisor

The anatomy of the nasolacrimal duct is described in Chapters 17 and 28. In the maxilla, the duct is enclosed in a bony canal that runs in a caudoventral direction through the maxilla to the apex of the 1st upper incisor (Figure 24.9). At this point the duct follows an S-bend, passing medially under the apex of the tooth and alongside the nasal septum, before its exit into the nostril through a tiny punctum, into the alar fold.

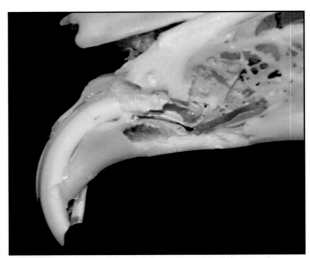

24.9 Relationship of the nasolacrimal duct to the apex of the 1st (large) upper incisor. The bone over the apex of the 1st maxillary incisor and part of the lateral wall of the bony canal that encloses the nasolacrimal duct have been removed from this prepared skull of a wild rabbit. The nasolacrimal duct has survived preparation as a strand of brown tissue that can be seen bending medially beneath the apex of the incisor. (Reproduced from *In Practice*, with permission)

Uncommon causes of dental abnormalities

Missing or supernumerary teeth

There can be variation in the number of teeth in the normal dental formula of any species and rabbits are no exception (Hillson, 2005). Missing or supernumerary teeth are not uncommon and may be more obvious on radiographs or prepared skulls (Figure 24.10) than on oral examination. They are rarely clinically significant.

Congenital prognathic abnormalities

Prognathism is a cause of malocclusion that affects only the incisors (Figure 24.11). It is evident from an early age and many breeders cull affected rabbits before they are old enough to be sold. There is evidence that some prognathic skull traits and resultant malocclusion have a genetic predisposition. Malocclusion can occur in any breed but appears to be

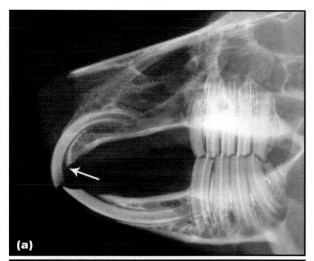

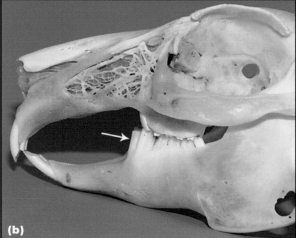

24.10 Rabbits with congenitally absent teeth or supernumerary teeth are occasionally encountered. **(a)** This skull radiograph shows the absence of the upper 2nd incisor (peg tooth) (arrow); this was a bilateral abnormality. **(b)** This skull shows a supernumerary mandibular premolar situated rostral to P1 (arrow). This was also a bilateral abnormality.

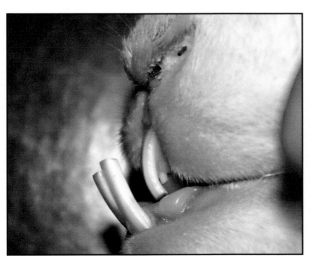

24.11 Congenital prognathism is a hereditary defect that only affects the incisors. It is evident from an early age and is usually due to a shortened maxilla, rather than an elongated mandible. The rabbit shown was a 6-month-old Netherland Dwarf.

more common in Netherland Dwarf rabbits, which are bred for their characteristic short-nosed head shape. There are varying degrees of malocclusion. In mild cases, the incisor teeth occlude edge to edge but remain short because they wear against each other. Once the rabbit is fully grown, this occlusal pattern does not change unless the rabbit develops other forms of dental disease. In rabbits with a large disparity between the lengths of the upper and lower jaws, the incisors never occlude and can become very long because they are not worn down by the opposing teeth.

Tooth fracture

Fractured crowns, especially of the incisors, are often the result of a fall or other trauma. The position of the tooth can alter and cause a malocclusion. Sometimes the broken fragment remains in place as the tooth regrows (Figure 24.12).

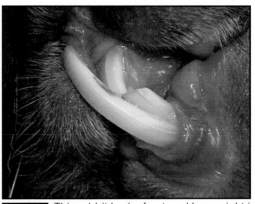

24.12 This rabbit had a fractured lower right incisor, which was broken below the gingival margin. The broken crown remained *in situ* and displaced the regrowing tooth, which was removed along with the broken fragment.

Jaw fracture

Jaw fractures seldom heal in perfect alignment, and they result in acquired malocclusion that alters the shape and direction of the teeth (Figure 24.13).

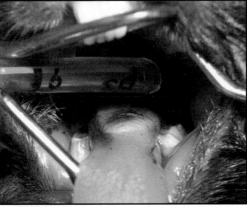

24.13 This 12-week-old rabbit had a mandibular symphyseal separation, which had allowed the left hemimandible to rotate inwardly and cause a malocclusion of the cheek teeth. The 1st lower premolar developed a spur that lacerated the tongue.

Neoplasia

Soft tissue tumours, odontomas and osteosarcomas can alter the position and occlusion of the teeth (Figure 24.14).

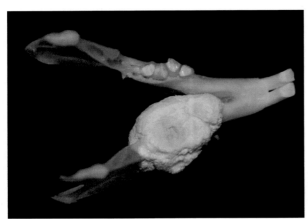

24.14 A prepared mandible from a rabbit that was euthanased because it was unable to eat. There was a rapidly growing large solid mass enclosing the teeth, presumed to be an osteosarcoma. Radiology of the chest showed metastases in the lungs.

Abscesses

Jaw abscesses are common in rabbits (see Chapter 29). Most are the result of dental disease but once infection has developed in the jaw, the resulting bone deformity can result in malocclusion.

Bone cysts

Large multicystic structures, containing serosanguineous fluid, can develop in the jaw and displace the teeth (Figure 24.15). Histologically, reactive inflammation may be present but the cause of these cysts remains unclear (Gardner *et al.*, 1997).

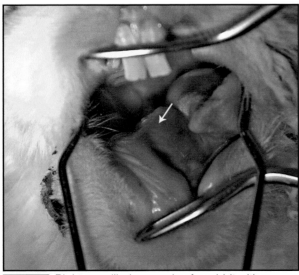

24.15 Right mandibular arcade of a rabbit with a large, rapidly growing polycystic mass in the mandible, which was enveloping the cheek teeth and displacing them (arrow). The rabbit was euthanased.

Progressive syndrome of acquired dental disease

The vast majority of dental disease seen in pet rabbits is due to progressive syndrome of acquired dental disease (PSADD). This syndrome affects the shape, position and structure of the teeth (Harcourt-Brown, 2006, 2007, 2009). The bone becomes osteopenic and the shape, structure and position of the teeth change. In the final stages of this syndrome, the teeth are either severely deformed and ankylosed into the bone (Figures 24.16 and 24.17) or disintegrating, with the roots resorbing into the bone. This syndrome can be staged. The features of each stage are summarized in Figures 24.18 to 24.21.

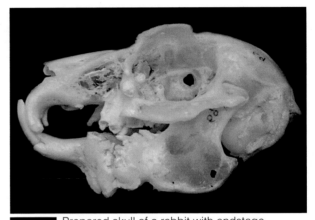

24.16 Prepared skull of a rabbit with endstage dental disease and dystrophic calcification with ankylosis. The skull shows many typical characteristics of endstage dental disease. The incisors are deformed and maloccluded. The apices of the upper 1st incisors have penetrated the palatine bone. The crowns of the cheek teeth are missing, eroded, deformed or maloccluded. The apices have penetrated the bone and are so ankylosed that it is difficult to distinguish between bone and dental tissue. The palatine bone, the calvarium and the mandible are transparent and osteopenic in comparison with the skull of the wild rabbit shown in Figure 24.3.

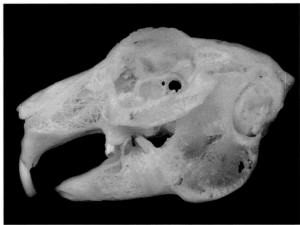

24.17 Prepared skull with endstage dental disease and osteopenia. The bone is thin and translucent and the few remaining teeth are distorted and deformed.

Site	Radiological and anatomical features		Significance
Incisors	Horizontal ridges in enamel signifying enamel hypoplasia. As acquired dental disease progresses, upper incisors become more curved. Occlusion of incisors may alter so that the tips of the lower incisors rest against upper 1st incisors rather than peg teeth. Pulp cavity can be reduced in size (white arrow). Apex of the 1st upper incisor can elongate and touch the palatine bone (red arrow)		Enamel hypoplasia is a sign of derangement in calcium metabolism as in other species. Elongation of the apex of the first upper incisor can block the nasolacrimal duct and cause epiphora
Line of palatine bone	Not as thick as in normal rabbits. Thinner at site of apex of 1st upper incisor (red arrow)		Loss of cortical bone is a sign of metabolic bone disease in other species
Apices of maxillary cheek teeth in alveolar bullae	Apices elongate to fill alveolus. Some may penetrate the bone of the alveolar bullae		No clinical signs may be seen in association with this change
Occlusal line	The occlusal line becomes uneven owing to alterations in the hardness of the teeth		Uneven cheek teeth may be seen during oral examination
Roots of cheek teeth	During PSADD, apical elongation occurs before changes to crowns. Loss of supporting alveolar bone at apex of tooth removes protective bony canal from mandibular alveolar nerve and exposes it to impinging dental tissue (white arrows). As dental disease progresses, apices penetrate cortical bone along ventral border of mandible (red arrow). Some teeth become more curved. Line of enamel at edge of tooth is lost and line of central enamel fold becomes thinner, disappears or becomes distorted. Interdental spaces start to widen. Apices of some teeth may penetrate ventral mandibular bone. Some teeth become distorted and deformed		Reluctance to eat hard food, notably hay, is often the first sign that owners notice. Exposure of the nerve to pressure when chewing hard food would make it hurt so the rabbit selects softer food. No obvious clinical signs associated with early changes to shape and structure of teeth. Food may become impacted in interdental spaces and observed during oral examination. Periapical abscesses can occur
Ventral mandibular border	Bone becomes thinner (red arrow). Swellings are present over elongated apices		Palpable swellings may be found during clinical examination

24.18 Signs of early dental disease. Apical elongation is the only sign that is present in all cases. Other signs may be seen in some sites in some rabbits.

Site	Radiological and anatomical features		Significance
Incisor crowns	Upper incisors become increasingly curved and lower incisors become less so. Change in shape and relative position of teeth results in malocclusion		In early stages, the function of incisors is impaired by blunt tips. Rabbit may have problems pulling dead hair from coat or biting through solid foods such as whole carrots or apples. In later stages, maloccluded teeth no longer meet and can grow quickly. Elongated crowns may be seen by owners. Soft tissue damage to the lips may result from long crowns
Apex of first upper incisor	In contact with or penetrating palatine bone (arrow)		
Line of palatine bone	Thinner than in normal rabbits especially at site of apex of first upper incisor		Evidence of generalized bone loss

24.19 Features of intermediate PSADD. Malocclusion is caused by alteration in the shape of the crowns. It may not be obvious on radiographs because they are two-dimensional images of three-dimensional objects. (continues) ▶

Site	Radiological and anatomical features			Significance
Maxillary cheek teeth	Shape of crowns alters and teeth become more curved			Curved teeth can develop spurs that dig into buccal mucosa inside cheek
Occlusal line	Uneven. Long crowns opposed by short ones			Impossible to say that all clinical crowns are long
Mandibular cheek teeth	Shape of crowns alters and teeth become more curved. Periodontal space widens. Apices of curved teeth penetrate bone (arrow). Teeth may rotate within the sockets			Curvature of teeth can result in spurs that lacerate tongue. In later stages, rotation of the 4th lower cheek tooth can cause spurs that dig into cheek. Infection can gain access to periodontal space

24.19 (continued) Features of intermediate PSADD. Malocclusion is caused by alteration in the shape of the crowns. It may not be obvious on radiographs because they are two-dimensional images of three-dimensional objects.

Site	Radiological and anatomical features			Significance
Incisors	The pulp cavities close. The shape of the crowns alters. Malocclusion is common. There is no enamel on the teeth. Loss of dentine occurs both supra- and subgingivally. Crowns may break off altogether			The teeth are no longer growing. Owners may be unaware of the severe abnormalities of the teeth. Maloccluded or absent crowns can make grooming or biting through hard food difficult
Apex of 1st upper incisors	Elongated apex has often penetrated palatine bone (arrow)			Complete occlusion of nasolacrimal duct can result in severe dacryocystitis. In some cases the nasolacrimal duct ruptures so tears can drain directly into the nasal cavity, and epiphora or dacryocystitis spontaneously improve or resolve
Line of palatine bone	Thin and often uneven			Evidence of osteopenia
Cheek teeth	Teeth can become deformed, curved and rotated. Some pulp cavities close and teeth stop growing. Elongated apices can calcify and become ankylosed in the socket. There is loss of enamel both in central enamel fold and peripherally. Roots may start to resorb and crowns can break off			The rabbit no longer develops sharp spurs that dig into soft tissue. General condition may improve. Can only eat soft food as teeth are not good enough to bite through hay. Crowns may break, usually just below gingival margin where they are no longer supported by alveolar bone. Loss of appetite and oral discomfort can occur when crowns break. Exposed crown can easily be removed and gum will heal

24.20 Signs of late dental disease. Not all of the teeth may be in the same stage of PSADD. Some normal teeth or teeth showing early changes can be interspersed with teeth showing late changes.

Site	Radiological and anatomical features	Significance
	Teeth in varying stages of disintegration. Many crowns missing, leaving smooth gums or remnants of teeth. Radiologically, teeth may be radiodense and ankylosed into bone or roots may be resorbing	Function of teeth is lost. Rabbit cannot eat hay or high fibre diet

24.21 Signs of endstage dental disease. Endstage dental disease does not mean the end of the rabbit's life. As in other species, rabbits can survive with absent or non-functional teeth (see Chapter 30).

Early changes

The first change to take place in PSADD is root (apical) elongation, which affects some or all the teeth. The elongated apices penetrate the bone at typical sites (Figure 24.22). Elongated roots of the cheek teeth may be palpated along the ventral border of the mandible. At this stage, owners are usually unaware of any dental abnormalities, although they may have noticed that their rabbit will not eat hay or other hard foods. This is due to elongated roots pressing on the sensory nerve supply as it enters the tooth at its apex. The bony canal that protects the mandibular alveolar nerve is no longer present (Figure 24.23). Any pressure on the teeth is likely to be painful, so the rabbit is reluctant to eat hay.

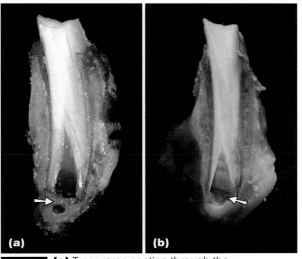

24.23 **(a)** Transverse section through the hemimandible of a rabbit without dental disease, showing the bony canal that encompasses and protects the mandibular alveolar nerve beneath the apex of the tooth (arrow). **(b)** Transverse section through the hemimandible of a rabbit in the very early stages of PSADD, showing the effect of alveolar bone loss and apical elongation. The mandibular alveolar nerve is no longer protected from pressure by the apex of the tooth (arrow). It is likely that this rabbit would have experienced pain if chewing hard food such as hay. Most owners offer hay to their rabbits but rabbits with the early stages of dental disease refuse to eat it. This is an effect, not a cause, of dental problems.

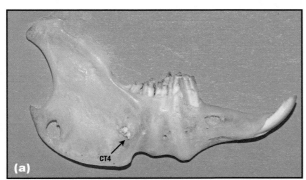

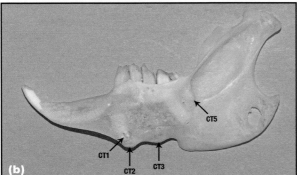

24.22 Apical elongation and sites of bone penetration. Apical elongation is one of the first changes to take place during PSADD. The elongated apices deform the bone and can penetrate the cortex at typical sites around the skull. **(a)** Lateral aspect. **(b)** Medial aspect.

Enamel hypoplasia also occurs and is manifested by horizontal ridges in the enamel, which are most obvious across the large upper incisors (see Figure 24.18). Another noticeable sign of early dental disease is epiphora caused by pressure on the nasolacrimal duct by the elongated roots of the upper 1st incisors (see Chapter 28).

Intermediate stages

Acquired malocclusion

The next stage of PSADD is acquired malocclusion due to alterations in the shape and position of the teeth, which changes the way they occlude and wear against each other. Not all the teeth may be affected to the same degree at the same time. At the outset of acquired incisor malocclusion, the upper incisors tend to become more curved and the lower incisors become straighter so that their tips no longer rest against the peg teeth but occlude with the tips of the large upper incisors instead. The chisel-shaped tips of the incisors become flattened as a result of abnormal wear. Eventually the tips of the incisors do not occlude at all and the crowns of the lower incisors protrude beyond the crowns of the upper ones. Once the teeth are out of occlusion, they will grow rapidly until the syndrome progresses to the next stage. The owners usually notice overgrown incisors, although many rabbits continue to eat unless the teeth are growing into their lips or nose.

Malocclusion of the cheek teeth also tends to follow a pattern. It usually begins with spurs on the 2nd, 3rd or 4th lower cheek teeth, which can lacerate the tongue and cause considerable soft tissue damage and distress to the rabbit. Anorexia, salivation and secondary gut stasis can be the result. These spurs are due to increased curvature of the teeth rather than elongation of the crowns (Figure 24.24). Curvature and spurs on the 1st lower cheek teeth are rare, probably because the apices of these teeth are adjacent to the root of the lower incisor, and are therefore supported. Curvature and spurs on the first two upper cheek teeth (maxillary premolars) often follow spurs on the lower cheek teeth. These spurs dig into the cheek and may penetrate the mucosa (Figure 24.25).

The clinical signs associated with spurs on the upper cheek teeth are less severe than those that are associated with spurs on the lower cheek teeth. Affected rabbits may chew in an abnormal manner or show mouthing because strands of food have become caught on the spurs. Some develop abscesses on the cheek because infection has been introduced through the puncture wound. During this stage, there is also loss of alveolar bone so the periodontal space widens (see Figure 24.24b), which also widens the interdental space, meaning that food can become trapped between the teeth. Infection can spread to the periapical area and abscesses can develop. In some cases the apices of the teeth continue to grow after they have penetrated the bone and abscesses form around them (see Chapter 29).

Rotation of the teeth

Later in the progression of the syndrome, the teeth may rotate within their sockets, which causes malocclusion. Rotation of the lower 4th cheek teeth can result in spurs that penetrate the inside of the cheek rather than the tongue (Figure 24.26); these spurs are easily missed during oral examination of the conscious rabbit. The last (tiny) lower cheek teeth can become elongated or loose and cause discomfort; they can be removed (see Chapter 27). Abnormalities at the caudal end of the molar arcade often cause so much discomfort that the rabbit will only chew on the opposing arcade to spare the painful side. The incisors can wear on a slant as a

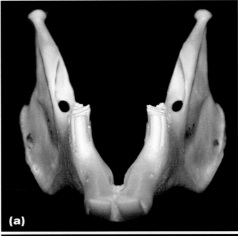

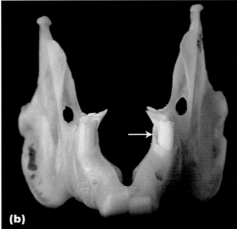

24.24 Curvature and spurs on the cheek teeth in prepared mandibles from **(a)** a wild rabbit and **(b)** a rabbit with spurs on both mandibular arcades. The cheek teeth of the wild rabbit point vertically. The cheek teeth of the rabbit with spurs are curved but the height of the teeth is similar to those of the wild rabbit. The apices are long and alveolar bone loss and widening of the periapical space is most evident on the left arcade (arrow).

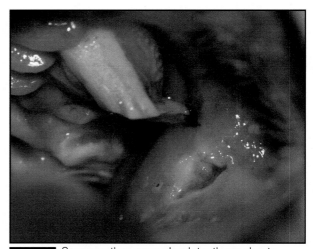

24.25 Spurs on the upper cheek teeth are due to increased curvature of the teeth rather than elongation of the crowns. Here, a spur on the 2nd upper premolar has penetrated the inside of the cheek. This can be a source of infection that results in an abscess in the cheek (see Chapter 29).

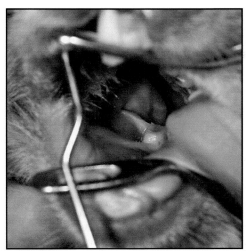

24.26 In the later stages of dental disease, loss of alveolar bone can allow teeth to rotate within the socket. The lower 4th cheek tooth may do this and result in a sharp spur digging into the cheek, which is painful. These spurs cannot be seen without a general anaesthetic. Even with the rabbit under anaesthesia, they are easily missed. It is important to examine each tooth carefully.

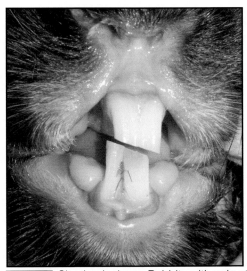

24.27 Slanting incisors. Rabbits with pain at the caudal end of the cheek teeth tend to chew on the other side of the mouth without closing the upper and lower arcade on the painful side. This leads to uneven wear of the incisors. The longer lower incisor is on the same side as the painful problem, so this rabbit's problem was on its right. It is often an abnormality of the tiny 5th (last) mandibular cheek tooth (M3). (Reproduced from *In Practice*, with permission)

result (Figure 24.27). Sometimes uneven wear can lead to a vertical point developing on the upper last cheek tooth that digs into, and ulcerates, the opposing gum. This can also be painful for the rabbit.

Dacryocystitis

Dacryocystitis is often associated with dental disease in cases where the elongated apex of the 1st upper incisor is occluding the nasolacrimal duct, which becomes infected and discharges pus into the conjunctival sac (see Chapter 28).

Late changes

Eventually the pathological changes that take place at the apices of the teeth destroy the germinal tissue, so the teeth stop growing. This can be mistakenly interpreted as a successful response to treatment instead of the passage of time. The pathological changes in the teeth do not take place simultaneously so some teeth are growing when others have stopped. Most of the teeth are uneven, misshapen or discoloured, although some can retain their normal structure and shape and continue to grow. Others remain as non-growing stumps which, if they occlude with an opposing tooth, can still be functional although the rabbit's ability to chew through tough food, such as stems of hay, is seriously impaired.

Endstage

Eventually, some or all of the crowns break off altogether, usually just below the gingival margin. The gum heals over the site where the crowns should be. At this stage the rabbit has no functional teeth and will require special care (see Chapter 30).

Causes of PSADD

There is controversy and debate about the aetiology and pathogenesis of PSADD. Genetic predisposition, inadequate dental wear and metabolic bone disease (MBD) are the most popular theories and it is probable that more than one factor is involved. At the time of writing, there are no published papers that show that insufficient dental wear is the cause of PSADD, although there are many articles, book chapters and conference proceedings that have put forward the theory. There is evidence that MBD is involved. This was the conclusion of the author's RCVS Fellowship thesis. A 7-year study of the skulls, radiographs, blood sample results and diet of pet rabbits with and without dental disease was conducted and a comparison made with wild rabbits. For the thesis, skulls from 172 rabbits were prepared and examined in detail. These were compared with the collection of 337 rabbit skulls kept at the Natural History Museum in London (Harcourt-Brown, 2006).

Although there is debate about whether lack of dental wear or MBD is the cause of acquired dental disease in pet rabbits, there is general agreement that the syndrome is due to incorrect feeding practices. It is linked with diets that are low in fibre and potentially unbalanced. Muesli mixes appear to be the worst offenders.

Insufficient chewing and lack of dental wear

Lack of hard or abrasive food and consequent reduced dental wear is often cited as a cause of overgrown teeth and malocclusion in pet rabbits. Many handbooks and leaflets on the care of pet rabbits suggest that twigs and branches should be provided for rabbits to gnaw on to wear their teeth down. Although it is plausible and logical to believe that insufficient dietary fibre would cause problems in a species that has evolved to eat a fibrous diet, there is little published evidence that this is the case. Various mechanisms have been proposed and all begin with the idea that insufficient occlusal wear results in elongation of the clinical crowns (Crossley, 2003; Capello, 2012). Crown length is difficult to measure in rabbits because:

- There is a lack of clear demarcation between the clinical and the reserve crown. Gingival hyperplasia or loss of alveolar bone affects the amount of tooth that is exposed above gum level
- There is a wide variation in the shape of the skull among rabbits of different breeds and sizes, which makes it impossible to standardize radiographs to measure crown height
- Uneven wear affects the occlusal relationship of the teeth, so a long tooth is usually opposed by a short tooth
- The length of the cheek teeth is affected by the occlusion of the incisors. If incisor malocclusion has developed to the point where the lower incisor occludes with the first upper incisor rather than the small peg teeth, the jaws are forced open so there is more space for the crowns of the cheek teeth to grow into
- Curvature of the teeth increases the length of the crown without altering its height.

Despite the problems associated with measuring the length of the exposed clinical crowns, if it is assumed that they are elongated because of inadequate dental wear, it is plausible that an increase in resting occlusal pressure on the teeth could result in bending of the clinical crowns and elongation of the reserve crowns (Capello, 2012). Lateral chewing movements could be affected so that spurs begin to form; elongation of the reserve crowns leads to apical deformity and impeded vascular support, so the teeth lose their ability to grow.

Underlying MBD

Calcium metabolism in rabbits: Rabbits have a high requirement for calcium owing to their high reproductive rate and the need for constant formation of new dental tissue. Laboratory investigations confirm that dietary calcium deficiency readily induces osteoporosis. Bone density studies using dual energy X-ray absorptiometry (DEXA) scanning show that demineralization of the vertebrae occurs after only 14 weeks on a low-calcium (0.1%) diet (Wu *et al.*, 1990). Another study showed that a dietary level of 0.6–1% calcium is required for optimum bone calcification (Norris *et al.*, 2001). Calcium deficiency is exacerbated by an inverse Ca:P ratio because calcium binds to phosphorus in the gut and because blood phosphorus levels stimulate a reciprocal fall in blood calcium, which stimulates parathyroid hormone (PTH) secretion and demineralization of bone. Therefore, foods such as cereals with an inverse Ca:P ratio are even more likely to induce MBD.

The calcium metabolism of rabbits differs from that of dogs, cats and humans. Calcium is absorbed readily in the gut of the rabbit, and the kidney regulates calcium balance by its ability to alter the amount that is excreted into the urine. It is normal for rabbits to pass large amounts of calcium in the urine, and this can cause problems if there is any underlying urinary tract problem (see Chapters 7 and 15). In any species, calcium can be absorbed from the intestine by two processes (Breslau, 1996):

- Passive paracellular diffusion, which depends on the concentration gradient between the intestinal lumen and the blood
- Active vitamin D-dependent transcellular transport, which is dependent on blood calcium levels.

In dogs, cats and humans, active vitamin D-dependent absorption is the main mechanism of calcium uptake from the gut, which means that calcium is absorbed according to demand. In rabbits, although active vitamin D-dependent uptake can take place, passive absorption is the main mechanism of intestinal calcium uptake (Bourdeau *et al.*, 1986). If intestinal concentrations of calcium are adequate or high, the amount of calcium that is absorbed is proportional to the amount of calcium that is present in the gut (Kamphues *et al.*, 1986), rather than the animal's calcium status.

However, if intestinal calcium levels are low, vitamin D is required to boost intestinal absorption in order to maintain blood calcium levels (Brommage *et al.*, 1988) and meet the animal's demand.

Efficient absorption of calcium from the gut is a way of meeting the rabbit's high calcium demand. The animal also recycles calcium because, as the teeth wear away, calcium is released into the gut, only to be absorbed again to lay down new dental tissue. This recycling process can only occur if there is sufficient calcium in the body in the first place. Low or marginal dietary calcium levels may be tolerated by rabbits with adequate vitamin D levels, because passive intestinal absorption can be boosted by active vitamin D-activated absorption, but if no vitamin D is present, this failsafe mechanism cannot occur. Vitamin D is obtained from the diet or from exposure to ultraviolet light. Wild rabbits enjoy basking in the sun but many pet rabbits are housed in hutches, sheds or houses and are not exposed to sunlight (Fairham and Harcourt-Brown, 1999). These rabbits rely on a dietary source of vitamin D. Vitamin D is not present in fresh vegetables or plants, although it might be present in sun-dried hay. However, because of unreliable weather conditions, there is a growing trend for drying hay artificially. Vitamin D is also important for other physiological processes. It is important in phosphorus metabolism and has a direct effect on bone mineralization.

Mechanism by which MBD causes dental disease: The visual and radiographic changes that take place in the teeth and the bones of the skulls of rabbits with PSADD show a disease mechanism that is characterized by progressive demineralization of the teeth and surrounding bone (Figures 24.28 and 24.29). The proposed mechanism is as follows.

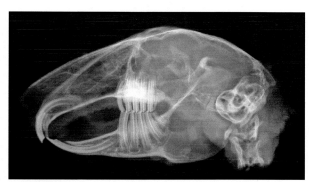

24.28 Radiograph of a sagitally sectioned head of a rabbit with healthy dentition. The lines of bone outlining the structures of the skull (the nasal bone, zygoma, mandible and calvarium) are straight and clear. The cortical bone along the ventral border of the mandible is thick. The palatine bone is straight and thick. The lamina dura can be seen outlining each tooth socket. Enamel can be seen outlining the teeth and the central enamel fold is evident in all the cheek teeth. (Reproduced from *In Practice*, with permission)

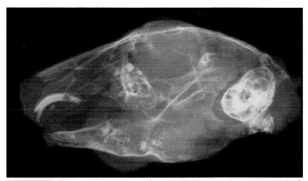

24.29 This radiograph of a sagitally sectioned head of a lop rabbit with advanced dental disease shows marked contrasts with Figure 24.28. Only a few remnants of dental structures remain. The lines of bone outlining the zygoma and mandible are thin, even in areas that are not subjected to any mechanical force during chewing. This skull is osteopenic, which is highly suggestive of metabolic bone disease rather than disuse atrophy, where bone loss would only occur in the parts of the skull that were subjected to mechanical strain during chewing.

1. Loss of alveolar bone supporting the apices of the teeth allows apical elongation to take place in response to the forces generated during chewing and biting.
2. Apical elongation causes compression of the nerves and germinal tissue at the apices of the teeth, which causes pain so that the rabbit does not wish to eat hard foods such as hay.
3. Insufficient calcium and changes within the germinal tissue lead to dental dysplasia, which leads to ridges in the enamel and uneven wear of the teeth.
4. Alterations in the shape of the teeth, such as curvature of the cheek teeth, develop because they are not adequately supported by bone. The change in shape is due to forces exerted on the teeth during chewing. Alveolar bone in rabbits is subjected to considerable strain during mastication (Weijs and De Jongh, 1977).

5. Curvature of the teeth results in abnormal contact and the development of malocclusion.
6. Loss of alveolar bone results in widening of the periodontal spaces and rotation of the teeth within the socket.
7. Demineralized, weakened teeth eventually fracture.

Evidence that MBD is the main cause of PSADD: There is supporting evidence for the hypothesis that MBD underlies dental disease in rabbits. Although there are only a few laboratory investigations into the relationship between calcium metabolism and dentition in rabbits, Kato (1966) found that rickets caused hypocalcification of the teeth, and Mellanby and Killick (1926) showed that a diet that was deficient in calcium and vitamin D caused 'poorly calcified alveolar bone and badly formed dentine' in rabbits. The paper shows radiographs of prepared mandibles that demonstrate root elongation and loss of cortical bone, similar to the signs seen in rabbits affected by PSADD. A study by the author showed significantly higher plasma PTH concentrations and lower total serum calcium concentrations in pet rabbits with advanced dental disease, in comparison with rabbits with normal teeth that were kept outside (Harcourt-Brown and Baker, 2001).

Inadequate dental wear does not explain the enamel hyperplasia and apical elongation that occur as early, rather than late, signs of dental disease in rabbits. These changes are most obvious in the upper first incisors, where ridges can be seen in the enamel and elongated apices often block the tear ducts and cause epiphora. This can occur when the length and shape of the incisor crowns are normal. The upper 1st incisor is not in contact with the lower incisors at rest in rabbits with normal dentition (see Figures 24.3 and 24.28), so apical elongation cannot be due to an increase in resting occlusal pressure.

Significance of the cause of acquired dental disease: Whether acquired dental disease is due to MBD or a lack of dietary fibre is not important when it comes to prevention. It is universally accepted that a high-fibre diet prevents most health problems in rabbits, including dental disease. However, the distinction is important when it comes to treatment and the decision about whether to perform repeated generalized coronal reduction or to be less invasive and only remove spurs and points that are causing soft tissue damage. Treatment of dental disease is covered in Chapter 26.

The role of muesli mixes
A statistically significant link between a diet of muesli mixes and dental disease in pet rabbits has been found (Mullan and Main, 2006). Muesli mixes (or some parts of them) are highly palatable to rabbits. They contain a mixture of cereals, legumes, pellets and extruded nuggets (Figure 24.30) and some brands include other items, such as locust beans or alfalfa. Dried peas, beans and cereals are the staple ingredients of muesli mixes. These ingredients are low in fibre so they provide little dental wear. They

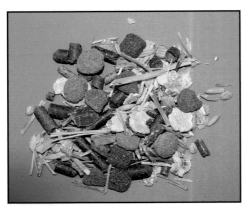

24.30 Muesli mixes such as this are not suitable as rabbit food.

are also deficient in vitamin D and calcium and have a highly inverse calcium-to-phosphorus (Ca:P) ratio, both of which are known to be contributory factors to MBD. Providing the diet as a mixture of ingredients allows selection of the most palatable items, and the two favourite ingredients that rabbits pick out from muesli mixes are maize and peas, which have a very low calcium content (Figure 24.31). The manufacturers know that the ingredients of muesli mixes are unbalanced in vitamins and minerals and attempt to overcome the problem by adding a vitamin and mineral supplement. The supplement is in powder form and is usually incorporated into the pellets to prevent the powder falling to the bottom of the bag. It can be incorporated into the extruded nuggets, but these are cooked, which denatures some vitamins so that more supplement is needed; most manufacturers prefer to incorporate the supplement into the pellets. Pellets are the least palatable ingredient to rabbits and are usually left uneaten in the bottom of the bowl, only to be discarded by the owner (Harcourt-Brown, 1996). As a result, the rabbit can easily consume an unbalanced, calcium-deficient diet that is mainly composed of peas and maize. Some manufacturers try to overcome the problem of calcium

deficiency by incorporating another ingredient, such as alfalfa, that is high in calcium to balance the calcium-deficient ingredients. Others attempt to coat the ingredients with supplement in a liquid form. Neither of these methods can guarantee that the rabbit consumes a diet containing sufficient calcium for the continual formation of new dental tissue.

Although muesli mixes are cheap, convenient, palatable, easy to store and are a popular diet for pet rabbits, they are not necessary and can cause dental disease, obesity and other health problems.

Prevention of dental disease

Prevention of dental disease starts at weaning, when the calcium requirement and a high-fibre diet are very important. Feeding muesli mixes to groups of young rabbits is inadvisable for many reasons. Instead of mixed rations, a pelleted or extruded concentrate is preferable and should be fed alongside an unlimited source of good quality hay or grass (Figure 24.32). Contrary to popular opinion, young rabbits can be fed on leafy green vegetables and garden plants from an early age (Figure 24.33). Exposure to natural daylight is also beneficial. It is the best way of maintaining optimal vitamin D levels. Grazing outside has the added benefit of a natural diet, as well as exposure to natural daylight. Rabbits with prognathic defects, usually Dwarf breeds, should not be bred from and, ideally, the parents should not be bred from again either.

Ingredient	Calcium content (%)	Phosphorus content (%)	Ca:P ratio
Peas	0.14	0.46	1:3
Maize	0.04	0.28	1:7
Oats	0.03	0.33	1:11
Wheat	0.06	0.33	1:5
Barley	0.07	0.39	1:6
Beans (kidney)	0.14	0.46	1:3
Apples	0.3	0.8	1:2
Carrots	0.37	0.32	1:1
Grass hay (Timothy)	0.19–2.5 0.5	0.11–0.8 0.3	1:<1–1:>3 1:<1
Grass	0.23–1.56	1.7–0.56	1:2–1:>3

24.31 Calcium and phosphorus levels of some ingredients of rabbit food. NB: It is recommended that rabbit diets contain 0.6–1% calcium.

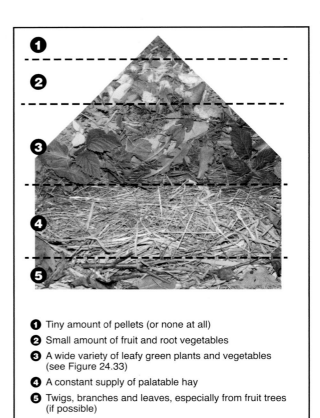

❶ Tiny amount of pellets (or none at all)
❷ Small amount of fruit and root vegetables
❸ A wide variety of leafy green plants and vegetables (see Figure 24.33)
❹ A constant supply of palatable hay
❺ Twigs, branches and leaves, especially from fruit trees (if possible)

24.32 The ideal diet for pet rabbits to prevent dental disease.

Vegetables		
• Broccoli – florets, stems, leaves • Brussels sprouts – peelings, stems and leaves • Cabbage • Cauliflower leaves	• Celery • Chicory • Chinese cabbage • Fennel • Kale	• Leeks • Romaine lettuce • Spinach • Spring greens • Watercress

Herbs		
• Basil • Chervil	• Coriander • Mint	• Parsley • Rocket

Byproducts from the vegetable garden		
• Carrot tops • Leaves and branches from fruit trees • Pea plants	• Strawberry, blackberry and raspberry leaves • Sunflower leaves	• Sweetcorn plants • Tops from celeriac, beetroot, artichokes or other root vegetables

Wild plants		
• Bramble (*Rubus fruticosus*) • Burnet (*Poterium sanguisorba*) • Chickweed (*Stellaria media*) • Cleavers (goosegrass) (*Galium aparine*) • Clover (*Trifolium*) • Coltsfoot (*Tussilago farfara*) • Comfrey (*Symphytum officinale*)	• Cow parsnip (hogweed) (*Heracleum sphondylium*) • Dandelion (*Taraxacum*) • Dock (*Rumex* spp.) • Grass • Ground elder (*Aegopodium podagraria*) • Groundsel (*Senecio vulgaris*)	• Knapweed (*Centaurea* spp.) • Plantain (*Plantago* spp.) • Shepherd's purse (*Capsella bursa-pastoris*) • Sow thistle (*Sonchus oleraceus*) • Vetches (*Vicia* spp.) • Wild chervil (*Anthriscus sylvestris*) • Yarrow (*Achillea milleforium*)

24.33 Leafy green plants that are suitable for pet rabbits. At least five different plants should be offered each day. NB: Although owners worry about plant toxicity, it is not a problem for rabbits that are given a choice of plants to eat, although it can be a problem if there is only a single houseplant on offer. Given a choice, rabbits do not eat poisonous plants or they are not susceptible to their toxins.

How to prevent dental disease in rabbits

The measures that prevent dental disease in rabbits mainly concern diet. Many of them also prevent obesity, reduce the risk of urinary tract and gastrointestinal disease and prevent boredom. Prevention of dental disease starts at weaning, when the requirement for calcium is high and long fibre is important.

The ideal diet for a rabbit with healthy teeth is shown in Figure 24.32. It should be:

• Palatable
• High in fibre
• Low in calories
• Balanced in vitamins and minerals, especially calcium, phosphorus and vitamin D
• Convenient and available for the owner.

This can be accomplished by:

• Avoiding any form of muesli mix. These diets are high in carbohydrate and low in fibre. Individual rabbits will select their favourite ingredients and eat an unbalanced diet
• Ensuring that a constant supply of good quality, palatable hay or grass (dried or fresh) is available at all times

• Feeding a wide variety of leafy green plants (see Figure 24.33). Contrary to popular opinion, young rabbits can be fed on leafy green vegetables and garden plants from an early age
• Restricting any food items that can be puréed such as fruit (e.g. apples, pears, bananas) or root vegetables (carrots, parsnips, beetroot, celeriac, swede, artichokes). Although rabbits eat these foods readily, the fibre in them is composed of small particles that are moved into the caecum where they are degraded by the caecal microflora and converted into volatile fatty acids and ultimately fat, so they predispose to obesity
• Avoiding or restricting pellets or nuggets. Although these foods are convenient and palatable and can be useful for rabbits with dental problems or when other food is scarce, they are not vital. If they are fed, only a small quantity is necessary. A small bowl can be offered once a day. Any food that is left can be removed after half an hour
• Excluding any starchy, sugary treats or human foods. Food nuggets can be used as a reward for training instead
• Avoiding any human food.

References and further reading

Ardran GM and Kemp FH (1958) A radiographic analysis of mastication and swallowing in the domestic rabbit: *Oryctolagus cuniculus*. *Proceedings of the Zoological Society of London* **130**, 257–274

Bhadresa R (1977) Food preferences of rabbits, *Oryctolagus cuniculus*, at Holkham sand dunes, Norfolk. *Journal of Applied Ecology* **14**, 287–291

Bishop MA (1995) Is rabbit dentine innervated? A fine structural study of the pulpal innervation in the cheek teeth of the rabbit. *Journal of Anatomy* **186**, 365–372

Blood DC, Studdert VP and Gay CC (2007) *Saunders Comprehensive Veterinary Dictionary, 3rd edn.* Saunders Elsevier, Edinburgh

Bourdeau JE, Shwer-Dymerski DA, Stern PA and Langman CB (1986) Calcium and phosphorus metabolism in chronically vitamin D-deficient laboratory rabbits. *Mineral Electrolyte Metabolism* **12**, 176–185

Breslau NA (1996) Calcium, magnesium and phosphorus. In: *Intestinal Absorption. Primer on the Metabolic Bone Diseases and*

Disorders of Mineral Metabolism, ed. MJ Favus, pp. 49–56. Lippincott-Raven, Philadelphia

Brommage R, Miller SC, Langman CB *et al.* (1988) The effect of chronic vitamin D deficiency on the skeleton in the adult rabbit. *Bone* **9**, 131

Cai JJ (1992) Effect of vitamin D overdosage on the tooth and bone development of rabbits. *Zhonghua Kou Qiang Yi Xue Za Zhi* **27**, 296–299 [in Chinese with an English abstract]

Capello V (2012) Small mammal dentistry. In: *Ferrets, Rabbits and Rodents: Clinical Medicine and Surgery*, ed. KE Quesenberry and JW Carpenter, pp. 452–471. Elsevier, St. Louis

Crossley DA (2003) Oral biology and disorders of lagomorphs. *Veterinary Clinics of North America: Exotic Animal Practice* **6**(3), 629–660

Fairham J and Harcourt-Brown FM (1999) Preliminary investigation of the vitamin D status of pet rabbits. *Veterinary Record* **145**, 452–454

Gardner DG, Bunte RM, Sawyer DR and Artwohl J (1997) Multicystic lesion of the jaw in a rabbit. *Contemporary Topics by the American Association for Laboratory Animal Science* **36**, 78–80

Harcourt-Brown FM (1996) Calcium deficiency, diet and dental disease in pet rabbits. *Veterinary Record* **139**, 567–571

Harcourt-Brown FM (2006) *Metabolic Bone Disease as a Possible Cause of Dental Disease in Pet Rabbits*. RCVS Fellowship Thesis (available in PDF form from the author)

Harcourt-Brown FM (2007) The progressive syndrome of acquired dental disease in rabbits. *Journal of Exotic Pet Medicine* **16**, 146–157

Harcourt-Brown FM (2009) Dental disease in pet rabbits. 1. Normal dentition, pathogenesis and aetiology. *In Practice* **31**, 370–379

Harcourt-Brown FM and Baker SJ (2001) Parathyroid hormone, haematological and biochemical parameters in relation to dental disease and husbandry in pet rabbits. *Journal of Small Animal Practice* **42**, 130–136

Hillson S (2005) *Teeth, 2nd edn.* Cambridge University Press, Cambridge

Hirschfield Z, Weinrab MM and Michaeli Y (1973) Incisors of the rabbit: morphology, histology and development. *Journal of Dental Research* **52**, 377–384

Horowitz SL, Weisbroth SH and Scher S (1973) Deciduous dentition in the rabbit (*Oryctolagus cuniculus*), a roentgenographic study. *Archives of Oral Biology* **30**, 517–523

Jubb KVF, Kennedy PC and Palmer N (1985) Bones and joints. In: *Pathology of the Domestic Animals, Volume 1*, pp. 2–131. Academic Press, London

Kamphues VJ, Carstensen P, Schroeder D *et al.* (1986) Effect of increasing calcium and vitamin D supply on calcium metabolism in rabbits. *Journal of Animal Physiology and Nutrition* **50**, 191–208 [in German with an English summary]

Kato J (1966) Effects of the administration of vitamin D2, D3, parathyroid hormone and calcium on hypocalcification of rabbit dentine and on changes in blood constituents caused by experimental rickets. *Gunma Journal of Medicine* **15**, 174–193

Lowe JA (1998) Pet rabbit feeding and nutrition. In: *The Nutrition of the Rabbit*, ed. C de Blas and J Wiseman, pp. 309–329. CABI Publishing, Wallingford

Mellanby M and Killick EM (1926) A preliminary study of factors influencing calcification processes in the rabbit. *Biochemical Journal* **20**, 902–926

Mullan SM and Main DCJ (2006) Survey of the husbandry, health and welfare of 102 pet rabbits. *Veterinary Record* **159**, 103–109

Ness AR (1956) The response of the rabbit mandibular incisor to experimental shortening and prevention of its eruption. *Proceedings of the Royal Society* **146**, 129–154

Norris SA, Pettifor JM, Gray DA and Buffenstein R (2001) Calcium metabolism and bone mass in female rabbits during skeletal maturation: effects of dietary calcium intake. *Bone* **29**, 62–69

Schwartz G, Enomoto S, Valiquette C and Lund JP (1989) Mastication in the rabbit: a description of movement and muscle activity. *Journal of Neurophysiology* **62**, 273–287

Shadle AR (1936) The attrition and extrusive growth of the four major incisor teeth of domestic rabbits. *Journal of Mammology* **17**, 15–21

Weijs WA and Dantuma R (1981) Functional anatomy of the masticatory apparatus in the rabbit (Oryctolagus cuniculus L.). *Netherlands Journal of Zoology* **31**, 99–147

Weijs WA and De Jongh HJ (1977) Strain in mandibular alveolar bone during mastication in the rabbit. *Archives of Oral Biology* **22**, 667–675

Wiggs RB and Lobprise H (1995) Dental anatomy and physiology of pet rodents and lagomorphs. In: *Manual of Small Animal Dentistry, 2nd edn*, ed. DA Crossley and S Penman, pp. 68–73. BSAVA Publications, Gloucester

Wu DD, Boyd RD, Fix TJ and Burr DB (1990) Regional patterns of bone loss and altered bone remodelling in response to calcium deprivation in laboratory rabbits. *Calcified Tissue International* **47**, 18–23

Yamada Y and Yamamura K (1996) Possible factors which may affect phase durations in the natural chewing rhythm. *Brain Research* **706**, 237–242

25

The dental examination

Vladimir Jekl

Oral/dental disease is the most common disorder encountered in small herbivorous mammals, including rabbits. The ability to recognize anatomical and physiological variations is necessary in order to understand disease pathophysiology and assess minor changes. Proper oral cavity examination and accurate diagnosis are the keys to appropriate treatment planning and prognosis. A paediatric laryngoscope or otoscope is used for a preliminary examination of the oral cavity. This is followed by a more detailed examination carried out under general anaesthesia using a rigid endoscope. Skull radiography and/or computed tomography (CT) is also recommended, together with bacteriology (for facial abscesses) and/or blood tests where indicated.

In some cases rabbits do not show any clinical signs of oral cavity disease, and it is recommended therefore that all rabbits presented should undergo oral cavity examination. Sedation or general anaesthesia is recommended for nervous rabbits, and for thorough oral examination.

Clinical history and examination

A complete history should be obtained from the owner to provide information about past and current problems, including any previous treatment. The onset of the current presenting problem should be described, such as whether it occurred gradually or suddenly. Special attention should be paid to the nutritional and mineral content of the diet because of the link between diet, calcium metabolism, dental disease and chewing problems (see Chapter 24). Apart from general history questions about eating and weight loss, particular questions associated with the presence of dental disease should include:

- Have the rabbit's eating habits changed?
- Does the rabbit prefer to eat softer foods (e.g. vegetables, fruits)?
- Does the rabbit refuse some parts of the diet (e.g. hay)?
- Is there any sign of the rabbit dropping food out of its mouth?
- Are there any signs of wet fur in the vicinity of the oral cavity?
- Is there any asymmetry in the face of the rabbit?
- Do you think that the rabbit's mouth smells different from usual?

- Is there a change in the size and appearance of the incisors?

A full clinical examination should be performed on all patients presented at the veterinary clinic, even for routine health checks. Non-specific general clinical findings commonly associated with oral cavity disease in rabbits are dehydration, poor body condition, unkempt hair, epiphora and ileus. Animals with cardiorespiratory disease require special attention, and acute life-threatening conditions should be addressed immediately.

Different forms of dental disease can induce signs of apathy, behavioural changes, anorexia, chewing disturbances, changes in food preferences and weight loss.

Epiphora (Figure 25.1) is commonly associated with apical elongation of the incisors or periapical pathology of the maxillary premolars or molars (see Chapters 24 and 28). In severe cases, wet dermatitis can occur as a result of chronic skin irritation. Incisor elongation may cause nasal discharge.

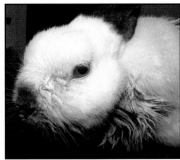

25.1 This rabbit is showing typical signs of dental disease. The epiphora was due to apical incisor elongation and nasolacrimal duct obstruction, and excessive salivation was associated with severe ulcerative stomatitis.

Oral pain due to stomatitis or malocclusion can cause lack of grooming, excessive salivation, a wet chin, wet fur on the front paws and changes in the size, consistency and quantity of faecal pellets. Oral pain may additionally cause pawing at the face.

Essential equipment for dental examination

Hand instruments
Standard dental equipment can be adapted for use in rabbits, although special instruments for rabbits and rodents are commercially available (Figures 25.2 to 25.4).

Hand instrument	Use in rabbits
Mouth gag	Essential instrument for intraoral inspection of the rabbit's long and narrow oral cavity. The two arms of a mouth gag, which open the mouth in a vertical direction, have two elliptical holes that fit the crowns of the maxillary and mandibular incisors. Mouth gags can be used only in anaesthetized rabbits because they interfere with chewing. Arm extension should always be performed very gently to avoid excessive stretching of the oral musculature, temporomandibular joint ligaments and cartilage, and to avoid fracture of the mandible or incisors. The mouth gag should be supported by an assistant in an optimal position (perpendicular to the examination table) to allow complete examination of the oral cavity by the clinician. In cases of abnormal incisor elongation, clinical crown adjustment is recommended before the insertion of a mouth gag. In rabbits with extracted or fractured incisors, a cheek dilator or eyelid retractor could be used as an alternative to allow vertical mouth opening (see Figure 25.4)
Cheek dilator	Available in different sizes; the instrument is chosen to fit the size of the animal. Dilators with longer blades are particularly useful in larger rabbits and allow proper cheek dilation. However, longer blades may hide buccal mucosa pathology, so it is necessary to examine the cheek teeth before insertion of the cheek dilator
Table-top gag	The rabbit and rodent table retractor/restrainer is a special platform for intraoral examination which acts as a mouth gag and positions the patient. This device allows the clinician to work alone (except for the anaesthetist). Not all practitioners like it
Paediatric laryngoscope	Use of a paediatric laryngoscope with incorporated light source is preferred by the author for intraoral inspection in both conscious and anaesthetized animals. The paediatric laryngoscope makes visualization of the teeth easier and can be used to push the tongue or cheek aside. Other suggested instruments are an otoscope, a bivalve nasal speculum, and a steel vaginal speculum with an additional light source
Otoscope	Recommended by other clinicians for intraoral inspection of conscious or anaesthetized animals. Gives additional magnification of the field of interest. Some lesions could be missed, owing to the narrow visual field
Dental spatula	Fine instrument of optimal size and shape for moving the tongue or cheek to one side. Curved blunt scissors are a useful alternative
Periodontal probe	Used to examine and evaluate gingival sulci, periodontal pockets, gingival recession or abscess cavities. Used for tactile examination of visible tooth surfaces and to evaluate tooth movement. The size of clinical crowns can be measured and compared. The William probe with line markings is most suitable for rabbits
Source of light	An external source of light, such as an operating light, penlight or headlamp, is necessary when a mouth cavity is evaluated. A light source is commonly incorporated in a laryngoscope, otoscope or vaginal speculum
Forceps	Small anatomical forceps with smooth tips are used to hold or depress the tongue while the lateral tongue surface and sublingual region are evaluated
Dental mirror	A small front-surface dental mirror is used for indirect visualization of the teeth and for illumination, especially in caudal parts of the oral cavity
Cotton buds	Helpful to clean the debris and saliva that accumulate in the oral cavity
Swabs and test tubes	Swabs and test tubes for microbiology and mycology, small biopsy tubes with 10% formaldehyde and micro slides for cytology should be prepared for obtaining samples for further laboratory investigation

25.2 Hand instruments used for examination of the oral cavity in rabbits.

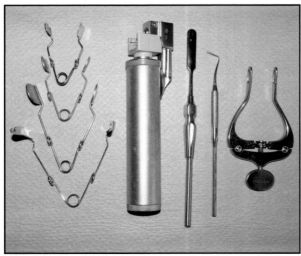

25.3 Special instruments for oral cavity examination include (from left to right) cheek dilators of different sizes, paediatric laryngoscope, dental spatula, periodontal probe and mouth dilator.

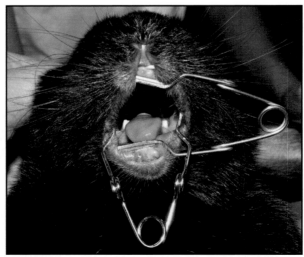

25.4 In rabbits with extracted or fractured incisors, horizontal opening of the mouth cavity is achieved with the use of a second cheek teeth dilator or eyelid retractor inserted between the upper and lower jaws.

The periodontal probe, dental spatula and dental handpiece are generally held in a modified pen grip. This provides maximum control of the instrument, precision, a wide range of movement and good tactile sensation for the clinician through the instrument (Figure 25.5).

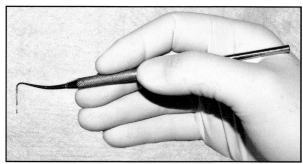

25.5 Each handheld instrument should be held between tips of the thumb and the index finger, which do not touch each other. The middle finger is used to guide the instrument and to detect tactile sensation. The pad of the finger, not the side, rests on the shank. The ring finger and little finger are placed in the patient's mouth, using an incisor or structures adjacent to the incisor as a fulcrum. This helps to support and stabilize the hand.

Endoscopic equipment

Endoscopic equipment used for oral cavity examination in rabbits is summarized in Figure 25.6.

Equipment	Use in rabbits
Rigid endoscope	Endoscopes with Hopkins rod–lens systems are most commonly used for oral cavity examination. Endoscopes of 18 cm working length, viewing angles of 30 and 70 degrees, and diameters of 2.7 or 4 mm allow easy handling and manipulation and are optimal for oral cavity examination
Protective sheath	Used for protection of the endoscope. Reduces accessibility to the buccal and lingual surfaces of the examined teeth. Limits manipulation of the endoscope within the oral cavity, so the author does not generally recommend its use for oral cavity evaluation in rabbits. A protective sheath with operating channel is recommended for surgical procedures or sampling, because it is possible to pass flexible instruments such as biopsy forceps precisely into the region of interest
Source of light	A xenon source of light with manual light intensity control provides illumination. The development of new sources of light based on light-emitting diodes (LEDs) offers promise
Endoscopic video camera	Very useful, as it allows better handling and field enlargement. The quality of the image is even better with the use of video-endoscopes, which have a charge-coupled device (CCD) chip located in the distal part of the endoscope
Otoendo-scopes	Can also be used for oral cavity examination. More robust but do not give an angle, which limits their use in small rabbits
Recording devices	Images and video can be recorded to the hard drive of a computer or another storage device. Lesions should be documented to evaluate progression and response to therapy and for consultation, discussion and client education

25.6 Endoscopic equipment used for examination of the oral cavity in rabbits.

Examination of the head, teeth and oral cavity in the conscious rabbit

Oral cavity examination should be performed in all rabbits after the general physical examination. Optimal assessment of a rabbit's head and teeth relies on familiarity with the normal anatomy of the rabbit skull and teeth, and with the physiology of chewing (see Chapter 24).

Oral cavity examination should involve the following.

- **Evaluation of facial symmetry and palpation of the jaws.** Signs of heat, discharge, crepitus and presence of lumps and bumps (Figure 25.7) should be noted:
  - Lateral and horizontal lower jaw excursion should be evaluated
  - Pain on manipulation of the jaws may be due to a jaw fracture, disease of the temporomandibular joint or retrobulbar pathology
  - Palpation of the ventromedial border of the mandible and zygomatic area could reveal bony swellings associated with apical teeth (tooth root) elongation or periapical pathology (see Chapter 24)
  - Palpation of the cheeks is not recommended before oral cavity inspection owing to possible coronal cheek teeth elongation with spike formation, which could cause unnecessary discomfort and pain if palpated
  - Palpation of submandibular lymph nodes and the chin scent glands may reveal inflammatory or neoplastic changes.

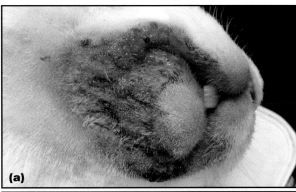
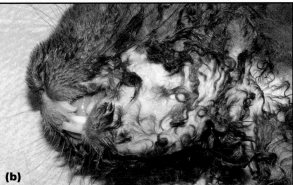

25.7 **(a)** Severe superficial dermatitis. **(b)** Swelling of the lower mandible due to a facial abscess.

- **Examination of external soft tissue and incisors**:
  - The lips are lifted with the thumb and forefinger and the nasal philtrum is examined for any inflammatory lesions, foreign bodies or traumatic injury
  - The mucosal surface, gingiva and gingival sulcus surrounding the incisors are evaluated for colour, presence of exudate, foreign bodies or any other lesions
  - The lower incisors should occlude with the secondary small incisors, which are behind the primary maxillary incisors. A sharp chisel-like cutting edge is present at the labial surface of the maxillary and mandibular incisors (see Chapter 24). The labial surface of the incisors is easily inspected and palpated. The healthy labial surface is white in colour and smooth on palpation, so any horizontal ridges and roughness are pathological (Figure 25.8).

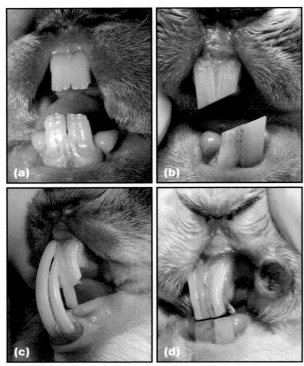

25.8 Different types of incisor pathology in the rabbit. **(a)** Horizontal ridges on the enamel surface indicate dysplastic changes of the germinal tissue of the tooth. **(b)** Oblique occlusal incisor surface and right mandibular shift. **(c)** Severe incisor malocclusion treated by improper crown trimming with nail clippers. **(d)** Elongated peg teeth may cause severe lip ulcerations.

- **Oral cavity examination.** The oral cavity of rabbits is long and narrow, which makes thorough clinical examination more difficult than in carnivores:
  - The premolars and molars form the uniform functional grinding unit: a relatively horizontal occlusal surface with transverse enamel folds. The enamel folds correspond to deep invagination of the enamel on the palatal side of the maxillary cheek teeth and the buccal side of the mandibular cheek teeth. They are filled with cementum-like material and are visible on the outside as developmental grooves. The enamel is thickest on the lingual surfaces of the maxillary cheek teeth and the buccal surfaces of the mandibular cheek teeth (see Chapter 24)
  - An otoscope can be used for conscious oral examination, although some lesions can remain undetected because of the limited visual field. It has the advantage of providing magnification. A bivalve nasal speculum allows broad-angle imaging and therefore gives a higher likelihood of detecting pathological lesions. In the author's experience, a paediatric laryngoscope gives a clear image of the buccal, occlusal and lingual surfaces of the premolars and molars. It provides depression of the tongue and separation of the cheeks from the teeth, which creates more space for visualization and detection of potential changes or pathology.
  - For conscious examination a rabbit is restrained manually. An assistant holds the animal's thorax, thoracic limbs included, and supports its back while the examiner holds the animal's head and retracts its upper lips with one hand while examining the oral cavity with the otoscope or laryngoscope in the other hand (Figure 25.9). An alternative is for the assistant to wrap the rabbit in a towel and hold it firmly and carefully against their body.

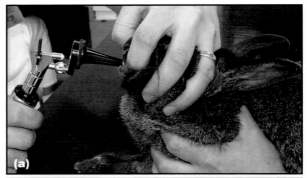

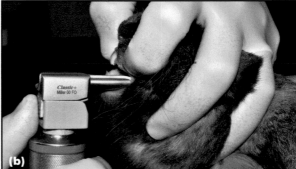

25.9 Oral cavity examination in the conscious rabbit can be performed with **(a)** an otoscope, **(b)** a paediatric laryngoscope or **(c)** a speculum. The rabbit's head is grasped in the left hand, the lips are lifted and the instrument is gently inserted. (continues) ▶

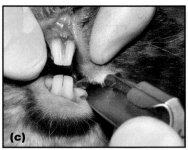

25.9

(continued) **(c)** Oral cavity examination in the conscious rabbit using a speculum. The rabbit's head is grasped in the left hand, the lips are lifted and the instrument is gently inserted.

WARNING
If any significant pathological change is identified in the oral cavity, the examination should be terminated immediately to avoid the risk of injury due to any unexpected movement during the conscious examination. If necessary, a thorough investigation of the oral cavity can be made with the animal under general anaesthesia.

Examination under general anaesthesia

Pre-anaesthetic considerations and patient positioning

A balanced approach to anaesthesia is indicated when conducting oral examinations and administering dental treatments to rabbits (see Chapter 1). Intravenous cannula placement and endotracheal intubation are optimal, especially in animals with impaired general health status. The patient is placed on a heating pad and is monitored throughout the procedure. Oxygen should be delivered via an endotracheal tube or nasal/facial mask during all procedures.

Anaesthetic gas delivery can be maintained by endotracheal tube or by nasal mask; each has advantages and disadvantages. The advantages of endotracheal intubation include precise delivery of the anaesthetic gas to the patient, prevention of gas leakage into the atmosphere, and provision of an airway to administer oxygen by intermittent positive pressure ventilation if necessary. An endotracheal tube can, however, restrict access to the oral cavity in small rabbits, and the use of a nasal mask may be preferred in some cases.

It is possible to use a commercially available small facemask designed for rodents, which can be applied over the rabbit's nostrils. A tight seal over the nostrils is maintained by a rubber diaphragm. Alternatively, a conical nasal mask, can be made from part of a plastic bottle. A diaphragm, which reduces the orifice diameter and gas leakage, can be made from part of a surgical glove (Figure 25.10). Nasal masks need to be held against the nostrils by the assistant throughout the dental procedure. Commercially available rodent anaesthetic circuits/facemasks are available that can be used for small rabbits and connected to a supply system for anaesthetic gas and to a gas exhaust system which safely removes the exhaled gases.

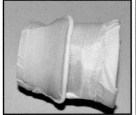
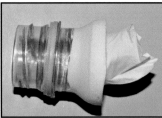
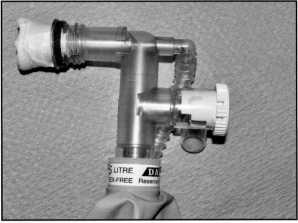

25.10 A customized nasal mask can be made from parts of a plastic bottle and a surgical glove; this minimizes gas leakage during dental procedures. If only injectable anaesthesia is used, oxygen can be administered via this small mask.

Oral cavity examination under general anaesthesia

General anaesthesia allows the practitioner to examine the oral cavity thoroughly, which minimizes the possibility of missing any oral pathology or iatrogenic injury. Endoscopic examination gives detailed visualization of pathological changes in the oral cavity and oropharynx of a rabbit. If inhalational anaesthesia is provided, the supply of the anaesthetic mixture is not interrupted during the oral cavity examination (see Technique 25.1).

Oral and dental records

It is good practice to keep accurate records of dental pathology and treatments. There are numerous ways of recording such data, with the simplest based on diagrams. Useful features of the dental protocol include the name and details of the owner, the animal's sex, weight and age, the date of oral cavity examination, illustrative images of dentition, tooth identification and coding systems. Dental charts also include pathological findings and performed procedures.

There are several methods of identifying teeth (see Chapter 24) and several systems can be used (Figure 25.11). A proper tooth identification sequence is helpful when discussing cases or writing case reports. Record charts of oral examination findings, endoscopic records, and X-ray or CT images serve as an essential clinical record for further therapy and treatment.

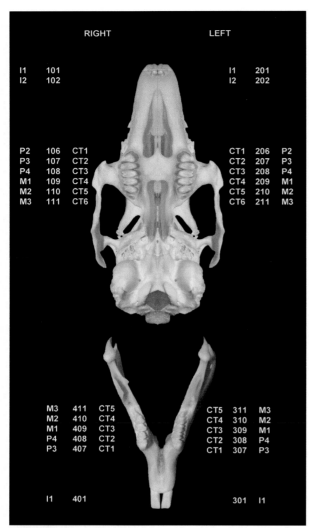

RIGHT					LEFT
I1	101			I1	201
I2	102			I2	202
P2	106	CT1	CT1	206	P2
P3	107	CT2	CT2	207	P3
P4	108	CT3	CT3	208	P4
M1	109	CT4	CT4	209	M1
M2	110	CT5	CT5	210	M2
M3	111	CT6	CT6	211	M3

M3	411	CT5	CT5	311	M3
M2	410	CT4	CT4	310	M2
M1	409	CT3	CT3	309	M1
P4	408	CT2	CT2	308	P4
P3	407	CT1	CT1	307	P3
I1	401			301	I1

25.11 A modified Triadan tooth numbering system is often used for identifying rabbits' teeth in the dental literature. However, many small mammal clinicians use a simplified nomenclature in which the premolars and molars are referred to by one common term: 'cheek teeth'. (CT = cheek tooth; I = incisor; M = molar; PM = premolar.)

Laboratory investigations

Several laboratory techniques can be helpful to investigate the aetiological background and primary or secondary infectious agents, and to direct medical or surgical treatment. Indications for laboratory investigations include skin lesions of the oral commissure and lips, any mass or discharge within the oral cavity, and facial swelling.

Cytological examination of swellings, discharges from eyes, nostrils and wounds, body fluids, or mouth and pharyngeal smears can give additional information about the nature and the aetiology of a process or clinical sign. Cytological samples can be obtained using a cotton swab or by aspiration from the mouth or lesion. A stained smear can give a good representation of the number and 'quality' of microorganisms present in a lesion. Aerobic and anaerobic culture should be performed in indicated cases to obtain as much information as possible.

Biopsy is one of the most reliable and informative diagnostic tools available, whether it involves cytology or incisional or excisional histopathology. With most lesions, a biopsy sample should be full-depth and include some of the normal margin.

Indications for radiography or CT scanning

Ideally, a complete radiographic study of the skull (see Chapter 4) should be performed in all cases of suspected or confirmed dental disease in rabbits. Bone loss, subgingival tooth crowns, apical elongation of the incisors, premolars or molars, periapical inflammation or jaw osteomyelitis may be seen on radiographs, and may not be revealed during physical or intraoral examination. Other common indications for skull or teeth radiography are head trauma and the presence of ocular discharge. Radiography is also commonly used in cases that require tooth extraction to evaluate possible inflammatory and dysplastic apical changes or ankylosis. Intraoral placement of dental films/sensors allows visualization of dental structures with minimal superimposition of other structures (see Chapter 3).

CT scanning is very helpful in cases of facial odontogenic abscesses or osteomyelitis because it allows exact lesion localization, proper surgical planning and determination of prognosis. CT images also allow evaluation of individual teeth and alveolar bone from several positions and angles (see Chapter 9).

Significant lesions and oral cavity diseases

Inherited diseases and variations

Mandibular prognathism (brachygnathia superior) is an inherited disease in some dwarf-breed rabbits, but it can also be seen in larger rabbits. Mandibular prognathism is an autosomal recessive trait. Abnormal elongation of the incisors is a result of abnormally large mandibles. This disease is seen in very young rabbits and should not be confused with acquired incisor malocclusion. Absence of second incisors or upper premolars is seen in some rabbits. No treatment is usually necessary.

Supernumerary incisors may appear between the 1st and 2nd incisors. This rare inherited condition is considered to be caused by a single recessive gene. Treatment is based on the clinical signs. If any incisor malocclusion is present secondary to tooth crowding, extraction of supernumerary teeth is indicated.

Achondroplasia, spina bifida with cleft palate and osteopetrosis are very rare conditions that may also be associated with oral cavity pathology.

Soft tissue diseases

Viral diseases

Rabbits with myxomatosis, which is caused by leporipoxvirus, commonly show clinical signs of apathy, anorexia, epiphora, blepharospasm, dyspnoea and fibrous swellings of the subcutaneous tissues throughout the body, typically on the eyelids and genitalia. Secondary respiratory infection is very common. The virus is transmitted via blood-sucking arthropods, including mosquitoes, fleas, lice, ticks and mites. Direct transmission is possible, usually by aerosol or direct contact. In some cases, the lips are swollen, with mild to severe haemorrhage in the gingiva or on the mucosal surface of the nasal philtrum (Figure 25.12). The severity of the lesions depends on viral strain and the immune status of the individual. The final diagnosis is based on clinical signs and on skin biopsy findings or post-mortem examination. In mild to severe cases, the animal is generally euthanased owing to the high contagiousness of the disease and progressive worsening of the clinical signs. In very rare cases and if only minor changes are present, the animal may be kept indoors and isolated from other rabbits. Any contact with vectors should be prevented and care should be taken to prevent mechanical transmission to other rabbits through contamination of clothing, dishes and other cage equipment. Supportive care and broad-spectrum antibiotics will prevent secondary bacterial infection. The best way to prevent myxomatosis is to control insect vectors and to use regular vaccination.

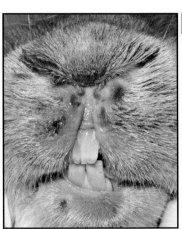

25.12
Superficial skin haemorrhages located on the lips and nasal philtrum in a rabbit with myxomatosis.

Oral papillomatosis (Figure 25.13) is caused by oral papillomavirus. The infection is transmitted through direct contact, with a high prevalence in young rabbits, and is reported sporadically in pet rabbits. This transmissible disease is characterized by slowly growing small white to pink wart-like sessile or pedunculate lesions, which are located behind the lower incisors, in the sublingual space or on the surface of the tongue. The polyps cause little or no discomfort and do not interfere with eating in most cases. Diagnosis is based on biopsy followed by histopathology, immunohistochemistry and electron microscopy. Therapy consists of surgical excision; or no treatment may be necessary. Most papillomas regress spontaneously within 2–3 months.

Bacterial diseases
Rabbit syphilis is caused by the spirochaete *Treponema cuniculi*. Characteristic lesions include ulcerative to crusting dermatitis of the genitalia,

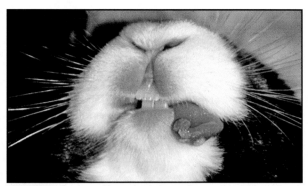

25.13 Oral papillomatosis in an 8-month-old female Dutch rabbit. The lesion was an incidental finding during oral examination when the rabbit was anaesthetized for ovariohysterectomy. There were no clinical signs. (Courtesy of Frances Harcourt-Brown)

perineum, nose and lips (Figure 25.14). Transmission is venereal or from mother to young. The diagnosis is based on clinical signs and on visualization of the organism in dark-field preparations of exudate from active lesions. Therapy is based on intramuscular administration of penicillin G (40,000 IU/kg q24h for 5 days, or 50–60,000 IU/kg once weekly for three treatments).

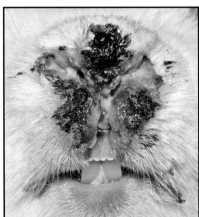

25.14
Rabbit syphilis affecting the nose and lips. Infected lesions caused by trauma can imitate this condition.

Deep dermatitis (Figure 25.15) is generally caused by multiple bacteria. Treatment consists of long-term antibiotic administration and local treatment with antiseptics.

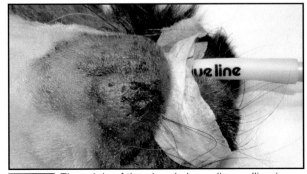

25.15 The origin of the chronic lower lip swelling in this patient was unclear. Histopathological examination of a skin biopsy specimen showed pyogranulomatous deep dermatitis of the lower lip.

Fungal diseases

Trichophyton mentagrophytes and *Microsporum canis* are the most common fungal species diagnosed in rabbits. Clinical signs include round alopecic regions with excessive crusting. The lesions typically occur on the ears, head and feet. The diagnosis is based on trichoscopy, skin scrapings mounted in 10% potassium hydroxide, and fungal culture. Treatment must include good hygiene and the client should be warned of the zoonotic potential of the disease.

Wet dermatitis

Superficial inflammation of the lips, oral commissure or chin (see Figure 25.7a) is a secondary condition, and is usually associated with excessive salivation and skin irritation due to dental disease, stomatitis, tongue infection or electrical burn injury (see below). Rarely, rabbits that are stained regularly with water from a drinking bottle, or those kept under conditions of poor hygiene, may also develop wet dermatitis. Greenish fur discoloration may be associated with *Pseudomonas aeruginosa* infection. Treatment is aimed at solving the underlying problem and supportive care.

Electrical burn injury

A rabbit that chews on live electric cables can burn its mouth. Electric shock can cause severe damage to the tissues of the mouth and may result in pulmonary oedema, characterized by breathing problems. The extent of damage depends upon the duration of exposure. Therapy consists of close monitoring of cardiorespiratory function and patient stabilization. A combination of non-steroidal anti-inflammatory drugs and opioids is used for analgesia. The wound and the oral cavity are washed with cold saline or chlorhexidine, with the use of an astringent agent (tannin). A first-degree burn causes the skin to become red, slightly swollen and painful. It usually heals in about 2–5 days. A second-degree burn is deeper and there is blistering. These burns are extremely painful. If there is no infection, healing is usually complete in 3 weeks. Immediately after the injury, it is difficult to assess the potential viability of the affected area. In these cases the wound is re-evaluated regularly until it is healed, and any superficial necrotic tissue is surgically debrided 2–10 days after the injury. In severe cases, oral force-feeding or feeding via nasogastric tube is necessary. Third-degree burns, which involve the full thickness of the skin and part of the subcutaneous tissue, cause very painful lesions that eventually form escharotic crusts. In such cases the rostral part of the tongue may need to be amputated, or plastic surgery of the lips or skin may be performed after formation of the final eschar. Antibiotics are administered in severe cases.

Tongue pathology

In addition to thermal injury, a wide range of diseases can affect the tongue. Like those of the gingiva, many problems of the tongue are extensions of oral problems, such as ulcerative stomatitis. Sharp spikes at the lingual surfaces of the mandibular premolars and molars commonly lacerate the tongue and cause erosions or ulceration. Scar formation is seen in severe cases, even after occlusal adjustment. Traumatic injury to the tongue due to foreign body penetration results in glossitis, with oedema of the tip of the tongue. Iatrogenic injury to the tongue or other soft tissues can occur owing to poor control of dental instruments (see Chapter 26). The clinical signs include anorexia, excessive salivation and chewing of the tongue. Intraoral examination shows that the tongue is swollen, hard on palpation, red to black in colour, with a necrotic mucosal surface and/ or erosive to ulcerative changes. In some cases nodules filled with pus are present.

In the case of actinobacillosis ('wooden tongue'), the tongue becomes indurated, shrunken and immobile (Figure 25.16). The diagnosis is based on oral cavity examination, histopathology, cytology and microbiological analyses. Therapy is similar to that for electrical burn injury; in severe cases surgical amputation of the rostral part of the tongue may be necessary. Tetracycline or tilmicosin are considered the antibiotics of choice.

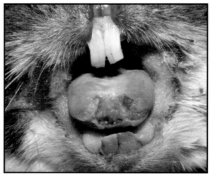

25.16
Lingual actinobacillosis.

Gingival disease

Gingival inflammation is characterized by increased redness, swelling, and bleeding of the gingiva on probing. Gingivitis in rabbits is usually secondary to periodontal disease or soft tissue laceration caused by sharp spikes on the premolars and molars.

Gingival hyperplasia involves proliferation of the gingiva as a result of chronic traumatic irritation or a chronic inflammatory process (Figure 25.17). If the proliferation affects the vicinity of the tooth, this hyperplastic tissue forms deep pseudo-pockets that are predisposed to food impaction, with secondary periodontal inflammation.

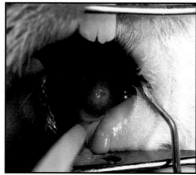

25.17 Local gingival hyperplasia due to chronic gingival irritation caused by elongated maxillary left premolars. Radiography and histopathological examination should be performed in such cases to exclude neoplasia.

Salivary gland disease
Salivary gland disease is a rare condition in rabbits and includes sialoadenitis and sialocele formation; the latter is a cystic structure that develops following salivary duct blockage. Inflammatory changes could be secondary to odontogenic abscessation or osteomyelitis. The diagnosis is based on clinical examination, aspirate examination and histopathology; therapy is surgical.

Chin gland disease
The rabbit chin gland (mental gland, submandibular gland) is a scent gland that is located under the chin (Figure 25.18). The most common disorder of these glands is inflammation and associated skin fistulation. This rare inflammatory process may be secondary to an odontogenic abscess, or primary, due to the presence of a foreign body. Therapy consists of surgical debridement and excision of the affected gland.

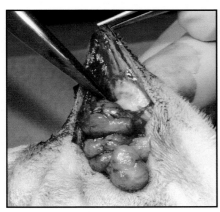

25.18 The chin scent glands are located in the intermandibular area (see Chapter 29).

Teeth and skull
A common consequence of acquired dental disease in rabbits is elongation and malocclusion of the incisors, premolars and molars. Periapical infection, with subsequent osteomyelitis and facial abscess formation, is much more prevalent in rabbits than in other herbivorous species with elodont dentition.

Particular dental diseases are described in detail in other chapters.

Neoplastic disease
Neoplastic lesions of the oral cavity can occur. They include fibroblastic osteosarcoma of the upper lip, mandibular and maxillary osteosarcoma, mandibular mucoepidermal carcinoma and ameloblastic fibroma. Odontomas, which represent abnormal development of dental tissues and consist of enamel, dentin and cementum, are considered to be pseudotumorous (hamartomatous) lesions and are seen in rabbits. Diagnosis is based on clinical examination, radiography, CT and histopathology. The therapeutic approach and prognosis depend on the tumour type.

References and further reading
Capello V (2006) The dental suite: equipment needed for handling small exotic mammals. *Journal of Exotic Pet Medicine* **15**, 106–115
Capello V, Gracis M and Lennox AM (2005) *Rabbit and Rodent Dentistry Handbook*. Zoological Education Network, Lake Worth
Crossley DA (2003) Oral biology and disorders of lagomorphs. *Veterinary Clinics of North America: Exotic Animal Practice* **6**, 625–659
Dorrestein GM (2007) Cytology and biopsies (histology) as diagnostic tools in oral cavity problems in exotic animals. *Proceedings of the CAZWV Veterinary Dentistry Conference on Exotic Pets, 4–6 May 2007, Brno, Czech Republic*, pp.29–30
Harcourt-Brown F (2002) *Textbook of Rabbit Medicine*. Reed Education and Professional Publishing, Oxford
Hirschfeld Z, Weinreb MM and Michaeli Y (1973) Incisors of the rabbit: morphology, histology and development. *Journal of Dental Research* **52**, 377–384
Jekl V, Hauptman K and Knotek Z (2008) Quantitative and qualitative assessments of intraoral lesions in 180 small herbivorous mammals. *Veterinary Record* **162**, 442–449
Jekl V and Knotek Z (2007) Evaluation of a laryngoscope and a rigid endoscope for the examination of the oral cavity of small mammals. *Veterinary Record* **160**, 9–13
Lennox AM (2008) Clinical technique: small exotic companion mammal dentistry – anesthetic considerations. *Journal of Exotic Pet Medicine* **17**, 102–106
Lindsey JR and Fox RR (1994) Inherited diseases and variations. In: *The Biology of the Laboratory Rabbit, 2nd edn*, ed. PJ Manning *et al.*, pp. 293–320. Academic Press, San Diego
Verstraete FJM and Osofsky A (2005) Dentistry in pet rabbits. *Compendium on Continuing Education for the Practicing Veterinarian* **9**, 671–684
Wiggs RB and Lobprise HB (1997) *Veterinary Dentistry: Principles and Practice*. Lippincott-Raven, Philadelphia

TECHNIQUE 25.1 ➜

TECHNIQUE 25.1:
Oral cavity examination under general anaesthesia

Patient positioning and preparation

General anaesthesia is required (see Chapter 1). Position the rabbit in sternal recumbency with its head and neck held horizontally. Ideally, mouth gags should be used because of possible iatrogenic injury to the temporomandibular joint, mandibles, incisors and gingiva.

Assistant

An assistant is required to hold the anaesthetic equipment and the horizontal mouth gag.

Additional instruments

- Mouth gag
- Cheek dilator
- Paediatric laryngoscope
- Dental spatula
- Light source (if not integral to instrument)
- Endoscopic equipment

Technique

1 The lips, oral cavity commissures and surrounding mucosal surface and skin are inspected thoroughly.

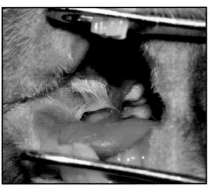

A hairy area is normal on the medial part of both lip commissures.

2 The mandible, maxilla and all other superficial skull bones are palpated for the presence of any irregularity or apical tooth elongation.

3 To perform the oral examination well and safely, it is necessary to open the rabbit's mouth in both horizontal and vertical directions:
- Special rabbit or rodent mouth gags are inserted between maxillary and mandibular incisors and the mouth is opened in a vertical direction
- Cheek dilators are used to open the mouth cavity in a horizontal direction
- An alternative to mouth gags is special table-top dental equipment designed for rabbits.

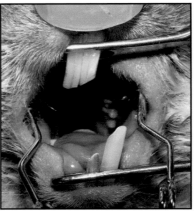

Oral cavity examination under general anaesthesia is facilitated by the use of mouth and cheek dilators. Oxygen flow to the nostrils of the patient is not interrupted during the procedure.

4 Intraoral inspection: Thorough oral cavity examination comprises a combination of evaluation of the teeth, periodontium, soft tissues and tongue, and data recording. Each tooth should be examined individually, along with its supportive structures. It is possible to examine the mouth cavity with the naked eye or with the use of rigid endoscopy. The author recommends using the same approach each time to avoid missing any pathology. Complete intraoral inspection consists of evaluation of:
- All surfaces of all maxillary and mandibular incisors, peg teeth included
- The dorsal part of the oral cavity, incisive papilla, palatine rugae, soft palate and gingiva
- The number of teeth
- The clinical crowns of all the teeth
- Tooth colour – brown pigmentation of the occlusal surfaces is normal and is caused by the presence of natural pigment in the herbivore's diet
- Tooth shape
- Tooth position
- Tooth structure, including the presence or absence of enamel or striations
- Fractures or resorptive lesions
- Clinical crown size
- Tooth surface
- Tooth mobility.

TECHNIQUE 25.1 continued:
Oral cavity examination under general anaesthesia

5 Gingival sulcus probing: The gingival sulcus is a space between the gingival margin and the tooth and can be up to 1 mm in depth for the premolars and molars in a normal rabbit. The periodontal probe is inserted gently and without force into the gingival sulcus, to the depth of the epithelial attachment. Any unnecessary force could cause damage to the epithelial attachment, and pain. Based on clinician preference, the teeth are palpated and the gingival sulci probed during the examination or at the end of the procedure.

6 Evaluation of the interdental spaces (the distance between two adjacent teeth).

7 Inspecting the right buccal vestibule. A dental spatula or paediatric laryngoscope can be used to push aside the buccal gingiva from the buccal teeth surfaces, which allows proper examination.

8 Evaluation of all the visible surfaces of right mandibular cheek teeth.

9 All the procedures are repeated on the left side of the oral cavity.

10 The tongue is pushed down to determine whether there are any sharp spikes on the labial parts of both mandibular arcades. If this pathology is present the affected side is evaluated and the other side is inspected after adjustment of crown size and occlusion. If no obvious pathology is present, the tongue is pushed aside with a dental spatula to allow proper visualization of the buccal gingival sulcus and gingiva.

11 The right lateral and right sublingual surfaces are examined while holding the tongue gently with anatomical forceps.

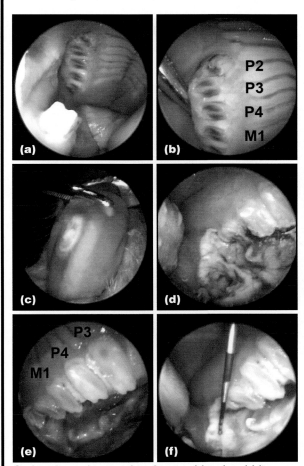

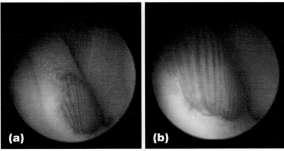

(a) On both ventrolateral sides of the tongue there is a red area near the lingual base which is normal, not pathological. **(b)** A more detailed view.

12 The soft tissues are evaluated for:

- Colour
- Swelling
- Hyperplasia
- Erosive and ulcerative lesions
- Gingivitis and stomatitis
- Food impaction
- Foreign bodies
- Purulent discharge.

Oral cavity endoscopy in a 3-year-old male rabbit. Examination revealed: **(a,b)** mild widening of interdental spaces between the premolars and molars in the maxillary right dental arcade; **(c)** lingual erosion; **(d,e,f)** severe stomatitis of the left buccal vestibule, and changes to the occlusal surfaces and buccal elongation of the entire left maxillary arcade. Palpation of the teeth and necrotic material did not show any association with odontogenic abscess.

TECHNIQUE 25.1 continued:
Oral cavity examination under general anaesthesia

Rigid endoscopy

The oral cavity examination is performed in the same way as described above, but the oral structures are magnified, which facilitates close examination of all parts of the oral cavity.

A viewing angle of 30 degrees allows visualization outside the axis of the endoscope. The field of view may be increased by rotation of the instrument, which makes it possible to examine all the parts of the oral cavity and oropharynx in detail. Surface lesions on the premolar and molar teeth and on the mucosal surfaces of the gingiva, tongue and hard palate may be detected. A viewing angle of 70 degrees provides excellent views of the mucosal or tooth surfaces, especially the ventral regions of the oral cavity, and in particular the occlusal surfaces of the mandibular teeth, the mucosal surface of the tongue and the caudal parts of the oropharynx.

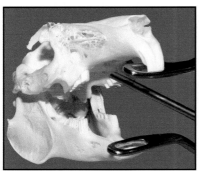

Endoscopy with the use of rigid endoscopes at 30 degrees (top) and 70 degrees (bottom) greatly enhances visualization of all intraoral structures.

1 With the endoscope held in a straight position, the mandibular and maxillary incisors are evaluated.

2 The soft tissues of the oral cavity and the maxillary cheek teeth are evaluated as described above. The author prefers to hold the endoscope in his right hand, while the periodontal probe or dental spatula is manipulated by the left hand.

3 Visualization of buccal or lingual cheek teeth surfaces and the cheeks is enhanced when the endoscope is rotated slightly (approximately 30–90 degrees), depending on the area of interest.

4 For evaluation of the occlusal surface of the mandibular cheek teeth and the dorsal lingual surface, the endoscope is rotated through 180 degrees.

5 The endoscope is used for direct tooth illumination and sometimes for transillumination, which is possible in some individuals. Transillumination allows evaluation of the tooth for colour changes (haemorrhage), opacity (non-vital teeth) and resorptive pathology (greater translucency).

6 Some common surgical interventions, such as the collection of biopsy specimens or swab samples, removal of foreign objects, intraoral wound debridement and correction of malocclusions in indicated cases, can be carried out under endoscopic control, which allows clear visualization of the operative site and minimizes the risk of iatrogenic injury.

7 Endoscopy can also be used in cases of periapical/odontogenic abscess to inspect the wound after debridement, or to allow the clinician to perform rhinoscopy and clean up the infection caused by odontogenic nasal fistulae.

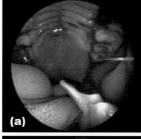
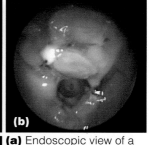
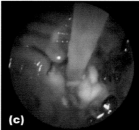

(a) Endoscopic view of a rabbit with obvious spike formation at the mandibular right 2nd cheek tooth. **(b,c)** Intraoral views of a rabbit with a retrobulbar abscess and flushing of the cavity with a tomcat catheter.

26

Treatment of dental problems: principles and options

Frances Harcourt-Brown

Rabbit dentistry is a controversial topic and many types of treatment have been described. At the time of writing, there are no published comparative studies that evaluate the success or failure of any particular dental treatment for rabbits and it is difficult to envisage how such a study could be conducted. As a result, treatment strategies are anecdotal and are based on dental techniques in other species and the perceived aetiopathogenesis of dental disease in rabbits, which is still unclear (although the sequence of events and pathological changes that take place are documented and described in Chapter 24). The purpose of this chapter is to discuss the indications for treatment and to describe the various techniques that are available in order to enable the practitioner to decide for themselves about their approach.

Considerations for treatment

Frequency of examination and treatment

Regular conscious dental checks are vital for any rabbit with a history of dental disease. The timing of these checks is dependent on the owner's needs, the progress of the rabbit's dental problems and the clinician's experience. The frequency of dental examination can be modified as the rate of progress of that individual pet's disease becomes apparent. Knowing what an individual rabbit's teeth looked like originally is an advantage. Keeping detailed records of dental procedures and taking skull radiographs are important to monitor the rabbit's progress (see Chapter 23).

Opinions differ about when rabbits with a history of dental disease should be booked in for treatment. One approach is to be proactive and perform elective dentistry before problems occur. An alternative approach is to rely on the owners to decide when treatment is necessary. Many owners are aware of the warning signs that indicate that their rabbit needs dental treatment and are often happier to bring the rabbit in for treatment as soon as it starts to show problems rather than to have elective treatment every few weeks.

The owner's wishes

Many owners are concerned about the effects of repeated anaesthesia and dental surgery on their pet. If dental pathology is detected, the decision to perform dental intervention can only be made with their support and understanding of the need for treatment. Prepared skulls, skull models, radiographs, photos or video recordings that were taken during previous dental procedures can be of great assistance during these discussions. The owner's trust in their veterinary surgeon's opinion is paramount because they are unable to examine their rabbit's cheek teeth for themselves and, to them, their rabbit may appear healthy. Cost is also an issue. In some cases, dentistry may be required every few months and the long-term cost of this is not inconsiderable. Euthanasia is an option that requires consideration for rabbits with dental problems. It is always a difficult decision because dentistry is usually successful in restoring the rabbit's appetite and alleviating other clinical signs. However, remission of signs may be short. Radiography and supportive care may also be necessary, which adds to the cost. Some owners cannot afford repeated treatment or feel that the discomfort the rabbit goes through prior to dentistry is unacceptable, so they opt for euthanasia. If they don't, any treatment plan requires their support and cooperation. Long-term management is required (see Chapter 30).

How much and what sort of dental treatment is necessary?

Examination of the oral cavity is an important part of any routine clinical examination of rabbits but it can be difficult to decide when a rabbit with dental pathology actually requires intervention. Dental treatment is always necessary for rabbits showing obvious signs of discomfort associated with their teeth, such as oral pain, salivation, eating difficulties, secondary dermatitis, weight loss or any disruption in normal behaviour. However, not all rabbits with dental pathology show signs of disease. Some rabbits can go through all the stages of the progressive syndrome of acquired dental disease (PSADD) without showing any obvious clinical signs and end up with non-growing or absent crowns that may be incidental findings during clinical examination (see Chapter 24). The visual abnormalities of the oral cavity that require treatment are shown in Figure 26.1; examination of the oral cavity under anaesthetic may be necessary for full visual assessment of the changes that are present.

Abnormality		Treatment and prognosis
Mandibular cheek tooth spur This is the most common indication for dentistry. Spurs are due to curvature of teeth and can cause considerable painful soft tissue damage to the tongue. The 2nd, 3rd and 4th mandibular teeth are most likely to be affected	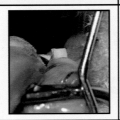	The spur can be removed easily with molar clippers or dental burrs. There is debate about whether occlusal adjustment is required (see text). If the teeth are still growing, the tooth can regrow in 4–6 weeks. If tooth growth is slowing, the interval is longer. Eventual cessation of tooth growth occurs in the majority of cases. Removal of the pulp arrests tooth growth and prevents recurrence. Extraction is difficult
Spur on a short crown This condition is unusual but is very problematical. It is easy to miss the abnormality on conscious oral examination. The condition is very painful because the spur impinges on the thin buccal mucosa	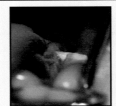	Molar clippers are safer than dental burrs for removing these spurs because of the proximity of soft tissue. Success of treatment can be short-lived, as the teeth are so curved that they only need to grow 1–2 mm before they impinge on the mucosa again; so repeat dentistry may be required in 2–3 weeks. Pulpectomy is indicated
Maxillary cheek tooth spur On the upper arcade, spurs most commonly form on the first two cheek teeth. Clinical signs may not be severe. The crowns can penetrate the mucosa on the inside of the cheek and cause discomfort or abscesses. Food can become caught around the teeth	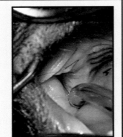	These spurs can be removed with molar cutters or dental burrs. In many cases the crown needs shortening and reshaping, and burrs may be preferable as they are less likely to shatter the tooth. Pulpectomy is not an option owing to the inaccessibility of the apex, but extraction is feasible and straightforward. The rate of growth of the maxillary teeth is slower than that of the mandibular teeth so these spurs tend to regrow slowly and require infrequent treatment. In the later stages of PSADD, fracture of the exposed crowns of these teeth is common; the fragment can easily be removed and the tooth will not regrow
Abnormalities of the last (5th) mandibular cheek teeth Elongation, mobility or deviation of these teeth can cause considerable soft tissue damage and pain. The changes cannot be seen during conscious oral examination	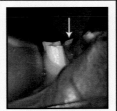	Elongated crowns can be trimmed with molar cutters. The teeth are small and can be transected without shattering. Mobile or displaced teeth can be extracted, although there is a real risk of haemorrhage that will need to be controlled. The prognosis is good after treatment. These teeth seldom seem to regrow to cause further problems
Mucosal pocket next to 1st and 2nd maxillary cheek teeth In some rabbits, deep pockets form alongside the upper mandibular cheek teeth. Impacted food collects in them	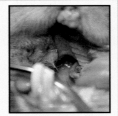	The crowns of the teeth that are adjacent to the pocket need to be shortened or the teeth can be extracted (see recommendations above for spurs on the maxillary cheek teeth)
Elongation of caudal mandibular cheek teeth Abnormal wear on a caudal mandibular cheek tooth can result in a pointed crown (white arrow) that digs into the opposing mucosa and causes ulceration (black arrow). This abnormality cannot be seen during conscious oral examination	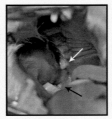	The condition is easily resolved by trimming the point off the mandibular cheek tooth with molar cutters or burrs
Erosive lesions Erosions can develop in the enamel, which may be filled with hyperplastic granulation tissue or gingival mucosa. These lesions are not painful and are a feature of late dental disease when the teeth are no longer growing	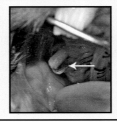	These lesions can be treated by trimming off the hyperplastic tissue and treating the crown. In many cases the crown will pull off because it has fractured or is about to fracture just below the gum line. Alternatively, it can be burred off

26.1 Abnormalities detected during oral examination that require dental treatment. (continues) ▶

Abnormality		Treatment and prognosis
Disintegrating broken crowns In the later stages of dental disease, the quality of the teeth is so poor that the crowns disintegrate and break at the level of the gum. Periodontal infection is common and there may be inflammation and pus around the tooth remnants	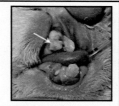	This condition is easily resolved by removing the loose tooth from the socket. In some cases involving disintegrating incisors, it can be helpful to transect the tooth below the gum margin so there is some loose gingiva to heal across the socket. It is vital to ensure that all fragments of tooth, no matter how small, are removed
Mandibular cheek tooth spur growing into the cheek In the later stages of dental disease, rotation of the teeth can result in spurs that deviate towards the cheek rather than the tongue. They usually develop on the 4th mandibular cheek tooth and can only be detected during thorough oral examination under anaesthesia	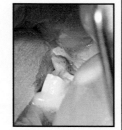	These spurs tend to form in the later stages of dental disease when tooth growth is slow. They can be removed with molar cutters or burrs, although cutters may be preferable because of the inaccessibility of the spurs and proximity of soft tissue. Regrowth is rare but if it the spurs do keep regrowing, pulpectomy is an option
Ulcerating mucosal flaps In rabbits with short crowns on the cheek teeth to keep the buccal mucosa in the correct position, flaps of mucosa can catch on the teeth and become hypertrophied, ulcerated and painful. Affected rabbits often spend time moving their mouths and salivating	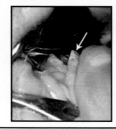	This is a difficult condition to treat. The flaps can be trimmed off, but in many cases long-term management is necessary because the rabbit is in the advanced stages of dental disease (see Chapter 30)

26.1 (continued) Abnormalities detected during oral examination that require dental treatment.

Establishing a treatment plan

A diagnosis of dental disease is made in any rabbit that shows any abnormality in the shape, structure or position of one or more teeth, including the section that is buried in the jaw. The surrounding bone may also be affected. Once the diagnosis is made, a treatment plan needs to be established, which can be difficult. Several types of dental pathology might be present in the same animal. Radiography, computed tomography (CT) and magnetic resonance imaging (MRI) are ancillary diagnostic procedures that can yield more information about the nature and extent of the dental abnormalities (see Chapters 4 and 9). The significance of the abnormalities needs to be assessed in order to decide on the treatment.

Treatment depends on the nature of the dental abnormality that is present. The aims of treatment are to:

- Alleviate pain and discomfort
- Reduce further problems and the frequency of dental intervention
- Avoid iatrogenic damage, i.e. to do no harm.

CASE EXAMPLE

This lateral view of the skull is from a 5-year-old male neutered Dwarf Lop rabbit presented for sudden anorexia that was fed on muesli mix, grated carrot and cereal treats. In the past he had undergone repeated shortening of the incisors with a dental burr. He had bilateral epiphora and had recently developed eating difficulties. He was anaesthetized to undergo oral examination and radiography, and to decide upon a treatment plan.

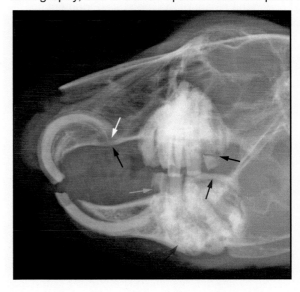

- There are generalized changes in all the teeth (malocclusion, apical elongation and dental dysplasia). The rabbit is showing typical signs of advanced dental disease. These changes are not reversible.
- The pulp cavities on the cheek teeth are not visible and it is difficult to identify individual

roots; there are no enamel lines or alveolar bone (green arrow), which means that the cheek teeth are no longer growing. Any spurs or elongated crowns on the cheek teeth will not regrow after treatment, which is beneficial.

- The incisors are misshapen and maloccluded, and the presence of an open pulp cavity (white arrow) suggests they are growing, albeit slowly. This may influence any decision to extract or reshape these teeth.

- There is apical elongation of the upper 1st incisors, with thinning and deformity of the palatine bone (purple arrow), which suggests blockage of one or both nasolacrimal ducts. If epiphora or dacryocystitis is present, the nasolacrimal duct should be flushed.

- There is an erosive lesion in the subgingival crown of the 1st mandibular cheek tooth (blue arrow). This tooth is not growing and will probably fracture in the not too distant future, but a decision is needed about whether to treat the erosion. The crown could be removed with a dental burr or left alone because it is unlikely to be a cause of discomfort.

- The 5th mandibular cheek tooth is very deformed and growing along the occlusal surfaces of the mandibular teeth (red arrow). Pus and food were collecting around it and the gingiva was inflamed, so the decision to treat this tooth is simple: the abnormal crown has to be removed to make the rabbit comfortable. The crown can be trimmed with burrs or clippers or the whole tooth can be extracted.

- The exposed crown of the 5th maxillary cheek tooth was mobile and it is probable that this was the cause of the rabbit's sudden eating difficulties. A fracture line can be seen (black arrow). This crown can be easily pulled off, which will ease the rabbit's discomfort.

- There is an area of radiolucency around a deformed root of a 4th mandibular cheek tooth, which indicates infection. The area of lucency is surrounded by a curved radiodense line (yellow arrow), which is probably the edge of a bony abscess cavity.

Establishing the treatment plan

Discussions with the owner
Euthanasia was considered, but the rabbit was not thin and had only recently developed eating difficulties. The owners were attached to him but funds were limited. MRI/CT scanning would have been ideal and informative but the cost of the procedure was prohibitive for the owners. Nearby facilities were not available. The owners opted for essential treatment.

Essential treatment
1. Remove the loose crown fragment from the 5th maxillary tooth.
2. Shorten and reshape the incisors with a dental burr or cutting disc.

3. Remove the elongated crown of the 5th mandibular tooth, either by trimming or extraction (see Chapter 27).
4. Remove any sharp edges or spurs that might impinge on neighbouring soft tissue. This can be done with handheld instruments or burrs.
5. Flush the tear ducts (see Chapter 28).
6. Cut out the muesli mixes and modify the diet to one that the rabbit is able to eat but that provides more fibre (see Chapter 30).

Optional treatment
1. Incisor extraction. This would resolve the incisor malocclusion but could be difficult: the lower incisors could be ankylosed into the bone. It might be easier to continue reshaping the upper teeth. An incidental consideration is that incisor extraction can make any future work on the cheek teeth difficult because it might be hard to keep a gag in place.
2. Treat the erosive lesion by removing the crown with a burr.
3. Investigate and treat the periapical abscess surrounding the 4th mandibular cheek tooth. At the time of examination the abscess was not clinically obvious. Ideally it should be treated but the surgery would be invasive, as the buried fragment of tooth would need to be removed. This procedure could be carried out if the abscess were to become a problem; meanwhile palliative treatment might be administered (see Chapter 29).
4. Coronal reduction. The aim of this treatment is to restore normal height and occlusal angle to the exposed crowns. It would not be successful in this case.
5. Long-term analgesia. It is difficult to know how much pain this rabbit will be in once the immediate problems of the broken and elongated crowns have been treated. It is probable that sensation is lost in the teeth without pulp cavities as the nerve supply to the tooth will have been lost, but there could be soft tissue discomfort. A trial course of oral meloxicam would allow the owner to decide whether their rabbit seemed 'happier' with analgesia and the decision to prescribe long-term analgesia could then be based on the owner's appraisal.

Treatment of fractured teeth and jaws

Fractured incisors can be the result of a rabbit falling on its face on to a hard surface or pulling at cage bars. If the incisors were normal before the trauma occurred, they may grow back to their normal shape and position. The rate of growth is 2–3 mm per week. It is important to keep shortening and reshaping the opposing incisors periodically, until the fractured teeth start to occlude with them again; otherwise an acquired malocclusion can develop. A burr or diamond cutting disc is required for this procedure.

Fractured cheek teeth are more serious than fractured incisors because malocclusion, periapical infection and abscesses can ensue. These cases need monitoring. Fractured cheek teeth may be the result of trauma or of chewing hard substances. Occasionally, splits in the exposed crowns of the cheek teeth may be encountered that will grow out (Figure 26.2).

Fractured jaws can be the result of periapical infection and abscessation (see Chapter 29) or the result of trauma. Treatment of jaw fractures is described in Chapter 22.

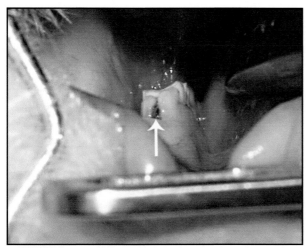

26.2 This 3-year-old male neutered rabbit was presented with acute anorexia. This longitudinal split in the crown of the 1st mandibular cheek tooth (arrow) was discovered during examination under anaesthesia. Only the exposed crown was affected, so the rabbit was treated with analgesia and nutritional support. He made a full recovery and the defect grew out over the following 6 weeks.

Treatment of incisor malocclusion

There are three options for treating incisor malocclusion:

- Trimming with handheld clippers
- Cutting and reshaping the teeth with dental burrs or a cutting disc
- Extraction.

The choice of treatment depends on the cause of the malocclusion and the stage of dental disease.

Extraction is often the best option in rabbits with incisors that do not occlude at all, but are still growing at a normal rate, because shortening or reshaping the teeth will only offer a temporary solution as the crowns rapidly regrow. Rapid regrowth occurs because the teeth are not subjected to any opposing pressure either at rest or during chewing. As there is no occlusal pressure, the teeth erupt and grow more quickly than those that are in occlusion (Ness, 1956).

Reshaping, rather than extraction, is indicated for teeth that are in partial occlusion (see Operative

Technique 26.1) or are only growing slowly because they are in the later stages of dental disease. Incisors that are affected by PSADD are often misshapen, so extraction is more difficult but may be unnecessary if the teeth have stopped growing.

Trimming with handheld clippers

Although this procedure is quick and easy, it is inadvisable to trim incisors with handheld clippers. There is little or no control over the final shape of the teeth and, if they are covered in healthy enamel (e.g. in cases of congenital malocclusion, or in the early stages of PSADD), the teeth will shatter and this leaves sharp edges that may expose the pulp cavity (Figure 26.3). Occasionally, in the later stages of PSADD (see Chapter 24), when the teeth may have little or no enamel, it can be quick and simple to trim a sliver of misshapen tooth with clippers (Figure 26.4) but it is never wise to transect the whole crown.

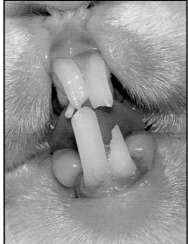

26.3 Owners sometimes trim their rabbit's teeth with nail clippers. This procedure is not recommended. Transecting the crown in this way can shatter the tooth and leave sharp edges and exposed dentine, as in this rabbit's left mandibular incisor.

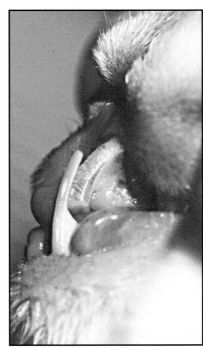

26.4 Although it is not acceptable to transect an enamelled crown with clippers, it is possible to remove slivers of tooth with handheld instruments. Molar cutters can be used without shattering the teeth. The long narrow section of the mandibular incisor shown here was clipped off.

Cutting and reshaping incisors with burrs or a diamond disc

The rabbit needs to be well restrained. Wrapping the rabbit in a towel and restraining it on its back to evoke a dorsal immobility response (see Appendix 4) can be effective. Some practitioners may prefer to sedate the rabbit.

The procedure (Figure 26.5) does not shatter the teeth and gives greater control over their final shape. The crowns should be reduced to as close to their natural shape as possible, bearing in mind that the pulp cavity may extend further than normal in overgrown incisors (Hobson, 2006). With the correct equipment, the procedure is quick and easy, although there is a risk of iatrogenic injury to surrounding soft tissues. The choice between a cutting disc and a burr depends on the practitioner and the equipment that is available. Both pieces of equipment can cause soft tissue damage, although this risk is higher with a cutting disc, especially if the crowns are completely transected. An alternative method is to use the disc to cut a deep groove in the crowns, at the desired height, and use molar cutters to snap through the remaining 0.5 mm or so. If burrs are used, a fissure burr is the most effective.

Another technique for correcting mild cases of incisor malocclusion where the upper and lower teeth are still in contact (Vladimir Jekl, personal communication) is described in Operative Technique 26.1.

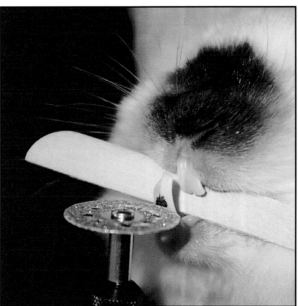

26.5 Cutting incisors with a cutting disc. Most rabbits will tolerate incisor shortening with power tools while they are conscious, although it is stressful for them. Some sort of gag is necessary to keep the mouth slightly open; a tongue depressor was used here but a 2 ml syringe is an alternative. The author prefers to make a deep groove in the teeth with a diamond cutting disc and then to snap the excess crown away by applying molar cutters across the groove. This reduces the risk of soft tissue damage from the disc as it goes through the tooth. The disc can also be used to smooth off any sharp edges that remain, although this is seldom necessary. Incisors can also be shortened with a dental burr.

Incisor extraction

This provides a permanent cure for malocclusion. In young rabbits with congenital malocclusion, or rabbits in the early stages of PSADD, the procedure is usually straightforward, although there can be complications such as regrowth of the teeth or abscess formation. Abscesses are usually due to a sequestrum of dead bone or an infected fragment of a tooth that was fractured or has regrown. Ensuring that the 'bleb' of germinal tissue is removed, and flushing and inspecting the sockets to ensure that all fragments of bone are removed, decreases the risk of complications. Extraction should be as atraumatic as possible but, in the later stages of PSADD, incisor extraction can be complicated by dystrophic calcification and ankylosis of the roots. It may be unnecessary if the teeth have stopped growing. Skull radiography can be helpful in the preoperative assessment of cases in order to assess the size of the pulp cavity to determine whether the teeth are still growing. Conditions that might cause complications, such as ankylosis or calcification of the incisor apices, may be evident (see Chapters 7 and 24). The technique for incisor extraction is described in Chapter 27.

Treatment of early signs of dental disease

Most rabbits in the early stages of dental disease appear to be healthy to their owners but clinical signs are evident, such as epiphora, palpable elongated apices of the cheek teeth, horizontal ridges on the enamel of the incisors or uneven wear on the cheek teeth (see Chapters 24 and 25). Although horizontal ridges may grow out, apical elongation and uneven wear are irreversible changes.

Recommendations for treatment of the early signs of dental disease range from conservative dietary management to elective generalized coronal reduction every 4–6 weeks. The choice of treatment depends on whether the practitioner believes that apical elongation is caused by lack of dental wear or by metabolic bone disease (see Chapter 25). Dietary management covers both options.

Dietary management

Rabbits in the early stages of acquired dental disease benefit from dietary modification to optimize their calcium, phosphorus and vitamin D status, and to increase their fibre intake. Many of these rabbits do not or cannot eat hay, owing to pressure on the nerve supply to the teeth, so offering them softer fibrous foods is important. Leafy green plants and vegetables are a good source of fibre. Grass and wild plants are ideal, especially if the rabbit has the opportunity to graze outside and bask in the sun so it can regulate its own vitamin D. Dried grass may be eaten in preference to hay because it is softer. Avoiding muesli mixes is essential, and restricting the amount of extruded or pelleted food is advisable. Dietary management of rabbits with dental disease is described in Chapter 30.

Generalized coronal reduction

Generalized coronal reduction is sometimes advocated for the treatment of early signs of dental disease, before clinical disease develops. Skull radiography and reference lines can be used to determine the height of the clinical crowns with a view to performing generalized coronal reduction (Boehmer and Crossley, 2009), though radiological assessment of crown height is unreliable because of the breed variation in head shape. The technique also requires perfect positioning for the lateral view of the skull. The recommendation for coronal reduction is based on the idea that insufficient dental wear and coronal elongation increases intraocclusal pressure and results in apical elongation, so reduction in the height of the exposed crowns should take pressure off the apices. In order to reduce the height of the exposed crowns, the occlusal surfaces from all the cheek teeth are removed, sometimes right down to the gum (Crossley and Aiken, 2003). The incisors are not reduced, even if epiphora is present. Generalized coronal reduction requires repeated general anaesthesia and impairs the rabbit's ability to chew hay because the enamel ridges are removed from the occlusal surface of the teeth. This procedure is invasive. It is recommended for rabbits that have been diagnosed with coronal elongation, which is a difficult parameter to assess both clinically and radiographically (see Chapters 4, 24 and 25).

Treatment of spurs on the cheek teeth

As acquired dental disease progresses, many rabbits develop markedly curved cheek teeth that form sharp spurs that lacerate the tongue or the inside of the cheeks (see Figure 26.1). These spurs can cause a great deal of pain and distress to the rabbit, and this is quickly resolved once the spurs are removed. However, any form of dentistry can only be palliative, and not curative, because of the irreversible change in shape of the affected teeth.

Anaesthesia is generally required to remove the spurs because of the anatomy of the mouth and the inaccessibility of the cheek teeth. Spurs can often form again quickly because rabbits' teeth continually erupt and grow and once the shape of the tooth has become curved, it will never straighten out and become normal. In most cases, progression of acquired dental disease means that a tooth with a spur will eventually cease growing and stop causing problems but it is difficult (or impossible) to predict which teeth will stop growing and when.

Spurs on the cheek teeth pose many problems for the rabbit, owner and veterinary practitioner, and as with any difficult condition in veterinary medicine, there are several approaches to treatment because there is no 'magic' cure. Treatment may be undertaken using handheld instruments or dental burrs (Figure 26.6). A comparison is given in Figure 26.7. There is also controversy over the need to reduce crown height rather than just removing the spurs. A

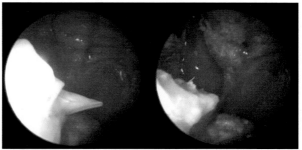

26.6 Endoscopic images of the intraoral examination of a 4-year-old rabbit before (left) and after (right) clinical crown adjustment with a dental burr. Dust from dental burring is seen in the area of the right maxillary arcades and soft palate. (Courtesy of Vladimir Jekl)

Advantages	Disadvantages	Conclusion
Dental burrs		
Good control over final shape of tooth Do not leave sharp edges Do not shatter teeth Do not cause longitudinal splits in teeth with enamel	Risk of causing soft tissue damage if moving burr touches lips, mucosa or tongue May expose innervated dentine if used for coronal reduction May cause thermal injury if used for extensive periods without water cooling Equipment can be bulky, especially if used with a guard; can be difficult to use in intubated rabbits Easy to get 'carried away' and forget that tooth is a piece of living tissue Equipment is expensive	Useful for removing spurs Useful for coronal reduction Higher risk of serious iatrogenic injury Need to be used carefully
Handheld instruments		
Quick procedure Short anaesthetic time Easy restraint Can be performed easily with rabbit intubated Equipment is cheap Serious iatrogenic soft tissue damage is unlikely No risk of thermal injury	Can shatter teeth and cause longitudinal splits if used on teeth with enamel (e.g. normal teeth or those in early stages of PSADD) May expose innervated dentine and pulp cavity if tooth shatters Less control over final shape of tooth	Useful for removing spurs Care is required in reducing crown height; only use in teeth with little or no enamel that are growing slowly or not at all Must never be used to transect the crowns of enamelled teeth that are growing

26.7 Comparison of using dental burrs and handheld instruments for spur removal.

comparison of spur removal and coronal reduction is illustrated in Figure 26.8.

Spur removal

During this procedure only the spurs or any other parts of the tooth that are causing soft tissue damage are removed. The procedure can be carried out using handheld instruments or with dental burrs

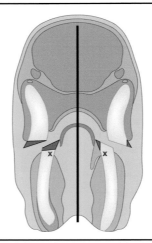

Coronal reduction
For this procedure the whole exposed crown is shortened, or even removed altogether by burring the exposed crowns down to the gum on both the upper and lower arcade. This procedure takes the teeth out of occlusion, which affects the function of the teeth postoperatively

Spur removal
For this procedure only the spurs are removed, so the length of the exposed crown is not altered and upper and lower teeth remain in occlusion and are functional

26.8   Coronal reduction *versus* spur removal. **X** marks the part of the tooth that will regrow to form a spur. This site is the same whether coronal reduction or spur removal is performed. Taking the teeth out of occlusion allows them to grow faster, so the spurs may grow back more quickly if coronal reduction is performed.

(see Operative Techniques 26.2 and 26.3) and is a simple safe technique for removing small sections of tooth that are causing soft tissue damage.

Coronal reduction

The aim of coronal reduction for the treatment of spurs is to restore the normal height and angle of the occlusal plane as closely as possible (Capello, 2012). The procedure must be conducted using dental burrs. Dental burrs in a straight nose cone are usually used to perform generalized coronal reduction. They may be air- or motor-driven and can be of high or low speed. Slow-speed handpieces require more pressure to achieve coronal reduction but do not generate as much heat as high-speed handpieces, which require water cooling. Tungsten, silicone, acrylic or diamond burrs are available in a variety of shapes and sizes. A flat fissure burr in a low-speed handpiece fitted with a burr guard is recommended by Crossley (2003).

Removing the pulp from problem teeth

Pulpectomy (see Operative Technique 26.4) stops the teeth growing so that they no longer develop spurs but still retain a functional crown. The bleb of pulp containing the germinal tissue is removed by opening the apex of the tooth where it protrudes through the mandibular bone. Pulpectomy can only be performed in teeth that are still growing and have accessible elongated apices (Figure 26.9). Fortunately, the teeth that commonly develop recurrent spurs are the 2nd, 3rd and 4th mandibular cheek teeth, which do have accessible apices (Harcourt-Brown, 1995). The apex of the last lower cheek tooth is impossible to gain access to because it penetrates the medial, rather than the lateral, aspect of the mandible and is therefore buried deep within the soft tissue. However, this small tooth can be extracted through the mouth. Pulpectomy for the incisors and maxillary teeth is not an option because their apices are not easily accessible.

Prior to pulpectomy, radiography is necessary to assess the apices and determine whether the teeth are growing or not. Open pulp cavities indicate growth. Absent or small pulp cavities indicate cessation or slowing of growth. The pulp cavities are visible on oblique views of the skull and pulp removal is only indicated for teeth with open pulp chambers (Figure 26.10).

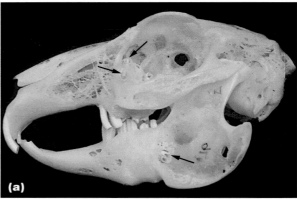
(a)

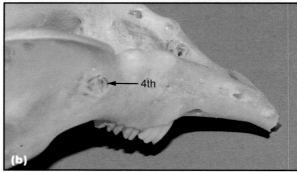
(b)

26.9   **(a)** Prepared skull of a rabbit with apical elongation of all the cheek teeth. The exposed apices and the pulp cavities can be seen in the orbit, lacrimal process and mandible. **(b)** The ventral aspect of a prepared mandible from a different rabbit shows the site of penetration of the 4th mandibular cheek tooth. Bulges at the apices of the 1st, 2nd and 3rd teeth could be palpated in the living rabbit along the ventral border of the mandible. (continues) ▶

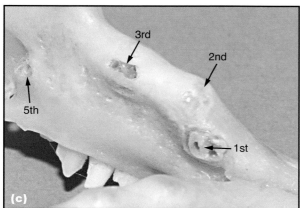

26.9 (continued) **(c)** The ventral aspect of the prepared mandible shows the sites of penetration of the apices of the 1st, 2nd, 3rd and 5th mandibular cheek teeth on the medial aspect. Bulges at the apices of the 1st, 2nd and 3rd teeth could be palpated in the living rabbit along the ventral border of the mandible.

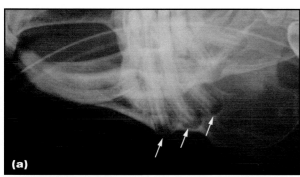

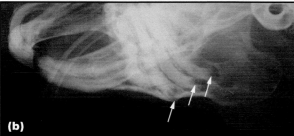

26.10 Oblique radiographic views of elongated apices to show the pulp cavities: **(a)** right and **(b)** left mandibular arcades of the same rabbit. The radiographs were taken with the rabbit on its back with its head extended and turned at approximately 45 degrees to the horizontal midline. On the right arcade there were spurs on the 3rd and 4th right mandibular cheek teeth. The pulp cavities can be seen as open structures on the right hemimandible. The pulp was removed from the 2nd, 3rd and 4th cheek teeth. On the left hemimandible the pulp cavities are smaller, indicating that tooth growth is slowing down. These teeth had been treated for spurs in the past but had none at the time of radiography, so the lingual edges were rasped and the apices left alone.

Extraction

Unlike incisor malocclusion, removal of misshapen cheek teeth is difficult, although there are some exceptions. The upper premolars and the 5th mandibular or 6th maxillary (tiny) cheek teeth can be removed via the oral cavity (Figure 26.11). Extraction is described in Chapter 27.

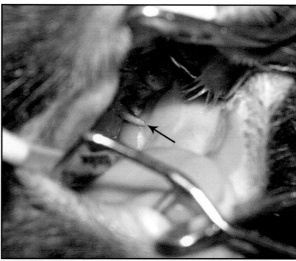

26.11 This 5-year-old neutered male Dutch rabbit was inappetent because food was caught round the elongated 6th maxillary cheek tooth, which was also impinging on the buccal mucosa inside the cheek (arrow). This tooth could be removed intraorally, although tooth fracture and haemorrhage are potential complications. An incidental finding was the absence of the crown of the 1st left maxillary cheek tooth, which had already broken off.

Treatment of mobile teeth

It is important to check teeth for mobility during dental examination. Increased mobility may be due to loss of supporting periapical bone, infection or crown fracture. Careful examination of the tooth and surrounding structures is necessary for the differential diagnosis. Radiography can be helpful. Loss of periapical bone is a common occurrence in PSADD and a mild degree of mobility can be ignored. Periapical infections require tooth extraction (see Chapters 27 and 29). Fractured crowns can be pulled off. It is common for diseased crowns to break as part of PSADD (Figure 26.12). They usually break just below the level of the gum and the crown can be pulled away easily.

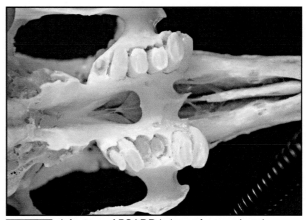

26.12 A feature of PSADD is loss of enamel and weakening of the teeth. The crowns often break just below the level of the alveolar bone where the tooth is no longer supported. On this prepared skull, two crowns on the left arcade (CT3 and CT4) had broken off in this way. The fractured occlusal section of tooth may be held in place by the gingiva but is mobile and can be a source of discomfort to the rabbit. The crown can be pulled off easily.

Treatment of periodontal disease

Examination of the periodontal pockets is described in Chapter 25. Primary infection is rare, so infection is usually secondary to exposed crown fracture or to foreign bodies that can be removed with a periodontal probe. Tartar is also rare but has been seen in a single case by the author (Figure 26.13); it was removed with a dental scaler. The presence of tartar was an indication that the teeth were no longer growing.

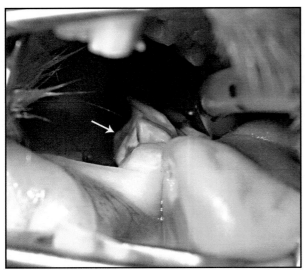

26.13 Tartar on the cheek teeth of a rabbit. This is the only case of tartar that the author has encountered in a rabbit. The tartar was easily removed with a dental scaler.

Iatrogenic damage from dentistry

Jaw injuries
Fractured jaws can be the result of tooth extraction, especially during abscess surgery (see Chapters 27 and 29). Jaw injury can also be due to the inappropriate use of gags, especially if the rabbit is lightly anaesthetized and moving its mouth in response to the presence of the gag. Opening the mouth wide with a strong gag can result in temporomandibular luxation if the rabbit tries to close its mouth. Surgical anaesthesia is always necessary when using gags.

Damage to the teeth
Dental procedures can damage the teeth. Inappropriate use of clippers can result in shattered teeth and leave sharp edges (see Figure 26.3). Inappropriate use of dental burrs can also cause severe damage to the teeth, especially if the burr is applied to the occlusal surface (Figure 26.14)

Penetrating injuries to soft tissue
Whether teeth are shortened with clippers or with dental burrs, there is a risk of iatrogenic damage. Care is required to prevent soft tissue damage from dental burrs as injuries can be serious and extend deep into the tissue (Figure 26.15). Extensive injuries can prove fatal but even minor lacerations of the tongue can be very painful postoperatively.

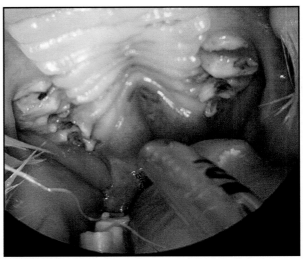

26.14 Damage due to inappropriate use of dental burrs. This rabbit was referred for treatment because he was undergoing dentistry every 3–4 weeks. He would only eat soaked nuggets and banana. Oral examination showed evidence of previous dentistry, including a deep groove along the right maxillary incisors that extended below the level of the gum.

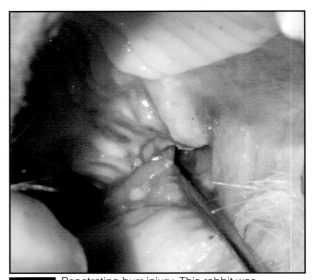

26.15 Penetrating burr injury. This rabbit was presented as a second-opinion case because it had not eaten since undergoing dentistry a week previously to remove a spur that was lacerating the tongue. After the procedure, the rabbit developed a flaccid swollen face extending across the cheek from the mandible to the zygoma. A probe inserted into the puncture wound in the angle of the jaw showed that the wound extended to a depth of 1.5 cm. The rabbit died. Wounds in this site, or lateral to the 1st upper cheek tooth, can be the result of a burr 'walking off' a tooth into the surrounding soft tissue.

During use of the burr, the soft tissue can be protected by dental spatulas and guards on the burr (Figure 26.16), minimizing the risk of injury. A common cause of soft tissue trauma is a burr 'walking off' the tooth. The use of a modified pen grip and gentle pressure on the burr reduces the risk of this happening. Slightly moistening the surface of the tooth with a damp cotton bud can also help (Hobson, 2006).

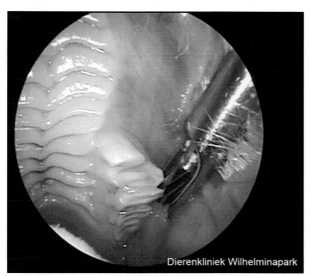

26.16 Guards are available to protect the surrounding soft tissue when using burrs during dentistry. (Courtesy of Evert-Jan de Boer)

Exposure of innervated dentine

In healthy cheek teeth two extensions of the pulp cavity are found, on either side of the central enamel fold, which taper towards the occlusal end of the tooth (see Chapter 24). Nerve fibres extend from these pulp cavities into the dentine and, at the occlusal end, there is a greater proportion of unmyelinated fibres, which are believed to be nociceptive (Bishop, 1995). In the early stages of dental disease, when the pulp cavities are open and the teeth are continuing to erupt and grow, innervated dentine may be exposed by extensive coronal reduction (Figure 26.17) or by transecting the crowns with clippers.

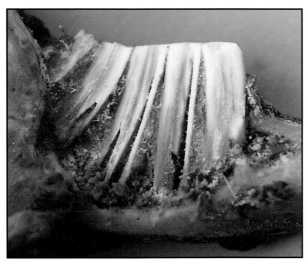

26.17 Post-mortem specimen showing the lateral aspect of a longitudinally sectioned hemimandible of a wild rabbit. It shows the relationship of pulp cavity to exposed crown after coronal reduction. The cheek teeth were burred nearly to the gum before the specimen was prepared. The rostral extension of the pulp cavity of the 2nd cheek tooth has been exposed to its extremity close to the occlusal surface. Nerve fibres will extend into the dentine from this site. (Reproduced from *In Practice*, with permission)

Removal of occlusal surfaces and interference with chewing

Coronal reduction takes the teeth out of occlusion and removes the occlusal surfaces. The effects of this procedure will vary according to the amount of exposed crown that has been removed and the stage of dental disease. In healthy rabbits and in those in the early stages of dental disease, the occlusal surfaces of the cheek teeth have sharp enamel ridges across them that are used to transect sections of hay, grass and other vegetation. Coronal reduction removes the occlusal surfaces, including the enamel ridges. It is often performed with the postoperative advice to change the rabbit's diet to include more hay, which is difficult for an animal that has had all the crowns and occlusal surfaces removed. In rabbits with teeth that are still growing, the crowns quickly regrow but it may be several days before the rabbit can eat again, and nutritional support and pain management are required during this period (Verstraete and Osofsky, 2005). If coronal reduction is conducted on rabbits in the later stages of dental disease, the teeth are no longer growing so they will never be functional, and the rabbit's impaired ability to eat fibrous food will be permanent (Figure 26.18).

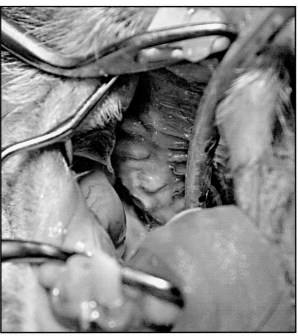

26.18 This rabbit had undergone generalized coronal reduction in the late stages of dental disease. The photograph only shows the left maxillary teeth but all four arcades were similar. No teeth were in occlusion. The rabbit was only able to eat softened, grated or shredded food.

Thermal injury

Thermal injury is a consideration when using power tools for dentistry, and a small study into the increase in temperature of rabbits' teeth during burring resulted in a recommendation to cool the teeth throughout the procedure (Schumacher,

2012). The heat that is generated does not need to penetrate the full depth of dentine into the pulp chamber to cause damage to tubules in the dentine and to affect blood flow in the pulp chamber (Allen *et al.*, 2004). Thermal injury can cause haemostasis, inflammation and thrombosis. The degree of injury is related to the temperature rise in the dentine and pulp, which depends on the length and extent of the burring procedure. Limiting the use of a burr to 3–4 seconds and dipping it in water to cool it between teeth should reduce or negate the risk of thermal injury. Cooling the teeth during the procedure is ideal but poses many difficulties in rabbits owing to limited access to the oral cavity. Not only does water reduce grinding temperatures but it also keeps the burr free of dental debris so it works more efficiently.

Abscesses resulting from dentistry
Penetrating injuries of the buccal mucosa can result in soft tissue abscesses around the head. Transecting or burring crowns to gum level can expose the pulp cavity and allow infection to gain access to the periapical area and cause an abscess (see also Chapter 29). The worst-case scenario is to perform generalized coronal reduction with clippers so that the teeth shatter and the pulp is exposed (Figure 26.19).

Haemorrhage
Two branches of the facial artery are situated underneath the buccal mucosa in the fornices close to the lateral aspect of the last cheek tooth. Penetration of these arteries during dental procedures can cause severe haemorrhage; care is therefore required when working in this area. Extraction of the last lower molar will often cause bleeding. Luckily, rabbit blood clots quickly, so

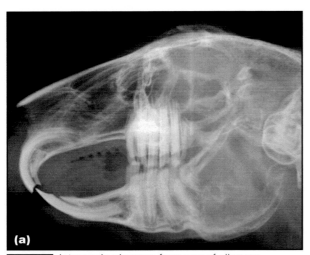

(a)

26.19 Iatrogenic abscess from use of clippers. **(a)** Lateral view of the skull of a rabbit that was presented as a second-opinion case because he had not eaten since dentistry was performed 3 days previously. The rabbit had a history of fast-growing recurrent dental spurs so the veterinary surgeon had attempted to increase the interval between dental procedures by removing all the crowns of the left arcade down to the gum. Molar clippers were used for the procedure. (continues) ▶

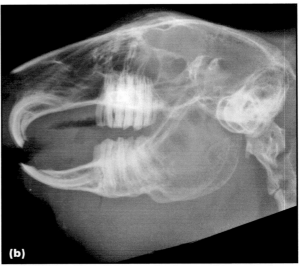

(b)

26.19 (continued) Iatrogenic abscess from use of clippers. **(b)** Despite antibiotics, analgesia and other supportive care, a large gangrenous abscess developed under the jaw over the next 3 days and the rabbit died. This case emphasizes the need for consideration of the effects of dentistry. Removing spurs from the edges of one or two teeth with molar cutters is completely different from cutting off the whole exposed crown, especially in teeth that are growing and have an open pulp cavity.

applying pressure for a few minutes with a swab or cotton bud is usually successful.

References and further reading

Allen ML, Baker GJ, Freeman DE *et al.* (2004) In vitro study of heat production during power reduction of equine mandibular teeth. *Journal of the American Veterinary Medical Association* **224**, 1128–1132
Bishop MA (1995) Is rabbit dentine innervated? A fine structural study of the pulpal innervation in the cheek teeth of the rabbit. *Journal of Anatomy* **186**, 365–372
Boehmer E and Crossley D (2009) Objective interpretation of dental disease in rabbits, guinea pigs and chinchillas. Use of anatomical reference lines. *Tierärztliche Praxis* **37**, 250–260
Capello V (2012) Small mammal dentistry. In: *Ferrets, Rabbits and Rodents: Clinical Medicine and Surgery*, ed. KE Quesenberry and JW Carpenter, pp. 452–471. Elsevier, St. Louis
Crossley DA (2003) Oral biology and disorders of lagomorphs. *Veterinary Clinics of North America: Exotic Animal Practice*, ed. DA Crossley, pp. 629–660. Saunders, Philadelphia
Crossley DA and Aiken S (2003) Small mammal dentistry. In: *Ferrets, Rabbits and Rodents: Clinical Medicine and Surgery, 2nd edn*, ed. KE Quesenberry and JW Carpenter, pp. 370–382. Saunders, St. Louis
Harcourt-Brown FM (1995) A review of clinical conditions in pet rabbits associated with their teeth. *Veterinary Record* **137**, 341–346
Harcourt-Brown FM (2006) *Metabolic Bone Disease as a Possible Cause of Dental Disease in Pet Rabbits*. RCVS Fellowship Thesis [available in PDF format from the author]
Harcourt-Brown FM (2009) Dental disease in pet rabbits. 2. Diagnosis and treatment. *In Practice* **31**, 432–445
Hobson P (2006) Dentistry. In: *BSAVA Manual of Rabbit Medicine and Surgery, 2nd edn*, ed. A Meredith and P Flecknell, pp. 184–196. BSAVA Publications, Gloucester
Ness AR (1956) The response of the rabbit mandibular incisor to experimental shortening and prevention of its eruption. *Proceedings of the Royal Society* **146**, 129–154
Schumacher M (2012) Thermal stress of teeth during dental treatment of pet rodents and lagomorphs – do teeth get too hot/overheated? *Proceedings of the 21st European Congress of Veterinary Dentistry, Lisbon*, p.62
Verstraete FJM and Osofsky A (2005) Dentistry in pet rabbits. *Compendium on Continuing Education for the Practicing Veterinarian* **27**, 671–684

OPERATIVE TECHNIQUE 26.1:
Reshaping maloccluded incisors: an alternative method
Vladimir Jekl

This approach is only used in cases where the incisors are in close contact.

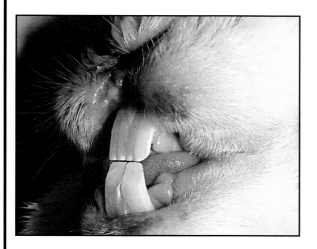
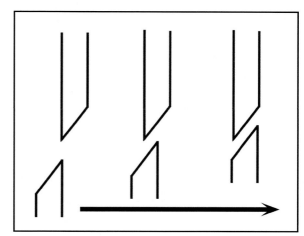

The incisor malocclusion is treated by adjusting the crown height and occlusal surface of the maxillary incisors with a high-speed precision dental handpiece or a diamond burr. The adjustment of the lower incisors is conducted so that their occlusal surfaces are parallel to the occlusal surfaces of the upper incisors.

This 'reverse occlusion' allows the upper incisors to work as the incline plane, resulting in lingual movement of the lower incisors and restoration of the physiological occlusion. The treatment should be repeated three to six times at 7-day intervals. As the mandibular incisors move lingually, physiological incisor occlusion is re-established. If the treatment is successful, no further treatment is necessary and incisor malocclusion is completely resolved. The author (VJ) has had a success rate of approximately 40% with this technique.

OPERATIVE TECHNIQUE 26.2:
Treatment of cheek tooth problems using handheld instruments
Frances Harcourt-Brown

Positioning and assistance

The procedure is conducted under general anaesthesia with the rabbit intubated. Endotracheal intubation gives greater control over the depth and length of anaesthesia and prevents jaw movement. It also prevents inhalation of dental fragments, blood or fluid. After intubation, the rabbit is placed in lateral recumbency while a gag and cheek dilators are inserted into its mouth. The rabbit is then repositioned to sternal recumbency for oral examination.

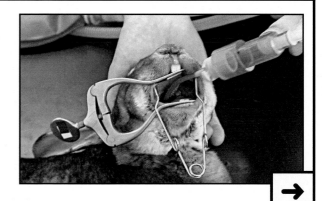

OPERATIVE TECHNIQUE 26.2 continued:
Treatment of cheek tooth problems using handheld instruments
Frances Harcourt-Brown

An assistant is needed to hold the head and make sure that the endotracheal tube remains in the correct position. The assistant holds the rabbit's head in a position that allows the light from a head torch or operating light to shine into the mouth so that the oral cavity can be examined and dentistry performed in a methodical fashion.

Instruments

- Gag
- Cheek dilators
- Curved scissors
- Long-handled molar cutters
- Diamond rasp (not ridged rasp)
- Crocodile forceps
- Crossley's molar extraction forceps
- Crossley's molar elevator
- Cotton buds
- Light source

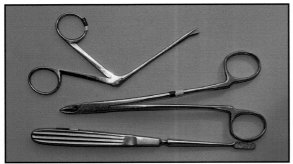

The most useful instruments: short-handled crocodile forceps (top) can be used to remove tooth fragments; long-handled molar cutters (middle) and a diamond rasp (bottom) are used to trim and rasp the teeth.

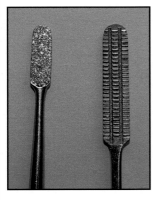

The rasp on the left is a diamond rasp that is extremely useful for smoothing off sharp edges quickly and atraumatically. The rasp on the right is a heavy, cumbersome, solid-ridged instrument that is ineffective and can cause trauma to the teeth and surrounding tissues, and is therefore not recommended.

Procedure

1 The soft tissues of the lips, gums, tongue, cheeks and oral mucosa are examined. Any swellings around the jaw are palpated. Any pieces of food that are wedged between or around the teeth are removed.

2 Each tooth is examined individually, systematically and carefully, ensuring that the occlusal, buccal and lingual surfaces are seen. The curved scissors are useful for pushing the lips and tongue to one side during the examination.

3 Each tooth is checked for mobility using a Crossley's molar elevator or a dental probe.

4 After the thorough oral examination has been conducted and dental problems identified, skull radiographs can be taken if necessary. The gag and cheek dilators need to be removed first.

5 After radiography (if done), the gag and cheek dilators are replaced and any parts of the teeth that are causing trauma to neighbouring soft tissue, such as spurs or sharp edges, are removed.

6 Long-handled molar cutters are used carefully to remove spurs, sharp edges or points. Spurs are usually removed with a single clip. The crowns are not transected, so the occlusal surface remains untouched.

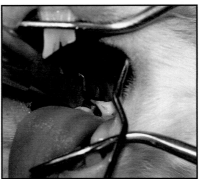

(Image reproduced from *In Practice*, with permission)

7 The fragments of teeth that have been removed are taken out of the mouth using crocodile forceps. Otherwise, the fragment can become embedded in the mucosa and cause ulceration and pain postoperatively.

8 Any sharp edges on the tooth are rasped with a diamond rasp.

→

OPERATIVE TECHNIQUE 26.2 (continued):
Treatment of cheek tooth problems using handheld instruments
Frances Harcourt-Brown

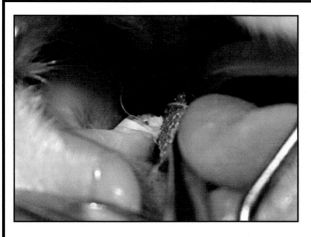

9 Long crowns are left alone unless they are causing soft tissue damage. These are usually wearing against opposing short crowns.

10 Any elongated crowns that are causing soft tissue damage are shortened to the required height by 'nibbling' the tooth with molar cutters rather than transecting it close to the gum. A diamond rasp can also be used to reduce crown height, especially if the tooth has little or no enamel on it.

11 Any loose crowns that are broken just below the gum margin can be pulled off with molar extraction forceps. These teeth are identifiable by their mobility. Sometimes they can be seen on radiographs (see Chapter 24). The gingiva surrounding the crown is often inflamed and may even be purulent. Once the fractured crown is removed, the gingival socket should be inspected for any residual fragments of tooth that need to be removed. Once the crown has been removed the tooth will not grow again.

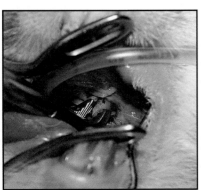

Using molar extraction forceps to remove a loose crown. (Image reproduced from *In Practice*, with permission)

12 If the upper premolars are elongated and mobile, extraction is considered depending on the condition and presence of the opposing teeth.

13 If the last lower cheek teeth are mobile or elongated, extraction should be attempted. If this fails because the crown breaks, the root can be left *in situ* and extraction attempted again at a later date if problems recur.

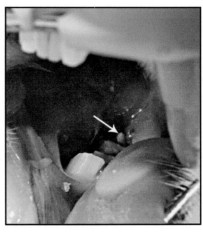

Mobile 5th mandibular cheek tooth. (Image reproduced from *In Practice*, with permission)

Postoperative care

- After dentistry, the mouth is carefully inspected again to make sure that no problems have been missed. Any fragments of tooth are removed with crocodile forceps and cotton buds. The edges of the teeth are checked again and any sharp edges are smoothed with the diamond rasp.
- Antibiotics (if necessary) and analgesics are given parenterally before the rabbit recovers from anaesthesia. The author's preference is meloxicam in all cases and trimethoprim/sulphonamide if there is soft tissue damage.
- Consideration is given to the rabbit's nutritional status before it recovers from anaesthesia. If the rabbit was not eating prior to the procedure, or its mouth is likely to be painful, food and fluid can be instilled directly into the stomach (see Chapter 2).

OPERATIVE TECHNIQUE 26.3:
Treatment of cheek tooth problems using burrs
John Chitty

Equipment

- Mouth gag
- Cheek dilators or dental table
- Metal dental spatula
- Low-speed high-torque dental handpiece and burr
- Burr guard if required
- Light source
- Cotton buds
- Mouth ulcer gel (e.g. Iglü or Orabase)

Burring equipment

A low-speed high-torque handpiece is appropriate for this procedure. Such handpieces are usually available for the polishing head of dental machines used in small animal practice. However, this author prefers using a modeller's grinding tool with a flexible handpiece.

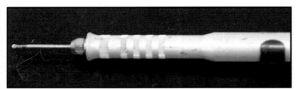

High-torque handpiece. (© John Chitty)

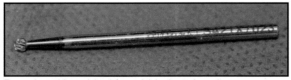

Rose-head burr ideal for rabbit dental work.
(© John Chitty)

Handpieces are available that hold burrs either straight or at a 90 degree angle. Choice should be based on availability and individual preference. Guards are also available (see below), although they may cause difficulties working. Use of these is down to individual preference. In all cases metal dental spatulas are essential for holding soft tissues away from the burr.

Using a burr has the following advantages:

- Dental procedures can be completed much more quickly than by using a file, especially if molars require shortening as well as spur removal
- It allows for more accurate 'shaping' of the teeth, which may enable longer intervals between dental procedures

- The burr does not result in 'shattering' of teeth with exposure of dentine and pulp that would allow introduction of infection
- If a high-torque handpiece is used, only very light pressure is required to remove spurs or shorten molars. This prevents excess pressure being applied to the germinal tissue of the tooth, resulting in altered tooth growth
- It is relatively easy to access and correct spurs on the buccal surfaces of the upper molars.

The following disadvantages are also pertinent:

- Molar therapy with a burr is very difficult with an endotracheal tube in the way. In dwarf rabbits, the lack of space in the mouth may make it impossible to use an endotracheal tube
- Working space inside the rabbit's mouth can be an issue, especially in dwarf breeds. In very tiny rabbits, it may be impossible to use a dental burr without causing soft tissue damage. In these cases it is better to use a file
- The equipment required is more expensive than clippers/files, though most small animal practices now have dental equipment adequate for these purposes
- Iatrogenic soft tissue damage is common if the technique is not performed with great care. Guards are available for dental burrs. However, these are cumbersome and may reduce working space and visibility within the rabbit's mouth. This author prefers to use an unguarded burr with the soft tissue protected with a dental spatula and cheek dilator
- It is easy to 'get carried away' and over-shorten teeth. This results in exposure of pulp/dentine and considerable pain and is more likely to introduce infection than to increase the length of time between dental procedures.

In summary, dental burrs can greatly facilitate molar procedures but should be used with great care.

Preoperative preparation

The timing of molar treatment may vary between cases (see text). In some cases it may be felt beneficial to anaesthetize the patient as soon as possible and remove spurs and then provide analgesia, fluids, supportive feeding and (if necessary) antibiosis postoperatively. In others, it may be felt beneficial to stabilize the rabbit with analgesia, supportive feeding and fluids preoperatively for up to 48 hours in order

→

OPERATIVE TECHNIQUE 26.3 (continued):
Treatment of cheek tooth problems using burrs
John Chitty

to reduce anaesthetic risks during the dental pro-cedure. This decision should be made on a case-by-case basis depending on the rabbit's condition and perceived anaesthetic risk (see Chapter 1).

Positioning and assistance

General anaesthesia is induced and maintained as appropriate. Intubation may be performed as space allows within the mouth.

There are two possible positioning aids, each with their advantages and disadvantages:

- EITHER the rabbit is placed in sternal recumbency and a gag and cheek dilators are inserted into the mouth, with an assistant holding the rabbit's head so that the light from a head torch or operating light shines into the mouth and enables the oral cavity to be examined
- OR the rabbit is placed on a dental table, which is an ingenious device with a gag and cheek dilators fixed to a table-top unit, enabling the angle of the unit to be adjusted to suit the operator.

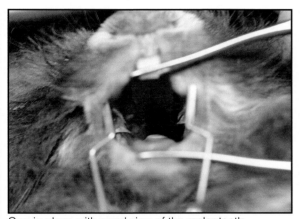

Gag in place with good view of the molar teeth.
(© John Chitty)

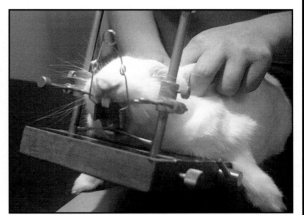

A rabbit on a dental table with its mouth open.
(© John Chitty)

Advantages	Disadvantages
Mouth gag and cheek dilators	
Inexpensive Easily fitted in the mouth Can be used with the rabbit intubated, so there is greater control over length/depth of general anaesthesia and protects airway from fluid and debris Easily cleaned/sterilized and long user life Mouth gags tend to be appropriate for all sizes of rabbit Cheek dilators come in a range of sizes for differently sized patients Enables an assistant to hold the rabbit's head in the correct position for the surgeon via the mouth gag; their spare hand can be used to hold the tongue	Giant rabbits are difficult for the assistant to hold (may require a second assistant) Some designs of gag are hard to close quickly; this is important if the rabbit starts to wake up during the procedure
Dental table	
Excellent visualization and working angle A flexible light may also be fitted to the unit, greatly facilitating the procedure Does not require an assistant to hold the rabbit Suitable for all sizes of rabbit	Fiddly and difficult to fit to the mouth; if using 'gas-only' anaesthesia the rabbit is normally waking up by the time the unit is fitted Hard to close the mouth in a hurry More expensive than routine gags and requires more maintenance

➡

OPERATIVE TECHNIQUE 26.3 (continued):
Treatment of cheek tooth problems using burrs
John Chitty

In all cases, iatrogenic damage to incisors (or mandibles/temporomandibular joints) is possible if the devices are used incorrectly, if anaesthesia is inadequate or if the gag is opened too far.

One major difficulty is accessing the molars in rabbits where the incisors have been removed. Both methods described rely on the mouth gag being fitted to the incisors; without these teeth, the gag tends to slip off and it is difficult to open the mouth adequately. Overall, the dental table works much better in such cases. However, gags and dilators can still be used, although it is better to use a gag that has a larger hole through which the incisors are normally placed; in some cases these may fit around the gums where the incisors were. Certainly these cases are difficult for a single assistant to hold and a second may be required to hold the tongue for the surgeon. Concurrent molar and incisor disease is common and the likelihood of future molar procedures should be considered when making the decision to remove incisors or simply to trim regularly.

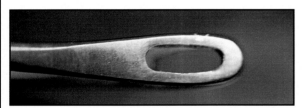

The large hole in this mouth gag can be placed over the gums where the incisors were. (© John Chitty)

Procedure

1 The tongue is held by the assistant.

2 After a thorough oral examination has been conducted and dental problems identified, skull radiographs can be taken if necessary. The gag and cheek dilators need to be removed first.

3 After radiography (if done), the gag and cheek dilators are replaced (or the rabbit is placed on the dental table) and any parts of the teeth, such as spurs or sharp edges, that are causing trauma to neighbouring soft tissue are removed. The metal spatula is held such that the burr does not contact soft tissue. Molar spurs are ground away or coronal height reduction may be performed as necessary. The amount of tooth removed is the same whether using hand

instruments (see Operative Technique 26.2) or a burr. Similarly, decisions on tooth removal may also be made at this time (see Operative Technique 26.2).

Potential complications

- Soft tissue trauma. Mouth ulcer dressings should be applied and analgesia and antibiosis administered. Haemorrhage should be arrested using pressure applied via cotton buds. Damage deep enough to cause excessive haemorrhage is rare when burrs are used.
- Exposure of pulp. This should not occur unless excessive coronal reduction has been performed. Analgesics and antibiosis should be administered until the tooth has healed.
- Thermal injury to dental tissues. This has been described in horses (Allen *et al.*, 2004) but not in rabbits and has not been seen by the author. Nonetheless it is a theoretical consideration if the burring technique is very poor.

Immediate postoperative care

Long-term dental care is discussed in Chapter 30. However, all dental cases will require some short-term care immediately after the procedure.

- Fluid therapy, especially for a prolonged procedure. This author (JRC) gives all dental cases a single subcutaneous bolus of isotonic saline at 30 ml/kg. Further fluid therapy is given depending on individual need.
- All cases require analgesia (see Chapter 2).
- Gut prokinetics: opinions vary on the benefit of giving prophylactic prokinetics; metoclopramide may be given according to individual need/clinician preference. In all cases, faecal output should be monitored.
- Antibiosis: indicated in all cases where there has been mouth ulceration or exposure of dentine/pulp. In the latter case, antibiosis should be continued for 5–7 days.
- Nutrition: critical care diets should be given until the rabbit is eating and passing faeces. This may mean that some cases cannot be discharged on the same day and require hospitalization for up to several days.

OPERATIVE TECHNIQUE 26.4:
Pulpectomy
Frances Harcourt-Brown

This technique is used to arrest the growth of selected teeth that are curved and continually develop spurs that grow into the tongue or buccal mucosa.

Preoperative assessment

- After the rabbit has been anaesthetized and intubated, the skull is radiographed, including right and left oblique views of the mandible.
- A thorough oral examination is conducted to identify the teeth with spurs that are causing problems.
- The fur is clipped from the ventral aspect of the mandible so it is easily visualized.
- The apices of the teeth that have spurs are identified by visual inspection and careful palpation of the jaw. Only teeth with open pulp cavities are candidates for surgery. These have been identified radiographically.

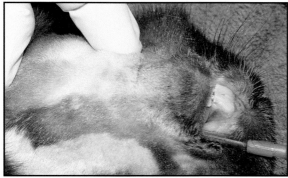

Palpation of the ventral border of the mandible to locate the swellings over the elongated apices of the teeth.

- The spurs on the affected cheek teeth are removed and the edges of the teeth rasped prior to pulp removal.

Positioning

The intubated, anaesthetized rabbit is placed on its back in a trough with its head extended.

Instruments

- 5" Crile and Halsted straight and curved artery forceps
- Martin splinter forceps
- 2 mm Debakey dissecting forceps
- 5" Adson dissecting forceps
- 5" Olsen–Hegar scissor/needle-holder
- 5" straight sharp/blunt scissors
- 4.5" straight strabismus forceps
- 6" Metzenbaum scissors
- No. 9 scalpel handle
- No. 15 scalpel blade
- 18–21 G hypodermic needles

Procedure

1 The surgical site is prepared.

2 Prior to making the skin incision the mandible is palpated again to identify the apices that are to be operated on.

3 Make an incision over the ventral border of the mandible.

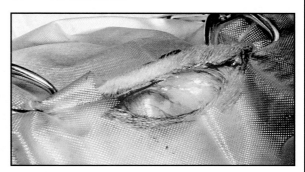

4 Dissect down to the mandibular bone and the swelling over the apex. There are no hidden structures and any blood vessels are obvious. The scent gland that is located under the chin may be encountered in some individuals, especially entire males. It can easily be pushed away from the incision.

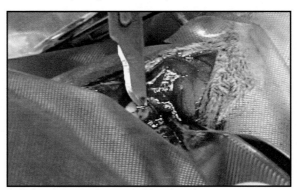

Soft tissues over the ventral border of the mandible.

OPERATIVE TECHNIQUE 26.4 (continued):
Pulpectomy
Frances Harcourt-Brown

5 Expose the swollen bone, which has often been penetrated by the elongated apex. Scrape away the periosteum over the swollen area. This will reveal either the apex of the tooth penetrating the bone or a circular area of thin reddish brown bone overlying the apex.

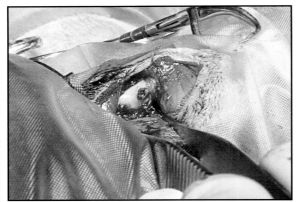

Elongated apex that has penetrated the ventral border. In many cases, the enamel on the circumference of the tooth and in the central enamel fold can be identified.

6 Lift and remove any residual bone over the apex. A scalpel blade may be used after drilling an initial hole with a hypodermic needle. The bone is soft or sometimes non-existent over the apex of the tooth.

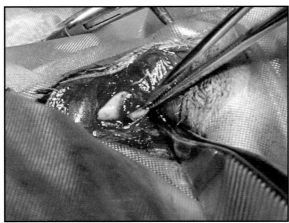

Any residual bone that is covering all or part of the apex of the tooth can be carefully removed.

7 Pick out the germinal tissue from the pulp chamber with a needle. There is sometimes some haemorrhage from the mandibular blood vessels but this soon stops if pressure is applied.

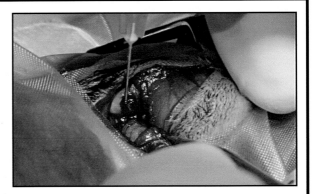

8 Examine the pulp tissue that has been removed. There should be two conical sections. If both are not present, keep exploring the apex of the tooth and the pulp cavities.

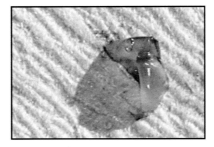

9 At the end of the procedure, flush the empty pulp cavities with methylated spirit to destroy any residual germinal tissue. Leave the hole in the bone open.

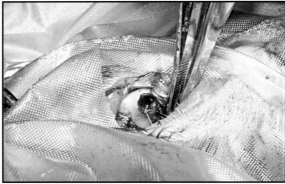

Postsurgical appearance of the apex of the tooth after the pulp has been removed.

10 Close the soft tissue and stitch up the skin wound.

Pulpectomy
Frances Harcourt-Brown

Postoperative care

Analgesia is required; the author uses meloxicam. Antibiotics may be given depending on the surgeon's policy; the author uses trimethoprim/sulphonamide.

Potential complications

Case selection is the main problem with this procedure. Teeth with open pulp cavities and apices that have penetrated the bone are straightforward. If the apices have not penetrated the bone, they may be difficult to locate and there is no pulp to remove from teeth in which the pulp cavities are closed.

There are few complications associated with the surgery. Occasionally the mandibular nerve is exposed but this does not seem to cause problems. Sometimes there may be postoperative swelling and seroma formation. In some cases the spurs on the teeth need to be trimmed again after 3–4 weeks before tooth growth ceases completely.

27

Tooth extraction

Will Easson

Tooth extraction in rabbits, compared with that in dogs and cats, is complicated by the anatomy of the mouth (Figure 27.1). The lips do not retract caudally nearly as far as in carnivores, so it is difficult to see all the surfaces of the teeth. While the broad principles of extraction are the same as in other species, access to the teeth, their attachments and their roots is more difficult and requires adapted techniques and equipment.

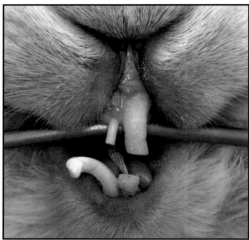

27.1 Access to the incisors is relatively straightforward, but access to the cheek teeth in rabbits can be a challenge for both visualization and access. These incisors show various stages of the progressive syndrome of acquired dental disease (PSADD; see Chapter 24). One crown has fractured beneath the gingiva, one is growing in a distorted shape and the others have stopped growing.

Relevant anatomy

The anatomy of the temporomandibular joint and the length of the mandible and maxilla conspire to restrict the gape of a rabbit's mouth (Figure 27.1). The orbicularis oris muscle prevents retraction of the lips caudally from the diastema and therefore access for incisor extraction is straightforward but access to the premolars is more restricted. Further caudally the teeth become even more difficult to access. The operating surgeon's sight is also restricted by the long oral cavity with a small opening. This means that the operator frequently has to use one eye, which compromises depth perception and visibility when looking along a row of closely abutting cheek teeth. To access the premolars and molars for extraction, long-handled instruments or an alternative method to gain access are required.

External access to the cheek teeth can be accomplished via the ventral mandible. In the healthy animal the cortical bone here is thick, with a smooth periosteum. Laterally the bone can be equally thick and smooth, but lingually the cortical bone is thinner. Overlying the lateral and medial aspects of the bone are the attachments and muscle bodies of the masticatory muscles.

Indications for extraction

The indications for tooth extraction and their advantages and drawbacks are summarized in Figure 27.2.

Indication	Advantages of extraction	Drawbacks of extraction
Incisors		
Congenital malocclusion and subsequent overgrowth Acquired malocclusion and overgrowth Selected cases of dacryocystitis (see Chapter 28)	Provides a permanent solution to the problem Removes the need for repeat trims Removes the possibility of periods of reduced fibre intake prior to each presentation for trimming Surgery is often cost-effective when compared with repeated trimmings over months or years	Removal of the incisors is frequently resisted by clients Requires a general anaesthetic with analgesics and antibiotics Regrowth is possible Postoperative infection is possible Impairs the rabbit's ability to pull out dead hair so owner will need to groom it regularly Cannot bite, so food will need shredding or grating (see Chapter 30) Makes subsequent dental work difficult because most techniques for opening the mouth for dental work rely on the presence of the incisors as an anchor for opening the jaws. Adapted equipment or techniques for using existing gear will be needed

27.2 Indications for, and advantages and disadvantages of, tooth extraction. (continues) ▶

Indication	Advantages of extraction	Drawbacks of extraction
Cheek teeth		
Mobility The origin of, or involvement in, abscessation Persistent overgrowth or spur formation of isolated tooth	Removes the discomfort associated with a mobile tooth Removes a source of infection in cases of abscesses Removes the immediate source of the problem, which can recur as often as monthly	The surgery is more complex and has a higher morbidity than reshaping or spur removal (see Chapter 26) In some cases the absence of a tooth may make the chewing action more difficult The jaw bone may remodel over time. This can change the spacing and alignment of the other teeth Requires a general anaesthetic with the attendant risks

27.2 (continued) Indications for, and advantages and disadvantages of, tooth extraction.

Incisors

Incisor malocclusion is the most common indication for incisor extraction because it is a permanent solution and should be considered in cases of recurrent 'overgrowing' incisors (Figure 27.3). Other solutions such as repeatedly trimming the incisors are frequently employed first, but can be unsatisfactory because the patient may experience eating difficulties for a period prior to presentation for incisor trimming. Each time the teeth overgrow, the interruption in food intake or a change in the quality of the food (reduction in fibre content owing to selection of food for ease of prehension and mastication) can predispose the patient to gastrointestinal hypomotility or gut stasis. Overgrown incisors can make prehension and mastication of food difficult and inhibit the chewing motion, and may contribute to unsatisfactory wear.

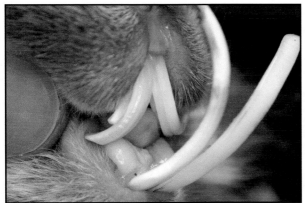

27.3 Malocclusion in rabbits can result in repeated overgrowth of the incisors, and extraction is indicated.

If clippers are used for incisor trimming, there is a risk of shattering the tooth, which could lead to abscessation. There is also potential discomfort from the pressure and jarring of the clippers. If burring or diamond cutting discs are used, there is a risk of trauma and laceration each time the procedure is performed, so incisor removal is a good alternative to these techniques. In the author's experience working in general practices, the extraction procedure is usually cost-effective for the owner when considering the cost of repeated trimming.

The possibility of incisor involvement should be investigated in rabbits showing persistent epiphora or dacryocystitis (see Chapter 28). Radiography can show incisor root pathology as a contributing factor to the dacryocystitis, and extraction of the incisors may help in the treatment of the epiphora or dacryocystitis, although this cannot be guaranteed.

Poor enamel quality is not an indication for extraction of the incisors in itself, but ridged or fragile/brittle incisor enamel can be an indication of incisor root disease and should stimulate the clinician to obtain skull radiographs.

Cheek teeth

Cheek teeth are generally preserved if possible; there are fewer occasions when extraction of premolars and molars is necessary compared with incisors. One of the most common indications for extraction of cheek teeth is involvement in abscessation. Any abscess around the head and neck of a rabbit should be evaluated radiographically (see Chapter 29). **All** involved cheek teeth should be extracted because the teeth can act as sequestra for the persistence of infection. This is usually performed at the same time as abscess surgery, using the extraoral approach (see below and Operative Technique 27.3).

Another indication for extraction of a cheek tooth is loss of attachment to the alveolar bone, which results in the tooth becoming mobile or even loose within the socket, which is uncomfortable for the patient (Figures 27.4 and 27.5). Extracting the tooth allows the patient to eat normally again soon after

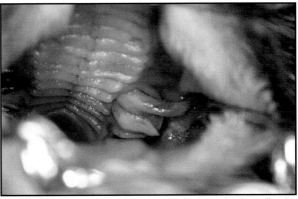

27.4 In this rabbit, the upper left premolar has tilted obliquely sufficiently to grow out laterally, causing regular trauma to the buccal mucosa. These teeth often become mobile, increasing the discomfort; there is evidence of occlusion with its mandibular counterpart on the tooth's palatal aspect. This tooth was extracted intraorally.

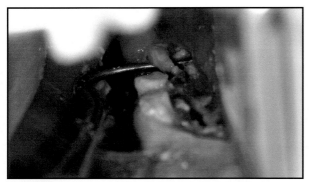

27.5 In this rabbit the last cheek tooth is tilted distally. It is contacting the mucosa at the back of the mouth, and should be removed.

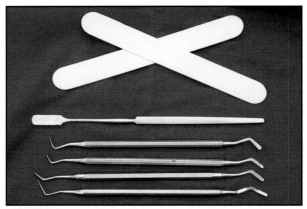

27.6 Wooden tongue depressors, metal rodent dental spatula, and various sizes and designs of molar luxators.

the procedure. Skull radiography is necessary to assess the rabbit's dentition before extraction. The intraoral approach is most commonly used in this case, and the upper first and lower last cheek teeth are the most likely candidates.

The author has also extracted molars where there has been a sole tooth repeatedly forming a 'spur' that traumatizes the tongue. Extraction was performed to avoid the use of repeated anaesthetics to trim a single tooth. In the small number of rabbits this has been performed in, the gap left is quickly closed by the neighbouring teeth.

Instruments for tooth extraction

- **Rodent dental table (rodent gag).** In this author's opinion, this gag (see Chapter 26) is essential for intraoral cheek tooth extraction because it holds the head firmly and at a continuously adjustable angle. If the patient has had its incisors removed it will still hold the jaws open but the incisory bones will slip off the crossbars. The author uses a combination of a heavy sandbag behind the patient's rump to reduce this, an assistant holding the head, and a shaped custom rubber coating (Sugru) over the crossbars.
- **Cheek pouch dilators/human 'Thudicum' nasal speculum/bivalve vaginal speculum.** The author finds that with all of the commercial 'cheek pouch dilators' the springs holding the blades open are too strong, which can cause them to flip out of the patient's mouth, as well as possibly traumatizing or overstretching the muscles and oral structures to which they are applied. The author's preference is for Thudicum nasal specula, which are made of springy metal and can be adjusted and bent as the situation requires. Their rounded solid metal blades also provide a degree of tissue protection against mishaps. Their malleable nature makes them gentler than the sprung wire type of dilator (see Chapter 25).
- **Wooden tongue depressors** (Figure 27.6). Their main use, when broken in to sections, is to be wedged behind the cheek pouch dilator blades to hold all the tissue out of the way and protect it.

- **Hypodermic needles and 1 ml syringes.** The hypodermic needles are used to sever the periodontal ligaments. The syringes are used as handles if required.
- **20 ml syringe and short catheter.** For flushing the operative site and cooling the bone and burr.
- **Scalpel blades.** A No.15 or No.15T scalpel blade is usually the right depth for rabbit teeth; other sizes do not match the size and shape of the teeth as well.
- **Crossley incisor luxator** (Veterinary Instrumentation, UK; Jorgensen Instruments, USA).
- **Crossley molar luxator** (Figure 27.7).
- **Crossley molar forceps.** The author has modified these to reduce the thickness of the jaws for greater precision (Figure 27.8). Vittorio Capello has designed a similar set, available from Precision Surgical in the USA.
- **Extraction forceps.** Designed by Frances Harcourt-Brown, these modified needle-holders (Veterinary Instrumentation, UK) assist in the removal particularly of incisors and small fragments.
- **Dental machine with >35,000 rpm air turbine-driven handpiece.** A range of spherical or teardrop-shaped tungsten carbide or diamond-coated burrs are best for bone burring. Some people use a rotary tool such as a Dremmel or a professional wall- or arm-mounted rotor with flexible shafts and foot pedals (which seem mainly to be sold for spinal surgery). Care must be taken when using these: the torque is higher than with a dedicated air-turbine dental unit.
- **Suction unit.** This makes removal of the debris produced by burring much easier.
- **Cotton-tipped buds.** With adrenaline, should be kept ready in case there is excessive bleeding from traumatized structures.

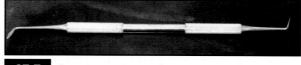

27.7 Crossley molar luxator.

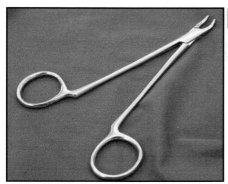

Crossley molar forceps.

Incisor extraction

Rabbit incisors are usually extracted using a 'closed' technique, accessing the root attachments using scalpel blades, hypodermic needles and/or a dedicated instrument (the 'Crossley incisor luxator'). The step-by-step procedure is described in Operative Technique 27.1.

'Open' techniques have been described for retrieving fragments of broken incisors, either laterally through the incisor bone, or rostrodorsally, where they may be obstructing the nasal passages.

It is wise to take radiographs of the incisors before starting surgery. This allows the identification of fractured incisors, abscesses, and teeth with particularly distorted shapes. This knowledge can and will help in decision-making when the surgeon is severing the periodontal ligament, much of which is done by touch. Taking radiographs after surgery confirms and records complete removal of the tooth, but is not always necessary.

Cheek tooth extraction

There are two access strategies for cheek tooth extraction: 'intraoral', i.e. access through the open mouth of the anaesthetized rabbit; and 'extraoral', i.e. through an incision made through the skin and accessing the tooth root through the cortical and alveolar bone.

Intraoral technique

Intraoral 'closed' cheek tooth removal is the most frequently used technique in the author's practice, but it can be demanding: the narrow gape of the rabbit, lack of access to the reserve crown and its attachment to the alveolar bone, as well as the close apposition of the abutting cheek teeth to each other, make selective removal without affecting the other teeth difficult. The author tends to use the intraoral approach for diseased mandibular teeth where the tooth itself is relatively loose (e.g. is involved in an abscess) and the clinical crowns of the adjacent teeth are not obscuring access. For maxillary teeth the intraoral approach is nearly always employed. Extraoral techniques can be employed later if the intraoral approach fails. This author will usually, at least briefly, try the intraoral

approach, even in cases where the tooth appears misshapen on radiographs, because it does not involve surgical preparation and breaching the skin. In the author's subjective opinion, postoperative morbidity seems less significant.

Intraoral techniques are usually relatively quick to perform, there is less preparation and the patient spends less time under anaesthetic. The technique does require long-handled instruments, some of which can be improvised, and some dexterity! It is most commonly used on the 1st premolars, owing to the relative ease of access; the further caudal the affected tooth, the less useful this approach becomes. The step-by-step procedure is described in Operative Technique 27.2.

Extraoral technique

Extraoral, 'open', cheek tooth removal is employed in cases in which intraoral extraction is not possible or practical. Examples include patients in which radiography of the teeth shows an indistinct periodontal ligament (ankylosis), fractured teeth, osteomyelitis or abscessation. Extraoral extraction is employed in the latter cases because of the reduced risk of iatrogenic fracture of the bone. There have also been cases where a single mandibular crown repeatedly forms a spur that traumatizes the tongue, but the surrounding teeth are otherwise clinically acceptable. To extract this errant tooth intraorally would involve risk of damage to the abutting cheek teeth, as well as being technically demanding.

The extraoral technique requires the availability of a drill with a bone burr bit to remove the cortical alveolar bone and expose the tooth root and unerupted crown. The drill can be as simple as a Dremmel or other rotary handpiece, or as sophisticated as a dedicated dental air-driven turbine handpiece. With the appropriate equipment the most difficult part of the extraoral approach is making the incision in the correct place. The step-by-step procedure is described in Operative Technique 27.3.

Complications

Infection
Infection and subsequent abscessation are ever-present threats with most dental and surgical procedures. Rabbits form abscesses full of a thick caseous material which is difficult to evacuate, and abscesses in general are difficult to resolve (see Chapter 29).

Preoperative preparation is important; cleaning the area with dilute chlorhexidine swabs or cotton-tipped buds is a logical way to reduce microbial contamination of the operative site. With both incisor extractions and the intraoral extraction of molars, cotton-tipped buds can be soaked in dilute chlorhexidine and used to cleanse the surrounding gingiva and crown. In this case sterility cannot be achieved, but the aim is to reduce contamination of the operative site. With the external approach to cheek tooth extraction full sterile technique should be used.

Perioperative antibiotics are recommended (e.g. potentiated sulphonamides or fluoroquinolones). In the author's practice they are given with the pre-medication (buprenorphine) a couple of hours before surgery, by subcutaneous injection. Sterilized instruments are used on one patient only. For external extractions, full surgical preparation of the patient and the site surrounding the surgical area is needed, and the use of sterilized drill bits, handpiece shrouds, gown and gloves is recommended.

Small pieces of fractured teeth or bone can act as sequestra for postoperative infection and it is important to check the extraction site and remove these at the end of surgery. Should signs of infection occur during postoperative monitoring and follow-up, these should be treated quickly and aggressively.

Bone fracture
Radiographs of the skull are often advisable prior to the tooth extraction procedure in order to assess the roots, identify all the affected teeth and assess the level of osteomyelitis. Areas of osteomyelitis are potential weak points in the bone, and should be borne in mind when selecting an extraction technique. If there is extensive osteomyelitis and abscess formation around a tooth, the forces that are to be exerted may cause bone fracture. An extraoral technique may actually carry a lower risk of a bone fracture despite the bone burring and removal. If the bone is fractured during the procedure, stabilization is not usually necessary to encourage the patient to start eating again after the surgery (see Chapter 29). It is important to continue with the surgery as far as possible to remove the intended teeth and allow the patient to recover, concentrating on multimodal analgesia, gastrointestinal stimulants and close monitoring (see Chapter 2).

Tooth fracture and retention of fragments
This is mainly a risk of incisor extraction but can be seen with molar extractions too. Retained fragments left *in situ* indefinitely run the risk of abscessation and osteomyelitis. After extraction, it is important to inspect the apex of the tooth for evidence of fractures. If the tooth has fractured, there are two options:

- If the tooth fractures early in the procedure without much mobility being achieved it may be possible to provide antibiotic cover, leave the socket open (as opposed to suturing the gingiva closed) and wait for the tooth to regrow. The author suggests advising the owner to schedule examination and radiographs under anaesthetic and re-extraction in about 4–6 weeks to give the tooth the chance to regrow. Before reattempting re-extraction, radiographs are needed to reassess the structure of the tooth
- The second option (also needed if there has been no regrowth in this time) is to remove the fragment in some way, either using delicate instruments or by changing technique (e.g. to an external approach through the ventral aspect of the mandible).

Retained germinal tissue and regrowth
When the tooth has been extracted the surgeon should also inspect the apex for the presence of germinal tissue. The presence of germinal tissue in the pulp cavity in the apex of the tooth means there is a risk of the tooth regrowing. The germinal tissue is a red/pink bleb of soft tissue in the hollow of the apex of the root. The surgeon can maximize the chance of removing the germinal epithelium with the tooth by pressing the tooth back into the alveolar socket and rotating it slightly before withdrawing it from the socket. Other techniques described include vigorous flushing with saline, suction of the apex of the socket with a syringe and Spruell needle, introduction of a stiff curette or probe into the alveolar socket as far as it will go (measured against the extracted tooth) and scraping the apex of the alveolar socket. Afterwards the socket should be flushed with a dilute saline or chlorhexidine solution. If there is a suspicion of some germinal tissue remaining in the socket, flushing with a small quantity of methylated spirit can be used to destroy it.

Overgrowth of the opposing tooth
This is not usually a problem with extracted molars, although it can happen in rabbits that have fractured several healthy mandibular teeth (see Chapter 26). Usually, the 'offset' arrangement of the molars where each molar occludes against two others, coupled with the jaw movement during mastication, means that even when one is removed the opposing tooth it still wears against others. Often there is some bone remodelling and movement of adjacent teeth which reduces the gaps left by extraction.

Other complications
Gut stasis, aspiration pneumonia and airway blockage are other possible sequelae to anaesthesia and dentistry in rabbits. Prevention of gut stasis is described in Chapter 2. Oral surgery produces a lot of debris. This should be cleared away during the procedure, making sure that saliva and flushing water do not pool in the mouth. Tooth fragments should always be removed from the oral cavity to avoid the possibility of airway obstruction and aspiration.

References and further reading

Bohmer E (2010) *Zahnheilkunde bei Kaninchen und Nagern: Lehrbuch und Atlas [Gebundene Ausgabe]. (Dentistry in Rabbits and Rodents: Textbook and Atlas)* Schattauer, Stuttgart [In German]

Capello V (2004) Extraction of cheek teeth and surgical treatment of periodontal abscessation in pet rabbits with acquired dental disease. *Exotic DVM* **12**(4), 31–38

Capello V (2004) Extraction of incisor teeth in pet rabbits. *Exotic DVM* **6**(4), 23–30

Capello V, Gracis M and Lennox A (2005) *Rabbit and Rodent Dentistry Handbook.* Zoological Education Network, Lake Worth

Harcourt-Brown F (1997) Diagnosis, treatment and prognosis of dental disease in pet rabbits. *In Practice* **19**, 407–427

Harcourt-Brown F (2001) *Textbook of Rabbit Medicine.* Butterworth-Heineman, Oxford

Harcourt-Brown F (2009) Dental disease in pet rabbits. 1. Normal dentition, pathogenesis and aetiology. *In Practice* **31**, 370–379

Harcourt-Brown F (2009) Dental disease in pet rabbits. 2. Diagnosis and treatment. *In Practice* **31**, 432–445

Harcourt Brown F (2009) Dental disease in pet rabbits. 3. Jaw abscesses. *In Practice* **31**, 496–505

Sayers I (2010) Approach to preventive health care and welfare in rabbits. *In Practice* **32**, 190–198

OPERATIVE TECHNIQUE 27.1:
Incisor extraction

Patient positioning and preparation

The procedure is carried out with the rabbit under general anaesthesia (see Chapter 1). Lateral or sternal recumbency may be used; the author prefers lateral recumbency. The surgeon will find it necessary to hold the patient's head to help change the angle of instruments, owing to the curvature of the tooth crowns.

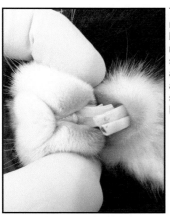

The patient is in lateral recumbency, with its head restrained manually by the surgeon, facilitating achievement of the angles necessary to sever the periodontal ligament.

Assistant

Not required.

Instruments

- No.15 or No.15T (dropped-tip) scalpel blade
- Hypodermic needles and 1 ml syringes: the bevel points of the hypodermic needles are used to sever the periodontal ligaments. The syringes are used as handles if required. Several will be needed: the needles must be bent to match the curvature of the tooth, and they quickly become blunt
- Crossley incisor luxator (sterile)
- Cotton-tipped buds (sterile)
- Extraction forceps (small)

Procedure

1 Using a cotton-tipped bud, swab the gingiva surrounding the incisor teeth with dilute chlorhexidine or povidone–iodine.

2 Sever the gingival attachment on all four sides of the incisor using a scalpel blade or hypodermic needle; this is done by gently pushing the scalpel blade between gingiva and tooth until bone is touched. It is sometimes possible to push the scalpel between the bone and crown enamel and start the next step.

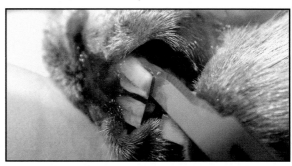

3 The scalpel blade or needle can be advanced deeper until it contacts the junction between the alveolar bone and the tooth.

4 Using either a Crossley incisor luxator, scalpel blade or hypodermic needle, manoeuvre the cutting edge between tooth and bone and cut along the peridontal ligaments on all four sides of the incisors. Take your time and be gentle.

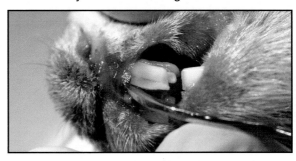

PRACTICAL TIP
While working on the axial surface (the surfaces between the two incisors), applying lateral pressure and holding for a few seconds (the author counts to 10), can help significantly loosen the incisors. If a scalpel blade is used, this pressure is applied after gently twisting the blade.

5 Gradually work your way along the enamel, remembering that the maxillary incisors curve more sharply than the mandibular incisors. You will probably need to use an angled hypodermic needle to work along the labial and palatal/lingual aspects of the incisors.

→

OPERATIVE TECHNIQUE 27.1 continued:
Incisor extraction

6 Once the tooth is loose (can be wobbled significantly using only gentle finger movements), with gentle pressure press the tooth *back deeper* into the socket and rotate it slightly in the socket. This step has been suggested to improve the chances of removing or damaging the germinal epithelium and thereby reducing the chance of tooth regrowth.

7 Grasp the tooth gently with forceps next to the gingival margin, and gently pull it out of the alveolar bone. The direction of pull is important – it must be along the direction of the tooth as it emerges from the bone. When extracting the maxillary incisors, the direction is usually perpendicularly ventral. The mandibular incisors are commonly about 45 degrees to horizontal by the time most are extracted. Put moderate, constant traction on the tooth; do not twist or rotate. Keep repositioning the forceps to keep the tips of the jaws next to the gingival margin.

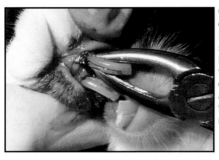

Correct angle of extraction is vital for success. Pulling along the curvature of the long axis of the tooth is necessary.

The tooth should come out in a few seconds. If not, repeat stage 3 onwards – particularly stressing the ligament. Patience and gentle handling at this point save time and fractured teeth.

8 Check the apex of the reserve crown for a small blob of pink soft tissue.

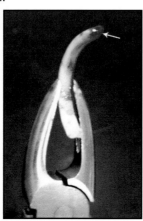

9 If this is absent, you will need to introduce a curette (a long curved hypodermic needle or the incisor luxator instrument can be utilized) and curette the alveolar cavity to destroy the germinal tissue. Some authors (Harcourt-Brown) suggest flushing the cavity. Strong suction with a syringe and a Spreull needle has also been described (Evert-jan de Boer).

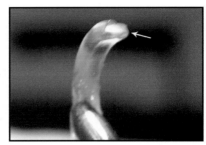

There is no germinal tissue at the end of this extracted tooth.

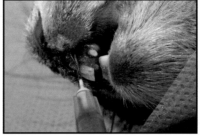

Curetting the socket.

10 Some authors (e.g. Capello) recommend suturing the gingiva closed. This author (WE) does not suture the gingiva closed but leaves it open to granulate: the alveolar socket is flushed with dilute chlorhexidine, then left to form a blood clot.

Postoperative care

- Particular attention to postoperative pain relief (and antibiotics where used) is maintained for 5 days using non-steroidal anti-inflammatory drugs (NSAIDs) by mouth. Checks are made as with the other techniques: a 24-hour check; then an oral examination at 3–5 days.
- Perioperative antibiotics are used by some authors where there is no infection already present. Trimethoprim/sulphonamides can be a useful alternative to the fluroquinolones that are more commonly used, although the fomer are, at least theoretically, not useful where pus is present.

➡

OPERATIVE TECHNIQUE 27.1 continued:
Incisor extraction

- Gastrointestinal stimulants such as cisapride, metoclopramide or ranitidine should be used to help maintain gastrointestinal motility throughout the recovery period. In most cases a single injection given between induction of anaesthesia and recovery is sufficient.
- Patients should be eating and defecating normally when fully recovered from the anaesthetic and in all cases within 12–24 hours.
- Dietary modification is necessary. Rabbits without incisors cannot bite chunks out of apples or carrots and have problems nibbling large leaves. Some authors recommend feeding chopped hay to help with prehension postoperatively but this is usually unnecessary as most rabbits learn to prehend and masticate blades of hay and grass without problems.
- Some help with grooming may be necessary for long-haired rabbits.

OPERATIVE TECHNIQUE 27.2:
Cheek tooth extraction: intraoral approach

Patient positioning and preparation

The procedure is carried out with the rabbit under general anaesthesia (see Chapter 1). Preoperative skull radiographs are taken. For the surgical procedure, the patient is placed in sternal recumbency and the jaws are held open by the rabbit dental table or by a rodent mouth gag held by an assistant. Gags, cheek pouch dilators or nasal specula are used to obtain the best view and access to the cheek tooth to be extracted.

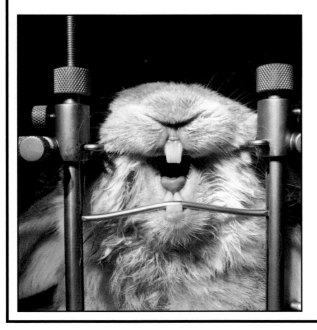

PRACTICAL TIP
Visualization and access are considerably enhanced by breaking about 2.5 cm off the rounded ends of a wooden tongue depressor. Wedge these down on either side of the molar arcade and use the cheek pouch dilator or nasal speculum to hold these apart. This clears the surgical field of soft tissue.

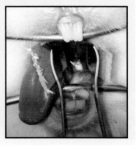

Assistant

Required to hold the rabbit's head and mouth gag in the absence of a rabbit dental table.

Equipment

- Crossley molar luxator
- Molar extraction forceps
- Hypodermic needles
- 1 ml syringes
- Sterile cotton-tipped buds
- Adrenaline 1:1000
- Sterile saline
- 10 ml syringe
- Catheter for flushing

OPERATIVE TECHNIQUE 27.2 continued:
Cheek tooth extraction: intraoral approach

Procedure

1 Remove any impacted food material from around the tooth – standard curved dental curettes and picks as used in dogs and cats are useful for this. Wipe the area with a dilute chlorhexidine-soaked cotton-tipped bud to clean the area.

2 Either use the sharp tips of a Crossley molar luxator, or bend hypodermic needles midway along at 90–100 degrees (the molar forceps are very useful for making this sharp bend).

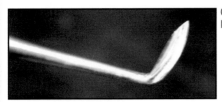
Crosley molar luxator tip.

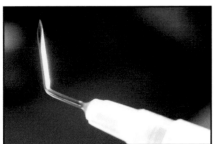
Bent needle.

3 Work the luxator between the tooth to be extracted and the adjacent teeth, applying gentle pressure for a few seconds each time towards the centre of the target tooth so as to stretch and sever the periodontal ligament.

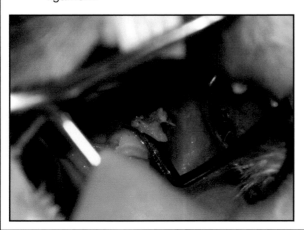

When using a needle, the straight edge should slide down the enamel, and the bevel should be away from the tooth, so different orientations are required for each aspect of the tooth. Needles become blunt quickly and should be replaced frequently.

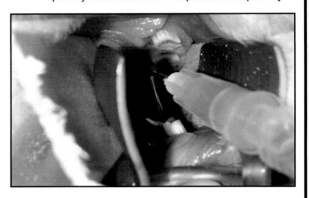

4 Work around the other three sides of the tooth in a similar manner. When doing this, bear in mind the orientation of the reserve crown: *mandibular* molars should go more or less straight down (ventrally) whereas the reserve crowns of *maxillary* molars are tilted slightly mesially although this varies in individual teeth. Apical elongation and pathology alter the shape of the tooth (see Chapter 24). With experience the surgeon will be able to use the preoperative radiographs to assist in feeling their way along the crown with their chosen luxator.

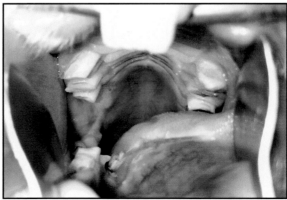
While the clinical and reserve crowns are perpendicular to the jaw bone in the mandible, the maxillary teeth are angled mesially, and this needs to be taken into account when severing the periodontal ligaments.

OPERATIVE TECHNIQUE 27.2 continued:
Cheek tooth extraction: intraoral approach

---

5 Once the tooth is loose in its socket, use either a small curved haemostat or the Crossley molar forceps to grasp it gently. Put gentle distracting traction on the tooth. Do not twist.

PRACTICAL TIP
It can sometimes help to use a finger placed on the lingual or palatal aspect of the incisors as a fulcrum, gently using the forceps as a lever. The author finds that this technique gives much finer control over the distracting direction and force.

Fairly minimal force should be needed. If the tooth does not come free quickly and with minimal force, repeat the luxation step. If the tooth is not coming out despite being loose in its socket, the surgeon should consider approaching the tooth root apex externally (see Operative Technique 27.3).

6 Once the molar has come free and been removed, examine the apex of the tooth for the presence of germinal epithelium. In the author's experience this usually comes with the tooth without any specific action being necessary. This is also to make sure that the tooth has been extracted entire and not fractured, leaving a potentially devitalized fragment *in situ*. Some practitioners recommend curetting the alveolar socket with a sharp implement then flushing with chlorhexidine to prevent regrowth of the tooth.

7 Some authors (Capello) mention suturing the alveolar opening once extraction is completed. This author has not found this to be necessary; the alveolar space becoming filled with a blood clot and then granulation tissue within a few days.

8 It is sometimes recommended to take postoperative radiographs. This will depend on the surgeon's confidence in how the procedure went. If the tooth was extracted in its entirety with germinal epithelium present and the crown intact then radiographs are probably not necessary, save to document definitively that the tooth was extracted. If there is any doubt, or if trauma to the adjacent teeth could have occurred, then postoperative radiographs should be taken.

Postoperative care

Postoperative pain relief (and antibiotics where used) is maintained for 5 days; postoperative checks are performed as for the other extraction techniques (see Operative Technique 27.1). General postoperative care is similar to other surgical techniques and is described in Chapter 2.

OPERATIVE TECHNIQUE 27.3:
Cheek tooth extraction: mandibular extraoral approach

Patient positioning and preparation

The procedure is carried out with the rabbit under general anaesthesia (see Chapter 1). The patient should be in dorsal recumbency. A trough and sandbags help with support in this position. The forelimbs should be secured in extension caudally. Masking tape can be used over the chin to stabilize the skull.

Clip the patient from the incisory area back to the caudal mandible or mid-throat, depending on which tooth or teeth are to be extracted. Prepare the area for aseptic surgery with scrub solution. Drape with a sterile drape.

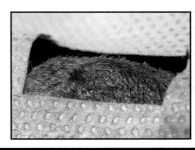

The ventral aspect of the mandible has been clipped and scrubbed. (Rostral is to the left of the picture; caudal to the right.)

OPERATIVE TECHNIQUE 27.3 continued:
Cheek tooth extraction: mandibular extraoral approach

Assistant

Will be needed to drip sterile saline over the cutting burr to cool it and flush away debris.

Equipment

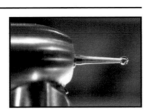

- High-speed burr for bone (tungsten carbide, diamond grit)
- Molar extraction forceps
- Hypodermic needles
- 1 ml syringes
- Sterile cotton-tipped buds
- Sterile saline
- 10 ml syringe
- Catheter for flushing

Procedure

1 Make an incision over the tooth to be extracted. An incision length of about 5 mm–1 cm is usual. You will need to dissect bluntly through thin muscle (and sometimes fat) to get to the bone surface.

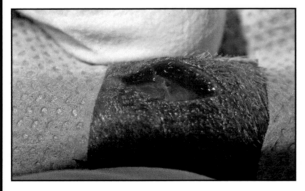

PRACTICAL TIP
Positioning the incision and making sure you are about to operate on the correct tooth is a valid concern, as you are about to incise the skin. You are often operating on teeth with roots producing a bulge in the ventral mandible and therefore palpation is usually sufficient. Having the radiographs available is helpful and having a metallic marker on them as a guide can help further; a hypodermic needle or self-adhesive X-ray marker can provide useful reference points for confidence.

2 Use the dental burr to remove cortex and open through the bone cortex to expose the root apex. The assistant should produce a steady drip of saline on to the operating site to cool the bone and flush away debris. Use the high-speed burr to remove cortical bone until you can see the apex of the root with surrounding periodontal ligament on all four sides Stop drilling once you are looking at the root end-on; it is surrounded by a thin darker coloured square demarcating the pulp chamber.

Note: There may be evidence of abscessation when you burr through the bone cortex. While abscesses are detailed elsewhere in this Manual (Chapter 29) the opportunity to remove infected tissue should not be missed, and should be accomplished before proceeding with the molar extraction.

3 The author uses hypodermic needles to work between the tooth and the alveolar bone, severing the periodontal ligament.

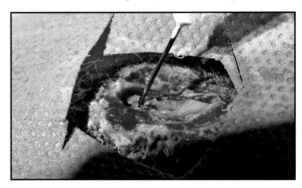

Scalpel blades or a Crossley molar luxator can also be used.

PRACTICAL TIP
The author sometimes finds that access is easier and quicker if some additional bone from the lingual aspect of the mandible is burred away. The bone is much thinner here than laterally.

4 The tooth is usually extracted using forceps, but sometimes it is easier to push it through into the mouth and pull it out from there.

OPERATIVE TECHNIQUE 27.3 continued:
Cheek tooth extraction: mandibular extraoral approach

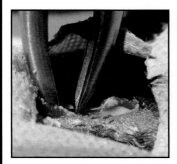 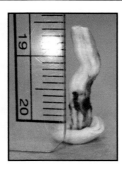

5 The author has recently started packing the cavity with carboxycellulose plugs (Traumastem) in the gap left by the absent tooth to prevent ingress and impaction of oral contents before healing.

6 Once you are ready to close the incision, flushing the area with saline should be considered; there is likely to be dust/slush from the burr of the bone, and if any contact was made with the oral cavity sterility may have been compromised. Any abscessation may also have compromised the sterility of the operation site. If sterility was maintained then simple closure of the soft tissues over the open bone is sufficient. If there was abscessation, consider marsupialization (see Chapter 29). The author closes using a monofilament absorbable suture (e.g. Monocryl) in the muscle, fat and subdermal layers. Postoperative radiographs should be taken if a fragmented molar was extracted, to verify and record that the entire tooth has been removed.

Postoperative care

- The author follows up the patient the next day to make sure it is eating, drinking and defecating normally, and to assess the effectiveness of pain medication.
- The next rechecks are at 3–5 days to assess the external wound, and then at 2 weeks to assess the tooth extraction site intraorally.
- A full oral examination under general anaesthesia is performed to assess the opposing molars and crown heights (with or without additional X-rays) after 6–8 weeks.

28

Dental-related epiphora and dacryocystitis

Richard Saunders

Definitions
- In *Saunders Comprehensive Veterinary Dictionary* (2007), **epiphora** (also occasionally referred to as illacrimation) is defined as 'an abnormal overflow of tears down the face, due usually to stricture of the nasolacrimal duct.' Overproduction of tears, typically due to ocular irritation, may mimic epiphora, but is technically referred to as hyperlacrimation.
- **Dacryocystitis** is strictly defined as inflammation of the lacrimal sac, although in common usage it involves other regions of the nasolacrimal duct, and usually involves bacterial infection as well as inflammation.

Anatomy of the nasolacrimal duct and related structures

Knowledge of the normal anatomy of the nasolacrimal duct, and the structures through which it travels, is required to investigate and treat rabbits with epiphora, dacryocystitis and chronic nasal discharge. There are specific anatomical points relating to the nasolacrimal duct and the nasal and ocular structures in the rabbit which must be understood. The anatomy of the nasolacrimal duct is illustrated in Chapter 17.

Lacrimal fluid from the eye drains into the ventral fornix of the lower conjunctival sac. From there, it passes into a single, relatively large (2–4 mm wide) slit-like to ovoid lacrimal punctum (Figure 28.1). There is no lacrimal punctum in the upper eyelid of the rabbit. The punctum is positioned on the inner aspect of the lower eyelid surface, approximately 3–5 mm from the medial canthus and 3–5 mm from the eyelid margin, and may be pigmented. A short (approximately 2–3 mm long) lacrimal canaliculus

runs ventrocranially into a dilated area, the lacrimal sac, which is located in a funnel-shaped fossa near the bony margin of the orbit, supported medially by the lacrimal bone. The duct then passes through the lacrimal foramen, and runs rostroventrally and medially through the maxillary bone (Burling *et al.*, 1991).

The nasolacrimal duct is lined by simple columnar epithelium with many mucus-producing cells. Proximally, the duct contains villous folds, thus expanding its internal surface area. The epithelium is highly vascular, with a rich lymphatic supply.

The lumen of the nasolacrimal duct varies along its length, with an average internal diameter of 2 mm. At two points, the duct both narrows to approximately 1 mm and diverts its course dramatically. At the most proximal of these two points, the duct curves rostrally as it exits the lacrimal foramen. Distally, it deviates mediodorsally as it twists around the apices of the 1st maxillary incisor, between the alveolar bone of the incisor and the nasal cartilage (see Chapter 24). Beyond this point its path continues medially and rostrally before exiting within the nasal vestibule, several millimetres inside the nares, at the ventromedial aspect of the alar fold.

Obstruction of the nasolacrimal duct at the proximal point described above tends to lead to distension of the lacrimal sac. Obstruction at the distal point generally creates distension of the entire duct proximal to that point, including the lacrimal sac.

The nasolacrimal duct resides in a longitudinal bony canal (Figure 28.2) within the maxilla (the canalis lacrimalis maxillae), closely associated with its medial aspect. It enters this canal at the proximal lacrimal foramen and exits at the level of the palatine bone, at the nasolacrimal duct flexure.

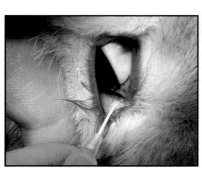

28.1
The single ventral lacrimal punctum, with an intravenous catheter entering it.

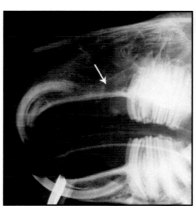

28.2
The bony lacrimal canal, through which the nasolacrimal duct is visible on this plain lateral radiograph (white arrow).

Aetiopathogenesis

Inflammation of the wall of the nasolacrimal duct and associated structures may occur in any species, and may be due to blockage by a foreign body, polyp, tumour or traumatic damage, or inflammation following accumulation of debris (e.g. sterile accumulations of lipid droplet material from the tear film; Marini *et al.*, 1996). Local vascular and lymphatic congestion can occlude the duct. While these conditions may occur in rabbits, they are the sole primary cause in only a minority of cases, usually at the least severe end of the spectrum. They may be progressive, with blockage of the nasolacrimal duct followed by inflammation and secondary bacterial (or less commonly fungal) infection.

Although it is common in some breeds of dog, lacrimal apparatus atresia has not been documented in the rabbit. Acquired eyelid deformities, following trauma or infection (including neonatal infections), may lead to closure of the lacrimal punctum through scarring.

The main cause of epiphora/dacryocystitis in pet rabbits is obstruction caused by tooth apex pathology (overlong reserve crowns impinging on the duct, soft tissue inflammation and infection, including abscessation). Expansile bone lesions (including osteomyelitis and bone remodelling) subsequent to dental pathology may occlude the duct. This may be complete or partial, and generally occurs following maxillary incisor disease, or cranial cheek tooth disease (typically involving the 1st and less commonly the 2nd maxillary cheek tooth).

Severe rhinitis, involving maxillary bone abscessation, is a less common alternative cause of nasolacrimal duct obstruction. Blockage of the duct with inspissated purulent material or scarring due to chronic or successive episodes of upper respiratory tract infections may occur.

Diagnosis

History

There is usually a history of acute, chronic, continuous or intermittent tear overflow, or purulent material from either end of the nasolacrimal duct (i.e. from one, or less commonly both, nares or eyes). This may wax and wane, and sometimes apparently self-cure completely following erosion of the nasolacrimal duct walls in the later stages of the disease.

Visual examination

A full ophthalmological and intraoral examination is advised in all cases of suspected epiphora or dacryocystitis. Instilling fluorescein dye into the eye may be used to assess the patency of the nasolacrimal duct, as well as to identify any corneal ulceration.

Clinical signs

Clinically, epiphora and dacryocystitis may be regarded as different stages in a continuum of disease, although there may be difficulty in differentiating them grossly. Expression of the material from the duct by lavage may reveal heterogeneous clear and grey material in epiphora; in contrast, it may not be possible to express material in cases of dacryocystitis. However, in most cases, differentiation is easy owing to the profuse purulent material that is present in cases of dacryocystitis.

Epiphora

This may vary in degree from clinically silent to significant overflow ventrally on to the face, resulting in large areas of unilateral or bilateral denuded fur and tear-staining or scalding of the skin, with or without secondary bacterial or fungal infection (Figure 28.3). Diagnosis may be complicated by the presence of a companion rabbit that grooms away the overflowing tears, preventing fur and skin damage, and obscuring the problem (Figure 28.4). Conversely, dermatitis or self-trauma of the affected area may occur secondarily, even with relatively mild disease. The eyelids themselves are usually not affected to any clinically significant degree.

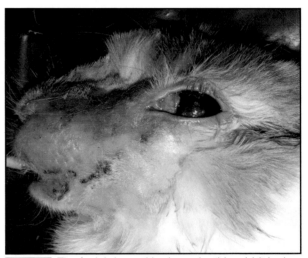

28.3 The facial dermatitis shown by this rabbit is due to tear overflow on to the fur and skin. (Courtesy of Frances Harcourt-Brown)

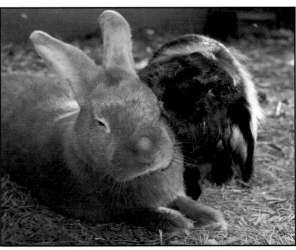

28.4 Mutual grooming is a part of the rabbit's social behaviour. (Courtesy of ME Buseth)

Dacryocystitis

This usually involves overflow of purulent material into the conjunctival sac, and on to the eyelids and facial skin in more severe cases (Figure 28.5). Differential diagnoses include primary bacterial conjunctivitis, or rhinitis/sinusitis in cases where there is purulent nasal discharge. It is possible for any or all of these conditions to occur simultaneously as a result of infection spreading from one site to another, or involving multiple areas of the head. Discharge is typically white to creamy, and of stringy to thick texture. Gentle pressure applied to the skin overlying the lacrimal sac, massaging or 'milking' material dorsocaudally towards the lacrimal punctum, may express material residing within the lacrimal sac, which may become visibly distended with pus.

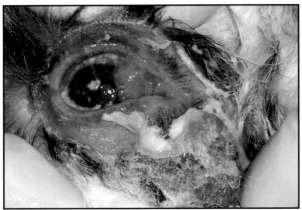

28.5 Severe keratoconjunctivitis, blepharitis and periorbital dermatitis secondary to dacryocystitis. (Courtesy of L Duckworth)

Nasolacrimal duct cannulation

Definitive diagnosis of epiphora or dacryocystitis requires cannulation of the duct(s) and lavage to express material from the distal punctum (or less frequently the proximal punctum). This procedure is described in Technique 28.1. The amount of pressure required to express material, and the nature of the material, are diagnostically and prognostically revealing. In some cases it may not be possible to flush the duct if it is totally occluded. If the wall is weakened it may rupture subcutaneously or into the nasal cavity, making it difficult to observe the expressed material. Cytology may be performed to demonstrate a cellular inflammatory response, and bacterial culture and sensitivity testing may be indicated for diagnostic purposes and selection of therapy.

Radiography and CT/MRI scanning

Radiography, including contrast studies (Figures 28.6 and 28.7) , or other imaging modalities such as computed tomography (CT; Figure 28.8) or magnetic resonance imaging (MRI; Figure 28.9) are useful in identifying the point or points at which there is occlusion of the duct(s), and identifying any causal pathology present, for example incisor or cheek tooth reserve crown elongation and associated bony reaction or osteomyelitis.

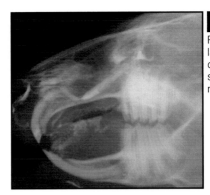

28.6 Positive-contrast lateral dacryocystograph showing the normal nasolacrimal duct.

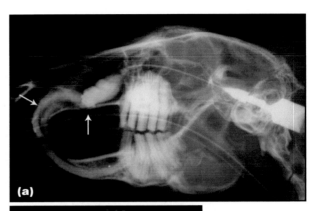

(a)

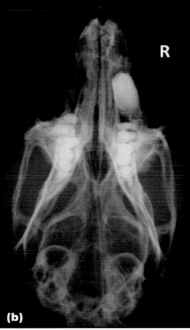

(b)

(Image reproduced from *In Practice*, with permission)

28.7 Positive-contrast study of a rabbit with dacryocystitis affecting the right eye. **(a)** On this lateral view, the nasolacrimal duct is filled with aqueous positive contrast medium (iohexol), showing that the nasal section of the duct has ruptured into the maxillary sinus (white arrow). There is pathology and apical elongation of the 1st incisor, which is distorting the maxillary bone and occluding the nasolacrimal duct. The tooth has no enamel or pulp cavity (yellow arrow). There is also deformity and apical elongation of the cheek teeth. **(b)** Dorsoventral view of the same rabbit. Iohexol had also been instilled into the left nasolacrimal duct, which was not obstructed. A thin line of contrast material can be seen in the nasal section of the duct. (Courtesy of Frances Harcourt-Brown)

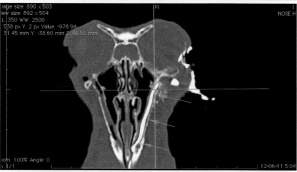

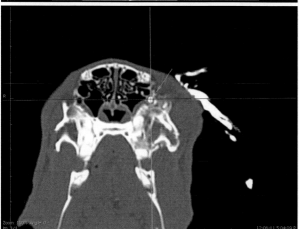

28.8 This contrast CT series shows three views (from top to bottom: sagittal, coronal, transverse) of the left nasolacrimal duct. The orange arrows mark the duct, filled with water-based contrast material. (Courtesy of Laura Crews)

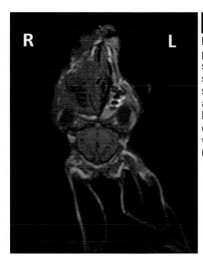

28.9 MRI scan (coronal plane) of a rabbit skull. There is severe rhinitis, sinusitis and associated bone lysis and dacryocystitis on the worst affected side (R).

Medical treatment

Treatment of epiphora and dacryocystitis depends on the underlying cause or causes. Flushing of the duct(s) is helpful in diagnosis, and in many cases of low-grade early epiphora a single flush of the affected duct(s) may be sufficient to clear a duct that is blocked with debris (either foreign material such as a grass seed or cellular material). In cases of more significant blockage, whether or not associated with inflammation of the walls of the duct, repeated gentle flushing over a period of several days may gradually achieve patency. Concurrent antibiosis (Figure 28.10) and/or anti-inflammatory therapy may help to reduce the occlusive effects of infection and inflammation around the duct or involving the walls of the duct, effectively widening the narrowed lumen and allowing lavage.

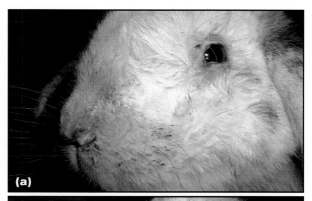

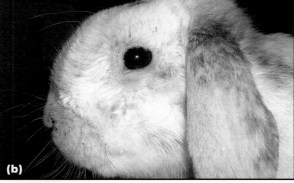

28.10 **(a)** Before treatment, there is significant purulent discharge from both ends of the nasolacrimal duct. **(b)** After systemic antibiotic treatment, mild epiphora remains.

Nasolacrimal duct flushing

Successful flushing (i.e. removing the material present in the duct, which should exit via the distal puncta) may not be possible if the duct is occluded along a significant portion of its length, or by thick tenacious pus, or by a resistant foreign body. It may also not be possible if the duct is externally occluded by dental pathology (either directly, in the form of overlong reserve crowns within the maxilla, or indirectly in the form of osteomyelitis or periapical infection arising from dental disease). However, rupture of the duct may occur with flushing, creating a new drainage exit into the nasal cavity (Figure 28.11). This can resolve the clinical signs of dacryocystitis and

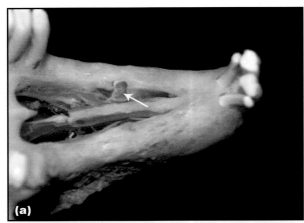

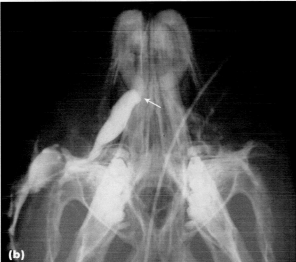

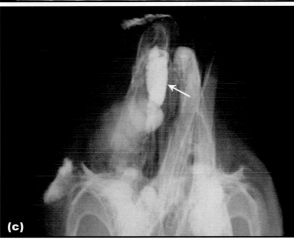

28.11 Erosion of the maxilla and spontaneous rupture of the nasolacrimal duct. **(a)** Prepared maxilla of a rabbit with advanced dental disease. The elongated apex of the incisor has curved towards the nasal passages and penetrated the bone (arrow). The site of this lesion can be seen in **(b)**, a dacryocystogram of a nasolacrimal duct blocked by an elongated curved incisor that has not penetrated the bone. Penetration of the bone and diversion on lacrimal fluid into the nasal cavity can be seen in **(c)**, a dacryocystogram of an anaesthetized rabbit with severe dacrocystitis. The iohexol has bypassed the distal section of the nasolacrimal duct, and can be seen in the nasal cavity; this improved drainage assisted in resolution of the clinical signs. (Courtesy of Frances Harcourt-Brown; (b) reproduced from *In Practice*, with permission)

epiphora. A proximal rupture, before the duct enters the canalis lacrimalis maxillae, is not as helpful because material from the duct enters the retrobulbar and periocular subcutaneous areas and this does not establish drainage.

Choice of flushing agents

The choice of flushing agents for the nasolacrimal duct is controversial and many different agents have been used. Some authorities believe that it is the physical action of flushing, removing any debris, preventing the inflammation produced by its presence and removing bacteria by physical cleaning, which is effective (Harcourt-Brown, 2009). It is therefore suggested that a sterile, non-irritant fluid such as water, normal saline or Hartmann's solution be used, at body temperature.

Others feel that it is worth applying topical antimicrobial agents directly at the site of the infection. These may be incorporated as part of the flushing solution, for example antibiotics, povidone–iodine or F10 (Health and Hygiene Pty, South Africa) can be added at a typical dilution of 1:250 with sterile water for injection. The solution can either be used to flush the duct or can be instilled into it to fill the duct after flushing. The products used should be non-irritant to tissues at appropriate dilutions.

Flushing frequency

A single flush of the affected duct(s), with or without topical treatment, may be sufficient in mild cases, e.g. of debris accumulation or foreign body obstruction, without significant inflammation or if the procedure is carried out vigorously under general anaesthetic (Harcourt-Brown, 2009).

Repeated flushing (along with topical and/or systemic antibiosis and anti-inflammatory therapy) may be carried out daily, or less frequently, until no purulent material is obtained. If initial flushing is unsuccessful, or if proximal duct rupture occurs resulting in exophthalmos, medical treatment should be used alone for approximately 1 week, before reattempting flushing.

Antibiotic therapy

Topical ocular antibiotic therapy may help to control secondary bacterial conjunctivitis, and a portion of the eye drops applied will make their way down into the duct, but this may be so little as to be insignificant in a case where the duct is partially or completely occluded. Topical ocular antibiosis alone cannot be advised except for the very mildest of cases, preferably following nasolacrimal duct flushing. The use of trypsin has been suggested, in order to break down proteinaceous deposits. A capsule of oral trypsin replacement product (e.g. Tryplase) is dissolved in 5–10 ml of normal saline and instilled into the duct; this is repeated after 48 hours. Acetylcysteine is preferred by this author to help break down purulent material within the duct, and a suggested regime is 1 ml (200 mg) Parvolex added to a 5.0–7.5 ml bottle of tear film replacement product or appropriate liquid topical antibiotic preparation (see wildpro.twycrosszoo.org).

Antimicrobial therapy should ideally be selected on the basis of recent culture and sensitivity testing. The vast majority of cases involve only bacterial growth, but fungal pathogens are possible. Both aerobic and anaerobic culture should be performed. Although *Pasteurella* spp. has often been implicated (Peterson-Jones and Carrington, 1988), a number of other bacterial pathogens may be cultured, e.g. *Staphylococcus aureus*. Anaerobes may also be recovered from this site, and may be a reason for treatment failure when antibiotics effective against aerobic bacteria alone are used. Gentamicin is generally effective against *Pasteurella* spp., and fusidic acid is usually effective against *S. aureus*. Other *Staphylococcus*, *Moraxella*, *Neisseria*, *Pseudomonas* and *Bordetella* spp. are also frequently cultured, but may sometimes be found in nasolacrimal duct culture from healthy rabbits, and so may be part of the normal flora (Marini *et al.*, 1996).

Long-term use of topical antibiotics may be required to control infection which develops secondarily to a narrowed nasolacrimal duct. If other pathogens are recovered, appropriate antimicrobial medication is advised. However, fungi can be found as opportunistic invaders and may be of no clinical significance.

Systemic antibiosis may be of more use than topical treatment in attaining effective tissue levels in the affected tissues if these are outside the duct, and may also help to achieve effective tissue levels in the duct wall. Use of both local and systemic antibiosis is advised in most cases. However, antibiotics alone are rarely effective in treating these syndromes, because the condition is not solely due to bacterial infection. They may achieve a clinical cure in cases of pure bacterial infection (e.g. following expulsion of foreign material), or in mild cases of external partial obstruction, where bacterial infection completes the obstruction.

Anti-inflammatory therapy

Topical or systemic anti-inflammatory therapy may be beneficial. Reduction in inflammation increases the lumen diameter and aids the flushing and removal of material. This may allow lavage of the duct where it was not previously possible. It may also help in cases where the lacrimal punctum is occluded due to conjunctival inflammation and it is not possible to cannulate the duct. Topical corticosteroids may be beneficial in this situation, although they should be used with caution. They may be effective in reducing conjunctival inflammation and permitting cannulation and flushing of the nasolacrimal duct. Topical non-steroidal anti-inflammatory drugs (NSAIDs) may also be used, but are considered less efficacious.

Systemically, NSAIDs are preferable to corticosteroids in rabbits, especially in those with possible subclinical upper respiratory tract infections. Analgesia may be required, especially in concurrent dental disease or severe facial pyoderma: NSAIDs or, less commonly, opioids may be utilized.

Ancillary treatment

Decongestants (e.g. pseudoephedrine) may have a place, used either topically or systemically, in reducing swelling around the duct. However, any effect they may have is temporary and rebound congestion may occur, worsening the condition, following cessation of treatment. Their use is therefore only advised in the short term, to assist in unblocking the nasolacrimal duct by flushing.

Supportive care and management

Skin scalding may be treated symptomatically by gently removing any crusted tear discharge manually, clipping and/or bathing the fur and skin, and cleaning the area with saline, warm water or dilute povidone–iodine, before drying it well and applying a barrier product such as lanolin or petroleum jelly.

If the rabbit is housed singly, the addition of a compatible companion rabbit, to provide mutual grooming, may help to alleviate facial skin scalding (see Figure 28.4; Venold and Montiani-Ferreira, 2007).

Dental treatment

Medical treatment of epiphora or dacryocystitis is unlikely to be successful if the underlying cause is constriction of the nasolacrimal duct by external inflammation or other pathology of dental origin. It is sometimes suggested that impingement of cheek teeth apices/roots on the duct can be relieved by shortening the clinical crowns. However, the tooth apices do not impinge directly on the duct and, if severe bone involvement is present, in nearly all cases the pathology is irreversible by this stage, even with removal of the affected teeth. If infection and bone distortion attributable to infection and osteomyelitis of the dental apex are the cause of the dacryocystitis, successful resolution of the underlying problem, including removal of the affected bone, may resolve the condition. Where this helps, it is probably due to the creation of new drainage pathways following removal of the involved tissues.

Extraction of cheek teeth via an intraoral approach may succeed only in removing the clinical crowns, or otherwise incompletely removing the whole tooth. This may leave a remnant which acts as the nidus for infection of the bone. Conversely, in some cases drainage of the nasolacrimal duct directly or via the nasal cavity may subsequently occur via the mouth. This is likely to be temporary until the site heals, and cannot in any case be recommended as a treatment option.

Pathology of the incisor apex is a common cause of epiphora/dacryocystitis. Incisor extraction may resolve nasolacrimal duct blockage by removing the reserve crown which is impinging on the duct, or allowing the periapical inflammation to resolve following removal. Again, the pathology may be refractory to extraction and the source of occlusion may remain, because bony changes are likely to be permanent (Harcourt-Brown, 2002a). It is difficult to advise incisor extraction solely to treat nasolacrimal duct blockage.

Surgical treatment

Surgical treatments to create an opening from the nasolacrimal duct into the nasal cavity are well described in human patients with epiphora/dacryocystitis, and are usually carried out endoscopically, but are not reported in the rabbit. They are unlikely to be practicable except as part of abscess removal, given the small size of the patient, and the difficulty of approaching the relevant area at the correct oblique angle via a nasal approach and keeping the new aperture from healing closed.

Marsupialization of the lacrimal sac

Some rabbits with severe dacryocystitis develop distended infected lacrimal sacs that become enlarged and dilated and constantly discharge pus into the conjunctival sac, causing chronic painful keratoconjunctivitis. The lacrimal sac is easily palpated cranioventrally to the medial canthus and readily expresses large amounts of pus through the lacrimal punctum. These cases are often associated with apical infection of the 1st incisor, so the whole nasolacrimal duct fills with pus. Extraction of the infected incisor is indicated alongside surgery to remove the pus and marsupialize the lacrimal sac; this can be effective in curing the keratoconjunctivitis, although the rabbit will always suffer from epiphora because the lacrimal punctum is removed during surgery and the lacrimal fluid cannot drain into the nose. The surgical procedure is described in Operative Technique 28.2.

Prognosis

Simple cases of internal luminal blockage with no underlying pathology have an excellent prognosis following treatment. Cases of obstruction partially due to pathology external to the duct carry a variable prognosis. As a rule, if they can be cleared with repeated flushing and medical treatment, and the dental pathology is managed, the prognosis is good.

If there is total intractable obstruction of the duct through permanent fibrosis resulting from inflammation, or impingement from tooth or bone pathology, the prognosis for resolution of the epiphora is hopeless unless a new aperture is created either therapeutically or by progression of the disease process, or the affected tooth or teeth are removed. Dacryocystitis may be controlled with medical therapy, and the skin disease resulting from epiphora may be managed.

In one study, 43% of rabbits made a full recovery with appropriate treatment (Florin *et al.*, 2009). Those rabbits that required longer courses of treatment, and those requiring systemic treatment, had a much poorer prognosis. However, whether the duct was patent or not on flushing made little difference to whether there was a successful outcome. Treatment duration may need to be long, with 6 weeks being typical, and it is common to underestimate the severity of the underlying disease issues in these cases.

References and further reading

Bauck L (1989) Ophthalmic conditions in pet rabbits and rodents. *Compendium on Continuing Education for the Practicing Veterinarian* **11**(3), 258–261, 264–266
Blood DC, Studdart VP and Gay CC (2007) *Saunders Comprehensive Veterinary Dictionary, 3rd edn.* Saunders Elsevier, St. Louis
Burling K, Murphy CJ, Curiel JS, Koblick P and Bellhorn RW (1991) Anatomy of the rabbit nasolacrimal duct and its clinical implications. *Progress in Veterinary and Comparative Ophthalmology* **1**, 33–40
Florin M, Rusanen E, Haessig M, Richter M and Spiess B (2009) Clinical presentation, treatment and outcome of dacryocystitis in rabbits: a retrospective study of 28 cases (2003-2007). *Veterinary Ophthalmology* **12**, 350–356
Harcourt-Brown FM (2002a) Dacryocystitis in rabbits. *Exotic DVM* **4**(3), 47–49
Harcourt-Brown FM (2002b) Ophthalmic diseases. In: *Textbook of Rabbit Medicine*, pp.292–305. Butterworth Heinemann, Oxford
Harcourt-Brown FM (2009) Dental disease in pet rabbits. 2. Diagnosis and treatment. *In Practice* **31**, 432–445
Hillyer EV (1994) Pet rabbits. *Veterinary Clinics of North America: Small Animal Practice* **24**(1), 25–65
Kern TJ (1997) Rabbit and rodent ophthalmology. *Seminars in Avian and Exotic Pet Medicine* **6**(3), 138–145
Marini RP, Foltz CJ, Kersten D *et al.* (1996) Microbiologic, radiographic and anatomic study of the nasolacrimal duct apparatus in the rabbit (*Oryctolagus cuniculus*). *Laboratory Animal Science* **46**, 656–662
Oglesbee B (2011) Epiphora. *The 5-minute Veterinary Consult – Small Mammal, 2nd edn*, pp. 407–409. Blackwell Publishing, Iowa
Peterson-Jones SM and Carrington SD (1988) Pasteurella dacryocystitis in rabbits. *Veterinary Record* **122**, 514–515
Venold F and Montiani-Ferreira F (2007) Selected ocular disorders in rabbits. *Exotic DVM* **9**(1), 32–37
Williams DL (2006) Ophthalmology In: *BSAVA Manual of Rabbit Medicine and Surgery, 2nd edn*, ed. A Meredith and P Flecknell, pp. 117–128. BSAVA Publications, Gloucester

TECHNIQUE 28.1:
Flushing the nasolacrimal duct
Richard Saunders

Patient preparation and restraint

- The author prefers to carry out initial superficial proximal nasolacrimal duct flushing under good manual restraint and topical local anaesthesia with proxymetacaine, rather than general anaesthesia. The rabbit may be wrapped in a towel with only the head exposed.
- Sedation may be employed in fractious rabbits, or those resenting the procedure.
- General anaesthesia is necessary if concurrent dental investigation or treatment is required or if dacryocystorhinography is performed. It is also necessary in order to pass a cannula through the lacrimal foramen into the nasal portion of the duct for flushing (Harcourt-Brown, 2009).

Equipment

- Intravenous catheters: 20 to 26 G, without wings. Although purpose-designed cannulas are available, intravenous catheters are the author's choice. The risk of corneal laceration or nasolacrimal duct puncture is significantly greater when using metal cannulas
- Syringes: from 2 to 5 ml, depending on handling preference and the volume of fluid required to flush the duct thoroughly; 2 ml may be insufficient in some cases, 5 ml is adequate in nearly every case. Larger syringes carry an increased risk of applying excessive pressure and rupturing the nasolacrimal duct
- Flushing liquid (warmed sterile normal saline or Hartmann's solution)
- Focal light source

Technique

1 A few drops of topical local anaesthetic are placed in the conjunctival sac(s) and left for a minute or so to take full effect.

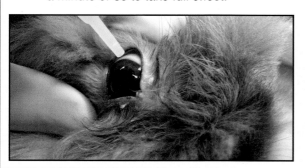

2 The single, medially positioned lacrimal punctum consists of an ovoid aperture, and access to it is best gained by entering it at a shallow angle, parallel to the long axis of the oval. If the punctum is obscured or filled with pus, manual expression of pus and cleaning it away will assist with visualization. The punctum is visualized by eversion of the lower eyelid using gentle fingertip handling only. It helps to place traction on the very edge of the lid, angling it ventrally and laterally away from the globe. Excessive traction on the eyelid is resented, and may also occlude the punctum; general anaesthesia or sedation may be necessary for these cases.

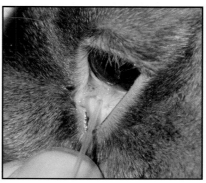

The punctum is identified in the ventral eyelid.

3 An appropriately sized cannula is selected, e.g. 24 G (0.56 mm) to 20 G (0.90 mm). If too narrow a gauge is used, it will not be possible to achieve sufficient pressure to flush the nasolacrimal duct, because the fluid will leak around the catheter. The tip of the cannula is introduced in a ventromedial direction until resistance is encountered. The presence of some topical local anaesthetic in the cannula may help to minimize discomfort on introduction of the cannula, this being one point at which some rabbits resent the procedure.

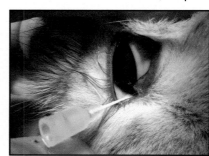

A suitable cannula is inserted into the punctum.

TECHNIQUE 28.1 continued:
Flushing the nasolacrimal duct
Richard Saunders

PRACTICAL TIP
If it is difficult to insert a cannula into the punctum because of the small size of the aperture, or because the rabbit keeps moving, sedation or anaesthesia should be employed. Excellent lighting, and magnification as necessary, will assist in the more difficult cases. If it is not possible to enter the punctum using the catheter selected, it may be possible to use a narrower catheter initially, progressing to a larger one once initial entry has been made.

4 A syringe, filled with sterile water for injection, saline or therapeutic agents, is connected to the cannula, and gentle pressure is applied until material appears from the nostril, or it is judged that the duct is blocked. Massaging the side of the face at the same time from the medial canthus downwards may help to break up purulent debris accumulations.

5 If no fluid can be instilled, withdraw the cannula by 1–2 mm, as the tip may be occluded in the acute bend at this point, and reattempt flushing.

6 Rabbits may resent the procedure at the point where fluid starts to emerge from the distal punctum, and reintroduction of the cannula may be required should they dislodge it. Subsequent flushing is usually tolerated.

7 Flushing is continued until fluid flows freely from the distal end of the duct in the ipsilateral nostril and there is no sign of purulent material present; it is repeated at intervals as necessary.

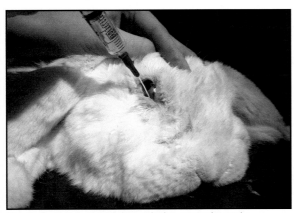

Sterile fluid is passed through the cannula and nasolacrimal duct until it flows freely.

Dacryocystography

Water-soluble contrast medium (e.g. 1–2 ml Conray 280, sodium/meglumine iothalamate) may be instilled at this point to demonstrate nasolacrimal duct narrowing or rupture using radiography, if necessary. Inhalation of the contrast medium, after passage through the duct, may create superimposition artefacts on the radiograph within the nasal passages, and should be avoided. Dilute preparations are easier to instil into the narrowed nasolacrimal duct; however, more concentrated solutions remain within the duct for longer, providing a clearer image with less risk of inhalation.

Notes and complications

Inability to enter the punctum
If this is not possible, this author prefers to treat the animal with topical (e.g. flurbiprofen, fucidic acid) and/or systemic anti-inflammatories and antibiotics (e.g. enrofloxacin, meloxicam) and to reattempt cannulation after approximately 1 week of treatment. If the duct is permanently stenosed as a result of local fibrosis, surgical reopening is unlikely to be permanently effective.

Inability to flush the duct
If no fluid emerges despite flushing in the conscious rabbit, repeating the process under general anaesthesia and advancing the cannula carefully through the lacrimal foramen allows pressure to be applied directly to the site of the blockage, rather than further dilating, and potentially rupturing, the lacrimal sac. A plastic cannula, rather than a metal one, must be used for this procedure. Systemic and topical treatment as above may help to resolve blockages caused by inflammation only, and medical treatment followed by reattempting the flush 1 week later may be tried.

Rupture of the duct
When flushing via a catheter placed superficially into the nasolacrimal duct, excess pressure may cause rupture of the duct at a point proximal to the stenosis or blockage, with fluid entering the retrobulbar space or collecting under the skin. Swelling around the eye or exophthalmos may result. This usually subsides without incident, although antibiosis and analgesia may be warranted. Rupture is less likely to happen when the catheter is advanced more deeply into the duct; if rupture does occur in this case, it is likely to be sufficiently distal to avoid the →

TECHNIQUE 28.1 continued:
Flushing the nasolacrimal duct
Richard Saunders

---

above problem and may actually assist drainage of the duct by creating a new aperture within the nasal cavity (see Figure 28.11).

Recurrence of copious amounts of pus
Where there is copious purulent material present, repeated attempts to flush the duct daily for several days may incrementally relieve the obstruction and allow full passage of fluid eventually. Addition of proteolytic or other materials to the flushing fluid may assist (see text). If all the above fail, radiography and reassessment of the sinuses and teeth, especially the maxillary incisors, is indicated. Some authors have described the use of large-diameter nylon suture material inserted through the punctum, to dislodge obstructions. Given that recalcitrant obstructions are likely to be extramural, this approach does not often work, and when it does, probably achieves its aim by creating a hole through the duct wall into the sinus or nasal cavity. Marsupialization of the lacrimal sac (see Operative Technique 28.2) is an effective way of diverting pus away from the lacrimal sac and treating the infection.

OPERATIVE TECHNIQUE 28.2:
Marsupialization of the lacrimal sac
Frances Harcourt-Brown

Indications

In some severe cases of dacrocystitis, pus is continuously produced in the lacrimal sac, which becomes very dilated and can be palpated as a soft swelling ventromedial to the lateral canthus. The eyelids may become glued together with pus.

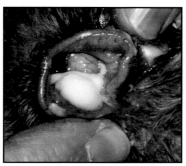

Applying digital pressure to the swelling will squeeze copious amounts of purulent secretion through the lacrimal punctum into the conjunctival sac.

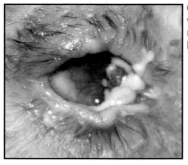

Constant contact with pus can result in a painful keratoconjunctivitis.

The condition is often associated with periapical infection of the maxillary 1st incisor, and extraction of the incisor may be indicated.

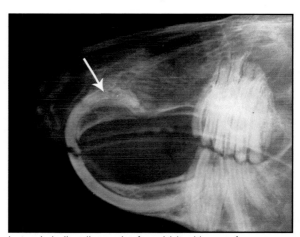

Lateral skull radiograph of a rabbit with a profuse unilateral ocular and nasal discharge and a palpably dilated lacrimal sac. There is radiopacity of the maxillary sinus and a fractured maxillary incisor (arrow). The root was infected and obstructing the nasolacrimal duct.

The aim of marsupialization of the lacrimal sac is to divert pus away from the eye and allow the infection to be controlled and treated.

OPERATIVE TECHNIQUE 28.2:
Marsupialization of the lacrimal sac
Frances Harcourt-Brown

Positioning and patient preparation

The rabbit is anaesthetized and intubated (see Chapter 1). Skull radiographs are taken and the nasolacrimal system and associated teeth are examined carefully. Local anaesthetic (proxymetacaine) drops are applied to the eye and instilled into the nostril because this is a very painful condition. Preparation for surgery can be very stimulating, especially if the rabbit is only lightly anaesthetized. Prior to surgery the discharge around the eyelids and conjunctiva is removed and the fur clipped from the face between the eye and nose. The nasolacrimal duct is thoroughly flushed to remove all the purulent material. Dacryocystography may be undertaken. The surgical site is prepared for surgery.

Equipment extras

- A blue (0.76 mm) irrigating cannula (Portex)
- Fine surgical kit
- Optical loupes (optional)

Procedure

1 The cannula is inserted through the punctum lacrimale into the lacrimal sac. The lacrimal sac is identified by palpation and a 5–8 mm skin incision is made over it. The landmarks that are used to identify the site of the lacrimal sac are the medial canthus of the eye and the zygomatic prominence.

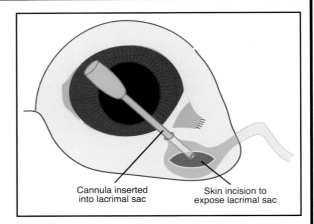

Cannula inserted into lacrimal sac · Skin incision to expose lacrimal sac

2 The skin is separated and the subcutaneous tissue is separated by blunt dissection to expose the lacrimal sac, which is close to the skin. The zygomatic salivary gland may also be exposed.

3 The wall of the lacrimal sac is grasped with dissecting forceps and tented. The loose tissue of the tented lateral wall of the lacrimal sac is trimmed away. The medial wall of the lacrimal sac is firmly attached and is not easily removed. It provides a barrier between the interior of the lacrimal sac (which is infected) and the retrobulbar space.

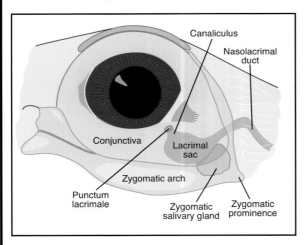

Canaliculus · Nasolacrimal duct · Conjunctiva · Lacrimal sac · Zygomatic arch · Punctum lacrimale · Zygomatic salivary gland · Zygomatic prominence

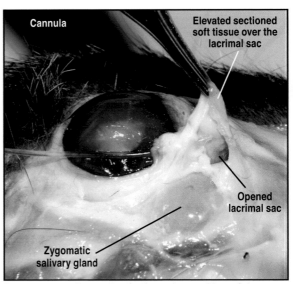

Cannula · Elevated sectioned soft tissue over the lacrimal sac · Opened lacrimal sac · Zygomatic salivary gland

Post-mortem dissection to show the position of the lacrimal sac.

OPERATIVE TECHNIQUE 28.2 continued:
Marsupialization of the lacrimal sac
Frances Harcourt-Brown

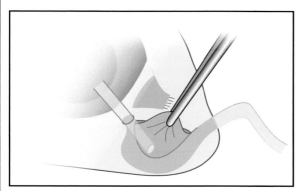

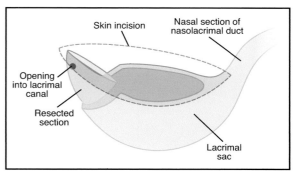

Lateral aspect of lacrimal sac to show resected section.

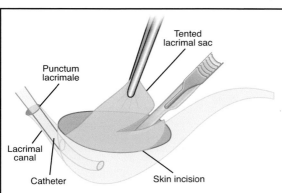

5 The remaining lacrimal sac is marsupialized by suturing its cut edge to the skin. The author uses 1.5 metric (4/0 USP) Vicryl Rapide (polyglactin) because the stitches can be wiped off and do not need to be removed. The marsupialized cavity leads into the nasolacrimal duct as it passes through the lacrimal bone and into the nasal passages.

4 Within the wall of the lacrimal sac, the opening into the lacrimal canal to the punctum is identified. The section of wall, including the opening into the lacrimal canal needs to be excised so there is no connection between the lacrimal and conjunctival sacs and pus can no longer discharge into the eye. Once there is no pus in the conjunctival sac, any keratoconjunctivitis rapidly responds to treatment.

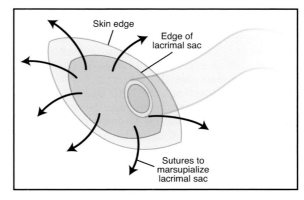

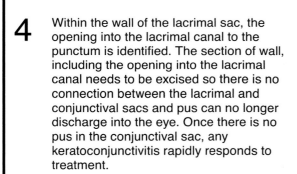

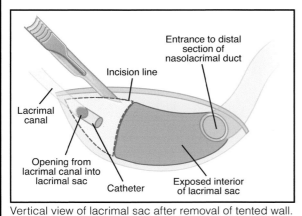

Vertical view of lacrimal sac after removal of tented wall.

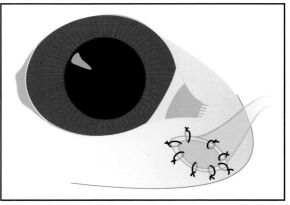

OPERATIVE TECHNIQUE 28.2 continued:
Marsupialization of the lacrimal sac
Frances Harcourt-Brown

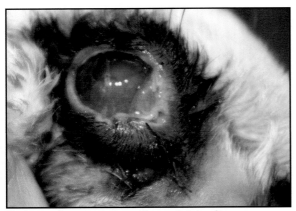

Postoperative appearance immediately after marsupialization.

Postoperative care

The conjunctiva and lacrimal sac are cleaned twice daily after instillation of local anaesthetic drops (proxymetacaine). Antibiotic eye drops (e.g. gentamicin) are instilled into both the eye and lacrimal sac after cleaning. Analgesia is indicated. The author's choice is oral meloxicam (0.3 mg/kg q12h) and tramadol (5 mg/kg q8h) for as long as necessary. Systemic antibiotics are also indicated. The author's choice is parenteral cefalexin (20 mg/kg) because it penetrates the aqueous humour. It is given by daily injections for 7–10 days. If the discharge from the marsupialized sac continues to be profuse, the rabbit may be sedated or anaesthetized again after 3–4 days to have a catheter inserted into the nasal section of the nasolacrimal duct so it can be flushed and cleared. After surgery, the keratoconjunctivis quickly resolves.

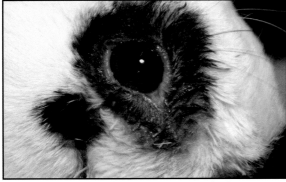

Same rabbit as above, 5 days postoperatively.

Long-term care

This procedure permanently blocks the nasolacrimal duct so the rabbit will always have a degree of epiphora, but this is minimal if there is no conjunctival irritation from infection. A bonded companion or dedicated owner may be required to keep the face clean. Any discharge from the eye should be lacrimal fluid, which can be milky in colour.

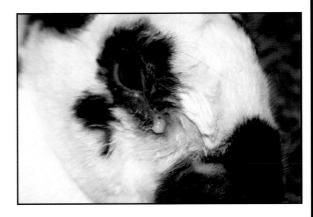

In the few cases where infection persists in the distal section of the nasolacrimal duct, purulent material may discharge through a fistula in the skin at the site of surgery. A catheter can be inserted to flush the duct. Repeat radiography and reappraisal of the source of infection is needed. Extraction of the maxillary first incisor is usually necessary.

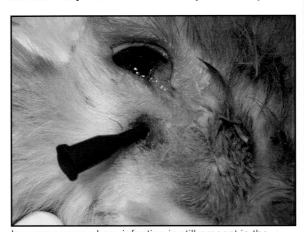

In some cases where infection is still present in the lacrimal duct, a fistula may form beneath the medial canthus. A cannula can be inserted to flush material through the duct and out of the nose.

29

Facial abscesses

Frances Harcourt-Brown and John Chitty

Facial abscesses are a common problem in pet rabbits, and rapid advances have been made in their successful treatment in recent years. Despite the large number of rabbit abscesses that are treated in general practice, there are very few published papers in the scientific literature. Four papers are available: two are single case reports (Ward, 2006; Martínez-Jiménez et al., 2007); the other two are small retrospective studies involving 13 rabbits or fewer (Remeeus and Verbeek, 1995; Taylor et al., 2010). The absence of a larger comparative study is not surprising because of the difficulties in comparing the outcome of treatment for abscesses that vary in severity, site and aetiology. In the absence of peer-reviewed studies, clinical treatment of facial abscesses in rabbits relies on the anecdotal experiences of referral clinicians. This chapter describes the recommendations of some of these clinicians, with the idea of informing the reader of the current state of knowledge and to present the management options that are available. The Editors are grateful to Brendan Carmel, Will Easson, Vladimir Jekl, Alessandro Melillo and Aidan Raftery for contributing their techniques and experiences in this chapter; their personal opinions and those of the Editors are referenced throughout the chapter by initials. The clinician is best advised to review the available options and choose the one that would appear to have the best chance of success with the facilities at their disposal and given the individual circumstances and needs of the patient and its owners, with the welfare of the patient as sole primary concern.

Aetiology of abscesses

Suppuration and abscess formation

The definition of an abscess is 'a localised collection of pus in a cavity formed by the disintegration of tissue' (Blood et al., 2007). Abscesses are the product of suppurative inflammation, which is a process that is characterized by the formation of large quantities of pus in response to invasion of tissue by pyogenic bacteria or, occasionally, fungi or parasites. Pus consists of inflammatory exudate, bacteria, cellular debris and dead phagocytes, predominantly neutrophils that migrate to the abscess as part of the host response to infection. Neutrophils contain lysosomal granules that contain enzymes that degrade and destroy bacteria; as these enzymes are released,

bacteria, neutrophils and dead tissue cells undergo autolysis to form pus. Initially, the suppurative process commonly causes local pain, anorexia, fever, toxaemia and a leucocytosis; as the process continues, a cavity containing the pus is formed, which becomes walled off from the surrounding tissue by a fibrous capsule, and the systemic effects subside. The effect of an abscess on the patient is determined in the initial stages by the pain and toxaemia that is generated, and later by the size and location of a chronic abscess that can put pressure on surrounding tissue.

Response to suppurative infection in rabbits

Rabbits differ from dogs and cats in their response to suppurative infection. Although the nature of the inflammatory response is influenced by the type and pathogenicity of bacteria involved, rabbits seldom show signs of acute inflammation in response to infections. Systemic signs such as pain, fever and toxaemia are unusual. Whether this is because rabbits hide signs of pain effectively or genuinely do not feel pain associated with infection is difficult to know. Chronic abscess formation and localized signs are more common. It is difficult to know why rabbits seem to be more susceptible to abscess formation than other species but it has been shown that their neutrophils have diminished bactericidal capacity in the presence of chronic infection (Bamberger and Herndon, 1990). Haematologically, rabbits do not develop marked leucocytosis after an acute infectious challenge (Toth and January, 1990). Instead, a change in the distribution of white cells occurs in response to infection, with a relative neutrophilia and lymphopenia (Toth and Krueger, 1989). A reduction in blood cellularity, with chronic anaemia, low white cell count and lymphopenia, occurs (Hinton et al., 1982) in response to any chronic disease and this is often the blood picture of pet rabbits with abscesses. Occasionally, a monocytosis may be seen.

Characteristics of the abscess capsule

The wall of an abscess cavity comprises a capsule of young connective tissue containing collagen fibres and blood vessels. Once the capsule is formed, neutrophils and other leucocytes continue to migrate into the abscess from blood vessels in the capsule. Antibodies that neutralize toxins and kill bacteria arrive at the site. Eventually the abscess capsule becomes thick and fibrous, being composed of fibro-blasts and inflammatory cells, with an inner layer of degenerating neutrophils (Chaffee *et al.*, 1975) (Figure 29.1). This fibrous capsule can have both advantages and disadvantages (Figure 29.2).

The abscess may expand along the line of least resistance and can rupture through the skin or into a body cavity, discharging pus, bacteria and toxins; or the capsule may remain intact and become so thick that it walls off infection from surrounding tissue. Even if the fibrous capsule is ruptured and the pus is drained, the cavity may fail to heal because the fibrous wall of the capsule is so rigid that it cannot collapse. Residual microorganisms along the inner surface of the capsule can proliferate and lead to renewal of infection.

Chronic abscesses are refractory to medical treatment because the fibrous capsule walls off and encloses the infection. Resorption of water from pus results in thick caseous material within the abscess cavity. By this time there is very little inflammation.

Bacteria involved in rabbit abscesses

A variety of aerobic and anaerobic bacteria have been cultured from dental abscesses in rabbits, and mixed infections occur. Gas production is a feature of some infections (Figure 29.3). Non-pathogenic contaminants, such as *Enterobacteriaceae* or *Bacteroides* spp. can be present, especially in abscesses that connect to the oral cavity. In other cases no bacteria are isolated, perhaps because the infection is so chronic that the bacteria have been eliminated, or because the wrong part of the abscess was cultured, or the sample was handled incorrectly.

Pasteurella multocida is the organism that is most frequently implicated in purulent infections. This bacterium has capsular polysaccharides that resist phagocytosis (Deeb, 1993). Other pyogenic bacteria that have been isolated from rabbit abscesses include *Staphylococcus* spp., *Pseudomonas* spp. and *Fusobacterium* spp. (Chaffee *et al.*, 1975; Dominguez *et al.*, 1975; Ward *et al.*, 1981). One study showed a predominant mixture of anaerobic Gram-positive rods, mostly *F. nucleatum* and *Actinomyces* spp., and aerobic Gram-positive cocci, particularly *Streptococcus milleri,* in a series of 12 abscesses that were cultured (Tyrell *et al.*, 2002). A more recent study cultured 30 different organisms, including haemolytic and non-haemolytic *Streptococcus* spp., *Acinetobacter* spp., *Escherichia coli, Enterococcus faecalis, Enterobacter cloacae, Proteus vulgaris, Staphylococcus* spp., *Pseudomonas aeruginosa, Bacteroides* spp., *Peptostreptococcus* spp., *Peptococcus* spp., *Mobiluncus mulieris, Micromonas micros, Parvimonas micra, Gemella morbillorum, Prevotella oris, Actinomyces* spp., *Clostridium butyricum* and *F. nucleatum* (Jekl *et al.*, 2012).

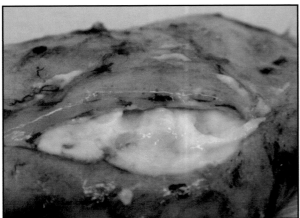

29.1 An abscess capsule is composed of fibroblasts and inflammatory cells, with an inner layer of degenerating neutrophils. In rabbits, the capsule can become very thick, forming an effective barrier between infection and surrounding tissue. Live bacteria are most likely to be present on the inner aspect of the capsule, which is the best site for taking samples for culture.

Advantages

- Provides a barrier that protects surrounding tissue from pyogenic bacteria
- Exposure of the inner surface of the capsule allows access to bacteria that can be killed by topical antibiotic therapy or, in the case of anaerobic infections, exposure to air and oxygen

Disadvantages

- Provides a physical barrier that encloses and harbours infection
- Hinders passage of antibacterial drugs into the abscess cavity
- Prevents rupture and drainage of pus, so the abscess can become large and compress adjacent tissues
- Does not collapse easily when punctured, so residual microorganisms along the inner surface of the capsule can lead to recrudescence of infection

Significance

- Removal of the fibrous capsule during surgery exposes neighbouring tissue to pyogenic bacteria but also removes tissue that can lead to recrudescence of infection
- In practical terms:
  - Removal of any parts of the fibrous capsule that are not attached to surrounding tissue is beneficial
  - Removal of capsule that is attached to surrounding tissue can expose healthy tissue to bacterial infection

29.2 Advantages, disadvantages and significance of a thick fibrous abscess capsule (see Figure 29.1).

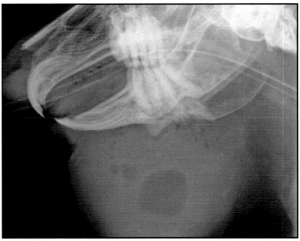

29.3 Some abscesses contain anaerobic bacteria that form gas. In the abscess shown here, a circle of gas can be seen in the centre of the abscess cavity.

Clinical features

Facial abscesses are characterized by a palpable swelling around the face. The swelling may be hard or soft, and painful or not painful. The skin may or may not be discoloured, and the swelling may have been present for days, weeks, months or even years. The swelling may have burst and discharged pus, or pus may be seen draining into the oral cavity if the swelling is squeezed (Figure 29.4).

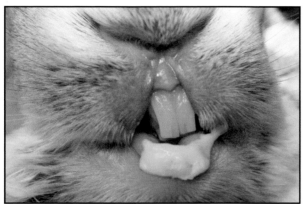

29.4 A simple but informative diagnostic procedure is to squeeze an abscess to see if, and where, pus can be expressed into the oral cavity. This is not easy to photograph in rabbits with abscesses involving the cheek teeth, but the rabbit shown here had a submandibular abscess involving the lower incisor and the first lower cheek tooth. Copious quantities of pus could be expressed from the incisor socket.

The site of the swelling is an important consideration, as it can help to identify the cause of a facial abscess. Many are related to dental problems, and the position of an abscess may give an indication of which teeth are involved (Figure 29.5).

In the case of retrobulbar abscesses (see later), the swelling may not be palpable but its presence is evident from the anterior displacement of the eye. Exophthalmos may be sudden if infection has eroded the retrobulbar venous sinus resulting in haemorrhage and haematoma formation (Figure 29.6).

Nerve damage

Abscesses around the head may be associated with facial nerve damage, with clinical signs depending on the site of the damage. Most dental abscesses affect the distal sections of the facial nerve that supply the skin on the cheek and lips. More proximally, the facial nerve may be affected by periapical infections of the caudal cheek teeth or by penetrating injuries inside the cheek. The blink reflex on the affected side may be impaired and this can result in keratitis.

Abscesses of the base of the ear often involve the most proximal section of the facial nerve, as it emerges from the stylomastoid foramen and runs across the lateral aspect of the tympanic bulla. Abscesses in this region are often associated with the swellings that are common in lop-eared rabbits with deformed ear cartilages (see Chapter 16). Rictus can be the result of facial nerve damage. It occurs when atrophy and fibrosis of the orbicularis

Site of abscess	Teeth likely to be involved	Clinical signs	Prognosis
Rostral mandible	Apices of 1st and/or 2nd mandibular cheek teeth and/or mandibular incisor	Mandibular swelling. Rabbit may appear to be unaffected by abscess	**Good:** Infected teeth are easy to remove, as access to apices is easy. Removal of a single incisor or cheek tooth seldom causes problems with elongation of opposing teeth, although their shape may change. The opposing teeth wear against remaining adjacent teeth
Caudal mandible	Apex of 4th mandibular cheek tooth	Swelling under masseter muscle part of cheek. Rabbit will often eat slowly and on one side of the mouth. Often swelling inside cheek on affected side that can make eating uncomfortable	**Good** but surgery might be difficult. Removal of infected teeth is hampered by masseter muscle, which is vascular, large and hinders visualization.

29.5 Clinical signs and prognosis of facial abscesses at different sites. (continues) ▶

Site of abscess	Teeth likely to be involved	Clinical signs	Prognosis
Caudal mandible or under throat	5th (tiny) mandibular cheek tooth	Pain in angle of jaw makes chewing painful. Swelling on caudal part of cheek. May extend to medial aspect of mandible under chin	**Guarded:** Lower 5th cheek tooth can deviate medially and penetrate mandible on medial aspect. The abscess may extend into submandibular structures which are difficult to access
On lateral aspect of cheek	Crowns of long curved maxillary 1st or 2nd cheek teeth that have penetrated mucosa of cheek	Affected rabbits may eat well	**Good:** Abscess can often be removed in its entirety or easily marsupialized. The elongated crown of the offending tooth needs to be shortened
Face anteroventral to medial canthus of eye (Reproduced from *In Practice*, with permission)	Maxillary 1st cheek tooth	Swelling on face below medial canthus of eye. Usually pus discharging from nostril, with dyspnoea and stridor. Associated with infection in maxillary sinus (see Chapter 16). May be pus discharging from punctum lacrimale and and associated keratoconjunctivitis	**Good** if infection is localized and arises from 1st upper cheek tooth that can be removed through the mouth. Gravity assists drainage of cavity into mouth **Poor** if infection has disseminated through nasal passages and sinuses. This is usually due to infection spreading from the roots of the upper 1st incisors or from periodontal infection from a foreign body in socket of incisor
Over zygomatic prominence ventral to the eye	2nd maxillary cheek tooth	Often localized abscess in rabbit that shows few other clinical signs	**Good:** Apex of tooth is accessible via zygomatic prominence. The tooth may be pushed into the oral cavity or removed through the mouth. Gravity assists drainage into mouth postoperatively

29.5 (continued) Clinical signs and prognosis of facial abscesses at different sites. (continues) ▶

Site of abscess	Teeth likely to be involved	Clinical signs	Prognosis
Retrobulbar abscess	Caudal (3rd, 4th or 5th) maxillary cheek teeth	Unilateral exophthalmos or swelling in orbit. May be mild or severe with associated panophthalmitis	**Good** if abscess can be drained without enucleation and infected tooth removed through the mouth **Poor** if infected teeth cannot be identified or infection is so extensive that it involves deep inaccessible bony structures
Around orbit, caudal to eye. (Hard to see elongated apex on radiographs because of superimposition of zygoma)	6th maxillary (tiny) cheek tooth	No exophthalmos. Swelling extending from beneath the zygomatic arch. Rare: usually infection involves other apices in alveolar bulla and causes retrobulbar abscess	**Good** if tooth can be removed. It is a small tooth that can be extracted through the mouth
Nose	Apex of maxillary incisors	Swelling on nose. Pus discharging from nostril. Dyspnoea. Stridor. May be severe dacryocystitis and keratoconjunctivitis (see Chapter 28). Can follow incisor removal or foreign body in 1st upper incisor socket	**Guarded:** Apices of teeth are accessible from lateral aspect of maxilla but infection may have extended into nasal cavity and maxillary sinuses. Distorted remnants of regrown incisors can be difficult to locate and remove
Chin	Apex of mandibular incisor	Swelling under mandible. May be few clinical signs other than problems biting through hard foods such as carrots. Pus may exude from socket (see Figure 29.4). Can follow incisor removal or foreign body in lower incisor socket	**Good:** Lower incisors are accessible and easy to remove. There are no important structures close to them

29.5 (continued) Clinical signs and prognosis of facial abscesses at different sites. (continues) ▶

Site of abscess	Teeth likely to be involved	Clinical signs	Prognosis
At base of ear	Unlikely to be related to teeth 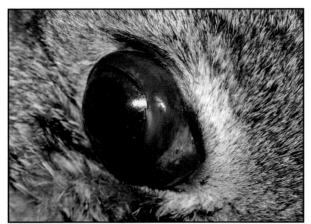	Common in lop-eared rabbits (see Chapter 16)	**Good** if is there is no nerve damage or middle ear infection. Abscess can be treated conservatively or by lateral wall resection **Moderate** if there is facial nerve damage (see Figure 29.7), which will be permanent **Guarded** if middle ear infection and vestibular signs are present (see Chapter 16)

29.5 (continued) Clinical signs and prognosis of facial abscesses at different sites.

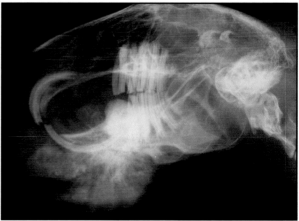

29.6 A large retrobulbar venous plexus is situated between the alveolar bulla and the globe (see Chapter 17). Erosion of this plexus by periapical infection can result in sudden haemorrhage behind the eye and marked exophthalmos.

oculi and zygomatic muscles occur. These muscles are innervated by the facial nerve, and muscle atrophy draws the affected side of the face back into a grimace. These rabbits have an asymmetrical face that looks odd (Figure 29.7) and they can have problems with mastication if food becomes trapped between the maxillary cheek teeth and the inside of the cheek.

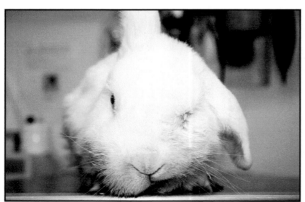

29.7 Rictus is a manifestation of nerve damage to the facial nerve, affecting the left side of this rabbit's face. Problems with mastication may arise if food becomes trapped between the maxillary cheek teeth and the inside of the cheek.

The mandibular nerve can be affected by abscesses that extend deep into the medial aspect of the mandible. These usually arise from the 5th mandibular cheek tooth. In rare cases, problems with mastication and swallowing may be observed. Affected rabbits may salivate profusely.

Differential diagnosis

Neoplasia and bone cysts are the major differential diagnoses and can be detected by radiography, ultrasonography or computed tomography (CT) or magnetic resonance imaging (MRI) (if available) or diagnosed from an aspirate of the contents of the swelling (Harcourt-Brown, 2009).

Differentiation of malignant bone neoplasia from osteomyelitis can be difficult. Both can show a mixed pattern of osteolysis and osteogenesis, with an interrupted periosteal reaction. Clinical history, palpation, aspiration and radiography can be more helpful than histopathology in the differential diagnosis. Speed of growth, a hard consistency and failure to aspirate pus are clinical indicators that a swelling on the jaw may be a tumour (Figure 29.8) rather than an abscess.

29.8 Lateral view of the skull of a 7-year-old rabbit with no previous history of dental problems. There was a hard, fast-growing mass on the mandible, which grew to be so large that it prevented the rabbit eating only 2 weeks after this radiograph was taken. Chest radiography confirmed metastases to the lungs and the rabbit was euthanased with a presumed malignant bone tumour.

Tapeworm cysts (Figure 29.9) can cause swellings on many parts of the body and may be mistaken for abscesses if they are on the jaw or behind the eye (Lloyd-Lucas and Jones, 2010). Ultrasonography (see Chapter 8) is extremely useful for differentiating tapeworm cysts from abscesses. One author (FHB) has encountered one *Coenurus serialis* cyst that grew in the sublingual tissue so that the tongue was enlarged and the enamel points on the cheek teeth were catching on it.

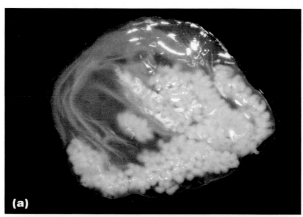
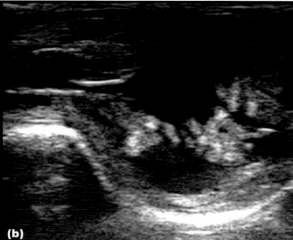

29.9 **(a)** A typical *Coenurus serialis* cyst. These cysts are an intermediate stage in the life cycle of *Taenia serialis*, a tapeworm found in dogs and foxes. Fresh herbage that has been contaminated by dog or fox faeces containing eggs is the source of infection. The cysts can be found in the subcutis around the face or on other parts of the body, such as the axilla or retrobulbar space. The swellings they cause can be mistaken for abscesses. The cysts are thin-walled fluctuating structures from which clear fluid is aspirated.
(b) Ultrasonography shows the presence of multiple scolices in the fluid-filled cavity.

Types of abscess

Primary infection
Although it has been reported in some of the older literature that primary bacterial infection is a cause of facial abscesses in rabbits, this is unlikely in pet rabbits. Most are due to secondary infection of tissue that has been damaged by another cause.

Periapical abscesses
Periapical abscesses are the most common type of jaw abscess and are usually associated with the progressive syndrome of acquired dental disease (PSADD) as described in Chapter 24. Periapical abscesses involve the apical enamel, dentine, pulp cavity, alveolar bone and the bone that surrounds the socket. Tissue damage at the site of bone penetration by elongated apices of the teeth predisposes the area to bacterial infection. Sometimes it is easy to see how the infection was introduced. For example, the periodontal space may be wide, so that food or a foreign body such as a splinter of wood (Figure 29.10) can become caught between the teeth; or a weakened tooth may split, which allows infection to track to the apex (Figure 29.11). In most cases it seems that secondary infection arrives via the bloodstream.

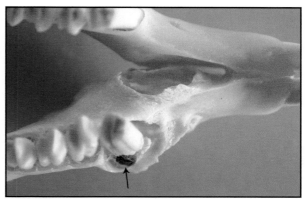

29.10 Occlusal view of a mandible of a rabbit that was euthanased because of a large mandibular abscess. The rabbit was in the initial stages of PSADD and there was alveolar bone loss resulting in wide periodontal spaces. A splinter of wood (arrowed) was discovered wedged in the socket of the 1st mandibular cheek tooth.

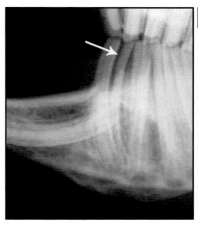

29.11 Periapical infections can be the result of trauma to the teeth from rabbits chewing on hard substances. This lateral view of the mandible shows a split 1st mandibular cheek tooth (arrowed) that led to the development of an abscess in the soft tissue at its apex.

Periapical abscesses fall into several categories:

- **Abscesses involving a single infected tooth root.** These abscesses occur at typical sites around the skull, where individual apices have penetrated the bone (see Figure 29.5)

- **Abscesses containing very elongated roots** that have penetrated the bone and continue to grow into the abscess cavity (Figure 29.12)
- **Abscesses with a bony capsule.** Some abscesses result in a proliferative bony capsule containing infected teeth (Figures 29.13 and 29.14)
- **Abscesses with subcutaneous fibrous tracts to distant sites.** Some periapical abscesses form fibrous tubes containing pus that can track to distant sites. These tracks may be single or multiple, tiny or large. The dewlap is the most frequent place for the abscess to become obvious (Figure 29.15)

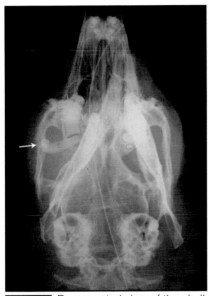

29.12 Dorsoventral view of the skull of a rabbit with a retrobulbar abscess. The elongated root of the 5th maxillary cheek tooth has penetrated the bone and continued to grow into the abscess cavity in the orbit (arrowed). Although this radiograph shows a true DV view of the maxilla, the mandible was deliberately pushed away from the side of the lesion to reduce superimposition of right upper and lower arcade so that the maxillary cheek teeth could be seen. (Reproduced from Harcourt-Brown (2009) with permission from *In Practice*.)

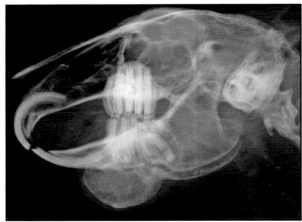

29.13 Lateral view of the skull with a localized bony swelling along the ventral border of the mandible. The swelling extended to the deformed apex of the lower 4th cheek tooth, which was the source of infection.

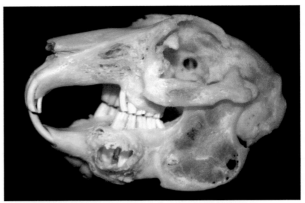

29.14 This prepared skull, from a rabbit that was euthanased because of bilateral mandibular abscesses, shows proliferation of the thin bone that enclosed an abscess capsule during life. Infection involved the apices of both the 1st and 2nd mandibular cheek teeth. If the rabbit had undergone surgery, it is probable that the root of the lower incisor would have been removed as its apex is immediately adjacent to the lower 1st cheek tooth on the medial aspect of the hemimandible and is often infected in abscesses at this site.

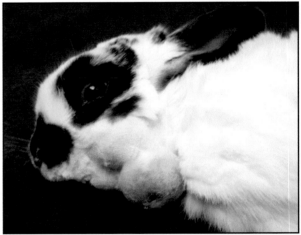

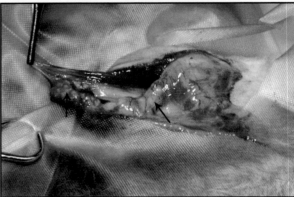

29.15 Some abscesses form subcutaneous tracks that branch out of the main capsule and extend into surrounding soft tissue (arrows). Pus may burst out of the track at a distant site. In the case of dental abscesses, the distant abscess is often under the chin or in the dewlap, where they form a discrete swelling that can be removed. Careful dissection will expose the track, which can be followed back to the infected tooth. The fibrous track can either be removed or opened and marsupialized. The decision depends on the extent of the fibrous track and how adherent it is to neighbouring tissues.

- **Generalized mandibular abscesses,** where infection appears to have spread through the cancellous bone of one mandible. In some cases the whole arcade of teeth may be infected and loose (Figure 29.16)
- **Generalized skull abscesses.** In some rabbits more than one arcade of teeth is infected (Figure 29.17).

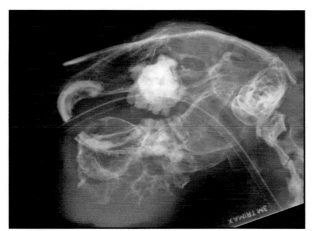

29.16 Lateral view of the skull of a rabbit with generalized mandibular abscesses. In the past, this rabbit had had extensive coronal reduction of the cheek teeth using dental burrs. Whether the infection was secondary to generalized pulp necrosis because of thermal injury, or whether it was due to spread of infection between teeth affected by PSADD, is difficult to prove. Thermal injury causes haemostasis, inflammation and thrombosis in the pulp. It is thought that exposure of the pulp cavity during burring was the cause of the mandibular abscesses in this rabbit. One author (FHB) has seen several similar cases.

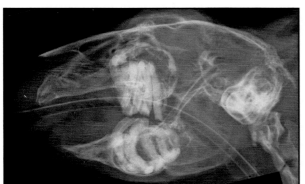

29.17 Lateral view of the skull of a rabbit with abscesses involving both mandibular arcades and one maxillary arcade. Her incisors had been removed on a previous occasion due to acquired malocclusion. The rabbit was of good bodyweight and appeared to enjoy life, although she could only eat softened food. Pus was discharging into the mouth from both mandibular arcades. Periodically, loose crowns could be pulled out via the oral cavity during her regular dental check-ups under anaesthesia. She would also have a 14-day course of parenteral penicillin/streptomycin on these occasions. This radiograph was taken when she presented with unilateral exophthalmos. Several loose crowns were easily removed from the upper arcade and the eye became less protuberant. The rabbit lived for a further 2 years with oral meloxicam each day. (Reproduced from Harcourt-Brown (2009) with permission from *In Practice*.)

Puncture wounds

Penetrating injuries from fight wounds, foreign bodies (Figure 29.18) or sharp points on the crowns of teeth can cause abscesses through introducing infection into the subcutaneous tissues. Elongated crowns can also penetrate the buccal mucosa and introduce infection into the soft tissue. The most likely teeth to develop spurs that can puncture the cheek are the 1st and 2nd maxillary cheek teeth. Penetrating injury results in an abscess on the side of the face (see Figure 29.5 and Chapter 24).

Fight wounds can result in abscesses on the face. They are usually encountered in entire rabbits, especially males, that are still housed with their siblings after they have reached sexual maturity; newly introduced rabbits may also fight. Signalment and clinical history usually suggest that a fight wound was the cause of the abscess, although radiography may be required to exclude the possibility of periapical infection.

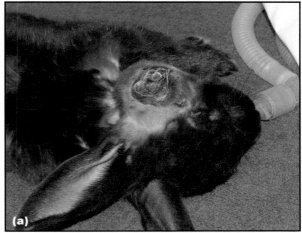

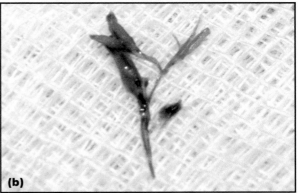

29.18 **(a)** This cheek abscess developed rapidly. There was skin necrosis over the abscess and the rabbit was inappetent. The position of the abscess does not identify any particular cheek tooth as a source of infection (see Figure 29.5) although the rabbit was suffering from advanced PSADD. The abscess was not identifiable on skull radiographs. Surgical exploration revealed a large quantity of liquid foul-smelling pus containing a large piece of hay **(b)** that presumably had been caught around a deformed tooth and penetrated the oral mucosa. The rabbit made a complete recovery after opening the abscess, removing the necrotic skin, draining all the pus and leaving the cavity open. A 10-day course of penicillin/streptomycin by subcutaneous injection was also given.

Iatrogenic abscesses

Iatrogenic abscesses can be a result of incisor removal. They usually form around a tooth that has regrown or a sequestrum of bone or tooth that has remained in the socket after removal (see Chapter 27). Incisor abscesses occur on the chin or nose (Figure 29.19; see also Figure 29.5).

Clipping teeth is often cited as a cause of periapical abscess because of the potential to expose the pulp cavity and allow infection to track through the tooth. This is difficult to prove, as elongated teeth that need shortening are already abnormal and most abscesses involve teeth that have never been clipped. However, exposure of the pulp cavity, either by clipping or burring, could easily introduce infection and in some cases radiography has suggested that this is the most likely cause (Figure 29.20).

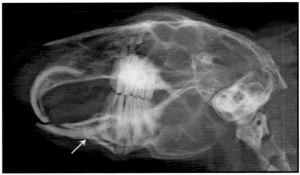

29.20 This lateral view of the skull shows an abscess at the apex of a mandibular incisor that was maloccluded. This was a rescue rabbit with no clinical history but the most plausible explanation for an abscess in that site was that infection had tracked through a pulp cavity that had been exposed during incisor clipping.

Ear base abscesses

Swellings at the base of the ear are commonly encountered in lop-eared rabbits due to cerumen bursting between deformed ear cartilages in the ear canal (see Chapter 16); infection may or may not be present. Abscesses at the base of the ear can also be due to penetrating wounds through the tympanic bulla. Cat bites or bites from other predators are the most common cause.

Diagnostic procedures

Imaging

If the facilities are available, CT/MRI scanning (see Chapter 9) is the most useful diagnostic procedure for the diagnosis and assessment of facial abscesses in rabbits. Ultrasound examination (see Chapter 8) may also be useful, especially for retrobulbar abscesses.

Radiography is essential for any rabbit with a facial swelling, especially if it is about to undergo surgery. The head needs to be carefully positioned for skull radiography so that a standard view is taken at the same angle each time (see Chapter 3). The lateral view yields the most information and a well positioned true lateral and dorsoventral view are the most useful views for overall assessment of the teeth and jaws, although other views can be useful (see Chapter 3). Oblique views can give valuable information about the apices of the cheek teeth but the outline of other structures can be difficult to interpret. Rostrocaudal views are difficult to interpret. Intraoral views can be very informative if dental radiography is available. Interpretation of skull radiographs is covered in Chapter 4.

In conjunction with clinical examination, skull radiography can give many diagnostic and prognostic indicators. It can be used to:

- Look for radiopaque foreign bodies such as needles
- Differentiate between abscesses, cysts and tumours

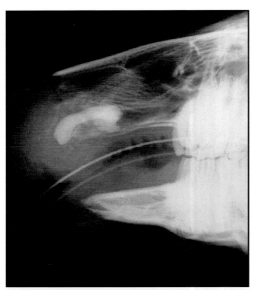

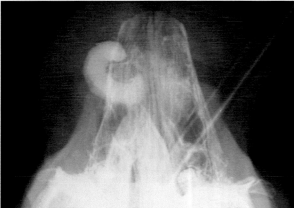

29.19 Lateral and DV views of the skull of a rabbit with a swollen nose, stridor and a nasal discharge. He was a rescue rabbit that had been adopted one year previously, with his incisors already extracted. One upper incisor had regrown to form a dysplastic remnant that was occluding the nasal cavity. There was severe osteomyelitis of the incisive bone and infection in the ethmoturbinates. The rabbit was eventually euthanased, despite extensive surgery to remove the tooth remnants and infected bone with prolonged courses of antibiotics. Recalcitrant infection had spread into the nasal passages and sinuses.

- Assess the stage of dental disease
- Assess which teeth are involved and the accessibility of those teeth
- Assess the number of teeth that are involved
- Assess whether opposing teeth are growing
- Give an idea of the shape and position of the teeth that need to be removed. This is invaluable during surgery when the radiograph can be examined once the abscess is open and some of the landmarks that can be seen on the radiographs can be seen in the abscess cavity.

Bacterial sampling

Knowledge of which bacteria are present and of their sensitivity to antibiotics can be helpful in confirming the diagnosis of an abscess and in the selection of antibiotics to treat it. Ideally, samples should be submitted for both aerobic and anaerobic culture.

False negative or erroneous results can be the result of attempting to culture pus. Swabs or needle aspirates of pus are rarely rewarding; there appear to be sufficient antibacterial elements in the pus to prevent bacterial growth in the laboratory.

It appears to be more rewarding to submit for culture a section of abscess wall obtained at surgery. If an incubator is available in the practice, a section of the abscess capsule can be wiped on a blood agar plate as soon as it is removed. This yields the causative organisms in most cases and sensitivity can be determined, although the plate may need to be submitted to a laboratory for definitive identification (FHB). This method is inexpensive but does preclude anaerobic culture.

Alternatively, some prefer to submit portions of removed tooth root and necrotic bone (VJ). It is important to discuss with the laboratory beforehand how the sample should be submitted.

Cytology

Cytological examination of another portion of the sample is useful to look for any bacteria that can be positively linked with the inflammatory response (JC). If bacteria are visible, their morphology and staining characteristics may provide some clues to their identity and likely antibiotic sensitivity.

Antibiotic therapy

Antibiotic therapy alone is unlikely to be curative for facial abscesses, although it is an adjunct to other treatments. Product authorization, the prescribing cascade and guidance on the use, and misuse, of antibiotics in small animal practice are all relevant to the use of antibiotics in rabbits. These topics are discussed in Appendix 1.

Tissue penetration

The thick fibrous capsule that is so characteristic of rabbit abscesses means that antibiotics cannot penetrate into the pus and that antimicrobial efficacy is impaired. Binding with purulent material can also inactivate some antibiotics, such as aminoglycosides and potentiated sulphonamides (Whittem

and Gaon, 1998). In order to be effective, antibiotic therapy needs to be combined with surgical drainage of the pus and removal of all infected tissue. Once the pus has been removed and the inner layer of the fibrous capsule exposed, topical application of antibiotics into the cavity is likely to be effective because the antibiotic comes into direct contact with the bacteria that are present on the inner surface of the capsule. Topical use also reduces selective pressure on gastrointestinal flora, and so is less likely to induce drug resistance (see *BSAVA Guide to the Use of Veterinary Medicines* at www.bsava.com) or antibiotic-associated diarrhoea. The risk of adverse effects, such as nephrotoxicity, is reduced by using an antibiotic topically, rather than systemically.

Susceptibility of pathogens

Ideally, culture and sensitivity testing should be performed in every abscess case to aid antibiotic selection. In practice, this can only be achieved if the case is managed surgically because a section of abscess capsule is the most reliable site from which to culture bacteria, and surgery is needed to collect the material.

A wide range of aerobic and anaerobic bacteria may be cultured from rabbit abscesses (see above), which can vary widely in their antimicrobial susceptibilities. In the study by Jekl *et al.* (2012) that cultured organisms present in abscesses in 30 rabbits, aerobic microbes were mostly sensitive to fluoroquinolones and beta-lactams and anaerobes were sensitive to metronidazole, penicillins and amoxicillin/clavulanate. In five rabbits, multi-resistant microbes (*Escherichia coli, Enterobacter cloacae, Proteus vulgaris, Pseudomonas* spp., *Streptococcus beta-haemolytica* group G) were found. Most of these microbial species, particularly *E. cloacae,* are important nosocomial pathogens.

Risk of antibiotic-associated diarrhoea

Antibiotic-associated diarrhoea is a risk when using antibiotics in rabbits. Although there are no published studies of the incidence of antibiotic-associated diarrhoea in rabbits kept as pets, there are anecdotal reports that antibiotic toxicity is a potential problem although it is not predictable or consistent. A study by Hara-Kudo *et al.* (1996) showed that a single intravenous high dose of a range of antibiotics could cause diarrhoea in rabbits, but morbidity was not 100% and varied with the class of antibiotic, aminoglycosides being the least likely to cause diarrhoea. Changes in the caecal microflora were found, with an increase in *Clostridium* spp., *Salmonella* spp., *Campylobacter* spp., *Staphylococcus aureus* and enteropathogenic *Escherichia coli.*

The pathogenesis of antibiotic-associated diarrhoea is complex. The caecal microflora is composed of a wide range of aerobic and anaerobic bacteria that play a key role in degradation of food to produce a range of metabolites that influence the survival and colonization of the bacteria within the ecosystem. Disruption of the normal microflora by antibiotics can allow pathogenic bacteria to proliferate and cause inflammation. The disruption in the enteric microflora also disturbs the metabolic function of the intestinal flora, which enhances water secretion and reduces water absorption, resulting in diarrhoea. Some bacterial species produce enterotoxins, notably *Clostridium difficile* or *C. spiriforme*, but not all rabbits harbour these pathogens. The pathogen and the disruption need to be present in the same animal to cause problems. Although it is counterintuitive, many of the pathogenic bacteria that cause antibiotic-associated diarrhoea are susceptible to the antibiotics that cause it; their spores are resistant, however, so the intestinal tract can be recolonized, and diarrhoea may then develop some time after the antibiotic has been withdrawn (Bartlett, 1992).

A review of the literature about adverse effects of antibiotics on rabbits kept in colonies (Morris, 1995) showed that the effects were inconsistent and varied with dose rate, route of administration and type of antibiotic. In many of the studies that showed adverse effects, antibiotics were used at high doses that would not be used in general practice. However, mortality for enteritis was 100% in rabbits that were given oral clindamycin or lincomycin at dose rates of 10–15 mg/kg q24h for 3 days. Ampicillin also induced enteritis in 50% of the rabbits that were given oral doses of 10 mg/kg q24h for 6 days. These dose rates are comparable with those used for oral preparations in dogs and cats. The LD_{50} for oral penicillin was 5.25 g/kg given as a single dose. This is considerably higher than the normal parenteral dose rate of 40 mg/kg.

Antibiotic options

As a result of their own experiences, each practitioner has their own opinion about the safety and efficacy of different antibiotics for the treatment of abscesses. Some options are given below (for drug doses see Appendix 1).

- **Fluoroquinolones** are available for veterinary use and some products carry authorization for use in rabbits. They will not penetrate abscess tissue and the older fluoroquinolones (enrofloxacin, marbofloxacin) are not active against anaerobes. They should penetrate surrounding tissues well, however, and systemic administration may be effective against abscess spread (JC). Topical use is indicated for cases where culture and sensitivity testing indicate that the organism will be susceptible. Ciprofloxacin is available as aqueous drops (Ciloxan, Alcon) that can be instilled into abscess cavities (FHB).
- **Trimethoprim/sulphonamide** preparations are unlikely to cause antibiotic-associated diarrhoea and may be given orally. They are inactivated by pus. However, although one study by Tyrell *et al.* (2002) showed only 7% of the organisms that were cultured were sensitive to trimethoprim/sulphonamide, some clinicians (JC) find this combination to be effective at reducing abscess spread and have not observed significant resistance.

- **Cephalosporins** may penetrate abscesses better than the drug classes above. Most clinicians use first-generation cephalosporins, though some prefer third-generation drugs (e.g. ceftazidime). Cephalosporins are active against a range of Gram-positive and Gram-negative organisms, including *Pasteurella* spp., and staphylococcal resistance to cephalosporins is less common than to penicillin.
- **Metronidazole:** where anaerobic infection is confirmed or suspected, this may be added to the regime.
- **Penicillin G** may be used as a long-acting injectable form at weekly intervals. Alternatively, a short-acting preparation may be used in combination with other antibiotics (e.g. metronidazole (WE, VJ) or marbofloxacin (AM, VJ) and given daily.
- **Penicillin/streptomycin** (Streptacare, Animalcare): one author (FHB) has used penicillin/streptomycin extensively for years in rabbits with purulent infections without adverse effects. It is her first choice. Penicillin is a narrow-spectrum bactericide that works synergistically with streptomycin against a wide range of pyogenic bacteria. It is effective against clostridial anaerobes and many of the bacterial species that have been cultured from rabbit abscesses (*Pasteurella, Staphylococcus, Streptococcus, Actinomyces*). Streptomycin is an aminoglycoside that is effective against *Pseudomonas* (Bishop, 2005) but is inactivated by pus. It. Although streptomycin is ototoxic in some species, there is no evidence for this in rabbits. Streptomycin has been described as completely harmless to rabbits (Gutschik *et al.*, 1982).
- **Gentamicin** is bactericidal and active against Gram-negative organisms and some Gram-positive ones, although purulent material binds and inactivates aminoglycosides, so gentamicin is only effective if all the necrotic material has been removed by thorough debridement. Gentamicin is not absorbed from the digestive tract, so oral administration is ineffective against facial absecesses. It does not cause disturbances in caecal microflora, so accidental oral ingestion of the antibiotic from an abscess cavity is not a problem. It is available as aqueous drops that can be used topically. It is one author's choice (FHB) for filling abscess cavities. Systemic administration is not recommended because of the risk of nephrotoxicity.
- **Azithromycin** reaches tissue concentrations higher than serum concentrations in rabbits. Taylor *et al.* (2010) found it to be safe and effective in four rabbits.
- **Chloramphenicol:** aqueous eye drops can be used as topical therapy for abscess cavities (FHB).
- **Clindamycin** and **lincomycin** are known to be of high risk for causing antibiotic-associated diarrhoea. Despite the effective antimicrobial properties of clindamycin, it is not recommended for rabbits (FHB) especially if it is placed (e.g. in

AIPPMA beads or as capsules) into cavities that open into the oral cavity.

- **Ampicillin** and **amoxicillin/clavulanate:** although these antibiotics carry a risk of inducing antibiotic-associated diarrhoea, they have been used parenterally on many occasions without any adverse effects by one author (FHB) when culture and sensitivity indicate a penicillin-resistant infection. The use of oral or topical formulations is not recommended. There are many anecdotal reports from owners of their rabbits developing diarrhoea and dying after they were prescribed oral paediatric ampicillin preparations.

Surgical management

Excision

As discussed in Chapter 11, abscesses (if well circumscribed) can be treated almost as tumours and excised completely. Although this may be possible for dental abscesses, it is unusual. For example, an abscess on the side of the face that has been caused by penetration of the buccal mucosa by a spur on an upper premolar may be removed completely. Circumscribed abscesses in the dewlap can also be removed, although most of them have a track that extends into a focus of infection in the bone that will need to be removed to prevent recrudescence.

Needle drainage

This is rarely, if ever, advocated as a major part of a treatment regime as the benefits of the insignificant amount of pus removed by this method are outweighed by the pain of the procedure and inflammatory response/possible contamination of surrounding structures. Some, however, may choose to reduce pressure on surrounding tissues

and improve comfort by needle drainage of a small quantity of pus. Some may also choose this method as a means of obtaining a sample for culture (and, of course, to confirm it is an abscess) – i.e. this is a technique that is only really useful in the presurgical management and diagnosis phase.

Lancing and flushing

Lancing abscesses and draining pus (in the manner of abscess therapy in dogs and cats) will rarely, if ever, achieve clinical cure as the nidus of infection remains, and it is very difficult (or impossible) to remove and drain such thick purulent material.

Surgical exploration of the abscess and removing all infected tissue

This is the treatment of choice for most authors in this Manual and in other books (e.g. Capello, 2012) although the surgery can be invasive and expensive, and repeated anaesthetic episodes may be necessary. Despite these problems most abscesses can be cured by surgery, although this does not prevent another abscess developing at another site on a future occasion. The prognosis depends on many factors (see later).

Preoperative planning

Preoperative assessment is very important. If available, CT scanning can be extremely useful but if facilities are not available radiography to identify the teeth that are involved and the extent of the abscess (see Figure 29.5). Palpation and visual inspection are also helpful. Other structures, notably nerves, nasal passages, ears, sinuses or the nasolacrimal apparatus, may be involved in the abscess. The important structures of the face that might be affected by an abscess or encountered during surgery are shown in Figure 29.21.

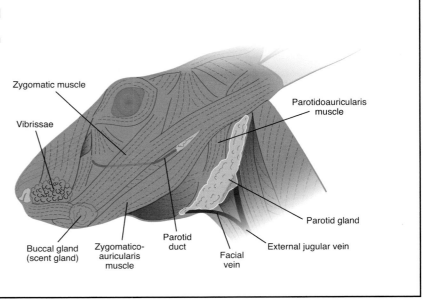

Superficial structures of the head
Rabbits have strong zygomatic and zygomaticoauricularis muscles that run from the edge of the mouth to the ear. They are innervated by the facial nerve.

Zygomatic muscle · Vibrissae · Buccal gland (scent gland) · Zygomatico-auricularis muscle · Parotid duct · Facial vein · Parotidoauricularis muscle · Parotid gland · External jugular vein

29.21 Important anatomical structures of the face. (continues)

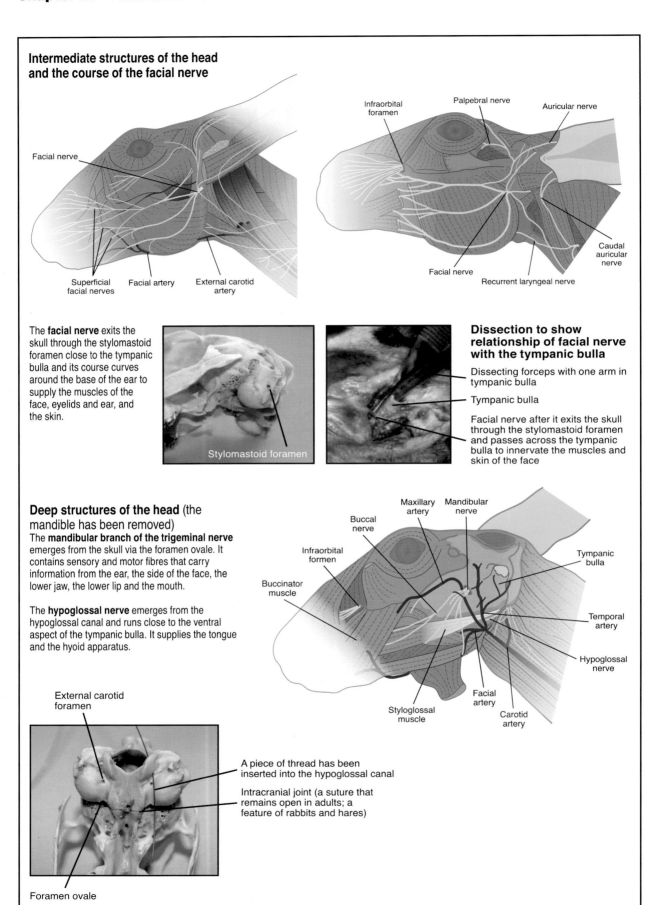

Intermediate structures of the head and the course of the facial nerve

Facial nerve

Superficial facial nerves

Facial artery

External carotid artery

Infraorbital foramen

Palpebral nerve

Auricular nerve

Caudal auricular nerve

Facial nerve

Recurrent laryngeal nerve

The **facial nerve** exits the skull through the stylomastoid foramen close to the tympanic bulla and its course curves around the base of the ear to supply the muscles of the face, eyelids and ear, and the skin.

Stylomastoid foramen

Dissection to show relationship of facial nerve with the tympanic bulla

Dissecting forceps with one arm in tympanic bulla

Tympanic bulla

Facial nerve after it exits the skull through the stylomastoid foramen and passes across the tympanic bulla to innervate the muscles and skin of the face

Deep structures of the head (the mandible has been removed)
The **mandibular branch of the trigeminal nerve** emerges from the skull via the foramen ovale. It contains sensory and motor fibres that carry information from the ear, the side of the face, the lower jaw, the lower lip and the mouth.

The **hypoglossal nerve** emerges from the hypoglossal canal and runs close to the ventral aspect of the tympanic bulla. It supplies the tongue and the hyoid apparatus.

Buccinator muscle

Infraorbital formen

Buccal nerve

Maxillary artery

Mandibular nerve

Tympanic bulla

Temporal artery

Hypoglossal nerve

Styloglossal muscle

Facial artery

Carotid artery

External carotid foramen

A piece of thread has been inserted into the hypoglossal canal

Intracranial joint (a suture that remains open in adults; a feature of rabbits and hares)

Foramen ovale

29.21 (continued) Important anatomical structures of the face.

Procedure
Once the abscess cavity has been opened (see Operative Technique 29.1) all the pus and necrotic tissue needs to be removed from the cavity. Debridement of deformed, infected alveolar bone is usually necessary. It can be difficult to differentiate bone from tooth; this is usually achieved by:

• Using a probe or other instrument, such as a scalpel blade (FHB), to assess the different texture of the tissue
• Visual examination
• Examining skull radiographs to orientate the position of the tooth roots.

Once the infected teeth have been identified, they are removed, either along with the necrotic bone via the abscess incision, or via the intraoral approach. The technique and instruments for molar extraction are discussed in Chapter 27. The choice between intraoral and extraoral extraction depends on the shape and mobility of infected teeth. Ideally, all infected tooth roots are identified and removed during removal of pus and debridement of the abscess cavity. The aim is to extract all the infected teeth. If a tooth is not mobile enough to be extracted through the cavity, small bone cutters can be used to section an infected tooth so that the distal section can be removed via the cavity and occlusal section via the mouth. Alternatively, in cases in which the infected root is less obvious, the oral approach may be used to extract the tooth (JC). However, if the intraoral route is chosen and the molar breaks, its root will require identification and removal via the incision. In some cases this may be simpler at a subsequent surgery. A decision is made either prior to, or at the end of, surgery, as to whether the abscess is to be marsupialized or closed. The technique for surgical treatment of abscesses and marsupializing the cavity is described in Operative Technique 29.1. Marsupialization is usually the preferred technique of the authors (FHB, JC) and AM.

Options for treating the abscess cavity after surgery
There are many techniques and products available for the treatment of abscess cavities once the pus has been removed, without or without infected teeth, bone or other tissue. Opinions vary between practitioners about the best approach. Not only does the choice depend on the personal preference and experience of the veterinary surgeon but it also depends on the site and cause of the abscess, the type and temperament of the rabbit, the commitment of the owner and, in some cases, financial constraints.

Repeated flushing of the cavity: Some authors prefer not to use topical therapy but to rely on flushing alone (WE). Chlorhexidine (0.05–1%), saline, 1:250 dilution F10SC (Health & Hygiene Pty) or dilute povidone–iodine solution may be used. Dilute (0.25–2%) iodine may also be used and may have some additional slight astringent effect that may assist in keeping the wound open (BC). Dilute

hydrogen peroxide can be used (AM) in the first days after surgery before the wound starts to granulate. During flushing, the rabbit's head should be angled downward to allow drainage of the fluid, as the debrided abscess is also open to the mouth. Other authors (FHB, VJ) avoid flushing abscess cavities but remove the contents with cotton buds and dressing forceps in the belief that flushing forces infected fluid deeper into the surrounding tissue and helps to keep any fistulae between the abscess cavity and the mouth open. Application of local anaesthetic into the abscess cavity (2–3 bupivacaine drops q8–12h) can make cleaning the abscess less painful (FHB).

Fill the cavity with topical preparations and leave it open: This option usually follows marsupialization of abscesses (see Operative Technique 29.1). The topical preparations are instilled after pus and tissue debris have been removed. Examples include the following.

• **Honey.** This is the authors' preference (JC, FHB). Honey has many healing properties (Mathews and Binnington, 2002). It decreases inflammatory oedema, attracts macrophages, accelerates sloughing of devitalized tissue, and provides a local cellular energy source so that a protective layer of protein is formed in the wound and a healthy bed of granulation tissue develops. Honey also has a deodorizing effect and has antibacterial properties due to its high osmolarity, acidity and hydrogen peroxide content. Studies have confirmed that honey accelerates wound healing in rabbits (Bergman *et al.,* 1983). The daily removal of the previous day's honey, flushing or cleaning the abscess cavity, and insertion of further honey into the abscess has the physical benefit of maintaining the marsupialization stoma for longer. Another advantage of honey is that its inadvertent passage into the mouth via tooth cavities will not cause problems. Nor will grooming of honey from the fur. However, some owners may find the need for daily cleaning of the cavity with cotton wool buds or swabs and packing with honey onerous.
• **Topical antibiotics.** Aqueous antibiotic solutions, such as gentamicin, ciprofloxacin or chloramphenicol eyedrops, can be instilled into the abscess cavity prior to the application of honey (FHB).
• **Aloe vera cream.** Topical instillation of an antimicrobial cream (e.g. HEALx Soother Plus, Harrison Pet Products) is recommended by some authors (Capello, 2009).
• **Intrasite gel** (Smith and Nephew). The gel rehydrates necrotic tissue and absorbs slough and wound exudate.
• **Potassium permanganate** ($KMnO_4$) can be used for topical treatment (VJ). It destroys bacteria and supports healing and granulation while keeping the wound dry. After the initial treatment it can be used in a diluted form with no adverse effects.

Pack the abscess cavity: Various products can be used to pack abscess cavities, on a temporary or permanent basis, and rely on release of antibiotic from the chosen product into the abscess cavity. The options are as follows:

- **Antibiotic-impregnated gauze strips.** This technique was described by Taylor *et al.* (2010). The choice of antibiotic depends on bacteriology and sensitivity. After lancing and flushing the abscess, the cavity is packed and the skin closed. The abscess is subsequently reopened weekly to remove the strips, flush the abscess and place fresh antibiotic-impregnated gauze strips. The procedure is repeated until the abscess resolves. It has been used to treat abscesses without removing infected teeth or bone. There may be many surgical interventions.

  A modification of this technique has also been used successfully by other authors (BC, AM). Following surgery, impregnated gauze strips (Figure 29.22) are placed, removed and replaced on a daily basis. This can generally be performed with the rabbit conscious, but may require sedation or light anaesthesia if extra curettage is required. Initially the cavity is packed with gauze impregnated with ceftazidime 20 mg/kg until results of culture and sensitivity testing are available from bacteriology, if performed. The cavity is flushed with saline and sometimes with dilute hydrogen peroxide prior to packing.

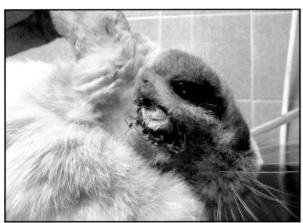

29.22 A gauze-packed abscess cavity. (Courtesy of A Melillo)

- **Poloxamer** (e.g. Pluronic PF-127) **gel infused with antibiotic** has been used recently with success and offers a useful alternative to antibiotic-impregnated gauze (BC). These substances are liquid when frozen or refrigerated and form a solid gel when brought to room temperature (so-called reverse-thermo nature). The gel is biodegradable and non-toxic. Poloxamers have been shown to be incorporated into cellular membranes, changing their microviscosity, and there is evidence that poloxamers can enhance healing in treatment of burns and other types of tissue trauma. They decrease bacterial adhesion and increase bacterial susceptibility to antibiotics (Hume and Gray, 2012). Water-soluble antibiotics can be added to the gel and the infused liquid packed into the marsupialized wound. The antibiotic elutes into the surrounding tissue over several days.

- **Hydrocolloid-based absorbent dressing** (e.g. Covidien, Smith and Nephew; Granuflex, ConvaTec) can be sutured directly around the wound and left in place for 3–5 days after surgery, after which time it can be removed (see Chapter 11).

- **Minocycline-containing dental gel.** Minocycline gel (e.g. Dentomycin, Henry Schein) is designed for packing infected periodontal pockets and can be inserted into areas of maxilla or mandible that have been debrided (JC). The gel hardens and slowly degrades, making it very suitable for this purpose. JC has used gel where significant bone debridement has taken place and yet the mandible has not fractured. The hardened gel may provide additional support for the weakened mandible. The abscess capsule is marsupialized and treated as described earlier.

- **Antibiotic-impregnated collagen sponge.** Medical collagen sponge designed for haemostasis can be packed into abscess cavities and soaked with antibiotic drops prior to closure of the wound (FHB). This technique gives high local levels of antibiotic without systemic side effects (Mehta *et al.,* 1996). Soft tissue swelling and seroma formation are potential postoperative complications after closure of the cavity. Swelling may be alleviated by using a Penrose drain if the cavity is large and deep, or by leaving a small gap in the suture line that will open to release serous fluid if pressure in the cavity builds up.

- **Antibiotic-impregnated polymethylmethacrylate (AIPMMA) beads.** Polymethylmethacrylate is used as bone cement in human and veterinary medicine and may be impregnated with antibiotics. Beads have been used to treat abscesses in rabbits (Hernandez-Divers, 2000). Postoperative swelling and seroma formation are potential complications after placement of AIPMMA beads. Another complication is recrudescence of the abscess; after all the antibiotic has leached out of the beads, they can act as nidi of infection, if pathogens are still present. The use of AIPMMA beads has largely been superseded by more degradable products.

- **Clindamycin capsule.** Implanting a clindamycin capsule, punctured with small needle holes, into an abscess cavity has been used by some to treat abscesses, despite the real risk of fatal antibiotic-associated diarrhoea if the drug were ingested because of leakage from the abscess site into the mouth or on to the skin, where the rabbit might ingest the antibiotic during grooming. This technique is not recommended.

• **Calcium hydroxide.** Previously, calcium hydroxide preparations have been inserted into abscesses (Remeeus and Verbeek, 1995). Opening/lancing of the abscess was performed, as described earlier, and purulent and necrotic material debrided. The cavity was then packed with calcium hydroxide and the capsule and skin closed using monofilament nylon. If this technique is used, care must be taken to avoid contact with the animal's soft tissues, as calcium hydroxide may induce considerable necrosis. This technique is not recommended.

Complications

Jaw fracture: In some cases, removal of necrotic bone and affected teeth will result in jaw fracture. Rabbits with PSADD tend to have osteopenic bone that is often infected at the site of the abscess. Jaw fracture is more likely in some sites than in others. Periapical infections of the lower 4th cheek tooth are the most likely to result in a broken jaw during surgery because the bone is very thin at this point. However, jaw fracture is not a terminal event. Most rabbits recover without any surgery, especially if the opposing arcade of teeth is functional (Figure 29.23). The postoperative period may be protracted, so syringe feeding (from the good side) is necessary for at least 7–10 days. It is not possible to repair such fractures easily (see Chapter 22). Most will heal in 14 days with conservative treatment, although jaw mobility and malocclusion can be long-term complications.

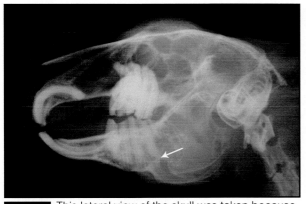

29.23 This lateral view of the skull was taken because the rabbit was suffering from epiphora. It was taken 3 years after the rabbit had undergone surgery for a mandibular abscess involving the lower 4th cheek tooth. The jaw had fractured during the surgical procedure, and the site of the healed abscess and fracture can be seen (arrow).

Fistula formation: After extraction of the cheek teeth, there is a hole from the mouth into the abscess cavity. For abscesses involving the maxillary teeth this is an advantage, as it allows drainage of infected material into the mouth. For abscesses involving the mandibular teeth it can be a problem, especially if the hole is large, as food can enter the abscess cavity. If the abscess is marsupialized, food and saliva can flow out of the wound and the skin

around the abscess site may become sore. In most cases, the gum heals over within a few days and the problem stops, but it may be necessary to stitch the gingiva to close the hole into the mouth. This can be difficult because of restricted access and visualization. Mucosal flap techniques have been attempted to close large deficits after multiple extractions but are not always successful (Ward, 2006).

Acquired malocclusion: Malocclusion can be a problem after extraction of infected teeth because the teeth adjacent to the abscess cavity rotate, shift or tip, and opposing teeth may grow into the gap. Ironically, these problems may be worse in rabbits with good dentition or those in the early stages of PSADD because the teeth continue to grow (see Chapter 24). A single tooth can be removed without problems because the rabbit learns to move its mouth so that the tooth is worn against the teeth that were adjacent to the one that was removed. If more than one tooth is removed, however, the opposing teeth can grow so long that they dig into the gum and need regular shortening under general anaesthesia (Figure 29.24). Overgrowth of opposing teeth is more of a problem after removal of the upper cheek teeth because the rate of growth of the mandibular cheek teeth is faster than the maxillary cheek teeth. Extraction or pulpectomy are options to prevent opposing teeth from growing (see Chapters 26 and 27). In the later stages of PSADD, tooth growth slows or ceases altogether so acquired malocclusion is less of a problem.

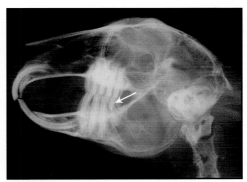

29.24 Lateral view of the skull of FHB's 7-year-old Dutch rabbit that had fractured a lower 4th cheek tooth by chewing on something hard in the garden. An abscess on the cheek developed and was cured by removing the fractured tooth in addition to the 5th mandibular cheek tooth which was displaced. Subsequently, the rabbit required dentistry every 6–8 weeks to shorten the opposing maxillary crowns that grew into a point that penetrated the mucosa (arrow). The rabbit was euthanased because of an intestinal lymphoma 18 months later.

Recrudescence: Recrudescence of an abscess is usually due either to premature closure of the cavity or to a focus of infection remaining in the jaw, usually an infected tooth or piece of infected bone. It is not unusual for rabbits with PSADD to have several infected teeth, however, and owners may interpret the development of a new periapical abscess as failure of treatment of a previous one.

Non-surgical management

Laser therapy

Some positive experiences with therapeutic lasers indicate that this technique may help to accelerate healing after abscess surgery (AM). Therapeutic lasers work on a wavelength from 630 to 905 nm (red to infrared) and have a biostimulant activity through several mechanisms:

- Enhancing ATP activity, with cell proliferation and therefore faster regeneration
- Increasing microcirculation and stimulating proliferation of endothelial cells. Hyperaemia is induced by the mild heat induced by the laser, which allows for more nutrients to be taken to the tissue, sustaining regeneration
- Reducing oedema, pain and other negative effects of inflammation, e.g. by inhibiting the production of leucotrienes and bradykinin.

Laser impulses are only effective on vascularized tissues and have little effect on any necrotic part of an abscess, but if the beam is applied along the margins of the lesions, it can stimulate healthy tissue. Laser penetration is seriously impaired by fur or dirt, so the target area needs to be carefully shaved and cleaned prior to the procedure.

Laser therapy can be used before, during and for 7–10 days after surgery. It is used for a few days prior to surgery in order to prepare the tissues and reduce potential postoperative complications such as necrosis or intraoral suture dehiscence. Postoperatively it speeds up tissue regeneration and healing.

Maggot therapy

One author (JC) has attempted therapy using sterile surgical blowfly larvae (Figure 29.25). These have been used in human as well as in other veterinary patients in the clearing of necrotic tissues (Bell and Thomas, 2001) and it therefore appears logical that

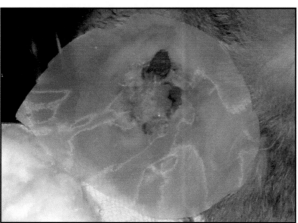

29.25 Maggots placed in an abscess cavity can be seen through the translucent semipermeable plastic sheet that will be sutured over the wound. As this cavity must be kept dark and damp, a gauze sheet is sutured over the plastic and impregnated daily with sterile saline. (© John Chitty)

they may be of some use in rabbit abscesses. Initial trials in JC's practice showed no obvious success, as maggots do not tolerate being in the presence of rabbit pus. If possible they would leave the area; this avoidance of rabbit pus has been seen both *in vivo* and *in vitro*, and may explain why rabbit abscesses are rarely, if ever, affected by myiasis. When prevented from escaping by the gauze sutured over the marsupialization stoma, the maggots invariably died after 2 days and without moulting to second or third stage larvae. However, the following advantages were seen:

- Rapid thinning of the abscess capsule – obvious even in a few days
- Rapid (<12 hours) liquefaction of purulent material (seen both *in vitro* and *in vivo*).

Thus, maggot therapy may yet have a place in management of these abscesses, though only after thorough debridement and removal of all purulent material such that beneficial effects may be seen on clearing of deeper necrotic material. The main difficulties with this therapy are:

- Owner and clinician distaste
- Expense of blowfly larvae and cost of repeated surgery to place larvae and remove them.

Palliative therapy

If surgery is not desired and the animal is not unwell then there are options for palliative therapy. These can be surprisingly successful on occasion, but, generally, are destined for failure at some point in the future; at that time owners can revisit their decisions.

Doing nothing

This is always an option *if the abscess is closed* – i.e. the abscess is not burst or draining into the mouth. It can be considered if the rabbit is well, eating and defecating normally and in good body condition. It should be stressed that 'doing nothing' really does mean doing *nothing*; lancing or needle drainage of the abscess (see above) are not considered when following this option, as they may either introduce further infection or induce an additional inflammatory response. The owner should be warned that the swelling may become quite large and will be unsightly. Alternatively, some small abscesses may not enlarge and eventually become walled off (Figure 29.26). Cheek tooth malocclusion can be a problem due to displacement of the teeth and may require intervention during the period of abscess management (see Chapter 26). Regular re-checks are essential to monitor progression of the abscess as well as checking bodyweight, body condition, molar condition and other signs of systemic illness.

WARNING
The decision to leave the abscess alone should be revised if the abscess bursts or the animal becomes uncomfortable.

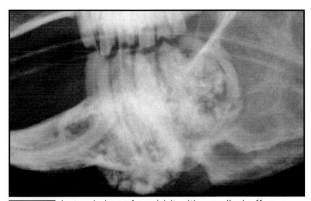

29.26 Lateral view of a rabbit with a walled-off abscess that never required treatment. This is a rare case. The pus has calcified granules in it. (Reproduced from Harcourt-Brown (2009) with permission from *In Practice*.)

Analgesia

Analgesia must be considered as a part of the palliative care regime (see Chapter 2).

Antibiosis

When to use this as part of the palliative therapy regime is largely down to the choice and experience of the clinician.

Some authors (e.g. FHB) believe that long-term antibiotics are never indicated; either the abscess is large and painful enough to require surgery or it is small and non-painful enough to be left alone completely.

Other authors (e.g. JC) believe that long-term antibiotic therapy can have a role in palliative care. The aim of the therapy is not to reduce the abscess, nor to remove it (although there are anecdotal reports of this occurring, especially with penicillin therapy, it is not wise to raise hopes unduly of a medical cure-all before embarking on therapy); rather, the aim is to prevent spread of the abscess to surrounding tissues. In most medical cases it is preferable to select antibiotics on the basis of culture and sensitivity testing, but accurate sampling (see above) is difficult (and will require 'disturbing' the abscess capsule). Empirical antibiosis is therefore usually employed. Drug choices are similar to those discussed earlier. An important consideration regards using antibiotics long term in these situations. While there is no evidence showing long-term antibiotic use increases risk of development of antibiotic resistance, measures should be taken to reduce the risk of this occurring:

- Avoid fluoroquinolones – unless indicated by culture/sensitivity or in some animals where drugs that require more frequent dosing or larger volumes may be difficult for owners to dose
- Avoid pulse therapy regimes
- Ensure a full dose of the drug is given at an appropriate dose rate via an appropriate route
- Avoid in-water dosing
- Reserve long-term antibiotic use for cases where the abscess enlarges or the abscess spreads without use of systemic antibiotic, and where surgical options are precluded by other criteria (see above).

Lancing and flushing

Periodic lancing and flushing can be considered as an adjunct to palliative care where surgery is not desirable but the abscess has burst, is draining into the mouth or is growing in spite of therapy. In some cases lancing and flushing may produce acceptable long-term results if well tolerated by the patient. In these cases long-term/permanent analgesia/antibiosis should be used alongside drainage of the abscess. The procedure is not curative and yet is invasive and likely to be non-cost-effective over the course of management, and so is hard to justify over more invasive surgery.

Euthanasia

Although the treatment of facial abscesses has progressed considerably in recent years and success rates can be good, some abscesses are not easy to treat. Therapy may require multiple surgeries and prolonged nursing, plus owner care and financial commitment. Some rabbits may be in such a debilitated state that they are unlikely to tolerate invasive surgery, or the owners may be unwilling or unable to afford the procedure or cope with the nursing their pet may require. In these cases, euthanasia should always be offered – alleviation of suffering is the prime concern and successful therapy can never be guaranteed. There are many prognostic indicators that may help in decision-making about euthanasia.

Prognosis

There a number of factors that affect prognosis of facial abscess, such as the cause, site and extent of the abscess and involvement of neighbouring structures. The prognosis for abscesses at various sites on the head in summarized in Figure 29.5. The likelihood of complications (see above) arising after surgery also affects the prognosis for the rabbit.

Site and extent

Maxillary abscesses, including retrobulbar abscesses (see later) tend to have a better prognosis than mandibular abscesses because the pus can drain into the mouth. The condition of the teeth on the contralateral side of the mouth is also very important. If these teeth are healthy and the rabbit can eat on that side, extensive surgery can be performed on the affected side without causing eating difficulties, which makes a big difference to the recovery of the rabbit postoperatively.

The extent of the abscess and the number of teeth that are involved is important. The prognosis is good for a well defined solitary abscess where infection has been introduced from a puncture wound or originates from a single tooth or tooth fragment (Figure 29.27) because the source of infection can easily be removed. In contrast, large bony abscesses involving more than one tooth are far more difficult to cure (Figure 29.28).

The involvement of surrounding structures, such as nerves, blood vessels or the globe can affect prognosis. For example, facial nerve injury

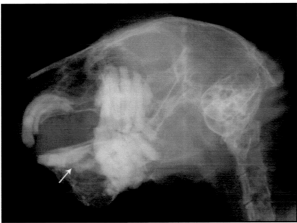

29.27 An example of an abscess with a good prognosis. Despite the evidence of advanced dental disease that can be seen on this lateral radiograph of the skull, the mandibular abscess that was present carried a good prognosis. The abscess was contained in a bony capsule. The calcified granules indicate that it was a longstanding chronic abscess. There is lucency around a single tooth fragment (arrow) that was easily accessible surgically. The tooth fragment was removed and the cavity marsupialized. The abscess did not recur, although the rabbit continued to have some dental problems. The fractured crown on an upper incisor was removed at the time of abscess surgery.

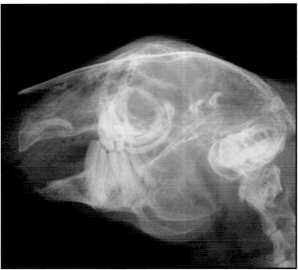

29.28 An example of an abscess with a bad prognosis. This 10-month-old rabbit was presented with a swollen nose, a purulent nasal discharge, salivation and anorexia. His incisors had been removed by the referring veterinary surgeon 2 months previously. Oral examination showed a spur on the 6th maxillary cheek tooth, curling round and penetrating the hard palate. The eye on the affected side was slightly exophthalmic. The lateral radiograph of the skull shows a generalized osteopenia. There is regrowth of a maxillary incisor, sinusitis and turbinate loss. The cheek teeth are grossly deformed (though some still have a central enamel fold) and they were still growing. The presence of a retrobulbar abscess was confirmed by aspirating pus from the retrobulbar space. The retrobulbar abscess and the abscess on the nose were treated at the owner's request but reappeared some weeks later. The rabbit was euthanased.

associated with dental abscesses may be iatrogenic or may be due to spread of periapical infections of the caudal cheek teeth or ear base abscesses. This can cause permanent facial nerve paralysis and eventual rictus (see Figure 29.7).

Concurrent disease

Concurrent disease affects the long-term prognosis of rabbits with facial abscesses. Anorexia and weight loss are non-specific signs of a number of diseases; it is easy to attribute these signs to an abscess if it is present but sometimes they are due to another disease, notably chronic renal failure. An indicator that this may be present can be seen on skull radiographs. Rabbits with renal disease have problems excreting calcium, so ectopic and dystrophic calcification commonly occurs (Harcourt-Brown, 2007). The hyoid bone is one of the sites that can become excessively calcified (Figure 29.29).

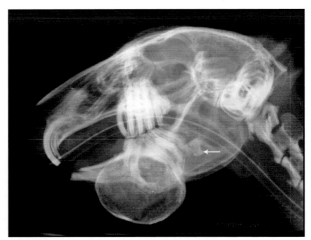

29.29 Mandibular abscess in a rabbit with chronic renal failure. This lateral view of the skull is well exposed, with good bone contrast. This is often a feature of rabbits with renal disease because they are unable to excrete excess calcium through their kidneys, and ectopic and dystrophic mineralization can be the result. The hyoid bone is calcified. Blood tests showed raised urea, creatinine, calcium and phosphorus levels but the owner still opted for surgery. The rabbit died postoperatively.

Temperament

The temperament of the rabbit, and that of its owners, are important prognostic factors. Rabbits that eat well and tolerate handling are more likely to do well than fractious, nervous rabbits because it is difficult for the owners to continue with the postoperative care. Rabbits with observant, dedicated owners who have time to deal with their rabbit will do better than rabbits belonging to busy or squeamish people.

Retrobulbar abscesses

Retrobulbar abscesses deserve special consideration, as the prognosis is often not as bad as many people might think. Although enucleation might seem the obvious course, it is only indicated if panophthalmitis has developed and the eye is painful and unsalvageable. The abscesses usually arise from the apices of the 3rd, 4th, 5th and occasionally the 6th maxillary cheek teeth, which are encased in the alveolar bulla on the anterioventral floor of the orbit. Apical elongation and infection result in an abscess that occupies the ventral part of the orbit and displaces the eye. The large retrobulbar venous sinus lies close to an abscess in this site; if infection erodes the blood vessel it may bleed and form a haematoma that suddenly pushes the eye further out of the socket (see Figure 29.6). Owners may not be aware that their rabbit has a retrobulbar abscess until the eye suddenly protrudes. At this point the eyelids do not meet over the cornea, so secondary damage to the eye occurs unless the condition is treated promptly.

Clinical signs

Rabbits with retrobulbar abscesses generally present with one or more of the following signs:

- Unilateral exophthalmos, with or without secondary changes to the globe
- Anorexia, reduced appetite and/or weight loss
- Discharge from the sinus, around the region of the lateral canthus of the eye
- Discharging pus inside the mouth from the 3rd to 6th cheek teeth.

Differential diagnosis

The differential diagnoses for *unilateral exophthalmos* are:

- Unilateral glaucoma
- Neoplasia (one author (FHB) has encountered two cases of lymphoma)
- Tapeworm cysts (the retrobulbar space is a common site for these to develop)
- Retrobulbar abscesses.

Diagnosis

Diagnosis is made through:

- Palpation: the abscess can often be palpated as a bulge under the eye, in the area medial to the zygomatic arch
- Examination of the oral cavity: abnormalities of the caudal maxillary cheek teeth may be seen and pus may be expressed into the mouth by applying pressure to the globe
- Skull radiography
- Ultrasound examination
- Tonometry, if it is difficult to differentiate between exophthalmos and glaucoma
- CT/MRI scanning.

Treatment options

Exposure of the abscess and removal of infected teeth

In one author's experience (FHB), most retrobulbar abscesses can be palpated in the ventral part of the orbit below the eye (Figure 29.30a). Once it is

located, the abscess capsule can be exposed by making a skin incision just above the zygomatic arch (Figure 29.30b). Blunt dissection is used to move the soft tissue and expose the abscess capsule, which can then be punctured and the pus aspirated with a syringe. Once the capsule has deflated, the surplus capsule can be trimmed away to expose the interior of the abscess cavity.

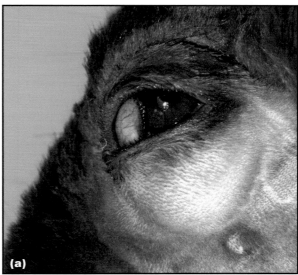

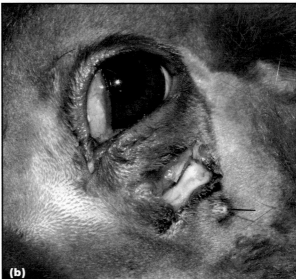

29.30 Retrobulbar abscess. The left eye of this rabbit had suddenly become grossly exophthalmic. A retrobulbar swelling was visible and palpable between the eye and the zygomatic arch **(a)**. Blood was aspirated from the swelling, as it was suspected that haemorrhage from the ophthalmic venous sinus behind the eye was responsible for the sudden marked exophthalmos and that infection from the abscess had eroded into the blood vessel. The globe of the eye looked normal. A discharging sinus adjacent to a maxillary cheek tooth was evident on oral examination and radiography confirmed the presence of elongated, deformed tooth roots in the retrobulbar space. **(b)** Exploratory surgery via an incision between the globe and the zygoma revealed the abscess capsule, which was opened to remove the pus. Two maxillary teeth were removed and the rabbit recovered without enucleation of the eye.

Residual pus is removed with cotton buds or a Volkmann's scoop and the infected teeth identified and removed in the same way as for other periapical abscesses. The periodontal attachments need to be broken down with elevators and the tooth removed via the abscess cavity or the mouth. Alternatively, the tooth may be sectioned and the fragments removed separately. Endoscopy may be used to aid visualization of the abscess cavity to identify and remove the infected teeth (Martínez-Jiménez *et al.*, 2007) The chances of a successful outcome for retrobulbar abscesses are greater if the infected teeth are removed, although this is not always possible.

Intraoral approach to the abscess

An intraoral approach can be used to drain and treat retrobulbar abscesses. Although examination of the surgical site is difficult in the anaesthetized rabbit, and impossible in the conscious rabbit, this approach does enable treatment without enucleation or damage to the eye.

1. After identifying the affected tooth roots from radiographs or CT scans, the mouth is examined and the gingival sulci of the 4th to 6th cheek teeth are thoroughly examined with a periodontal probe. Infected teeth tend to be mobile or displaced, and pus may be seen draining into the mouth alongside the infected tooth.
   - If there is sufficient pressure to cause exophthalmos then the probe will inevitably enter the abscess and pus will emerge; this confirms the best position (and affected tooth) for drainage.
   - On occasion there may be swelling caudal to the 6th cheek tooth. In these cases, the probe may be gently inserted into the most dependent part of the swelling. If pus emerges, the swelling may be enlarged.
2. The affected teeth are removed (see Chapter 27) using a No. 3 Hollenbach carver or Crossley molar luxator to break down the periodontal ligament and elevate the tooth, which can be grasped with molar extraction forceps and gently rotated to loosen and remove it. Haemorrhage can occur because of the proximity of the buccal artery or through inadvertent penetration of the retrobulbar venous sinus. Applying gentle pressure to the socket for a few minutes is usually effective in stopping bleeding.
3. After the teeth have been extracted, any residual pus can be removed with cotton buds, or some authors prefer to flush the cavity as thoroughly as possible using a catheter inserted into the empty socket cavity (see Operative Technique 25.1). This can be a difficult process, although retropulsion of the eye may be helpful.

Surgical drainage without removing all infected tissue

In some cases it is not possible to remove the infected tooth because of restricted access to the abscess cavity, or because the tooth breaks and a fragment is left embedded deep in the tissues below the eye. In these cases remission of the exophthalmos can be achieved by establishing drainage from the orbit into the mouth with a probe. Teaching the owners to massage and retropulse the eye twice a day facilitates drainage. In many cases the residual fragment loosens and becomes accessible if the exophthalmos returns, and surgical exploration is again required.

Enucleation

If the eye has been proptosed or has been exophthalmic for a long time then there may be considerable damage to the cornea. In some cases there may also have been sufficient pressure around the optic nerve and blood vessels such that the eye may no longer be functional (Figure 29.31). In these cases, it is simpler to remove the eye (see Chapter 17). The retrobulbar abscess may then be treated via the orbit in the same way as for other dental abscesses, although locating infected teeth within the socket can be difficult because of the remaining soft tissue in the orbit and because of the large venous sinus that can bleed profusely. The dorsal lobe of the deep gland of the third eyelid is white and soft and is easily mistaken for infected tissue. Recurrence of a retrobulbar abscess after enucleation can be distressing for the owner, as pus draining from an empty socket is cosmetically difficult.

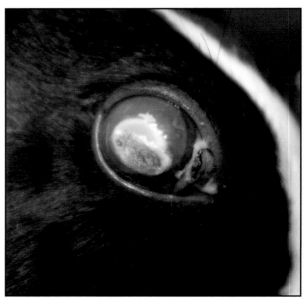

29.31 This exophthalmic eye would never be visual again and could only be a source of pain and discomfort for the rabbit. The eye was enucleated and the retrobulbar abscess treated by identifying and removing the infected teeth.

Postoperative care

Postoperative care depends on the technique that was used to treat the abscess.

- If the abscess cavity has been marsupialized and left open, options for treatment of the abscess cavity are similar to those for other facial abscesses, except that astringent preparations (honey, hydrogen peroxide, potassium permanganate) should be avoided because of the proximity of ocular tissue. Antibiotic drops can be used alone after cleaning the cavity.

- If the eye was not enucleated and drainage into the mouth was established, applying pressure to the globe once or twice daily expresses pus into the mouth. The owners can be taught to do this.

- Polyvinyl acetate sponges (e.g. Ear wicks, Dermapet) (AR) can be inserted and a drain placed to allow antibiotic delivery to the sponge twice daily. The drain may be sutured over the head, allowing easy access for owners to perform this task.

- If the abscess has been treated solely by the intraoral route, one author (AR) has found that these cases will often require regular anaesthetic episodes to keep the drainage hole open and to flush the abscess. Alternatively, the initial access may be used for temporary drainage and sampling, followed by systemic antibiotic therapy based on the bacteriology results. Even examination of the surgical site is difficult in the conscious rabbit, but this approach does it make it much more likely that the abscess can be treated without removal of, or damage to, the eye.

- Systemic antibiotic therapy, analgesia and daily cleansing of the wound is the same as for other facial abscesses.

References

Bamberger DM and Herndon BL (1990) Bactericidal capacity of neutrophils in rabbits with experimental acute and chronic abscesses. *Journal of Infectious Diseases* **162**, 186–192

Bartlett JM (1992) Antibiotic-associated diarrhea. *Clinical Infectious Disease* **15**, 573–581

Bell N and Thomas S (2001) Use of sterile maggots to treat panniculitis in an aged donkey. *Veterinary Record* **149**, 768–770

Bergman A, Yanai J, Weiss J et al. (1983) Acceleration of wound healing by topical application of honey. An animal model. *American Journal of Surgery* **145**, 374–376

Bishop Y (2005) *The Veterinary Formulary, 6th edn.* Pharmaceutical Press, London

Blood DC, Studdert VP and Gay CC (2007) *Saunders Comprehensive Veterinary Dictionary, 3rd edn.* Saunders Elsevier, Edinburgh

Calhoun JH and Mader JT (1989) Antibiotic beads in the management of surgical infections. *American Journal of Surgery* **157**, 443–449

Capello V (2009) Case report: Use of HEALx Soother Plus in postoperative treatment of a dental-related abscess in a pet rabbit. [Available at www.exoticdvm.com/mammal]

Capello V (2012) Small mammal dentistry. In: *Ferrets, Rabbits and Rodents: Clinical Medicine and Surgery*, ed. KE Quesenberry and JW Carpenter, pp. 452–471. Elsevier, St. Louis

Chaffee VW, James EA and Montali RJ (1975) Suppurative mandibular osteomyelitis associated with *Pasteurella multocida* in a rabbit. *Veterinary Medicine/Small Animal Clinician* **70**, 1411–1473

Deeb B (1993) Update for veterinary practitioners on pasteurellosis in rabbits. *Journal of Small Exotic Animal Medicine* **2**, 112–113

Dominguez J, Crase D and Soave O (1975) A case of pseudomonas osteomyelitis in a rabbit. *Laboratory Animal Science* **25**, 506

Gutschik E, Mortensen I and Møller S (1982) Experimental endocarditis in rabbits. 5. Results of long-term penicillin or streptomycin treatment of *Streptococcus faecalis* endocarditis and the effect of long-term exposure of healthy rabbits to the same drugs. *Acta Pathologica Microbiologica et Immunologica Scandinavica B* **90**, 25–35

Hara-Kudo Y, Morishita Y, Nagaoka Y, Kasuga F and Kumagai S (1996) Incidence of diarrhoea with antibiotics and the increase of clostridia in rabbits. *Journal of Veterinary Medical Science* **58**, 1181–1185

Harcourt-Brown FM (2002) Abscesses. In: *Textbook of Rabbit Medicine*, pp. 206–223. Butterworth-Heinemann, Oxford

Harcourt-Brown F (2007) Radiographic signs of renal disease in rabbits. *Veterinary Record* **160**, 787–794

Harcourt-Brown FM (2009) Dental disease in pet rabbits. 3. Jaw abscesses. *In Practice* **31**, 496–505

Hernandez-Divers SJ (2000) Mandibular abscess treatment using antibiotic-impregnated beads. *Exotic DVM* **2**, 15–18

Hinton M, Jones DRE and Festing MFW (1982) Haematological findings in healthy and diseased rabbits, a multivariate analysis. *Laboratory Animals* **16**, 123–129

Hume S and Gray L (2012) The use of enrofloxacin in poloxamer gel 407 (or Pluronic® F-127) to treat abscesses in rabbits and a guinea pig – case reports. *Proceedings, AAVAC/UEPV Conference, Melbourne*, pp. 245–246

Jekl V, Minarikova A, Hauptman K and Knotek K (2012) Microbial flora of facial abscesses in 30 rabbits – a preliminary study. *Proceedings, 22nd European Congress of Veterinary Dentistry, Lisbon*, pp. 133–135

Keel MK and Songer JG (2006) The comparative pathology of *Clostridium difficile* associated disease. *Veterinary Pathology* **43**, 225–240

Lloyd-Lucas A and Jones A (2010) Coenurus serialis cyst causing bone destruction in a rabbit. *Zoomed Bulletin – British Veterinary Zoological Society* **10**, 42–44

Martínez-Jiménez D, Hernández-Divers SJ, Dietrich UM et al. (2007) Endosurgical treatment of a retrobulbar abscess in a rabbit. *Journal of the American Veterinary Medical Association* **230**, 868–872

Mathews KA and Binnington AG (2002) Wound management using honey. *Compendium on Continuing Education for the Practicing Veterinarian* **24**, 53–60

Mehta S, Humphrey JS, Schenkman DI, Seaber AV and Vail TP (1996) Gentamicin distribution from a collagen carrier. *Journal of Orthopaedic Research* **14**, 749–754

Morris TH (1995) Antibiotic therapeutics in laboratory animals. *Laboratory Animals* **29**, 16–36

Remeeus PG and Verbeek M (1995) The use of calcium hydroxide in the treatment of abscesses in the cheek of the rabbit resulting from a dental periapical disorder. *Journal of Veterinary Dentistry* **12**, 9–22

Taylor M, Beaufrere H, Mans C and Smith DA (2010) Long-term outcome of treatment of dental abscesses with a wound packing technique in pet rabbits: 13 cases (1998–2007) *Journal of the American Veterinary Medical Association* **237**, 1444–1449

Toth LA and January B (1990) Physiological stabilization of rabbits after shipping. *Laboratory Animal Science* **40**, 384–387

Toth LA and Krueger JM (1989) Haematological effects of exposure to three infective agents in rabbits. *Journal of the American Veterinary Medical Association* **195**, 981–985

Tyrell KL, Citron DM, Jenkins JR and Goldstein EJC (2002) Periodontal bacteria in rabbit mandibular and maxillary abscesses. *Journal of Clinical Microbiology* **40**, 1044–1047

Ward GS, Crumrine MH and Mattloch JR (1981) Inflammatory exostosis and abscessation associated with *Fusobacterium nucleatum* in a rabbit. *Laboratory Animal Science* **31**, 280–281

Ward M (2006) Diagnosis and management of a retrobulbar abscess of periapical origin in a domestic rabbit. *Veterinary Clinics of North America: Exotic Animal Practice* **9**, 657–665

Whittem T and Gaon D (1998) Principles of microbial therapy. *Veterinary Clinics of North America: Small Animal Practice* **176**, 1095–1098

OPERATIVE TECHNIQUE 29.1 ➜

OPERATIVE TECHNIQUE 29.1:
Treating a dental abscess with marsupialization

The aim of marsupialization of a dental abscess is to remove all the pus and necrotic tissue, including infected teeth and bone, and leave an open cavity that can be cleaned daily. Although the basic principles are the same, there are variations in approach, which are described below with the author's initials after them.

Patient positioning and preparation

The rabbit is anaesthetized (see Chapter 1) and positioned so the abscess is accessible. Sandbags and a trough may be necessary. A dorsoventral and lateral radiograph of the skull, plus any other views that were taken should be available for inspection at any time during surgery. Before embarking on surgery, it is important to look in the mouth and examine all the teeth carefully, noting which crowns are loose and where any pus is coming from. The fur over the abscess site is clipped away and the skin prepared for surgery. The area is draped so that only the abscess is exposed. Sterile instruments and gloves are worn to minimize spread of infection.

Equipment

- 8 mm biopsy punch (JC)
- Rat-toothed forceps
- Olsen–Hegar needle-holders
- Mayo scissors
- Dressing forceps
- 20 ml syringe
- 2 metric (3/0 USP) polydioxanone or monofilament nylon suture material
- Swabs
- Cotton buds
- Volkmann's curette
- No. 3 Hollenbach carver or Crossley molar luxator
- Molar forceps
- Small bone cutters
- Adapted needle-holders to grasp tooth fragments (available from Veterinary Instrumentation, Sheffield) (FHB)
- No. 9 scalpel handle (FHB)
- No. 15 scalpel blade (FHB)

Procedure

1   The skin over the abscess is incised and the tissue over the abscess carefully dissected away to expose the abscess capsule.

2   Open the abscess.

Option A
The abscess can be opened with an 8 mm biopsy punch (JC) and the abscess wall sutured to the skin using polydioxanone or monofilament nylon. Four to six simple interrupted sutures normally suffice.

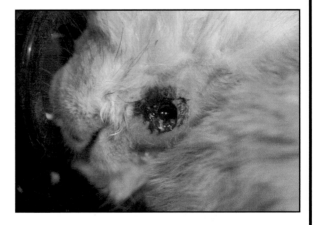

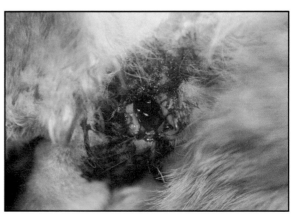

OPERATIVE TECHNIQUE 29.1 continued:
Treating a dental abscess with marsupialization

Option B
A small incision is made in the capsule, just large enough to insert a syringe tip to aspirate the pus. Squeezing the abscess at the same time as aspirating the pus facilitates removal.

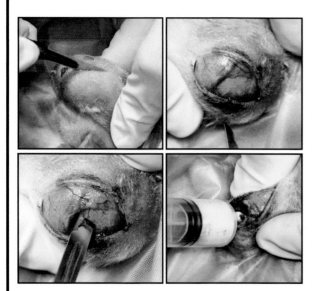

Once the abscess cavity has collapsed, a larger incision is made and the loose parts of the capsule are identified and removed (FHB). A section of the capsule can be used for bacteriological culture and sensitivity testing as organisms survive on the interior surface of the capsule.

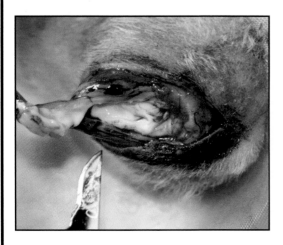

Once the interior of the abscess is exposed, residual pus is removed using cotton buds, dressing forceps or a Volkmann's curette. Bone cutters can be used to remove infected proliferative necrotic bone. Any remaining loose sections of capsule can be trimmed away to expose all of the interior of the capsule. Although pus and necrotic tissue can be flushed out of the cavity, it is not recommended as it can force infected fluid into adjacent soft tissue and disseminate infection further.

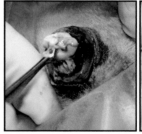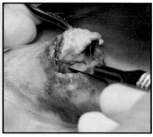

3 After the residual pus is removed with cotton buds, the cavity can be explored, looking for further pockets of pus and for infected teeth. It is important to follow abscess tracks (see Figure 29.15) and clear away all the pus and necrotic tissue to expose infected tooth roots. Localizing infected teeth can be difficult and skull radiographs are invaluable to orientate the abscess and identify tooth roots, which are often deformed, within the cavity. CT/MRI scans are extremely useful.

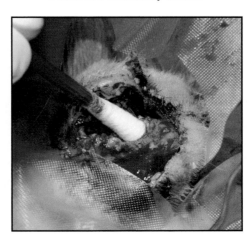

OPERATIVE TECHNIQUE 29.1 continued:
Treating a dental abscess with marsupialization

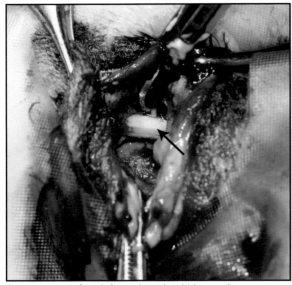

Appearance of an infected tooth within an abscess cavity (arrow).

4 Once they are identified, it is sometimes possible to remove infected teeth in their entirety through the abscess cavity. Extraoral cheek tooth extraction is described in more detail in Chapter 27. Alternatively the tooth can be sectioned with bone cutters; the distal section is then removed through the abscess cavity using adapted needle-holders and the rostral section may be removed through the abscess cavity (see below) or through the mouth.

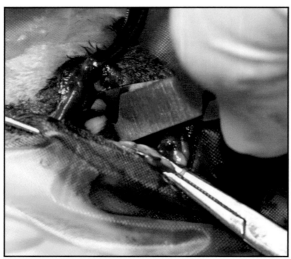

Sectioning the infected tooth root with bone cutters.

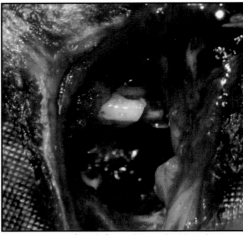

Appearance of an infected root that has been sectioned with bone cutters.

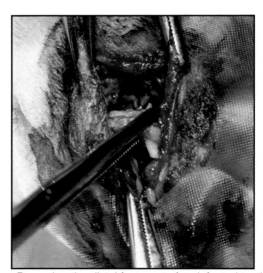

Removing the distal fragment of an infected tooth root with adapted needle-holders.

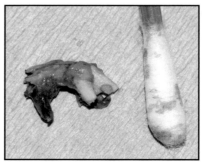

Appearance of distal fragment after removal.

OPERATIVE TECHNIQUE 29.1 continued:
Treating a dental abscess with marsupialization

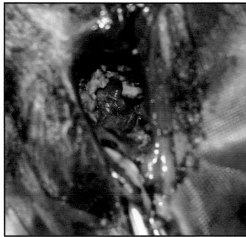

Appearance of cavity after removal of distal fragment.

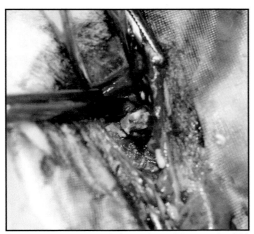

Elevating rostral tooth fragment with a scalpel blade.

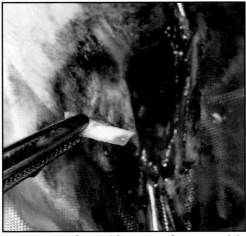

Appearance of rostral fragment after removal through abscess cavity.

5 If the abscess capsule was not opened with a biopsy punch and stitched to the skin at the outset of surgery, marsupialization needs to be completed after removal of the pus, excess capsule, infected bone and teeth. In order to do this, the abscess cavity is cleaned for a final time with cotton buds and any excess capsule trimmed away to the level of the skin, before stitching the skin and capsule together. If the abscess was large, surplus skin may need to be removed and some skin sutures placed to reduce the size of the wound.

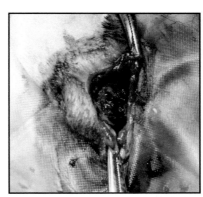

Appearance of abscess cavity after cleaning with cotton buds.

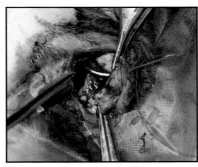

Suturing abscess capsule to skin.

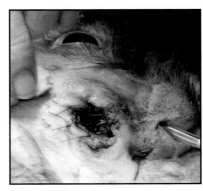

Appearance of marsupialized abscess at the end of surgery.

OPERATIVE TECHNIQUE 29.1 continued:
Treating a dental abscess with marsupialization

6 Once the abscess cavity has been marsupialized, bupivacaine can be instilled into the cavity and infiltrated into the surrounding tissue to provide local analgesia (FHB). The wound may be flushed and/or packed. A variety of techniques and agents are recommended by different authors (see main chapter text). Flushing the abscess cavity at the end of the procedure is controversial. Care must be taken not to flush purulent material deeper into surrounding tissues. The authors (FHB and JC) both use Manuka honey to pack the cavity. One author (FHB) also instills antibiotic drops, usually gentamicin.

7 At the end of surgery the oral cavity is inspected and any pus, blood or tooth fragments are removed.

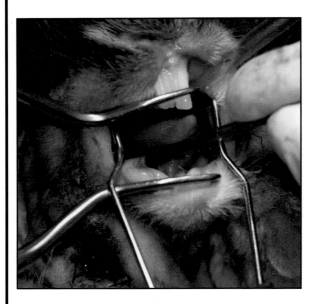

Consideration is given to the open tooth socket in the mouth. If there is a large hole, suturing the mucosa over the deficit will prevent food entering the abscess cavity and saliva leaking out of the wound. In some cases more fur needs to be clipped from the area around the abscess after surgery. This makes it easier to clean the skin postoperatively and prevents contamination of the fur with pus, honey or saliva.

PRACTICAL TIP
It is a good idea to show the nursing staff what has been done before the rabbit recovers from the anaesthetic, so that they know the site and extent of the wound; this helps them to clean the abscess cavity postoperatively or show the owners what to do.

8 Appropriate analgesia and antibiotics are given.

Postoperative care

A high standard of nursing care is essential, so hospitalization is usually necessary to observe the rabbit carefully, to ensure that all medication is given, to provide nutritional support, analgesia and comfort, and to clean marsupialized wounds effectively. Syringe feeding is often necessary, and prokinetic therapy is indicated for those rabbits that are not passing hard faeces or are only passing small faecal pellets. If the owners are able to manage the postoperative care and give injections, the rabbit can be sent home, although it should be checked after 48 hours.

The abscess cavity is cleaned once or twice daily by gently removing any pus or necrotic tissue with cotton buds and dressing forceps. The cavity is then packed with honey. One author (FHB) also instils antibiotic drops prior to the honey. Local anaesthesia can be maintained by instilling 3–4 drops of bupivacaine into the cavity once daily, 30 minutes before cleaning (FHB). Flushing the wound is not recommended as it may force fluid into the mouth and keep a fistula open.

Analgesia can be maintained with a combination of opioids and non-steroidal analgesics during the postoperative period, which may extend from 7 to 21 days depending on the size of the abscess and whether there is an open fistula into the mouth through the tooth socket.

The stitches are taken out of the skin after 5–14 days and the wound is checked every 7–10 days until it has healed. Antibiotic therapy is maintained until the wound has healed. Longer courses of antibiotics or repeated anaesthesia and re-curettage of the abscess may be necessary in cases that fail to heal completely after surgery. In those cases, another infected tooth root or an infected sequestrum of bone is usually delaying healing.

30

Management of chronic dental problems

Frances Harcourt-Brown

The treatment of diseased teeth has been covered in other chapters but there are other aspects of veterinary treatment that can improve the quality of life of a rabbit with chronic dental problems. In all but a small number of cases (such as traumatic fractures of healthy crowns or mild congenital incisor malocclusion), dental disease is an incurable and progressive condition. Once problems have started, the rabbit will never have perfect dentition so dental treatment can only be palliative. Management of the secondary problems greatly improves the quality of the rabbit's life.

Owner dedication

Despite the severe changes that have taken place in the teeth and surrounding jaw, many rabbits with dental disease appear to have a good quality of life (Figure 30.1).

Commitment from an owner is essential if a rabbit with chronic dental problems is to be managed successfully. Rabbits tend to hide signs of serious disease, so if the rabbit lives in a hutch or shed away from view any dental problems can easily be overlooked. The rabbit needs to be observed carefully and the owner must know what and how much the rabbit is eating and whether it is having problems chewing food. They also need to know if the rabbit is passing normal faeces and when it needs to be groomed or cleaned. All this takes time.

There may also be financial considerations. Repeated dentistry or treatment of abscesses can be expensive and if the owner cannot make the financial and time commitment to their pet, euthanasia should be considered. Euthanasia is preferable to ignoring the rabbit's dental problems until it develops a terminal crisis, such as starvation, hepatic lipidosis or flystrike.

In order to understand the commitment they are making to their rabbit, owners need to understand what is going on in their rabbit's mouth. They can only look at the incisors, but if the condition of the cheek teeth and the relationship of eye problems to dental disease are explained to them, committed owners can take on the management of their rabbit and improve its quality of life. Many owners are very happy and willing to do this, although it may take a long consultation to explain what is involved. Radiographs, photographs and prepared skulls are good educational material.

Frequency of oral examination and dental treatment

The health and demeanour of rabbits in the later stages of dental disease often improves as the teeth stop growing and spurs no longer dig into sensitive tissue. These teeth no longer have a nerve supply and are not painful. Some rabbits still need periodic dentistry but others cease to need dental intervention at all (Figure 30.2). Abscesses or odontomas are more common in rabbits with advanced dental

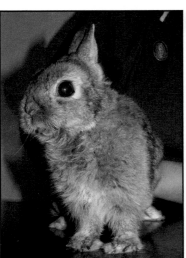

30.1 This 9-year-old rabbit has had dental problems all his life. He was born with incisor malocclusion and has had repeated treatment for spurs on the cheek teeth and recurrent abscesses. He has grooming difficulties. Despite these problems, he appears to have a good quality of life as a house rabbit and is a much loved part of the family.

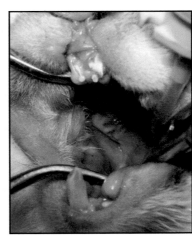

30.2 Endstage dental disease. This rabbit has no crowns at all on any of the cheek teeth; they have all broken off. Although this rabbit is free from oral discomfort, the inability to chew through fibrous foods has an impact on his health and welfare. This can be managed with dietary modification.

disease, so periodic clinical examination will be necessary. Skull radiography may need to be repeated on several occasions throughout the rabbit's life (Figure 30.3).

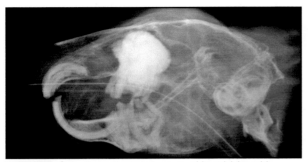

30.3 Odontomas are not unusual in rabbits with endstage dental disease. They are usually slow-growing solid tumours that may or may not add to the rabbit's existing dental problems. Surgery can be successful but is not always indicated.

Once the owner is aware of the warning signs of dental problems, the rabbit can be booked in when it needs treatment rather than electively. Observant owners are often able to detect the onset of dental problems from a change in their rabbit's behaviour and eating habits. The rabbit may appear lethargic and sit immobile in the same place for long periods of time. It may cease to be inquisitive and responsive or it may start to leave food or drop food uneaten. Some rabbits with dental problems refuse to drink from a sipper bottle or appear to be thirsty because they play with the bottle for long periods of time. These rabbits should be given a bowl to drink from. There is an argument that sipper bottles are never a good idea because it has been shown that rabbits prefer to drink from a bowl and will drink more if they do so (Tschudin *et al.*, 2011); this is also important for rabbits with urinary tract problems.

Treatment of secondary problems associated with chronic dental disease

Fractured crowns and sore gums
Cessation of tooth growth is a feature of the advanced stages of the progressive syndrome of acquired dental disease (PSADD) that is so common in pet rabbits. After the teeth have stopped growing and become deformed and demineralized, they often fracture just below the gum (see Chapters 24 and 26). The fractured crown remains in place, but is mobile and can be sore and cause eating difficulties. Periodontal infection is common. Pulling off the broken crown solves the problem because the gum can heal over. Occasionally, disintegrating crown remnants can protrude from a socket after a crown has eroded and disintegrated. Removing these remnants to below gum level, so the gum can heal, is usually successful. This can be done with the judicious use of molar cutters, ensuring that all fragments of teeth are removed (see Chapter 26). Postoperative antibiotics and analgesia are recommended.

Mucosal flaps
Another problem of advanced dental disease is the development of mucosal flaps in the space between upper and lower teeth that no longer occlude. The mucosa becomes hypertrophied (Figure 30.4) and any sharp edges on the teeth catch on it, causing ulceration and pain. These lesions can be difficult to treat. It is usually necessary to smooth or remove the neighbouring crown so it no longer catches on the mucosa. Sometimes the hypertrophied mucosa needs to be trimmed off. One method of removing thickened scarred hypertrophied mucosa is to crush the base of the tissue with rongeurs (or molar cutters) before trimming off the excess tissue. Crushing the tissue reduces haemorrhage and the likelihood of a gaping wound. Sutures can be placed but they may be uncomfortable postoperatively. Ideally the wound should be left to heal on its own, which takes 4–5 days.

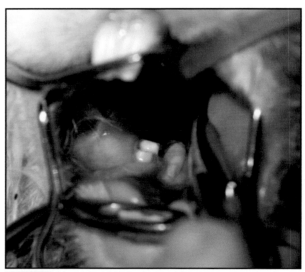

30.4 Hypertrophied mucosal flaps can develop in rabbits with short crowns on the cheek teeth. These flaps can catch on the teeth and become ulcerated and sore. Surgical removal is seldom successful on its own because the flaps quickly recur. Any sharp edges on the cheek teeth also need to be removed. In some cases, it is beneficial to reduce the height of the crowns so there is a bigger space between the upper and lower teeth, which prevents the flaps becoming compressed and damaged.

Choking
Choking is a hazard for rabbits with absent or non-occluding crowns, especially if they attempt to eat hay (Figure 30.5) or grass. Some rabbits that have never eaten hay in their lives will try to eat it when they are in the advanced stages of dental disease, presumably because the nerve supply to the teeth is gone and they feel no pain. Sadly, these rabbits do not have teeth that can cut through long strands, so they swallow the pieces whole. It is all too easy for a long strand to become lodged in the larynx or pharynx. For rabbits with no crowns on the cheek teeth, it is preferable to withhold hay and provide softer food instead (see later).

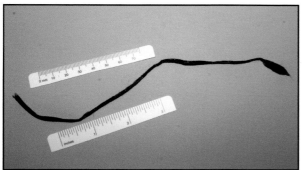

30.5 A piece of hay that was retrieved from a rabbit's mouth during a consultation. The rabbit had advanced dental disease and was presented with sudden-onset inappetence and profuse salivation. He made a complete recovery after the hay was removed. The stem was in the oesophagus and the seed head was caught around a deformed crown.

Dietary modification

Dietary modification is probably the most important aspect of managing rabbits with dental problems. The natural diet of the European rabbit, from which pet rabbits are descended, is grass, wild plants, tree leaves, bark and dried vegetation. The diet is seasonal, with fallen fruit or seeds at certain times of the year. The ideal diet for pet rabbits is one that mimics this natural diet. Good quality hay and/or grass, accompanied by leafy green plants and vegetables, is an acceptable substitute (see Chapter 24) but the rabbit has to have good teeth to be able to cut through the fibre. Rabbits with PSADD have impaired

ability to bite and chew fibre, so offering them a balanced diet that they can manage to eat (Figure 30.6) is an important part of their management.

Rabbits with apical elongation

Rabbits with apical elongation often find chewing hay painful and so do not eat it. Many owners of rabbits with dental problems say their rabbit 'has never liked hay'. Finding an alternative source of fibre is important. Grass and wild plants offer a good alternative and are softer. The dietary recommendations for rabbits in the early stages of dental disease are as follows.

- **No muesli mixes.** These diets seem to play a major part in the development of dental disease, obesity and other health problems in rabbits. They are not suitable for use as rabbit food (see also Chapter 24).
- **Freely available good quality hay or dried grass,** even though the rabbit may not appear to eat much. Dried grass is sold as an alternative to hay. It is softer and the stems are thinner. Some rabbits with dental problems that do not eat hay will eat dried grass.
- **Fresh grass.** This is softer than hay, so most rabbits with apical elongation will eat it. If possible, allow the rabbit to graze outside as much as possible and lie in the sun to synthesize and regulate its own vitamin D. If is not possible for the rabbit to go outside, fresh grass can be picked and brought in for the rabbit to eat.
- **Only a small amount of a pelleted or extruded food,** offered only once a day. This is optional

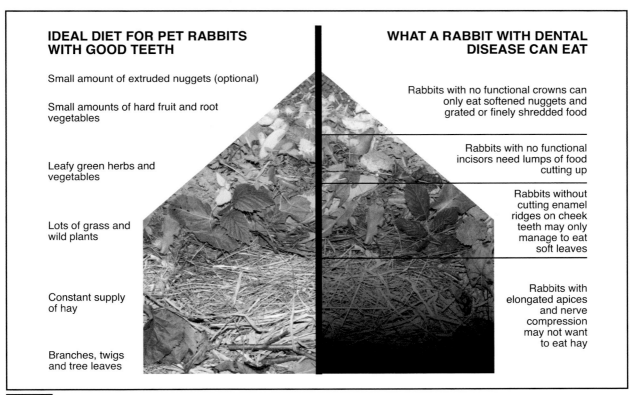

IDEAL DIET FOR PET RABBITS WITH GOOD TEETH	WHAT A RABBIT WITH DENTAL DISEASE CAN EAT
Small amount of extruded nuggets (optional)	Rabbits with no functional crowns can only eat softened nuggets and grated or finely shredded food
Small amounts of hard fruit and root vegetables	Rabbits with no functional incisors need lumps of food cutting up
Leafy green herbs and vegetables	Rabbits without cutting enamel ridges on cheek teeth may only manage to eat soft leaves
Lots of grass and wild plants	
Constant supply of hay	Rabbits with elongated apices and nerve compression may not want to eat hay
Branches, twigs and tree leaves	

30.6 Summary of dietary modification for rabbits with dental disease.

and can be excluded altogether if the rabbit is overweight and eats plenty of hay and a variety of leafy green plants.

- **A wide variety of leafy green plants and vegetables,** offered twice daily. A mixed diet including at least three different items each day is recommended because there may be problems if a single item is fed continually. Suitable plants are described in Chapter 24.
- **Restricted amounts of fruit and root vegetables.** These foods are low in indigestible fibre and can be fattening and cause soft caecotrophs. They include apples, pears and bananas, and carrots, parsnips, beetroot, celeriac and other root vegetables. The tops of these root vegetables can be fed.
- **No treats.** These include chocolate and yoghurt drops, biscuits, bread and sugary cereal treats.

Rabbits with absent, maloccluded or non-occluding incisors

Rabbits with non-functional incisors are unable to bite sections out of lumps of food, such as apples or carrots. However, they can still manage to transport pieces of food to the cheek teeth by using their tongue and lips. The lips on the lateral aspect of the mouth are folded inwards and have hair which helps with prehension of pieces of food. If the cheek teeth are healthy, once the food is between them it can be reduced to small pieces before it is swallowed. Rabbits with non-functional incisors only need to have their food chopped into manageable pieces. They can still eat hay and other fibrous foods.

Rabbits with advanced dental disease

Absent crowns or abnormal occlusion can affect the ability to prehend and chew food. Affected rabbits may take a long time to eat. These rabbits may not eat sufficient food to maintain their bodyweight so they lose weight.

These rabbits often cannot eat hay. Their teeth are not sharp enough to cut through it. They can usually eat leafy green plants, although harder foods such as broccoli or cabbage may need to be shredded or cut into small pieces so they are easier to eat. Nuggets of extruded food can help to maintain bodyweight. These diets are a compromise as far as dietary fibre is concerned, but they do offer a palatable balanced food that the rabbit can actually eat and digest. Many of these diets contain long fibre particles, although they will have been partially denatured by the cooking process.

Rabbits with endstage dental disease

Rabbits with endstage dental disease have serious problems with eating. They may have no crowns on the teeth at all or none that are in occlusion. Eating hay or hard food is not an option. Nuggets of extruded food are a lifeline because the rabbit can manage to survive on these diets, though the food may need to be softened. Although fruit is not ideal for rabbits because of its low indigestible fibre content, rabbits with endstage dental disease can be given some treat foods such as small pieces of

banana or apple. It is important to watch the weight of these rabbits. Nuggets, muesli mixes and soft foods such as bread, fruit and sugary treats are high in calories and rabbits that are fed on them can become obese. The amount of food may need to be restricted. Conversely, some rabbits with endstage dental disease become very thin. Eating without teeth is difficult and some rabbits can benefit from daily syringe feeding by their owners. Ground-up nuggets or recovery diets can be used.

Managing secondary complications of dental disease

Eye problems

Permanent or recurrent epiphora and dacryocystitis may be present in some rabbits with dental disease, especially in advanced cases with deformed, ankylosed tooth roots (Figure 30.7). Secondary conjunctivitis, keratitis or even corneal ulceration can be complications. Some cases are cured with treatment or resolve spontaneously, especially if the duct ruptures into the nasal passage so tears can drain into the nose (see Chapter 28). The cases that do not resolve are those in which the tear duct is completely obstructed, usually at the apex of the 1st upper incisor, by a deformed tooth root, or even an odontoma. Even if the tooth is removed, permanent distortion of the bone can leave the duct still blocked (Figure 30.8), so tears overflow from the conjunctival sac and soak the fur beneath the medial canthus of the eye. Facial dermatitis is a

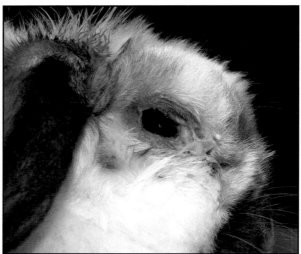

30.7 This rabbit has an obstruction to the tear duct at the apex of the upper 1st incisor. The photograph was taken after the instillation of proxymetacaine eye drops to provide local anaesthesia. Pus from the punctum lacrimale is leaking into the conjunctival sac and overflowing down the face. The fur is wet, matted and soiled. There is a spastic entropion. There was a corneal ulcer close to the punctum, although it is hidden by the lower eyelid in this photograph. These changes are typical of many cases of endstage dental disease. Eye ointment alone will not resolve them. Critical examination of the eye and determination of the aetiology is necessary before embarking on further procedures, which are described in Chapters 17 and 28.

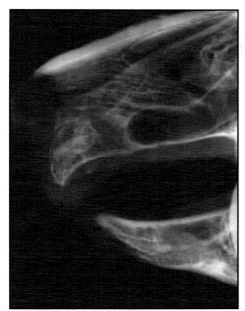

30.8 Lateral radiographic view of the rostral section of a sagitally sectioned head of a rabbit that had recalcitrant dacryocystitis. Although the tear duct cannot be seen, the bony canal that encompasses it is seen as a dilated tubular structure that was filled with pus. The nasolacrimal canal was still blocked, even though the incisors had been removed. A remnant of a peg tooth remains in the jaw.

painful sequel. The fragile skin easily becomes infected, especially if the tears are purulent as a result of infection in the nasolacrimal duct. This problem is incurable, but there are ways to manage these cases.

- **Reduce the amount of tears that are produced.** Fewer tears flowing down the face lead to less damp fur and a reduced risk of facial dermatitis. Tears are produced in response to corneal irritation; so ensuring that there is no irritation from dusty hay or particles/fumes from wood shavings can help.
- **Systemic and topical antibiotics.** Although antibiotic eye ointments may not cure the conjunctivitis, they can help to manage the infection, both in the eye and on the skin below the medial canthus. Fusidic acid (Fucithalmic) or chloramphenicol eye ointment are the author's favourite ointments. The choice of systemic antibiotics depends on the nature of any infection. Parenteral penicillin (or derivatives) or cephalosporins are used for purulent infections. Trimethoprim/sulphonamide or enrofloxacin are used for skin infections, either parenterally or orally. Antibiotics are given as a 7–10-day course at a therapeutic dose.
- **Clip away damp fur.** Regular removal of the fur from the face may give the rabbit an odd appearance but can help to treat the underlying skin infection. It is essential in cases of dacryocystitis, where the eyelids can become glued together by purulent exudates that need to be cleaned away from the eyelids and skin.

- **Examine the eye and consider surgery.** In some cases of chronic dacryocystitis, spastic entropion causes problems if the eyelids are in contact with the cornea. Surgery is indicated in these cases (see Chapter 17). In some cases of chronic dacryocystitis, the lacrimal sac becomes dilated and infected and can be palpated as a soft fluctuating structure below the medial canthus of the eye. Opening and marsupialization of the lacrimal sac (see Chapter 28) can be helpful in these cases because it diverts pus away from the conjunctival sac and allows the infection of the nasolacrimal duct to be treated with topical antibiotics directly on to the infected tissue. Systemic antibiotics are also required.
- **Massage the face near the medial canthus of the eye.** Applying pressure to the lacrimal sac can help to force tears out of the lacrimal sac into the duct and can improve drainage. Owners can be taught to do this on a regular basis throughout the day.
- **Provide a bonded companion** (see Chapter 28). Although owners can help to keep their rabbit's eyes and face clean, a bonded rabbit companion does a much better job. Rabbits spend a lot of time licking and cleaning their companion's eyes and face as part of their social behaviour. This can be a very satisfactory solution to the difficult problem of recalcitrant epiphora and dacryocystitis (see also Chapter 28).

Grooming difficulties

Dental problems interfere with grooming, either by impairing the rabbit's ability to grasp dead hair between the incisors or by making the tongue sore so the rabbit is reluctant to lick its skin and fur. The result is an accumulation of skin debris and parasites, such as the mites *Cheyletiella parasitovorax* and *Leporacarus gibbus*, in the fur. Moulting compounds the situation because it is difficult or impossible for the rabbit to remove dead hair from the coat. *Cheyletiella* causes pruritus and areas of heavy scurf.

Dental problems and impaired grooming also make it harder for rabbits to ingest caecotrophs, which often get caught in the fur under the tail. The caecotrophs may be softer and more liquid because a rabbit with dental problems has difficulty eating sufficient fibre. The result can be a soiled, wet, dirty mass of hair with infected skin beneath. Myiasis is an ever-present risk. These problems can be managed in a number of ways.

- **Providing bonded companions.** Bonded companions (Figure 30.9) will groom a rabbit with dental problems, which can help to remove dead hair from the coat to keep the eyes and ears clean. However, a companion is unlikely to clean the perineum and the area under the tail.
- **Clipping away all the wet and soiled fur.** All the fur around the tail and perineum, as well as that on the abdomen and inside the thighs, must be removed. Sedation may be necessary. The procedure is time-consuming but once the

427

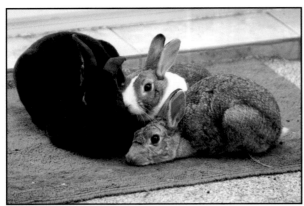

30.9 Provision of bonded companions for any rabbit has much to recommend it. Grooming the body, face and ears is part of their social behaviour and can be very beneficial for rabbits with chronic dental problems.

hair has been removed and the owners can see the anatomy of the region, they are often happy to keep the hair short with regular trimming (at least once a week). Providing them with a sharp pair of curved scissors is helpful. Simply bathing the area is not recommended and can be counterproductive because it leaves the fur damp and predisposes the underlying skin to infection.

- **Providing long-term analgesia.** Analgesics can be used to alleviate pain and inflammation in inflamed infected skin around the perineum. They also alleviate pain from spinal problems or arthritis, which are often present in older rabbits with advanced dental problems. Improving mobility can help the rabbit to groom and clean the perineal region. Oral meloxicam can be given indefinitely. It may be given once or twice daily, depending on the rabbit's response.
- **Providing enough space** for the rabbit to move away from soiled bedding to decrease the likelihood of caecotrophs sticking to the fur.

Soiled bedding should be removed regularly, maybe two or three times a day. Caecotrophs tend to be produced in the morning, so cleaning the litter tray or hutch at lunchtime helps to prevent caecotrophs from sticking to the fur.

- **Treating mite infestations.** Fur mites are easily treatable with a single topical dose of selamectin (8–16 mg/kg). All in-contact rabbits must be treated at the same time and any new rabbits must be treated before they are introduced.
- **Preventing flystrike.** Myiasis is an ever-present threat to rabbits with chronic dental problems, especially those with non-functional incisors that cannot groom dead fur or any deposited fly eggs from their perineal area. Myiasis can be prevented by vigilance. The perineal area must be kept clean and flies prevented from coming near the rabbit by keeping it indoors and using fly screens, fly traps and/or ultraviolet insect electrocutors. Various topical applications such as cyromazine (an insect growth regulator) or plant-based insect repellents containing octanoic and decanoic acid are available as preventive measures. Some products combine insect repellents with pyrethrum to kill adult flies and their larvae (Cousquer, 2006). However, none of these measures is a substitute for keeping the perineal area free of faeces and contaminated fur. The author uses a prophylactic monthly application of selamectin during the summer months for rabbits at a high risk of myiasis; this should kill any maggots that hatch from eggs that are deposited in the fur and cannot be removed by rabbits with non-functional incisors.

References and further reading

Cousquer G (2006) Veterinary care of rabbits with myiasis. *In Practice* **28**, 342–349

Tschudin A, Clauss M, Codron D and Hatt JM (2011) Preference of rabbits for drinking from open dishes versus nipple drinkers. *Veterinary Record* **168**, 190

Appendix 1

Formulary

John Chitty

This formulary is restricted to medications that are described in this Manual, and the doses are those used by the chapter authors. It is not intended as an exhaustive list of medications that can be used in rabbits, and further information on rabbit medications can be found in the *BSAVA Small Animal Formulary* and the *BSAVA Manual of Rabbit Medicine*.

Authorization and consent

As with many exotic species, few medicines are authorized for use in rabbits, and clinicians are advised to follow the prescribing laws adherent in their country (e.g. the Prescribing Cascade in the UK).

In the UK, informed consent should be obtained before use of non-authorized drugs. For exotic species (including rabbits), it may be appropriate for the client to sign a generalized consent to the use of non-authorized drugs on registration with the practice. This does not, however, remove the need for discussion of the reasons for using a particular drug and its possible side effects. For long-term use of a non-authorized drug, or where there is controversy over a drug's use (see below), specific written consent should always be obtained.

Some penicillin-containing injectable preparations available in the UK state a contraindication to use in rabbits on their data sheets. If the clinician deems these preparations appropriate, written informed consent for their use from the client is advisable.

Use of antibiotics in rabbits

There is considerable controversy over antibiotic choice in all species, owing to the widespread development of multi-resistant bacterial strains in human and veterinary medicine. Responsible antibiotic use is, therefore, a priority (see www.bsava.com for information on the PROTECT scheme).

In rabbits there are particular difficulties. For example, in the UK enrofloxacin is currently the only systemic (non-feed-additive) antibiotic authorized for use in pet rabbits. Under the Prescribing Cascade regulations, it is therefore appropriate for this to be the first choice for use in rabbits. However, other drugs may be prescribed in preference if the

veterinary surgeon believes that they may be more clinically effective, or to reduce the risk of the development of antibiotic resistance.

Ideally, culture and sensitivity testing should be utilized to determine antibiotic choice. In cases from which no bacteria are cultured, or where it is not possible to sample lesions directly, knowledge of likely bacterial isolates and their likely sensitivities may be of use in determining empirical therapy. Cytology of samples submitted for culture may also be helpful when there is no bacterial growth on laboratory culture, because the morphology of the bacteria may assist in presumptive identification and probable antibiotic sensitivity.

It is important with all drugs to use the correct dose rate and the correct route for an appropriate length of time. This is especially important where it is felt that 'important' classes of antibiotic (e.g. fluoroquinolones or third-generation cephalosporins) are essential. In-water dosing of fluoroquinolones in particular should be avoided, as should pulse therapy of these drugs.

In all cases, when antibiotics are prescribed for rabbits the likely effects of the drug (and dosage route) on the gut flora must be considered. Penicillin and its derivatives and cephalosporins are frequently advised for use in rabbits. However, care must be taken because gastrointestinal effects (including fatal diarrhoea) have been reported with these drugs. The following guidelines should be observed:

- Avoid oral use, or situations where rabbits may groom and therefore ingest a leaked drug (e.g. from an abscess or injection site)
- A high-fibre diet, including as much hay/grass as possible, may be appropriate while rabbits are receiving these drugs.

WARNING
Within the rabbit-owning community there are many anecdotal reports of the efficacy of penicillin, and some rabbit owners may wish to import long-acting penicillin injections. Importation of drugs in this manner is not legal in the UK. Veterinary surgeons are advised not to recommend this, nor to support the use of drugs obtained from other rabbit owners.

Appendix 1 Formulary

Drug name	Dose rate and route	Use/Comments
Antibacterials		
Amoxicillin/Clavulanate	7 mg/kg s.c. q24h	Can be used in cases of osteomyelitis where other antibiotics are ineffective. **Not for oral use**
Azithromycin	15–30 mg/kg orally q24h	
Cefalexin	15–20 mg/kg s.c., orally q12h	
Ceftazidime	100 mg/kg i.m., s.c. q12h	
Chloramphenicol	Topical, q12h	For eye infections and abscesses. Can be used as nasal drops
Ciprofloxacin	Topical, q12h	For eye infections and abscesses. Can be used as nasal drops
Enrofloxacin	20–30 mg/kg s.c., orally q24h 10–15 mg/kg s.c., orally q12h	Ineffective against anaerobes. Authorized dose rate 5 mg/kg orally or s.c. q12h
Gentamicin	Topical, q12h	For eye infections and abscesses. Can be used as nasal drops
Marbofloxacin	2 mg/kg orally, s.c., i.v. q24h	
Metronidazole	15–20 mg/kg s.c., orally q12h	
Penicillin G	40,000 IU/kg s.c. q24h for 5 days 50–60,000 IU/kg s.c. once weekly for 3 doses	Abscesses. Treponematosis. **Not for oral use**
Penicillin/Streptomycin	40 mg **penicillin** per kg s.c. q24h	Effective against anaerobes. Useful for purulent infections. **Not for oral use**
Procaine penicillin	40,000 IU/kg s.c. q24h	Can be used to treat treponematosis. Avoid intravascular injection. **Not for oral use**
Trimethoprim/Sulphonamide	30–40 mg/kg s.c., orally q12h	Inactivated by pus. Has been shown to decrease tear production
Analgesics		
N-Acetylglucosamine	25 mg/kg orally q24h for 14 days then every other day	For use in cystitis/hypercalciuria
Aspirin	100 mg/kg orally q8–24h	For mild pain; has some anti-inflammatory effects
Buprenorphine	0.01–0.05 mg/kg s.c., i.m., i.v. q6–12h	Opioid
Butorphanol	0.1–0.5 mg/kg s.c., i.m., i.v. q4h	Opioid
Carprofen	2–4 mg/kg s.c. q24h 1.0–2.2 mg/kg orally q12h	NSAID. Can cause injection reaction; ensure product goes into subcutaneous fascia not skin
Fentanyl	0.0074 mg/kg i.v. 12.5 microgram patch per 3 kg rabbit topically for 3 days	Do not cut patches. Hair growth can reduce efficacy of patch. May make drowsy as dose high when applied. Cover patch to prevent rabbit eating it
Fentanyl/Fluanisone	0.25 ml/kg s.c.	Used for sedation and analgesia
Flunixin meglumine	0.3–1.1 mg/kg orally, i.m., i.v., s.c. q12–24h	NSAID; limit use to 3 days
Flurbiprofen	1 drop topically q8–12h	Ophthalmic topical NSAID. May also be used intranasally
Ketoprofen	3 mg/kg i.m., s.c. q12–24h	NSAID
Meloxicam	0.2–0.5 mg/kg orally, i.m., s.c. q24h Up to 1 mg/kg s.c., orally q12–24h	NSAID. Higher doses suggested by pharmacokinetic studies and supported by some clinicians
Morphine	2–5 mg/kg s.c., i.m. q2–4h	Opioid
Nalbuphine	1–2 mg/kg i.m., i.v. q4–5h	Opioid
Naloxone	0.01–0.1 mg/kg i.m., i.p., i.v.	Opioid antagonist
Oxymorphone	0.05–0.2 mg/kg s.c., i.m. q8–12h	Opioid
Paracetamol	200–500 mg/kg orally 1–2 mg/ml drinking water	NSAID
Pethidine	5–10 mg/kg s.c., i.m., i.p., i.v. q2–3h	Opioid
Piroxicam	0.2 mg/kg orally q8h	NSAID
Tramadol	5 mg/kg i.v., s.c. q8h 5–15 mg/kg orally q8–12h	

Drug name	Dose rate and route	Use/Comments
Anxiolytics		
Diazepam	1–5 mg/kg i.m., i.v.	Pre-anaesthetic, tranquillizer. Benzodiazepine
Midazolam	0.5–2 mg/kg i.m., i.v., i.p., intranasal	Pre-anaesthetic, tranquillizer. Benzodiazepine
Prokinetics		
Cisapride	0.5–1 mg/kg orally q12h	
Domperidone	0.5 mg/kg orally q12h	
Metoclopramide	0.5–1 mg/kg orally, s.c. q12h	Effects mainly on stomach and small intestine. Lower end of dose range may have use as anti-nausea agent
Anti-ulcer drugs		
Ranitidine	5 mg/kg orally, s.c. q12h	Also prokinetic effect
Anti-adhesion drugs		
Pentoxifylline	2.5 mg/kg orally q12h for 3 days	
Verapamil	200 μg/kg orally, s.c. q8h for 3 days	
Miscellaneous		
Dantrolene	0.5 mg/kg orally q12h	For urethral spasm
Fenbendazole	20 mg/kg orally q24h for 28 days	For *Encephalitozoon cuniculi* infection
Hydrochlorothiazide	2 mg/kg orally q12h	Diuretic. Use in hypercalciuria
Potassium citrate	33 mg/kg orally q12h	Urinary alkalinizer. Monitor plasma potassium levels during therapy
Prazosin	0.25 mg/rabbit orally q12h	For urethral spasm

Appendix 2

A basic surgical kit for rabbits

John Chitty

- Scalpel handle for No. 15 blade
- Adson thumb forceps – rat-toothed
- de Bakey atraumatic forceps
- Iris scissors
- Metzenbaum scissors
- Towel clamps
- Allis tissue forceps
- Artery forceps – 2 straight; 2 curved; 2 fine Mosquito forceps
- Olsen–Hegar needle-holders
- Alm retractors or ring retractor
- Adhesive drapes (transparent or otherwise)
- Vascular clips and applicators very useful if available

For specialist instruments and equipment for more advanced surgical techniques (including orthopaedics) see individual Operative Techniques and chapters.

Appendix 3

A basic dentistry kit for rabbits

John Chitty

For keeping the mouth open:

- Rabbit mouth gag
- Cheek dilators
- Or a specialist table gag + cheek dilators

For 'manual dentistry' and tooth removal:

- Molar forceps
- Molar cutter
- Crossley molar luxator or No. 3 Hollenbach carver
- Crossley incisor luxator
- Adapted needle-holders to grasp tooth fragments (available from Veterinary Instrumentation, Sheffield)
- Diamond file
- Dental spatula
- Periodontal probes

For mechanical grinding of molar hooks and coronal reduction:

- High-torque low-speed dental head with rose-head burrs
- Dental spatula

To cut incisors:

- High-speed dental drill with cutting burrs
- Lip/mouth protector

Appendix 4
Dorsal immobility response in rabbits

Sally Everitt

Rabbits, along with many other prey species, may display fight, flight or freeze behaviour when they perceive a threat. It is thought that the freeze response is intended to deceive a predator into thinking that the animal is already dead and is believed to be an adaptive response to limit injury and allow the possibility of escape. This response has been described as a 'death feint', 'playing dead' or 'playing possum'.

A similar response may also be produced in the restraint of rabbits, most often by holding a rabbit in dorsal recumbency, with the head slightly below the body and stroking the abdomen until the rabbit is completely relaxed. In this condition the rabbit becomes immobile and does not appear to respond to mild noxious stimuli.

There has been some research into the physiological changes that take place in this condition; most studies are small and have produced varied and even contradictory results. Although animals in this state may at the time show bradycardia, reduced blood pressure and apparent lack of response to noxious stimuli, they may also show tachycardia and raised cortisol following the procedure, indicating that this is not a stress-free state.

This state has been variously described as 'hypnosis', 'trance', 'thanatosis' (playing dead) and 'tonic immobility', although all of these terms have problems in that they may suggest similarities with other physical or psychological states which cannot be substantiated. It may therefore be better to adopt a neutral descriptive term, e.g. dorsal immobility response.

There does seem to be variation between rabbits in the ease with which the dorsal immobility response can be induced and there may also be differences dependent on the experience of the handler and circumstances in which the animal is being handled. While the rabbit may remain in this state for some time it should also be remembered that they can come out of this state and 'take flight' very suddenly.

Veterinary surgeons sometimes use the dorsal immobility response to enable the rabbit to be examined or for minor, non-invasive procedures to be carried out. A document produced by the RSPCA and UFAW (*Refining rabbit care – A resource for those working with rabbits in research*; available at www.rspca.org) has advised that it is not acceptable to rely on the immobility response alone to 'facilitate any type of procedure that would normally require sedation, anaesthesia or analgesia'.

Whether it is appropriate to rely on the dorsal immobility response for radiography will depend on a number of factors, including the experience of the handler in using this technique, the positioning required, and the ability to ensure that the rabbit will not be injured if it regains mobility.

Index

Index